clinical pharmacy and therapeutics

eric t. herfindal

joseph l. hirschman

clinical pharmacy and therapeutics

edited by

eric t. herfindal, pharm.d.

Associate Clinical Professor of Pharmacy
Chairman, Division of Clinical Pharmacy
School of Pharmacy
University of California
San Francisco, California

joseph l. hirschman, pharm.d.

Assistant Clinical Professor of Pharmacy
School of Pharmacy
University of California
Director of Clinical Services
Health Application Systems
Consultant, PAID Prescriptions
Burlingame, California

with 34 contributors

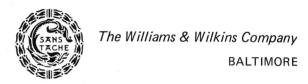

The Williams & Wilkins Company
BALTIMORE

Copyright ©, 1975
The Williams & Wilkins Company
428 E. Preston Street
Baltimore, Md. 21202, U.S.A.

Library of Congress Cataloging in Publication Data

Herfindal, Eric T Clinical pharmacy and therapeutics.

1. Pharmacology. 2. Therapeutics. I. Hirschman, Joseph L., joint author. II. Title.
[DNLM: 1. Drug therapy. 2. Therapeutics. WB330 H544c] RM300.H47 615 74-10913
ISBN 0-683-03959-8

Composed and printed at the
Waverly Press, Inc.
Mt. Royal and Guilford Aves.
Baltimore, Md. 21202, U.S.A.

To
Jere E. Goyan and Sidney Riegelman
whose continued support
made this effort possible.

foreword

On November 10, 1942, Sir Winston Churchill publicly announced the first encouraging news from the beleagured British forces still battling back from the disequilibrium born of having sustained the early onslaughts of World War II. To those attending the Lord Mayor's Day luncheon in London he explained, hopefully but cautiously, that the British Army had repulsed Rommel in North Africa. "Now this is not the end," declared Sir Winston. "It is not even the beginning of the end. But it is, perhaps, the end of the beginning."

I am pleased to introduce a clinical pharmacy book which seems to me to mark "the end of the beginning" of a new era for the profession. Originating with a new generation of practitioner-educators—by far the majority of contributors have academic appointments as well as service commitments—this volume incorporates the detailed technical knowledge and the strategy of its application in rational pharmacotherapeutics according to the perceived needs of these experienced practitioners.

Perhaps prophetically this book is, in part, the result of collaborative efforts by baccalaureate practitioners, physicians, and pharmacists who have professional masters degrees, but the major effort is carried by holders of the professional doctorate. In the years ahead all of us will hope and work for this sort of inter- and intraprofessional cooperation in optimizing pharmacy's contributions to improved drug utilization in health care, and we shall look to those practitioner-educators with doctoral level expertise to lead the way.

Most of the authors received their professional education in the pharmacy schools of California, a state which has provided more than its share of leadership in the new direction which the profession is taking. Encouragingly, we have many more years of leadership to anticipate from these authors; their mean age is 30.6 years.

This is not a book review; it is a foreword. and so I shall not attempt to characterize this volume's content except to remind the reader that it is a reference work, and therefore it is designed to provide an overview. Hopefully the material will provide instructor and student with an appropriate scope of each subject so that in-depth excursions into appropriate monographs, textbooks, and the primary literature can be facilitated and accomplished within an appropriate perspective.

Practitioner, student, and teacher will each find in this volume assistance in achieving an understanding and a comprehension of drug therapy phenomena useful in the practice of contemporary pharmacy. But for myself there is much more. Represented herein is the sort of initiative and personification of purpose that will enable the profession to redefine its concepts of contemporary practice.

The practitioner-educator has arrived on the pharmaceutical education scene to set new goals for professional practice and to influence the aspirations of our students for intellectual challenge and achievement in their services to society. The profession and, in the final analysis, all of society will be best served if those of us who are better established in academia will see this and all their other initial undertakings as the cornerstone upon which to build a strong and lasting profession. If we do this, if we can see in these devoted young people the potential for developing a clinical faculty which ultimately can be as productive as have been their counterparts in other health professions, then, indeed, we shall have seen" ... the end of the beginning."

Charles A. Walton, Ph.D.
San Antonio, Texas
February 24, 1975

preface

Clinical Pharmacy and Therapeutics is offered as a practical review of the diagnosis and treatment of diseases likely to be encountered by pharmacists. It has been prepared from the perspective of the pharmacist and pharmacy student and should serve as a bridge from the basic disciplines of pathology, biochemistry and pharmacology to the treatment of specific disease entities and not as a replacement for standard reference works in these areas.

For the pharmacist to be an effective therapeutic advisor to other health professionals, he must have an understanding of the pathology, etiology and diagnosis of diseases so that any therapeutic advice provided can be placed into a clinical perspective. In essence, we are advocating that the pharmacist be prepared to make therapeutic judgments. In doing so, the net result is one of synergy with the physician's viewpoints, thus improving the drug therapy rendered.

This spirit is reflected by all the contributors. The basic prerequisite for all contributors is that they be clinically experienced in the subject matter discussed. As a consequence, the material presented is based on the author's experience. All of the contributors are practicing pharmacists from a variety of professional environments. In addition to their regular practice, many are closely involved with phar-macy education. It is hoped that the reader of this text can benefit from the experiences of this outstanding group of pharmacists and extrapolate them to his own practice.

We have standardized for format within reasonable limits without inhibiting the flexibility of the various contributors. For those readers who wish to pursue any particular subject in greater depth, a list of references is included with each chapter.

Some of the chapters have previously appeared in the series "Current Therapeutic Concepts" published in the *Journal of the American Pharmaceutical Association,* but in most cases the material has been revised and updated for this volume.

We are grateful to the many colleagues who helped us prepare the manuscript. We wish particularly to thank Dr. Robert L. Day of the University of California School of Pharmacy, George B. Griffenhagen, Editor, and Leena Lassila, Associate Editor of the *Journal of the American Pharmaceutical Association* for their editorial assistance and encouragement.

We also wish to thank Donna Hoover and Alice Westbrook who labored long hours preparing the manuscript.

E.T.H.
J.L.H.

list of contributors

C. A. Bond, Pharm. D.
Assistant Clinical Professor of Pharmacy
School of Pharmacy
University of Wisconsin
Madison, Wisconsin

Douglas G. Christian, B.S.
Acting Assistant Chief
U.S. Veterans' Administration Hospital Pharmacy Service
San Diego, California

Ronald R. Conte, Pharm.D.
Clinical Pharmacist, Adult Health Center
San Francisco General Hospital;
Clinical Instructor of Pharmacy
School of Pharmacy
University of California
San Francisco, California

William A. Cornelis, B.S.
Staff Pharmacist
Providence Hospital
Southfield, Michigan

Richard F. de Leon, Pharm.D.
Associate Clinical Professor of Pharmacy
School of Pharmacy
Associate Director, Department of Pharmaceutical Services
University of California
San Francisco, California

Robert M. Elenbaas, Pharm.D.
Assistant Professor of Clinical Pharmacy
School of Pharmacy
University of Missouri—Kansas City
Kansas City, Missouri

Clarence L. Fortner, M.S.
Director, Clinical Research Pharmacy Service
Baltimore Cancer Research Center
National Cancer Institute
Baltimore, Maryland

Donald L. Giusti, Pharm.D.
Associate Professor of Clinical Pharmacy
Assistant Professor of Medicine
(Clinical Pharmacy)
Assistant Director of Pharmacy Services
College of Pharmacy
University of Cincinnati Medical Center
Cincinnati, Ohio

William R. Grove, B.S.
Deputy Chief, Baltimore Cancer Research Center
Clinical Research Pharmacy Service
Baltimore Cancer Research Center
Baltimore, Maryland

Philip D. Hansten, Pharm.D.
Assistant Professor of Clinical Pharmacy
College of Pharmacy
Washington State University
Pullman, Washington

Eric T. Herfindal, Pharm.D.
Associate Clinical Professor of Pharmacy
Chairman, Division of Clinical Pharmacy
School of Pharmacy
University of California
San Francisco, California

Joseph L. Hirschman, Pharm.D.
Director of Clinical Services
Health Application Systems
Burlingame, California

Robert J. Ignoffo, Pharm.D.
Assistant Clinical Professor of Pharmacy
School of Pharmacy
University of California
San Francisco, California

Marianne F. Ivey, B.S.
Assistant Professor of Clinical Pharmacy

School of Pharmacy
Department of Pharmacy Practice
University of Washington
Seattle, Washington

Fredric E. Jones, M.S.
General Manager, Internal Medicine Associates
Massachusetts General Hospital;
Associate in Medicine, School of Medicine
Harvard University
Boston, Massachusetts

Brian S. Katcher, Pharm.D.
Lecturer in Clinical Pharmacy
School of Pharmacy
University of California
San Francisco, California

Robert L. Kerr, Pharm.D.
Clinical Assistant Professor of Pharmacy
University of Maryland School of Pharmacy
Baltimore, Maryland

Mary Anne Kimble, Pharm.D.
Assistant Clinical Professor of Pharmacy
School of Pharmacy
University of California
San Francisco, California

Donald T. Kishi, Pharm.D.
Assistant Clinical Professor of Pharmacy
School of Pharmacy
University of California
San Francisco, California

Wayne A. Kradjan, Pharm.D.
Assistant Professor of Clinical Pharmacy
School of Pharmacy
University of Washington
Seattle, Washington

Robert H. Levin, Pharm.D.
Assistant Clinical Professor of Pharmacy

School of Pharmacy
University of California
San Francisco, California

Paul W. Lofholm, Pharm.D.
Chief of Pharmacy Services
Ross Valley Medical Clinic
Greenbrae, California

Rex S. Lott, B.Pharm.
Assistant Professor of Clinical Pharmacy
College of Pharmacy
Washington State University
Pullman, Washington

Robert K. Maudlin, Pharm.D.
Pharmacist and Educational Coordinator
Family Medicine Spokane
Spokane, Washington

Robert A. Miller, Pharm.D.
Director of Clinical Programs
Health Application Systems
Burlingame, California

Gary M. Oderda, Pharm.D.
Director, Maryland Poison Information Center
Instructor, Clinical Pharmacy
School of Pharmacy
University of Maryland
Baltimore, Maryland

Larry E. Patterson, Pharm.D.
Assistant Professor of Pharmacy
Clinical Pharmacist, Hematology Division, College of Medicine
Director, Drug Information Service, College of Pharmacy
The University of Nebraska Medical Center
Omaha, Nebraska

Peter M. Penna, Pharm.D.
Assistant Professor of Clinical Pharmacy

College of Pharmacy
Washington State University
Pullman, Washington

Perry G. Rigby, M.D.
Dean College of Medicine
University of Nebraska College of Medicine
Omaha, Nebraska

Barbara L. Sauer, Pharm.D.
Pharmacist
Pharmacare Services
Sacramento, California

Sam K. Shimomura, Pharm.D.
Assistant Clinical Professor of Pharmacy
School of Pharmacy
University of California
San Francisco, California

Gary H. Smith, Pharm.D.
Assistant Professor of Clinical Pharmacy
Director, Drug Information Service
School of Pharmacy
University of Washington
Seattle, Washington

Glen L. Stimmel, Pharm.D.
Assistant Professor of Pharmacy
University of Southern California School of Pharmacy
Los Angeles, California

David S. Tatro, Pharm.D.
Research Pharmacist
Division of Clinical Pharmacology
Department of Medicine
Stanford University School of Medicine
Palo Alto, California

Theodore G. Tong, Pharm.D.
Assistant Clinical Professor of Pharmacy
School of Pharmacy
University of California
San Francisco, California

Lloyd Y. Young, Pharm.D.
Assistant Professor of Clinical Pharmacy
College of Pharmacy
Washington State University
Pullman, Washington

table of contents

Section One/General

Section Two/Renal Diseases

Section Three/Gastrointestinal Diseases

Section Four/Cardiovascular Diseases

Section Five/Respiratory Diseases

Section Six/Endocrine Diseases

Section Seven/Rheumatic Diseases

Section Twelve/Neoplastic Diseases

Section Thirteen/Infectious Diseases

section 1

General

chapter 1

THE PHARMACIST IN THERAPEUTICS

Paul Lofholm, Pharm.D.

Pharmacy as a separate profession from medicine originated in Europe in the 13th Century when the Emperor of the Holy Roman Empire, Fredrick II of Hohenstaufen, issued a series of edicts separating the two professions. "A new profession of technicians rather than scientists was intended by the edict of 1240. What was called science remained with the physicians. At that time, medical knowledge was comprised of little more than some mutilated remnants of antique wisdom and the employment of these remnants within definite boundaries of a rigid medical and therapeutic doctrine."[1] For centuries after that pharmacy was taught and practiced as a technical aspect of medicine, not as an art and a science of its own.

During the 17th and 18th Centuries, the empirical and dogmatic pharmaceutical data were gradually replaced by scientific findings and reasoning because of the emergence of the basic sciences such as chemistry. Up until the last decade the various branches of pharmacy have been primarily concerned with the manufacture, procurement, preparation, distribution and control of drug products.

Recently, the concept of a "patient-oriented" approach in addition to the traditional "product-oriented" approach to pharmacy practice has emerged. The term "clinical pharmacy" is being used to describe this "new" role for pharmacists.

In effect, this is a recognition by pharmacists, physicians and other health professionals that the responsibility for health care can be effectively shared and that the pharmacist's contribution does not necessarily end when the medication is dispensed. As in other areas of health care, it has been demonstrated that properly trained technicians or assistants can assume many of the technical and repetitive functions involved in the dispensing, distribution and control of medications. No one involved in the practice or the teaching of clinical pharmacy would advocate that the profession relinquish its traditional responsibilities. In fact, the clinical practice of pharmacy is a modification and expansion of those activities which have been performed by pharmacists for centuries.

THE HEALTH TEAM

The health team is a management concept which declares that each provider (pharmacist, physician, nurse, physical therapist, etc.) has obligations to guarantee that optimal care is provided through cooperative efforts. In this environment, the participating members share information about the patient's current status, behavior, the objectives of therapy and the patient's prognosis. For example, the pharmacist may often be responsible to the team for the short run therapeutic management of the patient, communicating with the patient and evaluating his/her status at the time of prescription renewal services. The pharmacist may monitor therapy by ordering laboratory tests, alter therapy regimens or refer the patient to other team members. (S)He maintains records of his services and reviews them with other team members when appropriate. The team concept represents a significant departure from the traditionally fragmented health care system in that the pharmacist and the physician and other health professionals exchange information about the patient. While the team approach to care is not yet the rule, it is gaining momentum. One limitation to even faster acceptance is that pharmacists do not always have a practical therapeutic knowledge and the ability to apply it in practice. This text is designed to facilitate the gaining of a working base for increasing the pharmacist's participation in therapeutics.

THE PHARMACIST AS A THERAPEUTIC SPECIALIST

Recognizing the need to have a therapeutic specialist on the health care team, and building on the pharmacist's knowledge of chemistry and drug products, some schools of pharmacy have instituted modification of the traditional pharmacy curricula. For example, a decade ago courses in pathology and orientation to medicine were introduced. Today, these introductory courses have grown in sophistication to in-depth courses in clinical pharmacology and the treatment of disease. The pharmacy student of today commands a broader knowledge of therapeutics, pharmacology and their application to medicine. He has often been trained with medical and nursing students, he has made rounds with them and he has shared patient management responsibilities with them.[2] He comes to the health team environment ready to contribute his therapeutic expertise, and we see the metamorphosis of the pharmacist's role from dispenser of pharmaceuticals to therapeutic advisor in this circumstance. There has been a shift in academic emphasis from training the pharmacist as a specialist in drug products as chemicals to a specialist in drug products as pharmaceutical agents used in patients to treat disease.

The contemporary pharmacist has an understanding of the appropriateness of therapy and the ability to assess the benefit to risk ratio of drug therapy, and (s)he can suggest alternative medications when a patient's drug regimen requires change. The pharmacist applies pharmacological principles to the clinical situation, and then (s)he plans and monitors the drug regimen. With the numbers of pharmaceutical products available and with the increasing incidence of drug interactions and adverse drug reactions (ADR), it is clear that the need for the pharmacist as a therapeutic advisor on the health team is immediate.

The rest of this discussion is made keeping in mind that a major responsibility of a pharmacist will indeed be that of a therapeutic consultant on the health team and that the assumption of this role has already begun for some and is imminent for many others.

GENERAL PRINCIPLES OF THERAPEUTICS

The drug therapy process[3] sequentially outlines the process of making drug decisions and providing drugs to patients. It takes account of the complex relationship between patients, drugs and disease. Although it was originally conceived by Dr. Brian Katcher of the University of California, School of Pharmacy, as a vehicle to outline the major areas of failure in drug therapy and ways the pharmacist could reduce these failures, it turns out to be a useful guide to provide rational therapy to patients (Fig. 1.1).

PATIENT COMPLAINT

Generally the start of any mode of therapy begins with the patient. In most cases, a patient seeks medical help when symptoms arise which are perceived by the patient to be more than trivial. However, mass screening programs for diabetes, hypertension, tuberculosis and other diseases are successful in detecting disease before symptoms are noted by the patient. All practicing pharmacists are aware that a significant proportion of the population will delay seeking medical help and instead seek relief by self-medicating with nonprescription drugs and homemade remedies.

From the pharmacist's point of view many patient complaints are assumed to be drug-induced. The initial responsibility of the pharmacist is to prove or disprove this assumption. A drug history provides the initial insight as to possible drug-induced causes of illness. Chapters 3 and 9 describe the salient points of iatrogenic cause of peptic ulcer disease. Although patients may deny the usage of salicylates, a concentrated drug history effort on the part of the pharmacist can sometimes establish excessive self-medication with salicylates.

DIAGNOSIS

Although the pharmacist is trained to appreciate the physical diagnosis, (s)he by no means makes the diagnosis. (S)He depends on the physician for the diagnosis, then, knowing the diagnosis and background of the patient, the pharmacist can assist the physician in planning

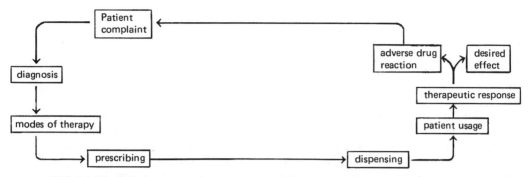

FIG. 1.1. The drug therapy process.
Adapted from B. Katcher, Failures in drug therapy.
Continuing Education in Health Sciences, University of California at San Francisco, School of Pharmacy, 1972.

a safe, effective and reasonable regimen for the patient.

Part of the diagnostic work-up should include questions about current and recent drug usage because drugs may mask disease. Drug usage may further complicate the usefulness of laboratory data by interfering with laboratory test methods and thus lead to erroneous results. For example, folic acid administration may improve the hematological status of a patient with pernicious anemia, but the progressive neuropathy may be masked, or the administration of salicylates may produce a false positive result when Clinitest tablets are used and again lead to a possible error in diagnosis.

MODES OF THERAPY

Drug therapy is only one of a number of methods of therapy that may be chosen. The question to be asked is, once the problem is diagnosed, which treatment modality should be used? Patient education, surgery, radiology, psychotherapy, reassurance or medication may be considered. The selection of the appropriate therapeutic modality is difficult. The benefits of therapy versus the risks of no therapy must be fully evaluated. However, the use of drugs to treat disease is frequently employed, and 65% of patients who go to the doctor receive at least one prescription drug.[4,5]

Drugs are relatively easy to use, especially for the ambulatory patient. They are generally safe and efficacious for the claimed indications, and they are relatively inexpensive. They usually do not require professional time to administer, or to monitor effects except in limited situations or when a serious adverse reaction occurs. They are highly promoted to the professions, and there may be significant patient pressure to use them. If they are used, many times the patient feels that something is being done for him, and that it was really worth it to see the doctor in the first place. The above reasons partially explain why six billion dollars are spent annually on drugs by the public.

PRESCRIBING

The clinician in making therapeutic decisions acknowledges the dynamic relationship between the patient, his disease and the drug. Furthermore, the decision includes not only the selection of the appropriate pharmacological agent but also the selection of the dosage form, route of administration, the frequency of administration, the dosage and the length of anticipated therapy. Only after the patient, disease and drug factors are studied can a rational therapeutic decision be made.

The selection of drug product involves a careful assessment of a number of parameters. Among the many factors to consider are age, sex, previous allergy, concurrent diseases, concurrent drug usage, gastrointestinal disease, renal disease, liver disease, pharmacogenetics and patient reliability.[6] A careful history will aid in discovering the significant patient factors. Furthermore, careful questioning of the patient should help establish the significance of any past drug reactions. One should clearly separate those patients who have experienced *expected* side effects from drugs versus those patients who in the past have experienced true idiosyncratic (nonpredictable) or allergic (non-dose-related) drug reactions. No patient should be denied optimal therapy because he experienced a predictable and preventable side effect.

The pharmacist should attempt to recognize and evaluate all factors which modify or limit the selection of the drug of choice. Some diseases preclude the use of certain drugs. For example, there is a risk of increasing the intraocular pressure in glaucomatous patients when certain drugs are administered (Chapter 34). Reserpine, indomethacin, corticosteroids and phenylbutazone increase the risk of peptic ulceration in patients with gastrointestinal disease. In a patient with several disease processes occurring coincidentally, one may need to assess therapeutic priorities in selecting which conditions to treat.

Pharmacists should have a basic knowledge of the efficacy and safety of the medication in terms of percentage of cure or improvement versus percentage of side effects which occur. Based on the experience of the pharmacist as validated by scientific fact, (s)he should have a series of "drugs of choice." Alternative therapy should likewise be established with a clear understanding as to why a particular drug is classified the way it is. Furthermore, the selection of any drug must be tempered by the expertise and background of the health team caring for the patient. If a particular physician is more familiar with belladonna tincture than propantheline, the pharmacist should be prepared to translate this choice to any therapeutic equivalent which is more familiar to the team.

Judgments on therapeutic efficacy in the clinical sense are difficult to make. Many conditions which are treated are self-limiting and, no matter what is prescribed, the patient improves. Therefore, without scientifically planned trials, many therapeutic regimens appear to be useful, not because of the pharmacological intervention but because of the natural course of the disease.

The pharmacist should also recognize that when patients are acutely ill, or complications preclude the use of the "drug of choice" or the primary drug has failed, greater risks are taken if more toxic drugs are prescribed. In doing so, the total patient must be kept in focus. Is therapy better than no therapy? For example, when a patient has a life-threatening infection, parenteral aminoglycoside antibiotics are often

prescribed when it is well known that they could produce permanent ototoxicity; on the other hand, these antibiotics are inappropriate for trivial infections.

Dosage is very critical if there exists a minimal dosage requirement for a therapeutic effect, and if a higher dosage of that same drug impairs ambulatory function or produces undesirable side effects. Patients on subtherapeutic levels of the drug will not experience the therapeutic advantage of therapy and patients on excessively high dosages may not be able to walk, care for themselves, work, drive automobiles, eat, sleep or perform other functions consistent with their lifestyle. In considering these factors, the patient is often begun on conservative (low dose) therapy which may be subtherapeutic. All too often there is no increase in the dosage, but rather the drug is discontinued, and then the patient is given a new prescription.

The dosage and frequency of administration have a scientific basis (pharmacokinetics)[7] and are based on the drug's relative rate of absorption, the volume of distribution, the rate of metabolism and the rate of excretion. Ideally, the dosing frequency is equal to the therapeutic half-life of the drug. As a rule, it will take 7 half-lives for a drug to be eliminated from the body. Although it is very useful to have pharamacokinetic data available, it is at present technically difficult to measure drug levels in the body except for a limited number of drugs like digoxin, quinidine, diphenylhydantoin, barbiturates and alcohol. Therefore, frequency of dosing decisions are often based on published data, previous clinical experience or tradition. However, the pharmacist with knowledge of drug kinetics can design dosing schedules to improve efficacy and/or reduce side effects. For example, because of diazepam's long half-life, it is often beneficial to prescribe this drug at bedtime as a single dose. Clinically, there are likewise advantages to giving sedative tricyclic depressants (amitriptyline) in larger doses at bedtime to promote sleep and lessen daytime side effects instead of giving smaller, more frequent doses.

The route of administration of medication is determined by the drug's site of action, the rate at which the patient requires the drug's effects and the patient's health status. Most drugs are administered orally because of convenience to the patient. However, the rate and extent of absorption (physiological availability) varies between pharmacological agents and their chemical forms, the physiological status of the absorption site and the nature of the dosage form administered. In fact, there is a greater variability in absorption from patient to patient than from tablet to tablet. If the oral route cannot be used because of gastrointestinal disease or nausea, the rectal route may be preferred. Local conditions or diseases limited to a particular area are often treated directly, *e.g.*, topically. For rapid action, parenteral and perhaps intravenous administration is required. For example, intramuscular diphenylhydantoin should not be used because of its unpredictability of absorption; therefore, intravenous therapy is preferred. By the oral route penicillin VK is absorbed better than penicillin G; therefore, penicillin VK is the drug of choice to treat susceptible infections when the oral route is desired.

DISPENSING

The dispensing phase of the drug therapy process includes analysis of the order, the selection of the drug product and the tailoring of the medication to meet the lifestyle of the patient. The pharmacist either compounds the product himself or else he selects a manufacturer's product which meets his standards, is physiologically available and is reasonable in cost. All drug products are assumed to meet the government's standards for safety and efficacy although they may vary widely in cost. Cost is not generally a valid criteria for quality.[8] Given the drug standards as they exist today, criteria to validate drug quality need only be applied where there has been a consistent demonstration of nonequivalence such as with digoxin. Where available, dissolution rates, dosage form composition, product assay data, lot-to-lot assay variability and *in vivo* drug level studies are helpful in demonstrating uniformity in drug product response. In many cases, the pharmacist can offer less costly therapy in a variety of therapeutic situations. Every effort should be made at the time of dispensing medications to select the most economical and efficacious drug products available.

PATIENT USAGE

Dosage form, taste, time of administration and frequency of administration must be properly tailored to the patient to promote compliance and thus ensure that the expected therapeutic outcome is achieved.

The problems of self-administration of medications by patients are extraordinary. Suppositories have been taken orally, antibiotic suspensions have been instilled into ears and therapeutic problems develop because patients are not informed as to the kind of medication they are taking, how to use it or how it acts in the body. As a rule patients do not read labels.[9] This does not mean that labeling is unnecessary. It does mean that the pharmacist should give detailed verbal instructions to all patients with new prescriptions, and that he should quiz patients getting renewals as to their knowledge of their drug therapy.

Often patients discontinue their medication because they feel better or they feel that the drug is no longer effective. The apparent basis for this action is how they perceive their illness. Patients need to know when medication is for symptomatic relief and when medication is for treatment of the disease. For example, every effort should be made to keep tuberculin reactors on isoniazid for the appropriate length of time. Similarly, the same effort should be directed to patients who are under treatment for hypertension.

THE THERAPEUTIC RESPONSE

The final step in the drug therapy process is an evaluation of the response to the medication. Most patients will improve. Some will experience ADR; 15 to 30% of hospitalized patients experience ADR while in the hospital.[6] The ADR rate for patients on medication in the community is unknown, but it may be as high as 15%. One of the roles of the pharmacist on the health team is to minimize the ADR rate through identification of potential drug problems before drugs are prescribed and dispensed.

CONCLUSION

The drug therapy process describes a series of interdependent variables which must be accounted for before, during and after evaluating therapeutic responses. The processing of therapeutic decisions in the above format should help all those making therapeutic decisions to have an objective in mind, to analyze the benefits versus risks of using pharmacological agents as a treatment modality and to select the most rational therapeutic regimen for the patient.

With a sincere interest in patients and their health and with a suitable training in therapeutics, any pharmacist can make a significant contribution to the health team and to patient care. It is imperative that every pharmacist strive to create an awareness in the minds of patient and physician as to his/her capabilities and responsibilities. Traditionally, patients have relied on themselves to understand therapeutics. Tradition seldom changes unless nudged by cold hard facts. While the competent physician may realize that there are problems in drug therapy, (s)he may not be aware of the fact that the pharmacist can be of assistance. For this reason pharmacists must exert every effort to equip themselves fully with the tools of therapeutics. And that is what the remaining chapters in this book are all about.

REFERENCES

1. Urdang, G.: Introduction to American pharmacy. In American Pharmacy, Ed. 5, p. ix, edited by J. B. Sprowls, Jr., J. B. Lippincott Co., Philadelphia, 1960.
2. Herfindal, E. T., and Levin, R. A.: Clinical pharmacy training in an outpatient clinic. Am. J. Pharm. Educ., 36: 72, 1972.
3. Katcher, B.: Failures in drug therapy. Continuing Education in Health Sciences, University of California at San Francisco, School of Pharmacy, May 3, 1972.
4. Stolley, P. D., Becker, M. H., Lasagna, L., McEvilla, J. D., and Sloane, L. M.: The relationship between physician characteristics and prescribing appropriateness. Med. Care, 10: 17, 1972.
5. Stolley, P. D., and Lasagna, L.: Prescribing patterns of physicians. J. Chronic. Dis., 22: 395, 1969.
6. Smith, J. W., Seidl, L. G., and Cluff, L. E.: Studies on the epidemiology of adverse drug reactions. Ann. Intern. Med., 65: 629, 1966.
7. Wagner, J. G.: Biopharmaceutics and Relevant Pharmacokinetics, pp. 51, 327. Drug Intelligence Publications, Hamilton, Ill., 1971.
8. Goyan, J. G.: Generic Equivalency and Therapeutic Efficacy. Statement read before the Subcommittee of Health, Education and Welfare Services, Interim Committee on Ways and Means, California State Assembly, November 22, 1966.
9. Schwartz, D., Wang, M., Zeitz, L., and Goss, M.: Medication errors made by elderly, chronically-ill patients. Am. J. Public Health, 52: 2018, 1962.

chapter 2

DRUG INTERACTIONS IN PERSPECTIVE

Philip D. Hansten, Pharm.D.

The adverse effects resulting from the combined effects of two or more administered drugs are collectively termed "drug-drug interactions." Many people in pharmacy have seen the prevention and detection of these adverse drug interactions as a major activity of the pharmacist. Indeed, patient drug profile information potentially available to the pharmacist along with his training in pharmacokinetics and drug action makes him the most suitable health professional to assume this responsibility. Although drug interactions thus constitute an area in which pharmacists might make contributions to decreasing untoward drug effects, we must not concentrate on this one topic to the exclusion of other important areas such as adverse reactions to single drugs and patient education.

IMPORTANCE OF DRUG INTERACTIONS

There exists a wide range of opinion concerning the importance of drug interactions as a cause of morbidity and mortality. A definitive and comprehensive study to detect the impact of all drug interactions (including interactions in which one drug is inhibited) has not yet been done in any specific patient population. However, the studies which have been done have given us some insight albeit within the limitations of the methods used.

The Boston Collaborative Drug Surveillance Program reported with an initial group of patients that 22% of reported adverse drug reactions were due to drug interactions,[1] while their subsequent, more extensive information including acute disease hospital patients yielded a figure of 6.9%.[2] As they properly pointed out, many interactions could have gone unrecognized and thus not included in their calculations. Another study done in a private community hospital indicated that 3 of 2,422 patients developed significant drug interactions for an incidence of 0.12%.[3] However, as the authors correctly stated, the design of the study probably did not allow detection of all drug interactions occurring in the patients studied.

Several epidemiological studies on the incidence of adverse drug interactions in patients receiving oral anticoagulants have appeared.[4-6] Although the methods of study varied, two conclusions were common to all three studies:

1. Patients on oral anticoagulants frequently receive potentially interacting drugs.
2. Although the potential for interaction is high, evidence of actual interaction was detected in about 5 to 10% of the total patients receiving oral anticoagulants.

Evidence available to date strongly indicates that the same situation is seen in other types of drug interactions: a considerable number of patients receiving interacting combinations with perhaps a few percent of the total patient population manifesting detectable signs of drug interaction.

Although evidence is accumulating that drug interactions are not as frequently a problem as originally suspected, the pendulum should not swing back to our previous state of ignorance and indifference. Deaths do occur as a result of drug interactions,[2, 7-10] and the collective impact of interactions involving inhibition of drug action is essentially completely unknown. Thus, drug interaction might well be considered an unknown portion of the general problem of unwanted drug effects. Interactions should certainly be studied and discussed, but not to the exclusion of attention to other important drug problems such as adverse reactions to single drugs, improper dosing with renal or hepatic impairment and patient education.

DETERMINATION OF CLINICAL SIGNIFICANCE IN SPECIFIC PATIENTS

The inability of health professionals to assess the potential clinical significance of specific interactions in individual patients has been a major impediment to the understanding of drug interactions. This difficulty appears to have arisen from lack of attention to the many patient factors and drug administration factors which may affect the outcome of the interaction. The specific conditions under which the interacting drugs are given are frequently more important than the theoretical clinical significance of the interaction itself. The following discussions consider some of the patient factors and drug administration factors which can be important in evaluation of the clinical significance of drug interactions in specific patients.

PATIENT FACTORS

Diseases

It is well known that diseases can affect the response to drugs, and this applies to drug interactions as well. Diabetics are more likely to develop anabolic steroid-induced hypoglycemia[11] and triamterene-induced hyperglycemia and hyperkalemia.[12] Patients with primary open angle glaucoma do not manifest the typical interaction seen between dexamethasone and diphenylhydantoin.[13] There are many other examples in which the patients' diseases may affect the clinical consequences of drugs given alone or in combination.

Renal Function

Since the kidney is involved in the excretion of many drugs and their metabolities, it would seem likely that impaired renal function might predispose patients to the development of drug interactions. For example, it has been proposed that renal impairment may increase the likelihood of an ethacrynic acid-warfarin interaction owing to the increased blood levels of ethacrynic acid and resultant increased displacement of warfarin from plasma protein binding.[14] The possible increased incidence of nephrotoxicity following the combined use of cephalothin and gentamicin is also probably more important in patients with pre-existing renal impairment.[15,16] Although it is commonly appreciated that drug excretion may be impaired in renal disease, it should also be remembered that the metabolism of some drugs appears to be impaired in uremic patients.[17] Finally, it should be remembered that patients with nephrosis may have hypoalbuminemia, a factor which also may affect the outcome of drug interactions.

Hepatic Function

It has been assumed that interactions of drugs which undergo hepatic metabolism would be more important in patients with liver disease. However, few examples of this phenomenon have appeared. It seems likely that in most cases, liver function must be severely impaired before drug metabolism is affected in a clinically significant way. It should also be remembered that severe liver disease may result in other conditions which can affect the outcome of drug interactions such as hypoalbuminemia and hypoprothrombinemia. Diphenylhydantoin may be an example of a drug which is more likely to be involved in significant interactions in the presence of liver disease. This may be due to impaired diphenylhydantoin metabolism and possibly competition between bilirubin and diphenylhydantoin for plasma albumin binding.[18,19]

Serum Protein Levels

Since many drugs are bound to a considerable extent to serum proteins (primarily albumin), one might expect drug actions and interactions to be affected by serum protein levels. In particular, interactions involving displacement of drugs from plasma protein binding sites might be expected to be most important in patients with hypoalbuminemia. In 1968, Anton presented evidence that adverse reactions and drug interactions may be more frequent in patients with lower serum albumin levels.[20] Lewis et al.[21] subsequently presented evidence to indicate that the frequency of side effects to prednisone is doubled in patients with serum albumin levels below 2.5 g/100 ml. The response to curare and other drugs may also be affected by serum protein levels.[22]

Urinary pH

Many commonly used drugs are weak acids or weak bases and as such have the potential for variable urinary excretion rates depending upon the pH of the urine.[23] Weak acids such as salicylic acid tend to be excreted more rapidly as the urinary pH increases since they are more ionized and reabsorption across the renal tubular cell is thus decreased. Conversely, weak bases such as amphetamine are more un-ionized as urinary pH increases, thus increasing renal tubular reabsorption and decreasing urinary excretion. However, it should be remembered that only some of the drugs within the pKa range for pH-dependent urinary excretion (acids: pKa 3 to 7; bases: pKa 7 to 11) will show this property in a clinically significant way. If less than 20% of the active drug is normally excreted in the urine or if the unionized form of the drug is not sufficiently lipid-soluble, the urinary excretion of the drug is not likely to be very sensitive to changes in urinary acidity.[23] Thus, when evaluating the role of urinary pH in drug excretion, one must consider a number of factors including properties of the drug molecule itself, all normal routes of metabolism and their ability to compensate for decreases in urinary drug excretion and the organ function of the specific patient under consideration.

Dietary Factors

In most patients receiving interacting drugs in this country, diet appears to play a minor role in the clinical outcome. However, it has been proposed that the interaction of some drugs (eg. antibiotics, salicylates, etc.) with oral anticoagulants may be the most significant in patients with an impaired vitamin K intake.[24] It also appears that the osteomalacia following combined anticonvulsant therapy may be more likely to occur in patients with low vitamin D intake.[25] Other examples will certainly be uncovered with additional research, and determination of the over-all impact of diet on drug interactions must await further study.

The related topic of drug-food interactions is receiving increased attention, and the reader is referred to the several reviews on this topic.[26-28]

Environmental Factors

The extensive number of chemicals to which we are exposed in our air, water and food have the potential for affecting our response to drugs and thus may affect the clinical outcome of drug interactions. Insecticide exposure has been shown to be associated with increased drug metabolism,[29],[30] probably a result of hepatic microsomal enzyme induction by the insecticide. Evidence is also accumulating that smoking and breathing urban air can increase drug metabolism.[31-33]

Pharmacogenetic Factors

The topic of pharmacogenetics is becoming quite important to the understanding of drug action in man, and there is little doubt that susceptibility to the adverse effects of many interactions is at least partly genetically determined. Pharmacological studies have confirmed what had been suspected for many years: that blood levels of drugs vary considerably between individuals. This has been shown for procainamide,[34] nortriptyline,[35] phenylbutazone[36] and several other drugs. It has also been proposed that the degree of hepatic microsomal enzyme inducibility may be genetically determined.[37] It has further been postulated that some patients may have a genetically determined decreased capacity for aromatic hydroxylation, a process involved in the metabolism of a number of commonly used drugs. Finally, although it has long been known that race may predispose patients to adverse drug reactions, there is increasing evidence that drug metabolism may show racial differences.[38],[39]

For some drug interactions, pharmacogenetic factors have already been shown to play a very significant role in the outcome of interactions. For example, Brennan et al.[40] have shown that genetically "slow" metabolizers of isoniazid also receiving diphenylhydantoin (DPH) are more likely to manifest elevated DPH blood levels and signs of DPH toxicity.

Age

If one looks at the ages of the patients involved in reported drug interactions, it quickly becomes obvious that these patients tend to be older. There are a number of reasons for this. First, and most obvious, older patients receive more drugs. Secondly, these patients receive more of the type of drugs known to be involved in interactions (e.g., oral hypoglycemics, oral anticoagulants, antihypertensives). Finally, elderly patients tend to have more diseases, poorer kidney function and a less adequate diet than the general population, all factors which

may predispose to interactions as discussed above.

Drug Administration Factors

Sequence of Administration. The order in which the interacting drugs are prescribed is one of the more important determinants of the clinical significance of drug interactions in specific patients, yet it is frequently overlooked in practice. The patient stabilized in an oral anticoagulant or oral hypoglycemic drug who is then given a drug which affects this balance is much more likely to be affected adversely by the interaction than a patient who is already receiving the interacting drug and is subsequently titrated with the anticoagulant or hypoglycemic agent. This simple and seemingly obvious fact has been neglected in both epidemiological studies and clinical pharmacological studies of drug interactions. In addition to the above considerations of patients on drugs which are titrated, many other interactions are affected by drug administration sequence for various reasons. The dangerous hypertensive episodes following the concomitant administration of monoamine oxidase inhibitors (MAOI) and indirect acting sympathomimetic agents occur when the sympathomimetic is administered to a patient already receiving an MAOI, not with the reverse order of administration. Kaolin-pectin (Kaopectate) impairs oral lincomycin absorption if the kaolin-pectin is given 2 hr after lincomycin, but it is without effect if given 2 hr before the lincomycin.[41] The probable importance of sequence of administration for any given interaction can usually be deduced by considering the mechanism of the interaction, along with other information such as the pharmacology of the drugs involved and pertinent patient factors.

Route of Administration. Some interactions, such as the inhibition of oral tetracycline absorbed by antacid preparations, are obviously route-dependent and can be avoided by changing routes or adjusting dosing schedules. It is now becoming apparent that oral absorption interactions are more frequent than previously suspected,[42-44] and thus route will be a factor to be considered in an increasing number of interactions. It should be noted that route of drug administration can be important in interactions not involving absorption. For example, a patient receiving MAOI who is subsequently given a standard oral dose of phenylephrine is likely to manifest a greater reaction than if the phenylephrine were given intravenously.[45] The proposed explanation for this phenomenon is as follows. Since phenylephrine is metabolized by monoamine oxidase (MAO) in the liver and intestine, the response to normal oral doses of phenylephrine is markedly enhanced. Intravenous doses of phenylephrine are smaller than oral because of decreased exposure to hepatic and intestinal MAO; thus previous inhibition of MAO would not be expected to result in a markedly enhanced response to standard parenteral doses of phenylephrine.

Duration of Therapy. There are many situations in which duration of drug therapy is important to the evaluation of an interaction in a specific patient. The majority of interactions require concurrent administration of the drugs for at least several days before the adverse effects of the interaction can be seen. Thus, for interactions involving enzyme induction, inhibition of monoamine oxidase and many others, duration is an important consideration. Failure to account for duration of therapy has resulted in confusion in epidemiological studies and in clinical pharmacological studies of drug interactions. For example, the known interaction between guanethidine and tricyclic antidepressants was not detected by some investigators who did not wait long enough to see inhibition of the antihypertensive effect of guanethidine.[46,47]

Dose of Drugs. As a general rule, the adverse effects of interactions are more likely to occur following larger doses. This is especially true for interactions involving competitive enzyme inhibition, plasma protein binding displacement and pharmacological effects of drugs. In some cases, the character of an interaction may change considerably at different doses. For example, barbiturates appear to enhance the metabolism of therapeutic doses of tricyclic antidepressants, while the adverse effects of toxic doses of tricyclic antidepressants appear to be enhanced by barbiturate administration.[35,48]

Dosage Form. A few interactions have been reported in which dosage form of the drugs may affect the outcome of the interaction. There is evidence that sustained release forms of phenylpropanolamine are less likely than the standard oral dosage form to produce a severe hypertensive reaction in patients receiving an MAO inhibitor.[49] As another example, propantheline administration has been shown to enhance absorption of one brand of digoxin tablets but to have no effect on digoxin administered as a liquid.[42] This is presumably because the liquid form is nearly completely absorbed even in the absence of propantheline.

APPLICATION OF DRUG INTERACTION INFORMATION IN IMPROVING PATIENT CARE

In order to perform a service to patients by preventing and detecting drug interactions, the pharmacist must do more than have a few drug interaction books on the shelf of his library. Obviously, patient medication profiles of some type must be kept in order to detect the patients potentially at risk. The pharmacist must continue to read original journal articles on drug interactions rather than depending completely on the compilations of others. An efficient and effective method of getting drug interaction information to the physicians of the patients involved must be developed. It is becoming apparent that a written form of communication to the physician is sufficient for the majority of interactions, with more rapid notification required only occasionally. Finally, it must be realized that the morbidity and mortality of adverse reactions and drug interactions cannot be reduced by passive and occasional attention by the pharmacist. Programs must be carefully developed, and extra time and energy must be expended if the results are to match the verbiage on drug interaction monitoring by the pharmacist.

REFERENCES

1. Borda, I. T., Slane, D., and Jick, H.: Assessment of adverse reactions within a drug surveillance program. J. A. M. A., 205: 645, 1968.
2. Boston Collaborative Drug Surveillance Program: Adverse drug interactions (editorial). J. A. M. A., 220: 1238, 1972.
3. Puckett, W. H., and Visconti, J. A.: An epidemiological study of the clinical significance of drug-drug interactions in a private community hospital. Am. J. Hosp. Pharm., 28: 247, 1971.
4. Starr, K. J., and Petrie, J. C.: Drug interactions in

patients on long-term oral anticoagulant and antihypertensive adrenergic neuron-blocking drugs. Br. Med. J., 4: 133, 1972.

5. Koch-Weser, J.: Hemorrhagic reactions and drug interactions in 500 warfarin-treated patients (abstract). Clin. Pharmacol. Ther., 14: 139, 1973.

6. Kleinman, P. D., and Griner, P. F.: Studies of the epidemiology of anti-coagulant-drug interactions. Arch. Intern. Med., 126: 522, 1970.

7. Shapiro, S., Slone, D., Lewis, G. P., and Jick, H.: Fatal drug reactions among medical inpatients. J. A. M. A., 216: 467, 1971.

8. Arch, R., and Kissane, J. (editors): Clinicopathologic conference: hypertension and the lupus syndrome. Am. J. Med., 49: 519, 1970.

9. MacDonald, M. G., and Robinson, D. S.: Clinical observations of possible barbiturate interference with anticoagulation. J. A. M. A., 204: 97, 1968.

10. Lloyd, J. T. A., and Walker, D. R. H.: Death after combined dexamphetamine and phenelzine (letter). Br. Med. J., 2: 168, 1965.

11. Landon, J., Wynn, V., and Samols, E.: The effect of anabolic steroids on blood sugar and plasma insulin levels in man. Metabolism, 12: 924, 1963.

12. Walker, B. R., Capuzzi, D. M., Alexander, F., Familiar, R. G., and Hoppe, R. C.: Hyperkalemia after triamterene in diabetic patients. Clin. Pharmacol. Ther., 13: 643, 1972.

13. Becker, B., Krupin, T., and Podos, S. M.: Diphenylhydantoin and dexamethasone-induced changes of plasma cortisol: comparison of patients with and without glaucoma. J. Clin. Endocrinol. Metal., 32: 669, 1971.

14. Sellers, E. M., and Koch-Weser, J.: Displacement of warfarin from human albumin by diazoxide and ethacrynic, mefenamic and nalidixic acids. Clin. Pharmacol. Ther., 11: 524, 1970.

15. Bobrow, S. N., Jaffe, E., and Young, R. C.: Anuria and acute tubular necrosis associated with gentamicin and cephalothin. J. A. M. A., 222: 1546, 1972.

16. Opitz, A., Herrmann, I., Herrath, D., and Schaefer, K.: Akute niereninsuffizienz nach gentamycin-cephalosporin-kombinationstherapie. Med. Welt., 22: 434, 1971.

17. Reidenberg, M. M., James, M., and Dring, L. G.: The rate of procaine hydrolysis in serum of normal subjects and diseased patients. Clin. Pharmacol. Ther., 13: 279, 1972.

18. Kutt, H., Winters, W., and Scherman, R.: Diphenylhydantoin and phenobarbital toxicity. The role of liver disease. Arch. Neurol., 11: 649, 1964.

19. Rane, A., Lunde, P. K. M., Jalling, B., Yaffe, S. J., and Sjogvist, F.: Plasma protein binding of diphenylhydantoin in normal and hyperbilirubinemic newborn infants. J. Pediatr., 78: 877, 1971.

20. Anton, A. H.: The effect of disease, drugs and dilution on the binding of sulfonamides in human plasma. Clin. Pharmacol. Ther., 9: 561, 1968.

21. Lewis, G. P., Jusko, W. J., Burke, C. W., and Graves, L.: Prednisone side-effects and serum protein levels. A collaborative study. Lancet, 2: 778, 1971.

22. Stovner, J., Theodorsen, L., and Bjelke, E.: Sensitivity to tubocurarine and alcuronium with special reference to plasma protein pattern. Br. J. Anaesth., 43: 385, 1971.

23. Weiner, I. M., and Mudge, G. H.: Renal tubular mechanisms for excretion of organic acids and bases. Am. J. Med., 36: 743, 1964.

24. O'Reilly, R. A., and Aggeler, P. M.: Determinants of the response to oral anticoagulant drugs in man. Pharmacol. Rev., 22: 35, 1970.

25. Hahn, T. J.: Anticonvulsive therapy and vitamin D (letter). Ann. Intern. Med., 78: 308, 1973.

26. Pierpaoli, P. G.: Drug therapy and diet. Drug Intell. Clin. Pharmacy, 6: 89, 1972.

27. Krondl, A.: Present understanding of the interaction of drugs and food during absorption. Can. Med. Assoc. J., 103: 360, 1970.

28. Faloon, W. W.: Drug production of intestinal malabsorption. N. Y. State J. Med., 70: 2189, 1970.

29. Kolmodin, B., Azarnoff, D. L., and Sjoqvist, F.: Effect of environmental factors on drug metabolism. Decreased plasma half-life of antipyrine in workers exposed to chlorinated hydrocarbon insecticides. Clin. Pharmacol. Ther., 10: 638, 1969.

30. Poland, A., Smith, D., Kuntzman, R., Jacobson, M., and Conney, A. H.: Effect of intensive occupational exposure to DDT on phenylbutazone and cortisol metabolism in human subject. Clin. Pharmacol. Ther., 11: 724: 1970.

31. Keeri-Szanto, M., and Pomeroy, J. R.: Atmospheric pollution and pentazocine metabolism. Lancet, 1: 947, 1971.

32. Boston Collaborative Drug Surveillance Program: Clinical depression of the central nervous system due to diazepam and chlordiazepoxide in relation to cigarette smoking and age. N. Engl. J. Med., 288: 277, 1973.

33. Keeri-Szanto, M., Muir, J. M., and Remington, B.: Smoking reduces the effectiveness of narcotics (abstract). Clin. Pharmacol. Ther., 14: 139, 1973.

34. Koch-Weser, J.: Pharmacokinetics of procainamide in man. Ann. N. Y. Acad. Sci., 179: 370, 1971.

35. Alexanderson, B., Evans, D. A. P., and Sjoqvist, F.: Steady-state plasma levels of nortriptyline in twins: influence of genetic factors and drug therapy. Br. Med. J., 4: 764, 1969.

36. Whittaker, J. A., Evans, D. A. P.: Genetic control of phenylbutazone metabolism in man. Br. Med. J., 4: 323, 1970.

37. Vessell, E. S., and Page, J. G.: Genetic control of the phenobarbital-induced shortening of plasma antipyrine half-lives in man. J. Clin. Invest., 48: 2202, 1969.

38. Jeanes, C. W. L., Schaefer, O., and Eidus, L.: Inactivation of isoniazid by Canadian Eskimos and Indians. Can. Med. Assoc. J., 106: 331, 1972.

39. Arnold, K., and Gerver, N.: The rate of decline of diphenylhydantoin in human plasma. Clin. Pharmacol. Ther., 11: 121, 1970.

40. Brennan, R. W., Dehejia, H., Kutt, J., Verebely, K., and McDowell, F.: Diphenylhydantoin intoxication attendant to slow inactivation of isonaizid. Neurology, 20: 687, 1970.

41. Wagner, J. G.: Pharmacokinetics. I. Definitions, modeling and reasons for measuring blood levels and urinary excretion. Drug Intell. Clin. Pharmacy, 2: 38, 1968.

42. Manninen, V., Apajalahti, A., Melin, J., and Karesoja, M.: Altered absorption of digoxin in patients given propantheline and metoclopramide. Lancet, 1: 398, 1973.

43. Nimmo, J., Heading, R. C., Tothill, P., and Prescott, L. F.: Pharmacological modification of gastric emptying: effects of propantheline and metoclopramide on paracetamol absorption. Br. Med. J., 1: 587, 1973.

44. Consolo, S., Morselli, P. L., Zaccala, M., and Garattini, S.: Delayed absorption of phenylbutazone caused by desmethylimipramine in humans. Eur. J. Pharmacol., 10: 239, 1970.

45. Elis, J., Laurence, D. R., Mattie, H., and Prichard, B. N. C.: Modification of monoamine oxidase inhibitors of the effect of some sympathomimetics on blook pressure. Br. Med. J., 2: 75, 1967.

46. Gulati, O. D., Dave, B. T., Gokhale, S. D., and Shah, K. M.: Antagonism of adrenergic neuron blockade in hypertensive subjects. Clin. Pharmacol. Ther., 7: 510, 1966.

47. Ober, K. F., and Wang, R. I. H.: Drug interactions with guanethidine. Clin. Pharmacol. Ther., 14: 190, 1973.

48. Noble, J., and Matthew, H.: Acute poisoning by tricyclic antidepressants: clinical features and management of 100 patients. Clin. Toxicol., 2: 304, 1969.

49. Cuthbert, M. F., Greenberg, M. P., and Morley, S. W.: Cough and cold remedies: potential danger to patients on monoamide oxidase inhibitors. Br. Med. J., 1: 404, 1969.

chapter 3

DRUG-INDUCED DISEASES

Robert K. Maudlin, Pharm.D.

The cure is worse than the disease.
Philip Massinger

Today, one might revise Philip Massinger's quote to "One man's cure is yet another man's disease." Probably no one should be more aware of this than today's pharmacist. Since he is responsible for providing the pharmaceutical agents that are prescribed for nearly 75% of all patients leaving a physician's office, the pharmacist must be aware of the responses his patients may experience from these agents. The pharmacist not only needs to know that the medication and its dosage are proper for his patients, but he also must be aware of what unwanted reactions might occur as a consequence of that therapy.

It is reported that 2.9 to 3.7%[1, 2] and possibly as high as 5% of hospital admissions are attributable to drug reactions, and that 18 to 30% of hospital patients will have a reaction to their medication before they are discharged.[3] It is estimated that in excess of 3% of all hospital deaths may be attributable to drugs. We would be naive if we assumed that the percentages reported were indicative of the total number of drug reactions occurring. Obviously the difference between the reported number and the actual number of reactions occurring in our hospitals must be large. Just as obvious is the fact that more drug reactions go unnoticed in the community than in our hospitals.

If the majority of these reactions were unpredictable owing to hypersensitivity or idiosyncratic reactions or were unavoidable owing to side effects from medications that have to be given, then we would just have to suffer the consequences. However, these situations make up only 20 to 30% of the reactions. The vast majority are totally predictable.

Many pharmacists don't have to review the literature to find such reports; first hand experience has provided them with more than enough examples. Yet the pharmacist has the last say before the patient gets the medication and is in the ideal position to prevent the 70 to 80% of drug reactions that are predictable and preventable. Through careful drug histories and family medication records the pharmacist undoubtedly could play a major role in the prevention of these reactions.

The various means by which drugs may induce diseases are overdosage, drug interactions, secondary effects, idiosyncracy and hypersensitivity. Generally, a drug reaction appears when the concentration of a given drug exceeds a certain threshold in the body. However, other drugs (drug interactions), underlying disease or enzyme deficiencies (idiosyncratic reactions) may turn a "normal dose" into an "overdose" leading to toxicity. No drug has a single pharmacological effect, and often those effects not being used therapeutically appear as side effects. These effects are termed secondary effects, and they may be so distressing as to necessitate terminating therapy. Hopefully these secondary effects will be attributed to the patient's drug and not as an extension of his underlying pathology. Finally, the unpredictable hypersensitivity or allergic reaction is independent of the dosage given, and likewise the symptoms are independent of the pharmacological properties of the drug.

Nonetheless, if a pharmacist were to step back and take a close look at all of these classes, hopefully he could prevent many of these reactions from occurring in his patients.

OVERDOSAGE

In years past when one envisioned the term "overdose," probably the immediate thoughts were that the physician prescribed too large a dose or that the patient took too many tablets. It was felt that if you adhered to the normal dose, you were pretty safe except in the obviously large or small patient. Now, however, the normal or average dose concept is being seriously questioned. Many factors influence the plasma concentrations of drugs—absorption, distribution, protein and tissue binding, metabolism and excretion. These factors are capable of changing normal doses into subtherapeutic doses or overdoses. A good example of this may be seen with diphenylhydantoin. The dose is usually 4 to 5 mg per kg of body weight (usual-

ly prescribed as 300 mg per day for convenience). It is now reported that this dosage will give blood levels that vary by as much as 4- to 7-fold.[4-7] This becomes quite important when you consider that the therapeutic index for diphenylhydantoin is quite small. Clinically effective plasma concentrations are in the 10 to 15 μg per ml range, and toxic effects may be seen above 15 μg per. In fact, 25% of patients taking the drug exhibit adverse reactions above 25 μg per ml. The reasons for these wide variations in blood levels appear to stem from several factors. Diphenylhydantoin is metabolized in the liver where it undergoes parahydroxylation. Some persons have been found to lack the hydroxylating enzymes to do this, which may predispose them to toxicity at normal doses. In contrast to this, persons could metabolize the drug too rapidly, leading to low levels of the drug. Recently, it has been suggested that serum levels may be altered by differences in the plasma diphenylhydantoin concentration at which enzyme induction occurs or differences in the level at which rate-limiting enzyme reactions become saturated.[8] The change may also be due to variations in absorption, which is relatively slow and occurs mainly in the upper portion of the intestine. Liver disease interferes with the metabolism of diphenylhydantoin. Other drugs such as bishydroxycoumarin, isoniazid, aminosalicylic acid and disulfiram inhibit the metabolism of diphenylhydantoin. On the other hand, phenobarbital enhances the metabolism of diphenylhydantoin.

Certainly a major cause of therapeutic failure and unexplained low plasma levels of diphenylhydantoin is failure of patients to take their medication. Up to 75% of the "refractory" patients have unreliable intake of drugs.

Other factors influence patient response to normal dosages of drugs. For example, we normally see congestive heart failure patients maintained on 0.25 to 0.50 mg of digoxin daily. Yet a patient with impaired renal function or one with hypokalemia may exhibit digitalis toxicity at this dosage. A patient with normal renal function loses, by various routes, about 35% of the digoxin in the body per day. The maintenance dose is meant to replace that loss. On the other hand, in the anuric patient only 14% of the digoxin in the body is lost per day.[9] Therefore, if the normal dose of 0.25 to 0.50 mg is continued in the presence of this anuria, drug accumulation and inevitable digitalis toxicity ensue. An increase in cardiac sensitivity to digoxin associated with hypokalemia is well documented. Animal studies have shown that hypokalemic dogs show toxicity after receiving 39% less digoxin than dogs with normal potassium levels.[10] The importance of this to a pharmacist lies in the fact that many of his patients on digoxin also are taking diuretics that deplete potassium. Administration of the thiazide diuretics, furosemide, ethacrynic acid or chlorthalidone results in large loads of sodium being presented to the renal tubules for excretion. Increased sodium-potassium exchange results, leading to marked increases in potassium excretion. It has been suggested that these diuretics are the most important predisposing or precipitating factor in digitalis toxicity today. Patients on both medications should always have their potassium levels monitored closely. Three alternatives are available to restore potassium in the presence of continued digoxin-diuretic therapy, dietary replacement, potassium-sparing diuretics or potassium chloride supplementation. The choice depends mainly on selecting an approach that will adequately restore potassium to normal levels, one which the patient will adhere to and one that is economical.

In the above examples systemic drug reactions were noted. However, local adverse effects to the systemic administration of drugs also occur. All pharmacists are aware of the gastrointestinal irritation associated with aspirin ingestion. This adverse effect is probably the major reason we have so many different aspirin preparations on the market, and it certainly is the nucleus for most of the aspirin advertising on television and radio and in magazines. About 5% of people ingesting aspirin complain of heartburn after a single dose. More serious than this heartburn is the gastric bleeding or ulceration that may occur. It is widely reported that 70% of the people taking 3 g of aspirin per day bleed 2 to 6 ml and 10% lose more than 10 ml per day.

Acid appears to be essential for aspirin-induced gastrointestinal bleeding. The pKa of aspirin is 3.5 implying that 50 percent of the drug is in the nonionized, lipid soluble, readily absorbable form at a pH of 3.5. At a pH of 2.5, 91 percent of the drug is in this form. Therefore the acid environment of the stomach promotes aspirin absorption. Once aspirin is absorbed into the gastric mucosal cell it encounters a pH of 7 whereas the surface of the gastric lumen has a pH of 2. Ionization occurs in the mucosal cell while a high concentration gradient of nonionized drug exits on the mucosal surface. Subsequently aspirin accumulates in the cell. This apparently disrupts the mucosal membrane barrier allowing hydrogen ions to back-diffuse into the mucosa. The result is cell damage, erosion, exfoliation and bleeding. Support for the necessity of acid comes from the finding that fecal blood loss and mucosal hemorrhages are significantly less common in achlorhydric subjects than in normal subjects following the administration of aspirin. Evidence showing that the addition of antacid buffers to aspirin tablets and aspirin solutions reduces fecal blood loss also implies the necessary role of acid. Gastroscopic studies have revealed that the oral administration of aspirin and acid will cause more mucosal erosions and bleeding than the administration of acid alone and that by replacing the acid with sodium bicarbonate the erosions and bleeding can be significantly reduced. Importantly the amount of blood loss with aspirin is reduced in direct relation to the buffer capacity of the formulation. Therefore it seems reasonable to assume that a local effect of aspirin in combination with acid is involved in inducing occult gastrointestinal blood loss.

Studies reporting gastrointestinal bleeding following intravenous administration of aspirin seem to lack continuity. Species specificity may explain this as mucosal erosions and bleeding are commonly reported in studies on rats but not in studies on guinea pigs, rabbits and dogs. As mentioned in my article, studies in man have failed to show that the intravenous administration of aspirin in normal doses causes blood loss above the normal levels (0.17-1.7) ml/day.[11]

Currently there are no commercially available tablet formulations of aspirin that will significantly reduce gastrointestinal bleeding. Studies are underway with aspirin tablet and solution formulations in combination with calcium carbonate, magnesium carbonate and magnesium oxide which apparently will markedly reduce these ulcerogenic properties.[12, 13] Until better formulations are available, pharmacists should recommend to their patients with gastrointestinal intolerance to aspirin (but who must take the drug) that the tablets be crushed and suspended in about 15 ml of water and this mixture added to a full dose of a non-aluminum-containing liquid antacid.

From these examples it is hoped that the idea of a normal dose for all patients be held as a relative phenomenon. There is no normal dose at which therapeutic effects are derived at which no adverse effects occur.

DRUG INTERACTIONS

The occurrence of drug interactions is certainly not new. However, there is a new awareness on the part of pharmacists who are recognizing the impact that these interactions have on patient response to drug therapy. All pharmacists owe it to themselves and to their patients to have a basic understanding of drug interactions and to have ready access to drug interaction information.

Because of the complexity of this subject, it is felt to be beyond the context of this discussion to cover it adequately. The author would, however, like to make reference to the book that he feels best covers this subject. *Drug Interactions* by P. D. Hansten (Lea and Febiger, Philadelphia, 1973) is complete, up-to-date, easy to use and economical. For a more detailed discussion of the mechanisms of drug interactions one may want to supplement, but not replace, this book with Hartshorn's *Handbook of Drug Interactions* (Don E. Francke, Cincinnati, 1970). These two books will give any pharmacist good back-up reference to supplement his own basic knowledge.

SECONDARY EFFECTS

No drug has but a single pharmacological effect. Drugs are used for one or a number of their beneficial effects, while those undesirable effects that cannot be avoided are often considered to be side effects. It is these unavoidable, bothersome effects that will be considered as secondary effects. Immediately such examples come to mind as the sedation accompanying antihistamine therapy in patients with colds, the loss of potassium or extracellular fluid contraction following thiazide diuretic therapy in treating hypertension, the Parkinson-like tremors due to phenothiazines during psycho-

therapy and the marked central nervous system depression following reserpine.

Narcotic analgesics cause significant respiratory depression in patients even in dosages considered to be too small to cause sleep or disturb consciousness. Apparently this depression is due to a decreased responsiveness of the brain stem to increases in carbon dioxide. This effect is dose-related. Nausea, secondary to these analgesics, is often referred to by patients as an allergic reaction. In reality this has little to do with an allergy but instead is due to a direct stimulation of the chemoreceptor trigger zone and sensitization to transmission from the vestibular apparatus. At equianalgesic doses, probably all narcotic analgesics will cause nausea and vomiting.

Thiazide diuretic therapy can lead to hyperuricemia and/or changes in carbohydrate metabolism in certain patients. The effect of these diuretics on uric acid appears to be biphasic in nature such that intravenous administration leads to uricosuria, while chronic oral therapy leads to uric acid retention and hyperuricemia (nearly 50% of the patients treated will show serum uric acid levels above 7 mg%). The actual mechanism by which this occurs is not fully understood, but these diuretics cause extracellular fluid contraction, and the decrease in renal tubular secretion of uric acid may be secondary to this. Ethacrynic acid, furosemide, chlorthalidone, acetazolamide, triamterene and the mercurial diuretics have also been implicated in causing hyperuricemia. The thiazides exhibit both pancreatic and extrapancreatic actions in causing hyperglycemia in certain patients. *In vitro* there is a reduction in glucose utilization, and the degree of this reduction increases as the dosage increases. Also, *in vivo*, patients who exhibit hyperglycemia while on thiazides have a decreased insulin response. Clinically, there appears to be little or no elevation in fasting blood sugar or evidence of glycosuria in nondiabetic patients. However, in diabetics or prediabetics there is increased hyperglycemia. In diabetic patients the thiazides may antagonize the hypoglycemic effect of the antidiabetic drugs.

It is not generally known that therapeutic doses of salicylates are as potent as some of the sulfonylureas and phenformin in lowering blood glucose levels in both diabetics and nondiabetics. The salicylates rank just behind alcohol and the antidiabetic drugs in causing hypoglycemia in children and adults.[14] This hypoglycemic effect is not due to enhanced insulin release or to increased sensitivity to insulin, but it may be due to increased utilization of glucose by peripheral tissues and a decrease in carbohydrate synthesis.

A secondary effect of the aminoglycoside antibiotics (streptomycin, kanamycin, neomycin and gentamicin) and the polymyxins (polymyxin B and colistin) is respiratory depression due to neuromuscular blockade. Apparently this problem occurs most commonly in patients with renal impairment, in patients receiving concomitant muscle relaxers, in those receiving the drug intravenously or intraperitoneally and in those receiving an overdosage. This respiratory paresis and paralysis may appear quickly and without premonitory manifestations. Even cessation of drug therapy when toxicity appears by no means assures protection from neurotoxicity or reversibility of all manifestations of the neuromuscular blockage. It is controversial whether calcium chloride or neostigmine is the best antagonist; however, one should provide mechanical support, regardless of the agent used.

A final example of drug secondary effects leading to disease is diphenylhydantoin-induced folic acid deficiency leading to megaloblastic anemia. Apparently dose-related, it has been shown that 60% of patients on long term diphenylhydantoin therapy exhibit folate deficiency.[15] Serum vitamin B_{12} levels are usually not altered. Certainly all of these patients do not manifest megaloblastic anemia; however, such anemia was noted in 0.50 to 0.75% of patients who had been taking diphenylhydantoin for 6 years. The low folate levels and clinical anemia do respond to folic acid therapy. In the past, investigators recommended therapy with 5 to 15 mg daily to restore levels to normal; however, some advocated dosages as high as 25 mg per day. Recently it has been found that 0.1 mg results in adequate hematological response in patients with uncomplicated folate deficiency and that doses greater than 1.0 mg do not enhance the hematological effect. However, this assumes complete absorption, and such is not the case when diphenylhydantoin is being administered concomitantly. Therefore, in these patients the dose should be 0.5 to 5.0 mg daily, adjusted according to the patient's serum folate levels. Of major interest is the recent recognition that the administration of folic acid to patients taking diphenylhydantoin leads to a reduction in serum diphenylhydantoin to below therapeutic levels. In some patients this had led to loss of seizure control. Folic acid interferes with the absorption of diphenylhydantoin to a degree, but it is probably more important that there is an increased metabolic conversion of diphenbyhydantoin to its metabolite parahydroxyphenytoin. Confronted with this dilemma, it becomes important to monitor serum diphenylhydantoin levels when folic acid is administered concomitantly. In order to avoid this complex problem, some authorities are now advocating that all patients started on diphenylhydantoin should receive supplemental folic acid. It is interesting to note also that other anticonvulsants such as primidone and phenobarbital have also been reported to lower serum folate levels.

Therefore, it is not unusual for one to find that disease is not of pathological origin but instead is due to a secondary drug effect. This has caused many clinicians to ponder; when I see patients in my office, the true dilemma that faces me is not which drug to start, but instead which drug to discontinue.

IDIOSYNCRASY

"Idiosyncrasy" is a term many think should be abandoned as it has countless connotations attached to it. However, for the lack of a better term, I have chosen it to refer to the unusual drug reactions that cannot be explained by the inherent properties of drugs themselves but instead by some altered characteristic within the patient taking the drug. This alteration may be temporary or permanent and therefore should be differentiated from true allergic reactions.

Drugs have been shown to induce hemolytic anemia in certain patients. Some of these patients have been found to have a deficiency of erythrocyte glucose 6-phosphate dehydrogenase (G-6-PD). This deficiency is noted in 10 to 15% of black American males and also in whites from the Mediterranean area. Glucose 6-phosphate dehydrogenase is responsible for converting glucose 6-phosphate to 6-phosphogluconate in the first step of the pentose phosphate pathway. This reaction is coupled with the reduction of nicotinamide adenine dinucleotide phosphate (NADP) to the reduced form (NADPH). In the red cell NADPH maintains glutathione in the reduced form. Drugs, such as those listed in Table 3.1, increase the rate of oxidation of glutathione, thereby increasing the demand for red cell NADPH. Patients with a G-6-PD deficiency are unable to provide adequate amounts of NADPH. Oxidized glutathione accumulates and the integrity of the red cell membrane is altered resulting in hemolysis.[4]

Drugs that are metabolized or concentrated in the liver have prolonged levels in patients with impaired hepatic function. During the first 3 to 4 weeks of life, neonates fail to conjugate chloramphenicol with glucuronic acid because of inadequate amounts of glucuronyl transferase in the liver. Also during the first 2 months of life, renal function is poor, which results in inadequate excretion of the unconjugated drug. Accumulation of chloramphenicol to toxic levels occurs in neonates on about the 4th day of treatment leading to the inhibition

of protein synthesis and increased levels of amino acids.[16] Such increases in amino acids and possibly elevations in serum ammonia levels may be responsible for the poor feeding patterns, regurgitation and abdominal distention seen initially in these patients. Following these initial signs and over the next 12 to 24 hrs., hyptonia, hypothermia and shallow, irregular respirations appear, leading to an ashen gray cyanosis. This "gray baby" syndrome is fatal in 40% of the neonates. The dosage of chloramphenicol must be no larger than 25 mg per day in children less than 1 month of age.[17] In addition, this drug must be used with caution in women in labor since toxic effects have also been noted in their newborn.

This same deficiency of glucuronyl transferase plays an important role in the occurrence of kernicterus (hyperbilirubinemia) in the neonate following sulfonamide therapy. Bilirubin is a normal breakdown product of hemoglobin. In adults it is generally conjugated in the intracellular smooth endoplasmic reticulum of the liver to a water-soluble glucuronide which is excreted in the bile. Neonates have a limited ability to do this owing to their enzyme deficiency. Kernicterus develops when there is an increase in free unconjugated bilirubin in the blood. This fat-soluble pigment is taken up by nerve cells and other tissues leading to uncoupling of oxidative phosphorylation. Cell death follows. The clinical picture of kernicterus is one of severe jaundice, somnolence, failure to feed, cerebral irritation, rigidity and head retraction. In excess of 50% of the babies die. If they survive, their future may hold cerebral palsy, deafness, seizures or mental retardation. Sulfonamides come into play because of their ability to displace unconjugated bilirubin from its binding sites on albumin. The mature liver would rapidly conjugate (detoxify) this bilirubin, but the neonate's liver is unable to do this. Sulfonamides should be avoided in pregnancy at term and during nursing because these drugs readily cross the placenta and are excreted in breast milk. However, since premature birth is a possibility at any time during the last trimester, sulfonamides should be avoided throughout the last trimester. Exchange transfusions have traditionally been used to manage hyperbilirubinemia, but this technique rarely decreases the bilirubin level to even half its pretransfusion level. Recently, phenobarbital therapy has been

TABLE 3.1 Drugs Capable of Inducing Hemolytic Anemia in Glucose 6-Phosphate-Deficient Individuals[a]

Antimalarials	Sulfonamides
Primaquine	Sulfanilamide
Pamaquine	Sulfacetamide
Pentaquine	Sulfapyridine
Quinacrine	Sulfisoxazole
Quinine	Salicylazosulfapyridine
Quinocide	Sulfamethoxypyridazine
	Sulfones
Analgesics and antipyretics	Thiazolsulfone
	Sulfoxone
Acetylsalicylic Acid	Diaminodiphenylsulfone
Acetanilid	
Acetophenetidin	
Antipyrine	Others
Aminopyrine	Naphthalene
	Phenylhydrazine
	Dimercaprol
Nitrofurans	Probenecid
	Chloramphenicol
Nitrofurantoin	Quinidine
Nitrofurazone	Trinitrotoluene
Furazolidone	Vitamin K
Furaltadone	

[a]Reprinted from Melmon, K. L., and Morrelli, H. F.: Clinical, Pharmacology, p. 541. MacMillan Co., New York, 1972.

found to be effective in lowering bilirubin levels. Apparently, it enhances glucuronidation by inducing hepatic microsomal enzymes, and it also produces more receptor protein for bilirubin conjugation. The dosage of phenobarbital used is 5 mg administered every 8 hr beginning 6 to 8 hr after delivery for 3 to 5 days until serum bilirubin levels fall to below 10 mg%. This effect continues for approximately 2 days after stopping therapy.[18]

HYPERSENSITIVITY

When the term "hypersensitivity" is mentioned, one almost invariably thinks of penicillin allergy. The prevalence of penicillin allergy is estimated at between 1 and 3% of all patients that receive the drug. Estimates from skin tests with penicillin G or penicilloyl polylysine would tend to make one think that the prevalence is higher (5 to 10%); however, less than half of these patients actually react to challenge with penicillin.[19] Probably only 0.1% of allergic persons exhibit anaphylactic reactions to the drug. *In vivo* penicillin is metabolized to penicillanic acid, and this reacts with the lysine groups of tissue protein to form penicilloyl-protein conjugates. Approximately 95% of all penicillins that react with proteins follows this path of degradation. Therefore, penicillolyl-protein conjugates are considered the "major" haptenic determinants of penicillin allergy.[20] All penicillins must be considered to be cross-reactive; however, the frequency of allergic phenomena occurring between penicillins may not be the same. For example, anaphylaxis rarely occurs except to the natural penicillins G and V.[21] This is explained by the recent identification of a proteinaceous antigen with penicilloyl specificity found in commercial penicillin. One microgram or less of this antigen can evoke the anaphylactic response in sensitized persons. Since the proteinaceous residue is removed in preparing the semisynthetic penicillins, this may explain why anaphylactic-type reactions rarely occur with these penicillins.[22] It is not rare to be confronted with the problem of whether to give penicillin to a patient with a history of penicillin allergy. A drug history by the pharmacist should be able to resolve the type of allergic reactions the person experienced in the past. If a true penicillin allergy cannot definitely be ruled out, then alternative therapy (if it will suffice) should be selected. If penicillin must be given, then skin tests with penicilloyl-polylysine and/or a minor determinant mixture (MDM), if available, should be done. A wheal-and-flare reaction will occur within 15 min if "positive." Recent evidence indicates that a negative reaction to both of these implies the patient can take penicillin without an immediate or anaphylactic reaction, and the likelihood of late reactions are not much greater than in patients with a negative history of penicillin allergy.

SYSTEMIC LUPUS ERYTHEMATOSUS

Possibly the most classic drug-induced disease is systemic lupus erythematosus (SLE). This disorder has reportedly been initiated or unmasked by more than 30 drugs. The implicated drugs do not seem to share any common characteristic either chemically or pharmacologically. This has led some authorities to attribute drug-induced SLE to an allergic response. However, doubts are created when one reviews the following criteria for an allergic reaction.

1. There must be a sensitizing dose.

2. The allergic response is different from the pharmacodynamic reaction of the drug or from any manifestation which represents accumulation of the drug.

3. Once a person is sensitized, even minute amounts of the drug will cause a prompt reaction.

4. Withdrawal of the drug will cause remission of the manifestation although at variable rates.

5. Sensitivity persists indefinitely.

However, recent evidence has shown that immune responses to hydralazine[23, 24] and to procainamide[23] have been detected in patients with drug-induced disease. In the case of hydralazine, circulating antibodies to native deoxyribonucleic acid (DNA) were found. In procainamide-lupus syndrome no such antibodies were noted; however, antibodies to denatured DNA and nucleohistone were found. These findings support the theory that at least in the cases of hydralazine and procainamide a unique hypersensitivity reaction may be occurring. Other authorities have advocated that drug-induced

SLE represents the activation of a latent lupus diathesis (genetic predisposition).[26] Supposedly this diathesis remains latent until unmasked by an agent with this potential, *e.g.,* drugs, sunlight etc. According to these investigators, persons who spontaneously contract SLE have a greater or more superficial diathesis, and therefore it is more easily uncovered. Doubt is shed on this theory when one considers that the incidence of overt SLE is only 1 in 8,000 to 1 in 25,000 while recent evidence shows that 50% or more of patients taking procainamide develop antinuclear antibodies (ANA) and 20% show clinical SLE. This high incidence of SLE following procainamide therapy appears to be too great to be the mere unmasking of a latent predisposition. The final offering for the mechanism by which drugs induce lupus is the generalization "by their peculiar pharmacological properties.[27] Though this is an obvious oversimplification and explains little, it probably adequately summarizes most of our existing knowledge.

Clinically idiopathic SLE runs a chronic course characterized by periods of remission and exacerbation and involves multiple organ systems. The symptomatology is diverse, as might be expected of such a disease. Fever, arthralgias, skin lesions, pulmonary infiltrates, pericarditis, glomerulonephritis and central nervous system abnormalities have all been frequently documented.

The pathological basis for this widespread involvement is thought to be due to the "deposition of complexes of anti-DNA antibodies and DNA in small vessels and in renal glomerular capillaries. The deposition of these antigen-antibody complexes leads to the fixation of complement, which in turn, becomes activated; this leads to release of chemotactic factors, activation of the kinin system, and so on. Thus, all tissue damage—in skin, in small blood vessels, in the kidney—is related to the presence of anti-DNA-DNA circulating in the blood."[28]

Laboratory findings, though not diagnostic in themselves, are essential for a final diagnosis of SLE. No single laboratory finding is present in all patients with lupus and absent in all patients without the disease. Therefore, one must seek positive results in multiple tests. Fluorescent ANA is positive in virtually 100% of the patients (1 or 2% may be repeatedly negative). Although the ANA test is positive more often than any other test in lupus patients, its usefulness is somewhat limited by the fact it is also positive in many other diseases. The LE cell test is more specific than ANA but also less sensitive, occurring in 60 to 85% of patients with lupus. About 15% of patients will show a false positive VDRL test result. Antibodies to erythrocytes, platelets, lymphocytes and ribosomes have been found. Decreased complement levels have been noted, and these fluctuate inversely to the levels of DNA antibodies. Thirty percent of patients with lupus have a positive rheumatoid factor.

The drug-induced syndrome closely resembles the clinical picture of overt lupus, though there are some noteworthy differences. Investigators have devoted much time to developing these differences into explanations of why the drug-induced disease cannot be the same as the idiopathic variety. Age of onset is often used to differentiate the two entities. The average age of onset of idiopathic lupus is 26 years compared to between 40 and 50 years for drug-induced. However, the onset of drug-induced SLE is limited by the age of the population in which the drug is being used; therefore, age is not a valid index for comparison or differentiation. The lower incidence of central nervous system and renal abnormalities in drug-induced lupus is also used to differentiate the two entities. Yet this may be explained by the fact that in drug-induced disease the inducing factor is quickly removed on withdrawal of the drug. It becomes more difficult to explain why pulmonary involvement occurs more commonly in drug-induced SLE than in the idiopathic disease. The finding that the vast majority of pulmonary involvement is induced by procainamide and not by other lupus-inducing drugs may imply, however, that the population receiving procainamide (older patients with possible underlying heart disease) may be the actual reason for this difference. The final major difference between the lupus syndromes rests in the fact that the drug-induced form is apparently reversible. Early reports in the literature claimed that withdrawing the drug which induced the syndrome would result in a prompt reversal. A different light has been shed on the subject when long term follow-ups have been done. Many reports have shown that the clinical or laboratory manifestations of drug-induced SLE have persisted for as long as the patients have been followed.[29,30] Alarcon-Segovia and his co-workers[26] had follow-ups for 9 years and reported 67% of their patients still showed manifestations at the study's conclusion. They concluded that this condition is not reversible and only marked improvement occurs. At best the difference between the naturally occurring disease and the drug-induced form is marginal.

Of the drugs that have been associated with lupus probably the greatest evidence has been compiled with hydralazine, procainamide, isoniazid (INH) and several anticonvulsants (diphenylhydantoin, mesantoin, trimethadione, primidone and ethosuximide). Other drugs have also been implicated, but the relationship is not well established. Table 3.2 lists drugs reported to have an association with the onset of SLE. Some of these drugs may be falsely associated with SLE, as they no doubt were given to patients with symptomatology consistent with pre-existing lupus.

Antimicrobials

The first documentation of a drug causing lupus appeared in 1945, when the sulfonamides were implicated.[31] Subsequent reports have implicated such antimicrobials as streptomycin, griseofulvin, penicillin and tetracycline, although the evidence implicating all of these drugs is unconvincing. For example, in the case of penicillin, the report involves six patients who already had diagnosed SLE or had symptoms of the disease at the time of penicillin administration.[32] In one tetracycline study, an 8-year-old female ingested 12 250-mg capsules that were outdated. A reaction ensued which the authors claimed simulated lupus over a 3-day period (skin rash, erythema following exposure to sunlight).[33] A photosensitivity reaction to degraded tetracycline is a distinct possibility in this case and not drug-induced SLE. A second report, equally unconvincing, was offered by Domz.[34]

Hydralazine

In 1953, the first report of hydralazine-induced lupus appeared.[35] Subsequently over 200 cases have been recorded. The frequency of SLE in patients taking hydralazine varies from 2 to 13%. However, if the same criteria were used to diagnose this drug-induced lupus as that used for spontaneous SLE, then the frequency would be no more than 1 to 2%.[36]

Apparently there is some relationship to dosage and duration of therapy and the induction of lupus. Initially it was felt that if the dosage could be kept below 400 mg per day the chance of toxicity would be minimized. Later reports suggested that the daily dosage should be kept below 200 mg. Most recently Alarcon-Segovia et al.[26] reported on 19 patients who developed lupus at dosages below 200 mg per day (75 mg in one patient). In the same study it was reported that 13 patients developed lupus while taking hydralazine for less than 30 days. The general consensus remains, however, that the likelihood of developing lupus following hydralazine therapy is greater if the dosage is high and therapy is maintained for a long time.

A factor that may contribute to the above finding is that persons who develop hydralazine-lupus are slow acetylators of the drug, which leads to their developing high levels of hydralazine for longer periods than normal.[37] The same study noted that persons not developing lupus were fast acetylators of hydralazine.

Characteristically, the symptoms, particularly those of rheumatoid arthritis, usually diminish and disappear on discontinuing hydralazine. As mentioned earlier, this caused many investigators to conclude that the hydralazine syndrome was different from SLE; however, in long term follow-up studies of these patients certain characteristics of the disease have remained.

TABLE 3.2:
*Drugs Reported to Be Associated with
the Onset of Systemic Lupus Erythematosus.*

Hydralazine	Streptomycin
Procainamide	Griseofulvin
Isoniazid	Oral contraceptives
Diphenylhydantoin	Methylthiouracil
Mesantoin	Propylthiouracil
Trimethadione	Chlorpromazine
Primidone	Guanoxan
Ethosuximide	Penicillamine
Aminosalicylic acid	Phenylbutazone
Methyldopa	Oxyphenbutazone
Tetracyclines	Reserpine
Penicillin	Corticosteroid withdrawal
Sulfamethoxypyridazine	Gold compounds
Sulfadimethoxine	Vitamins
Sulfadiazine	

It is thought that lupus, at least in part, is a hypersensitivity response to hydralazine. Antibodies to hydralazine and native DNA have been found in patients with the syndrome. The titers of these antibodies were found to parallel the severity of disease.

Procainamide

Procainamide was first introduced as an antiarrhythmic in 1951. It was not until December, 1962, that the first report of its relationship to SLE appeared.[38] Approximately 50% of persons taking procainamide developed antinuclear antibodies (though some report this to be as high as 83%),[39] and 20% of the patients had high enough titers to develop clinical symptoms of lupus erythematosus. Most of the patients who develop ANA do so within 3 to 6 months of the onset of therapy.

The level of dosage or the duration of therapy does not seem to play a significant role in procainamide-induced lupus. The genetically determined rate of acetylation in the liver may play some yet undetermined role — but it may be significant that the drug is acetylated.

The clinical pictures of procainamide-lupus and the idiopathic disease are similar. However, in the drug-induced disease there does appear to be less renal damage and more pulmonary involvement. The significance of this remains to be determined and may only represent the removal of the stimulus in the former and the select population that is exposed in the latter.

The mechanism of procainamide-lupus remains unknown — a recent report showing the presence of antibodies to single-stranded DNA, nucleohistone, red cell membranes and certain immunoglobulins in exposed patients implied that some type of hypersensitivity reaction may be involved. Yet the same study reported no evidence of antibodies to native DNA.[25]

Isoniazid

The first reported case of INH-induced lupus was in 1966, and since that time more than 20 cases have appeared in the literature. Antinuclear antibodies have been noted in 20% of the patients on antituberculosis therapy as compared to 4% of untreated tuberculosis patients.[40] The incidence of INH-lupus has been estimated at 0.1% of all treated tuberculosis patients.[36] INH, by implication, is assumed to be the inducing agent when the studies refer not specifically to this drug but instead to antituberculosis therapy. For this reason, streptomycin and aminosalicylic acid may be drugs capable of inducing lupus.

The mechanism by which INH induces lupus remains unknown. This drug, like hydralazine and procainamide, is acetylated in the liver. As with hydralazine, there appear to be "fast" and "slow" acetylators of INH. The role this plays in INH toxicity remains to be elucidated.

Anticonvulsants

The first report of a lupus-like syndrome following anticonvulsant therapy was in 1953. Since that time mainly the hydantoins, but also trimethadione, ethosuximide, and primidone have been implicated. The frequency with which the syndrome occurs has been reported to be as high as 8%. Patients reported to have developed SLE following anticonvulsant therapy have generally been treated for many months or years.

Convulsive disorders are recognized as manifestations of central nervous system involvement of SLE. Thus the relationship between a drug administered to a patient with a convulsive disorder to the subsequent development of lupus is difficult to establish. A thorough knowledge of the etiology of the convulsive disorder will hopefully prove valuable in determining if such a relationship exists.[41]

In patients developing this SLE syndrome while taking anticonvulsants, the clinical picture of the disease will generally reverse on withdrawing the drug. One must then consider what would happen to the control of the patient's seizures if the suspected offending anticonvulsant(s) were withdrawn. Alternative drugs do exist to manage convulsive disorders and a trial with another anticonvulsant agent should be tried while the patient is closely observed for reversal of the SLE syndrome. Phenobarbital is an alternative anticonvulsant. The dosage is 1 to 5 mg per kg per day, and because of its long half-life (approx. 5 days) it will take about a month to reach a steady state tissue distribution at a constant dosage.

Miscellaneous Drugs

The oral contraceptives have been reported to have a relationship to SLE. The incidence must be low considering the millions of women taking oral contraceptives and rarity of lupus. Nineteen incidents were found, but many of these cases already had diagnosed SLE and the administration of birth control pills merely resulted in a flare-up of symptoms. Of interest is the fact that clinical and laboratory signs usually reversed on stopping the pills. Also the oral contraceptives are given to the same female population (20- to 29-year olds) in which spontaneous lupus appears, and the cyclic nature of active disease could be confusing. A definite relationship has not been established between the oral contraceptives and lupus, but they should be used with caution, if at all, in women with existing disease.

Methyldopa has been implicated in activating lupus in two patients.[42] Both patients were elderly females with atherosclerotic heart disease, congestive heart failure and hypertension. A positive Coombs test, positive LE prep and a positive rheumatoid factor were used to diagnose lupus. All tests but the Coombs reversed within 6 months when methyldopa was stopped.

Chlorpromazine was reported to have induced lupus in one patient.[43] Following 17 months of therapy (400 mg per day) the clinical picture of lupus emerged, including arthralgias and positive ANA and LE prep. All symptoms and serological abnormalities were normal some 2 months after stopping therapy. Rechallenge with chlorpromazine led to reexacerbation of the disease. It would still be easy to disregard the phenothiazines since the clinical picture in which they are used could very well be the central nervous system involvement of lupus. A closer look should be taken at previous reports of phenothiazine-induced SLE and at the patients taking these drugs.

Phenylbutazone and oxyphenbutazone have both been suggested as inducers of lupus. Owing to the scarcity of existing reports, it becomes extremely difficult to conclude whether these drugs induced lupus or whether the arthralgias these drugs were used to treat were symptoms of pre-existing disease.

Pencillamine, thiouracil derivatives and guanoxan also have been associated with lupus erythematosus.

Drug-induced lupus erythematosus has been discussed in detail because it represents a classic drug-induced disease. However, drug-induced lupus cannot be explained by looking at the chemical structure or the pharmacological properties of the offending agents. Yet if a common denominator could be found among these drugs, the key to SLE might be found.

The intent of this discussion has been to make pharmacists aware that virtually every drug has the potential to induce disease in their patients and that this can occur even in "normal" doses. The pharmacist is at the strategic interface between a patient and his drug: an interface which may lie between a patient and his disease.

REFERENCES

1. Caranasos, G. J., Stewart, R. B., and Cluff, L. E.: Drug-induced illness leading to hospitalization. J.A.M.A., 728: 713, 1974.
2. Miller, R. R.: Hospital admissions due to adverse drug reactions. Arch. Int. Med., 134: 219, 1974.
3. Seidl, L. G., Thorton. G. F., Smith, J. W., and Cluff, L. E.: Studies on the epidemiology of adverse drug reactions. III Reactions in patients on a general medical service. Johns Hopkins Med. J., 1, 119: 299, 1966.
4. Melmon, K. L., and Morrelli, H. F.: Clinical Pharmacology: Basic Principles in Therapeutics. The MacMillan Co., New York, 1972.
5. Kutt, H., Winters, W., Kokenge, R., and McDowell, F.: Diphenylhydantoin metabolism, blood levels, and toxicity. Arch. Neurol., 11: 642, 1964.
6. Loeser, E. W.: Studies on the metabolism of diphenylhydantoin (Dilantin) Neurology, 11: 424, 1961.
7. Gibberd, F. B., Dunne, J. F., Handley, A. J., and Hazleman, B. L.: Supervision of epileptic patients taking phenytoin. Br. Med. J., 1: 147, 1970.
8. Arnold, K., and Gerber, N.: The rate of decline of diphenylhydantoin in human plasma. Clin. Pharmacol. Ther., 11: 121, 1970.
9. Jelliffe, R. W.: An improved method of digoxin therapy. Ann. Intern. Med., 69: 703, 1968.
10. Marcus, F. I., Nimmo, L., Kapadia, G. G., and Goldsmith, C.: The effect of acute hypokalemia on the myocardial concentration and body distribution of tritiated digoxin in the dog. J. Pharmacol. Exp. Ther., 178: 271, 1971.
11. Cooke, A. R., and Gouston, K.: Failure of intravenous aspirin to increase gastrointestinal blood loss. Br. Med. J., 3: 330, 1969.
12. Leonards, J. R., and Levy, G.: Safe and effective therapy with aspirin. Drug Ther., 2: 78, 1972.
13. Leonards, J. R., and Levy, G.: Reduction or prevention of aspirin-induced occult gastro-

intestinal blood loss in man. Clin. Parmacol. Ther., 10: 571, 1969.

14. Seltzer, H. S.: Drug-induced hypoglycemia. Diabetes, 21: 955, 1972.

15. Baylis, E. M., Crowley, J. M., Preece, J. M., Sylvester, P. E., and Marks, V.: Influence of folic acid on blood phenytoin levels. Lancet. 1: 62, 1971.

16. Ingall, D., Sherman, J. D., Cockburn, F., and Klein, R.: Amelioration by ingestion of phenylalanine of toxic effect of chloramphenicol on bone marrow. N. Engl. J. Med., 272: 180, 1965.

17. Goodman, L. S., and Gilman, A.: The Pharmacological Basis of Therapeutics, Ed. 4. The MacMillan Co., New York, 1970.

18. Young, C. Y., Tam, L. S., Chan, A., and Lee, K. H.: Phenobarbitone prophylaxis for neonatal hyperbilirubinemia. Pediatrics, 48: 372, 1971.

19. Smith, J. W., Johnson, J. E., and Leighton E. C.: Studies on the epidemiology of adverse drug reactions. N. Engl. J. Med., 274: 998, 1966.

20. Levine, B. B., Fellner, M. J., and Levitska, V.: Benzylpenicilloyl-specific serum antibodies to penicillin in man. J. Immunol., 96: 707, 1966.

21. Geyman, J. P.: Anaphylactic reaction to oral penicillin. Calif. Med., 114: 87, 1971.

22. Stewart, G. T.: Penicillin allergy. Clin. Pharmacol. Ther., 11: 307, 1970.

23. Hahn, B. H., Sharp, G. C., Irvin, W. S., Kantor, O. S., Gardner, C. A., Bagby, M. K., Perry, J. M., Jr., and Osterland, C. K.: Immune response to hydralazine and nuclear antigens in hydralazine-induced lupus erythematosus. Ann. Intern. Med., 76: 365, 1972.

24. Heine, W. I., and Greidman, H.: Hydralazine lupus syndrome associated with a possible antihydralazine antibody. J. A. M. A., 182: 726, 1962.

25. Blomgren, S. E., Condemi, J. J., and Vaughan, J. H.: Procainamide-induced lupus erythematosus. Am. J. Med., 52: 338, 1972.

26. Alarcon-Segovia, D., Worthington, J. W., Ward, L. E., and Wakim, K. G.: Lupus diathesis and the hydralazine syndrome. N. Engl. J. Med., 272: 462, 1965.

27. Axion.: Drug-induced lupus syndromes (editorial). Br. Med. J., 1: 193, 1970.

28. Rothfield, N. F.: Treatment of systemic lupus erythematosus. Drug Ther., 1: 61, 1971.

29. Shulman, L. E., and Jarvey, A. M.: The nature of drug-induced systemic lupus erythematosus. Arthritus Rheum., 3: 464, 1960.

30. Hildreth, E. A., Biro, C. E., and McCleary, T. A.: Persistence of the 'hydralazine syndrome.' J. A. M. A., 173: 657, 1960.

31. Hofman, B. J.: Sensitivity to sulfadiazine resembling acute disseminated lupus erythematosis. Arch. Dermatol. Syph. 51: 190, 1945.

32. Gold, S.: Role of sulfonamides and penicillin in the pathogenesis of systemic lupus erythematosus. Lancet, 1: 268, 1951.

33. Sulkowiski, R., and Haserick, J. R.: Stimulated systemic lupus erythematosus from degraded tetracycline. J. A. M. A., 214: 152, 1964.

34. Domz, C. A., McNamara, D. H., and Holzapfel, H. F.: Tetracycline in lupus erythematosus. Ann. Intern. Med., 50: 1217, 1959.

35. Morrow, J. D., Schroeder, H. A., and Perry, H. M., Jr.: Studies on the control of hypertension by hyphex. II Toxic reactions and side effects. Circulation, 8: 829, 1953.

36. Lee, S. L., Rivero, I., and Siegel, M.: Activation of systemic lupus erythematosus by drugs. Arch. Intern. Med., 117: 620, 1966.

37. Perry, H. M., Jr., Tan, E. M., Carmody, S., and Sakamoto, A.: Relationship of acetyl transferase activity to antinuclear antibodies and toxic symptoms in hypertensive patients treated with hydralazine. J. Lab. Clin. Med., 76: 114, 1970.

38. Ladd, A. T.: Pracainamide-induced lupus erythematosus. N. Engl. J. Med., 267: 1357, 1962.

39. Whittingham, S., Mackay, I. R., Whitworth, J. A., and Sloman, G.: Antinuclear Antibody response to procainamide in man and laboratory animals. Am. Heart J., 84: 228, 1972.

40. Cannat, A., and Seligmann, M.: Possible induction of antinuclear antibodies by isoniazid. Lancet, 1: 185, 1966.

41. Sparberg, M.: Diagnostically confusing complications of diphenylhydantoin therapy-review. Ann. Intern. Med., 59: 914, 1963.

42. Sherman, J. D., Love, D. E., and Harrington, J. F.: Anemia, positive lupus, and rheumatoid factors with methyldopa. Arch. Intern. Med., 120: 321, 1967.

43. Dubois, E. L., Tallman, E., and Wonka, R. A.: Chlorpromazine-induced systemic lupus erythematosus. J.A.M.A., 221: 595, 1972.

chapter 4

TERATOGENICITY AND DRUG EXCRETION IN BREAST MILK (MATERNOGENICITY)

Robert H. Levin, Pharm.D.

In 1930, a prepartum pelvic x-ray was linked to the birth of a malformed human child.[1] In 1940, maternal rubella infection was conclusively found to be the cause of congenital blind and deaf children.[2] However, interest in human teratology remained low until the 1960's. The years 1960 to 1962 saw the emergence of over 10,000 cases of congenital anomalies attributed to one drug—thalidomide.[3],[4] Surprisingly, there is still very little research to date in this area.

Teratogenesis means "the origin of a monster, and the disturbed growth process involved in producing a monster."[4] This is the traditional meaning, but currently there is a broader meaning. Any abnormality that occurs in a newborn infant, whether it is a major congenital malformation, *e.g.,* phocomelia, hydrocephalus or a minor congenital anomaly, *e.g.,* acid-base imbalance or central nervous system depression, is considered teratogenic.[2]

Since these abnormalities occur in the fetus, the mother acts as the initial carrier of the teratogenic insult. With maternogenic effects the mother again acts as the initial exposure to the offending drug and conveys it to the infant through breast feeding. Maternogenic as defined here are those drug-induced effects occurring in an infant and produced through breast feeding. The adverse or allergic effects caused by medications given directly to an infant either orally or parenterally are not considered to be in the context of this discussion.

NORMAL PHYSIOLOGY

During gestation the embryo or fetus is contained in a relatively protected environment. It is encased in the uterus, surrounded by amniotic fluid and nourished through the placenta. The uterus and amnionic sac afford a physical barrier against trauma or abuse. The placenta acts as a digestive tract, a lung, a kidney, a liver and a gland.

The placenta (Fig. 4.1), a dark red, spongy, mucous-type tissue, can be depicted as a large stagnant pool of maternal blood through which the fetal circulation, which can be thought of as an upside down candelabra, interplays. Maternal and fetal blood normally do not mix. However, there are occasionally unexplained fetal cells found in maternal serum. Nutrients, oxygen and essential hormones transfer from the maternal blood into the fetal blood via the fetal circulatory system. The placenta exchanges fetal carbon dioxide for maternal oxygen and metabolizes and purges endogenous fetal compounds.

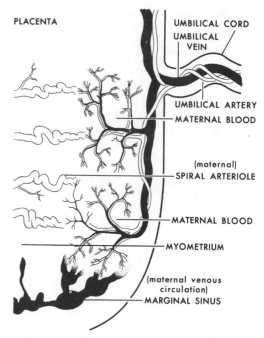

FIG. 4.1. Maternal and fetal circulation in the human placenta. *(Adapted from Netter.)*

The so-called "placental barrier" is a myth.[5] With few exceptions, all endogenous and exogenously administered compounds passively diffuse, or in some cases they are actively transported across the placental membrane. However, large ionized molecules such as heparin, insulin, curare, protamine and succinylcholine are very poorly, if at all, transported across the placenta. There are other factors that alter the permeability of compounds across the placental membrane: the size and thickness of the placenta, placental enzymes, the rate of placental blood flow, placental age, serum protein binding of compounds, a compound's lipid-water solubility, pH characteristics and concentration gradients between mother and fetus.[6] These characteristics of compounds are comparable to those discussed under drug excretion in breast milk.

The growth of the embryo or fetus roughly parallels the enlargement of the uterus and placenta. The placenta occupies around 30% of the internal steadily expanding uterus and at birth weighs about 1 pound. An average infant at birth weighs about 7 pounds. In the first 15 days of gestation the embryo is undifferentiated and increasing in size by general cell proliferation. After 15 days the cells begin to differentiate into germ layers. Specialized cells develop and proliferate to form eventually the fetus' organs, skin, limbs, heart, brain or other organs. This organ differentiation is well under way at 30 to 40 days and is fairly complete at 60 days.[7] From 60 days until birth the organs will mature, begin to function and at birth will be able to support life adequately.

The kidneys of a full term infant function at about 30% of their adult level.[5,8] They will mature to adult level at approximately 9 to 12 months of age. Most pediatricians consider the kidneys mature enough to handle medications normally at 1 to 2 months of age. Prior to 1 month of age, medications dependent on renal excretion must be given in reduced quantities or at longer dosing intervals.

The liver of the full term infant metabolizes a few endogenous compounds at birth and most compounds by 3 days of age. Liver function is adequate within a few weeks to metabolize all routine medication.[5,8] Other bodily systems mature at different times throughout childhood, but their immaturity has little effect on medication absorption, utilization or elimination.

EMBRYOGENESIS

The development of an embryo into an infant is a complicated, intricate process. There are a number of etiological processes that interplay in this development:[3] genetic determinants by Mendelian law account for 25% of the process, and genetic mutants by chromosomal abnormalities account for 3%; physiological and unclassified factors account for 69%; and finally environmental factors such as trauma, infection, x-rays, and chemical teratogens (drugs) account for 3%. This interplay is better appreciated through the use of an analogy.

Fraser[9] likened embryogenesis to the building of a ship. Both begin with a set of plans. The shipbuilder uses drawings and words carried on blueprints. The genes of a human are the specific instructions determining the characteristics of deoxyribonucleic acid (DNA), the master protein. These instructions are carried on chromosomes, and man has 23 pages of blueprints in 2 volumes, 1 from the mother and 1 from the father.

The building materials utilized for a ship consist of wood, steel, canvas and other components while in a human these materials are amino acids, protein and other components converted into protoplasm and cells by instructions from DNA. These instructions are translated by messenger ribonucleic acid (mRNA) which acts like a foreman to relay commands to the ribosomes, or workmen.

The building of the ship occurs in a protected environment, a shipyard, where safeguards are utilized to protect against rust, corrosion and other types of damage. The fetus is protected in the uterus from trauma, damage, environmental changes and external chemicals.

There are numerous chances for errors to occur in both shipbuilding and embryogenesis. Structural errors or malformations occur in ships when a mistake occurs in the blueprints. Even a typographical error might cause a ship's structure to be placed wrong, not made at all, not made at the proper time or made in the wrong shape. Similarly, a mutant gene might cause a malformation in a fetus by altering normal protein structure or by altering the normal rate of protein synthesis. An extra page of blueprints or part or all of a page missing will cause confusion and errors to occur during ship construction. Analogously, chromosomal aberrations (broken, unattached, misattached) can lead to genetic defects such as mongolism.

Finally, there are, in both, multifactorial problems. The ship may be rejected over-all because of "a lot of little things," e.g., green wood, skimpy caulking or incorrectly fitting sails. In humans, multifactorial problems are the leading cause of malformations and the most difficult to analyze and prevent.[4] Frequently, the mother has taken a few drugs, contracted an infection, received an x-ray or possibly fallen. Any one of these might be implicated, making it extremely difficult, if not impossible, to delineate a single cause. Each of these teratogens can cause indirect or direct fetal damage.

A teratogen can affect maternal tissues, the placenta, or embryonic tissues to cause either indirect damage to the fetus by affecting the mother first or direct fetal damage. Physiological changes in the mother can have profound effects on the fetus.[10,11] For example, decreased maternal renal function because of nephrotoxicity will lead to maternal and fetal uremia and the occurrence of toxic effects in the fetus. Changes in maternal serum glucose, electrolytes or acid-base balance will also be transmitted to the fetus possibly causing serious problems.

Trauma or toxicity to placental tissue, an indirect teratogenic effect, produces necrotic, nonfunctioning tissue.[10] The fetus may become toxic because of a buildup of endogenous by-products, lack of nutrients and lack of oxygen. The fetus may also become hypoxic owing to placental vasoconstriction and concomitant decreased perfusion produced by excess maternal serotonin or catecholamines. Drugs which produce effects on the fetus itself are classified as direct teratogens. Thalidomide is the classic example. Thalidomide interferes with normal fetal metabolism by acting as a competitive antagonist of glutamine, glutamic acid or folic acid.[12] It is also metabolized to derivatives of glutamine or glutamic acid, possibly interfering with fetal metabolic pathways. These direct fetal effects, without adverse effects on the mother, account for the severe anomalies caused by thalidomide.

PATHOGENESIS

Drugs are teratogenic only at specific times during embryogenesis (Table 4.1). Thalidomide serves as an excellent example to illustrate the pattern of pathogenesis of anomalies. Through collection of data from many mothers of "thalidomide babies" congenital defects were traced to a specific number of days between conception and thalidomide ingestion.[13]

Day 21-22: Absence of external ears, paralysis of cranial nerves

Day 24-27: Maximal phocomelia (flipper limbs)

Day 28-29: Severe reduction deformities of lower limbs

Day 34-36: Hypoplastic thumbs and anorectal stenosis

Fortunately, a number of lessons were learned from the thalidomide tragedy[3]:

1. A drug may have inoccuous effects in an adult but can be very damaging to a fetus.

2. It is extremely difficult to test for human teratogenesis in animals.

3. With epidemic proportions of a malformation occurring it required an extensive period of time to elucidate the teratogen.

4. It would be more difficult to find a teratogen with a low incidence of malformations.

5. It was difficult to collect retrospective data.

It is now mandatory (1962 Federal Food, Drug and Cosmetic Act) to test for teratogenicity of drugs in animals prior to their approval.[14] This is done even though animals are not the ideal model because they have a different genetic makeup, different reproductive processes, different metabolic pathways, different sensitivities or different body requirements than humans. The doses used in animals are generally much higher, and the route of administration is generally different. Animal studies, however, have elucidated a few significant principles to allow us to make some generalizations concerning the teratogenicity of drugs (Fig. 4.2). In order for a drug to elicit teratogenic effects it must be administered: at the proper dose (very high doses cause fetal death, low doses produce no effects); at the specific

TABLE 4.1
Teratogenicity during Embryogenesis

Days of Gestation	Cell Differentiation and Teratogenic Effects
<15	No differentiation of cells (germ layers formed). Embryo can be killed if enough cells are killed. Otherwise no teratogenic effects are seen.
15-25	Central nervous system differentiation occurs.
20-30	Precursors to axial skeleton and musculature occur and limb buds make appearance.
24-40	Major differentiation of eyes, heart and lower limbs.
60	Organ differentiation well under way and in many areas completed.
90	Differentiation complete and maturation occurring.
>90	Little susceptibility to the occurrence of congenital malformations.

1. A teratogen may exert its effect on a developmental structure up to the time of its critical differentiation.
2. A single teratogen may produce a variety of abnormalities.
3. A variety of teratogens may produce similar abnormalities.
4. Teratogenic abnormalities may be indistinguishable from hereditary malformations.
5. Effect of a single teratogen may vary in different species and in different genetic strains of some species.
6. Most congenital anomalies result from interaction of genetic and environmental factors.

FIGURE 4.2
Teratogenic Principles Arrived at
Through Animal Experimentation[15]

stage of embryonic development for teratogenic effects to occur; to a specific species strain; by a particular route of administration; to a host which is intrinsically susceptible. Karnofsky[16] succinctly summarized these data as "any drug administered at the proper dosage, and at the proper stage of development to embryos of the proper species — and those include both vertebrates and invertebrates — will be effective in causing disturbances in embryonic development."

INCIDENCE

The ingestion of medications by pregnant women is a common occurrence. Nelson and Forfar[17] reported that 97% of 1,369 pregnant women took at least one prescription drug during pregnancy. Also, 65% of these women self-administered over the counter (OTC) drugs, mainly analgesics and antacids. Of these women, 458 gave birth to infants with congenital abnormalities consisting of 175 major abnormalities (congenital heart disease, hydrocephalus, limb deformities) and 283 minor abnormalities (predominantly harelips). The normal occurrence of abnormalities for this population would be 26 to 40 (2 to 3%) infants.[2] The authors found no definite causes for their high rate of abnormalities but did recommend the avoidance of all prescription and OTC drugs, especially those with teratogenic potential, *e.g.,* amphetamines, barbiturates, narcotic cough medications, iron or sulfas. They recommended that supplements of vitamin C and folic acid be given to all expectant mothers.[5]

In another study, Peckham and King[18] reported that 92% of 3,072 pregnant women took at least 1 drug during pregnancy, and 21% of these took greater than 5 drugs. The average drug intake was 3.6 drugs per pregnancy and consisted of predominantly prenatal vitamins, diuretics, antihypertensives, analgesics, sedatives, hypnotics, antihistamines, antinauseants and antiobesity agents. Other studies have corroborated the thesis that pregnant women do consume as many, if not more, medications than nonpregnant females. This prolific ingestion requires pharmacists, physicians, nurses and other members of the health care team to be aware of those medications with possible teratogenic effects.

TERATOGENS IN THE FIRST TRIMESTER

The time of fetal organogenesis is the critical time for teratogenic gross malformations to occur (Table 4.2). Numerous drugs have been implicated in this trimester as teratogens, but only a few have unequivocally been shown to be teratogenic, such as aminopterin and thalidomide. Other medications have only been implicated in causing fetal malformations.

Antineoplastic agents like nitrogen mustards, folic acid inhibitors and cyclophosphamide have been implicated as teratogens. These medications are potent metabolic inhibitors and would be expected to cause malformations in humans as they do in animals. Other metabolic inhibitors that have been causally implicated are steroids, salicylates, phenylbutazone and chloroquin.

Abuse drugs are another group of potential teratogens. Amphetamine and phenmetrazine have been implicated in causing cardiac anomalies. Lysergic acid diethylamide (LSD) and chlorpromazine have been shown to cause chromosomal abnormalities and possible fetal malformations. The effects of chromosomal damage on mutation or teratogenesis cannot be ascertained for certain for at least a generation, but it seems prudent to strongly urge pregnant females to avoid these medications especially during the first trimester.

TABLE 4.2
Examples of Teratogenic Drugs[a]

Drug	Adverse Effects	Stage of Pregnancy	Significance	Ref.
Analeptics				
Dextroamphetamine sulfate	Transposition of great vessels, biliary atresia	First trimester	More evidence needed	19,20
Phenmetrazine	Skeletal and visceral anomalies	4th-12th week	One report only More evidence needed	21,22, 23
Serotonin	Multiple anomalies of skeleton and organs	4th-12th week	More studies needed	21
Analgesics				
Alphoprodine	Thrombocytopenia	Near term	More studies needed	24
Heroin	Respiratory depression, withdrawal symptoms	Near term	Fairly well documented	21,25, 26,27
Methadone	Prolonged withdrawal	Term	Fairly well documented	28
Morphine	Neonatal death	Near term	Needs more studies	1,2,21,25
Salicylates	Neonatal bleeding, thrombocytopenia	Near term	Needs more studies	15,24
Anesthetics (inhaled)				
Cyclopropane, ether, halothane	Neonatal depression	Near term	Established	27
Anesthetics (local)				
Lidocaine	Neonatal depression	Near term	More studies needed	27
Mepivicaine	Fetal bradycardia	Near term	Not established	29,30
Procaine	Neonatal depression	Near term	More studies needed	27
Anticoagulants				
Sodium warfarin	Fetal death, hemorrhage	Throughout pregnancy	More studies needed	14,21, 27,31
Antidiabetics				
Chlorpropamide	Prolonged neonatal hypo-glycemia, anomalies	Throughout pregnancy	More evidence needed before implication	32,33
Tolbutamide	Congenital anomalies, hypoglycemia	Throughout pregnancy	More evidence needed	15,34
Antiepileptics				
Diphenylhydantoin	Cleft gum, lip or palate	1st & 2nd trimesters	Fairly well documented	14,21

TABLE 4.2—*Continued*

Drug	Adverse Effect	Stage of Pregnancy	Significance	Ref.
	Syndactyly, polydactyly, microcephaly, anencephaly, neonatal bleeding	Near term	Fairly well documented	35-39
Primidone	Neonatal bleeding	Near term	Fairly well documented	24
Antihistamines Diphenhydramine	Thrombocytopenia	Near term	More studies needed	24
Promethazine	Thrombocytopenia	Near term	More studies needed	24
Anti-inflammatory agents Cortisone	Cleft palate	Very early in gestation	More studies needed	22,23, 40
Indomethacin, phenylbutazone	Thrombocytopenia	Near term	Fairly well documented	24
Antimalarials Chloroquine	Deafness	Throughout pregnancy	More studies needed	40
Primaquin (and other drugs causing hemolysis in G-6-PD deficient infants)	Hemolytic anemia	Near delivery	One case; more study needed	40
Quinine	Deafness, thrombocytopenia	Throughout pregnancy	More studies needed	40,41
Antimicrobials Chloramphenicol	Gray baby syndrome and death	Near term	Fairly well documented	21,25 42-44
Isonicotinic acid Hydrazide	Retarded psychomotor activity	Throughout pregnancy	More studies needed	45,46
Nitrofurantoin	Hemolysis	Near term	Not established; more studies needed	21,25 31
Novobiocin	Hyperbilirubinemia	Near term	More study needed	21,25,31
Streptomycin	8th nerve damage, micromelia, hearing loss, multiple skeletal anomalies	Throughout pregnancy	Debatable; more studies needed	21,31,32
Sulfonamides (long acting)	Hyperbilirubinemia and kernicterus	Near term	Fairly well documented	21,31, 42,45,47
Tetracyclines	Inhibition of bone growth, discoloration of teeth, micromelia, syndactyly	2nd & 3rd trimesters	Fairly well documented	15,42, 43

TABLE 4.2–*Continued*

Drug	Adverse Effect	Stage of Pregnancy	Significance	Ref.
Antimitotic agents				
Podophyllum	Fetal resorption, multiple deformities	1st trimester	More studies needed	21
Antineoplastics				
Amethopterin	Abortefacient, retarded growth, cleft palate, cranial anomalies, encephaloceles	1st trimester	Fairly well documented	21,25 32,48, 49
Aminopterin	Abortefacient, retarded growth, cleft palate, cranial anomalies, encephaloceles	1st trimester	Known teratogen	21,25,32, 40,48, 50,51
Busulfan	Possible anomalies	1st trimester	More studies needed	21,25, 32,48
Cyclophosphamide	Severe stunting, fetal death, extremity defects	1st trimester	More studies needed	21,25, 32,48
Antithyroid agents				
Methimazole	Goiter and mental retardation	From 14th week on	Fairly well documented	21
Potassium iodide	Goiter and mental retardation	From 14th week on	Fairly well documented	21,43,52
Propylthiouracil	Goiter and mental retardation	From 14th week on	Fairly well documented	21,53
Radioactive iodide	Congenital hypothyroidism	From 14th week on	Fairly well	30
Depressants				
Alcohol	Vacuolization of bone marrow cells, neonatal depression, decreased birth weight	Throughout and near delivery	More study needed	27,54
Barbiturates and other hypnotics	Respiratory depression, hemorrhage	Near deliver	Fairly well documented	14,27, 39
	Malformations	1st & 2nd trimesters	More study needed	55,56
Thalidomide	Phocomelia, hearing defect	28th-42nd day	Known teratogen	15,21,25, 48,57
Diuretics				
Thiazides (Hydro- chlorothiazide, chlorothiazide, methylclothiazide)	Thrombocytopenia, neonatal death	Latter part of pregnancy	One report only; evidence lacking	43,58
Hormonal steroids				
Androgens	Masculinization, labial fusion and clitoris enlargement	Throughout pregnancy	Well documented	15,22,30 43
Estrogens (stilbestrol)	Masculinization, labial fusion, clitoris enlargement and adenocarcinoma	Throughout pregnancy	More evidence needed	14,15, 43,59, 60

TABLE 4.2—*Continued*

Drug	Adverse Effect	Stage of Pregnancy	Significance	Ref.
Oral progestogens	Masculinization, labial fusion and clitoris enlargement	Throughout pregnancy	Fairly well documented	15,30, 43,59
Immunizations (live) Measles vaccine	Infected fetus	Throughout pregnancy	Needs more study	61
Mumps vaccine	Infected fetus	Throughout pregnancy	Needs more study	61
Rubella vaccine	Congenital rubella, anomalies	Throughout pregnancy	Fairly well documented	61-63
Smallpox vaccine	Fetal vaccinia	Throughout pregnancy	Fairly well documented	61,64
Social drugs – Legal Nicotine and smoking	Small babies, early birth, irritable	Throughout pregnancy	Probably significant	21,23, 40
Social drugs – illegal LSD	Chromosomal damage, stunted offspring, other malformations	1st trimester	Could be significant, more studies needed	65-68
Tranquilizers Chlordiazepoxide	Thrombocytopenia	Near term	More studies needed	24
Diazepam	Thrombocytopenia	Near term	More studies needed	24
Imipramine	Thrombocytopenia	Near term	More studies needed	24
Nortriptyline	Bladder distension, depression	Near term	More studies needed	69
Phenothiazines (in general)	Retinopathy, urinary retention, extrapyramidal reactions,hyperbilirubinemia	Close to delivery	More studies needed	40,70, 71
Chlorpromazine	Chromosome changes, possible goiter, thrombocytopenia	Throughout pregnancy; near term	More studies needed	24,72 73
Prochlorperazine	Thrombocytopenia	Near term	More studies needed	24
Reserpine	Nasal blockage	Near term	More studies needed	23,43, 74,75
Vitamins Vitamin A	Retarded growth, intracranial hypertension	Throughout pregnancy	In large doses· only	76,77
Vitamin C	Scurvy	Near term	More study needed	14

TABLE 4.2—Continued

Drug	Adverse Effect	Stage of Pregnancy	Significance	Ref.
Vitamin D	Excessive blood calcium, mental retardation	Throughout pregnancy	In large doses only	40,41
Vitamin K analogs	Hyperbilirubinemia, kernicterus	Near term	In large doses only	15,23, 43,78
Pyridoxine	Withdrawal seizures	Near term	More study needed; high doses needed	14
Miscellaneous Acetophenetidin	Methemoglobinemia	Near term	More studies needed	30
Cholinesterase inhibitors	Transient muscular weakness	Throughout pregnancy	More studies needed	30
Glyceryl guaiacolate	Thrombocytopenia	Near term	More studies needed	24
Hexamethonium bromide	Neonatal ileus and death	Throughout pregnancy	More studies needed	12,40
Lithium carbonate	Possible goiter toxicity	Throughout pregnancy	More studies	73,79

[a]Modified from Ref. 80 with permission.

The antihistamines, antinauseants, meclizine, cyclizine, chlorcyclizine and buclizine have been shown to be teratogenic in animals.[40] The evidence for their teratogenicity in humans, however, is contradictory and not at all conclusive.[3,40] The Central Nervous System (CNS) depressants also have been inconclusively implicated. Barbiturates, diphenylhydantoin and lithium in some studies seem to induce increased adnormalities.

THROUGHOUT PREGNANCY

Most antimicrobials are safe to take during pregnancy (Table 4.2). However, the aminoglycosides (especially streptomycin) and quinine have caused deafness, and tetracyclines are known to cause enamel staining and decreased bone growth. The use of novobiocin and sulfonamides near term have caused elevations in bilirubin at birth; chloramphenicol has caused gray baby syndrome; and nitrofurantoin has induced hemolysis.

Oral anticoagulants may cause hemorrhage in utero or at birth. Discontinuing them 1 week before delivery and utilizing herparin, if needed, will avoid neonatal hemorrhage.

Oral antidiabetics such as tolbutamide and chlorpropamide have been implicated in causing fetal malformations in the first trimester and physiological changes in the last trimester. Excessive doses causing hypoglycemia in both mother and fetus are potentially damaging as is maternal overdosage with insulin. Insulin used for psychiatric shock treatment has also been implicated as a teratogen.[72,81]

Hormonal agents cause physiological changes in the fetus. The antithyroid drugs propylthiouracil, potassium iodide or radioactive iodide can produce fetal goiters if employed in the second or third trimester. Androgens and progestins will cause masculinization of female fetuses which may or may not be reversible. Diethylstilbestrol (DES) has been shown to cause vaginal adenocarcinoma in young women exposed to it in utero because their mothers were given DES for the prevention of miscarriage.

Social drugs like tobacco and alcohol in

excessive amounts have led to infants with decreased birth weights. Also, tobacco causes the infants to be more irritable, and alcohol induces transient hematological changes.

Vitamins, which are almost routinely taken during pregnancy, are not without toxicity. Excessive vitamin A has been known to cause increased intracranial pressure and other symptoms of hypervitaminosis A. Hypervitaminosis D has been observed and consists of hypercalcemia and mental retardation. Large maternal doses of vitamin C have induced scurvy (a rebound phenomenon) shortly after birth. Large maternal doses of pyridoxine have subjected neonates to withdrawal seizures after birth. Finally, water-soluble vitamin K analogues given in large doses to mothers shortly before delivery have produced kernicterus.

PRIOR TO DELIVERY

Problems caused by vitamins, anticoagulants and antibiotics have been discussed. CNS depressants may cause severe respiratory depression at birth. Barbiturates, narcotics, tranquilizers (both minor and major), anticonvulsants and general anesthesia all have this potential. In addition, the fetus habituated to barbiturates and/or narcotics will go into symptoms of withdrawal at birth. Reserpine has induced neonatal nasal stuffiness, a serious problem in infants who breathe only through their nose. Mood elevators such as nortriptyline have caused depression and severe bladder distension in neonates. Finally, neonatal bleeding has been caused by the maternal ingestion of a number of drugs: salicylates, thiazides, indomethacin, promethazine, diphenhydramine, chlordiazepoxide, diazepam, chlorpromazine, imipramine, prochlorperazine and glyceryl guaiacolate.

DISCUSSION

The fact that a drug is taken by mothers who have abnormal infants does not necessarily mean that it is teratogenic.[17] If a mother contracted a disease which in itself was teratogenic and a drug was taken to treat that disease, the drug may be wrongly implicated as the teratogen. A prior congenitally abnormal fetus may produce symptoms in the mother, and she may treat herself for these symptoms with a drug which later may be wrongfully implicated. The early weeks of pregnancy are implicated in 10 times as many fetal abnormalities as the later trimesters. These fetuses are usually stillborn or aborted, but if a drug is used to prevent this abortion, it could be implicated at birth as a teratogen.

In contrast, it has been reported that some mothers who are deficient in folic acid or vitamin C and are not supplemented have an increased rate of fetal abnormalities.[17]

DRUGS EXCRETED IN BREAST MILK

After delivery, drugs no longer gain access to the infant through the placenta. However, medications ingested by the mother may be passed to a nursing infant through the breast milk. In this way, the infant may be exposed to a wide variety of foods and medications.

NORMAL BREAST PHYSIOLOGY

The breast is composed of glandular, fibrous and adipose tissue and rests on a bed of connective tissue. The glandular tissue is composed of 15 to 20 lobes arranged radially around the nipple. Strands of fibrous tissue connect the lobes, and adipose tissue occupies the space between and around the lobes. Each lobe is divided into several lobules and connected by areolar tissue, blood vessels and ducts (Fig. 4.3a). Each lobule contains a small lactiferous duct. Eventually these lactiferous ducts unite and form a single main canal for each lobe. These 15 to 20 main canals each become dilated and form a reservoir (sinus lactiferous) for milk storage and finally merge and pass through the nipple.

The functioning part of the breast is the alveoli or acini (sacs) in the lobule (Fig. 4.3b). It is in the acini epithelium that milk is produced and secreted into the lactiferous ducts. Drug excretion from the blood occurs in capillary beds, through the acini epithelium into the lactiferous ducts.

NORMAL COMPOSITION OF MILK

The composition of milk is determined by the mammary gland with little or no external

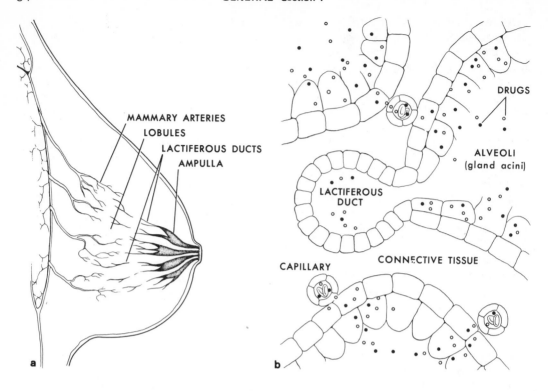

FIG. 4.3. a. Cross section of breast. b. Magnified cross section of a lobule depicting drugs entering alveoli from capillaries. *(Adapted from* Nutrition Today, *vol. 5, no. 4.)*

bodily control[83]. The milk occurs in three forms: colostrom, transitional or mature milk. Colostrom, which serves as a precursor for milk, may be expressed from the breasts as early as the 4th month of pregnancy, but it usually appears after parturition. It is scanty the 1st few days after birth, becomes well established on the 3rd or 4th day and usually continues no more than 5 days. It has, however, been known to continue for as long as 10 days. Colostrom is a transudate consisting primarily of serum albumin (3 to 5%) and cast off epithelium (colostrom corpuscles) which have undergone fatty degeneration. It has a higher specific gravity than mature milk (1.030 to 1.060 compared with 1.026 to 1.036) and also a higher average pH (7.7 compared with 6.8). It is richer in vitamin A, sodium, potassium and other minerals but lower in sugar and fat. Colostrom will be quickly modified by the mammary gland into transitional milk.

Transitional milk is produced within the 1st week of breast feeding. It usually lasts for a few weeks during which time it achieves a moderate increase in fat and sugar and a gradual decrease in proteins and minerals. Milk finally takes on a stable or mature character near the end of the 1st month of lactation.

Mature maternal milk, along with normal infant nutritional stores, is a complete dietary source for the first 4 to 6 months of life. To avoid deficiencies, it must be supplemented with food after 6 months, but it can be utilized as a protein supplement for a number of years.

Mature milk has between 0.9 and 1.6% protein, 2 to 6% fat, and 6.5 to 8% lactose. The composition of milk at the beginning of a feeding is highest in protein and lowest in fat. This is reversed toward the end of the feeding. What effect this might have on excretion of drugs is unknown. However, it is known that the difference between milk at pH 6.8 and blood at pH 7.4 will influence the excretion of drugs into breast milk.[84]

Once established, mature milk will vary little in composition.[83] Providing the mother has an adequate nutritional food intake, her diet can be quite varied without affecting milk composition or volume. A deficient maternal diet will first cause a decrease in milk quantity but will not affect milk composition unless the mother's tissue stores are depleted. A decreased water intake will cause maternal thirst before it affects milk production.

CONTROL OF MILK PRODUCTION

The initiation and maintenance of milk production has not been adequately studied. The evidence regarding the roles of physiological and endocrine factors in lactation is contradictory.[82,85-87] As previously mentioned, lactation usually begins about the time of birth or shortly thereafter. Its inhibition during pregnancy is assumed to be the result of the occurrence of high estrogen and/or progesterone levels. The effects of estrogen on milk secretion are dose-dependent. At low endogenous levels occurring postpartum, milk secretion occurs whereas at high doses (diethylstilbestrol or parenteral estrogens given postpartum), lactation is inhibited. In most women, low dose oral contraceptives do not decrease lactation even when given immediately postpartum.[88] It is thought estrogens may work partly by affecting prolactin (lactogenic factor) from the anterior pituitary.

Prolactin is presently under extensive investigation in an effort to delineate its true role during pregnancy and lactation.[85,86] During pregnancy, prolactin along with estrogen, progesterone and human growth hormone aids in breast development. It achieves high concentrations during pregnancy and during breast feeding, but it is in low concentration after birth in the absence of breast feeding. Interestingly enough, if breast feeding is complete, successful and unrestricted the high levels of prolactin achieved have been reported to be contraceptive.[89] This contraceptive effect is seen only in primitive societies and has not been observed in America, where formula supplements are frequently given.

The posterior pituitary, in addition to the anterior pituitary, is involved in and stimulated by an infant breast feeding.

Infant → stimulation of →
nursing   nerves in nipple

⌐→ anterior pituitary → prolactin production
| → lactation (milk production)
└→ posterior pituitary → oxytocin release
   → "letdown" reflex

The release of oxytocin by the posterior pituitary initiates the "letdown" reflex (Fig. 4.4). Oxytocin stimulates the expression or ejection of milk from the breast whereas prolactin stimulates milk production. The letdown reflex is responsive to other internal and external factors. The actions and sounds associated with nursing can initiate this reflex. In contrast, distractions such as fright, pain and emotional distress can inhibit milk expression. It is hypothesized that high levels of the catecholamines, adrenalin and norepinephrine produced in the latter circumstances cause a vasoconstriction in the mammary circulation which prevents oxytocin from reaching the contractile cells.[87] Medications, in excessive doses which also release endogenous catecholamines, e.g., amphetamines and most decongestants, may interfere with milk secretion.

QUANTITY OF MILK PRODUCED

The quantity of milk produced is dependent upon the demands of the infant. If the infant's demand is increasing, milk supply will adjust accordingly within 2 days and vice versa. The actual secretion of milk is a discontinuous process. During feeding there is increased milk secretion due to the depletion of milk stores. In all probability, drugs would also be excreted into milk in larger amounts when the milk is being actively secreted. To derive the total quantity of drug ingested (measured as mg per 100 cc or mg %), it is necessary to know the quantity of milk ingested by the infant. This is dependent on the age and weight of the infant (Table 4.3).

DRUG EXCRETION

There is a decided lack of information concerning the excretion of drugs into milk.

Infant nursing → stimulates nerves in nipple → afferent stimuli through nerves → posterior pituitary → release of oxytocin → efferent stimuli via blood → mammary blood circulation → contraction of minute contractile cells of alveoli → express milk into ducts → lactiferous sinus → available to infant.

FIG. 4.4. *Letdown reflex.*

TABLE 4.3
Quantities of Milk Ingested[83]

Amount at each feeding[a]	Age
ml	weeks
20- 45	1
30- 90	2
40-140	4
60-150	6
75-165	12
90-175	16
120-225	24

[a]Feedings are usually every 3 to 4 hr; quantity consumed dependent on infant's weight.

This is probably due to the difficulty in carrying out experimental observations in nursing mothers; the complicated analytical procedures required for many drugs and a general lack of interest in this subject by most researchers. Furthermore, the majority of scientific data available is generally from uncontrolled, unsophisticated studies. Most original work was done over 20 years ago and consists largely of case reports. However, within the last few years, there have appeared a few original articles regarding drugs excreted in breast milk.[90-92] Many animal studies have been done, but it is difficult to extrapolate these results to humans. What information, then, can the pharmacist utilize to form meaningful judgments concerning the safety of drugs in the nursing mother?

Unless contrary information exists, it can be assumed that any drug orally administered to and absorbed by the mother will be excreted in her milk. For a majority of drugs and foods the concentration achieved in the milk is insufficient to elicit any clinical symptoms in the infant. There are some drugs, however, that are excreted in sufficient quantities to cause observable and sometimes serious effects in the infant. The excretion of drugs is dependent on the following physiochemical characteristics: the pH gradient between plasma and milk, the

pKa or the degree of ionization of the drug, the lipid-water solubility characteristics of the drug, the distribution of the drug by body transport mechanisms and the concentration gradient of diffusable drug between plasma and milk.

The normal pH of blood ranges between 7.35 and 7.45 with an average of 7.4 The average pH of milk is 6.8 with a range of 6.5 to 7.4.

The pKa is the negative log of the dissociation constant of an acid. The more a compound dissociates to release hydrogen ions the more acidic it is and the smaller will be the value of its pKa. A strong acid such as salicylic acid has a pKa of 3.0, whereas a weak acid such as phenobarbital has a pKa of 7.4. The relationship of pH and pKa is represented by the Henderson-Hasselbach equation:

$$pH = pKa \text{ (of acid)} + \log \frac{(salt)}{(acid)}$$

for acidic compounds, and

$$pH = pKa \text{ (of base)} + \log \frac{(base)}{(salt)}$$

for basic compounds. This formula is also used when determining physiological acid-base balance where

$$pH \text{ (7.4)} = pKa \text{ (6.1)} + \log \frac{(HCO_3^-)}{(H_2CO_3)}$$

This equation is reduced to the familiar ratio of $HCO_3^-/H_2CO_3 = 20 : 1$. It is important to remember that when pH = pKa the concentration of salt and acid in solution is equal. Since the pH and pKa are logarithmic relationships, each unit change of pH reflects a 10-fold change in relative concentrations of acid and salt forms. When exposed to body fluids of differing pH separated by a physical membrane, an acid or base will accumulate in the fluid in which it is most ionized and where most soluble. Serum concentrations of erythromycin with a pKa of 8.8 will have about 15 times more salt (ionized) than base (un-ionized). When erythromycin is secreted into milk with a pH of 6.8, the ratio of ionized to un-ionized molecules is 100 : 1. Therefore, the concentration of erythromycin in milk should be 6 times its concentration in serum, and in fact this relationship has been shown experimentally.[93] In general, basic drugs are excreted in higher concentration in milk, whereas acidic drugs are less concentrated in milk.

Diffusion across a concentration gradient also plays a role in drug excretion. A drug with a high lipid solubility will diffuse very poorly into breast milk but will attain a high level of concentration in fat depots. A highly ionized large molecule such as heparin, insulin or protamine will also diffuse extremely poorly across cell membranes. To achieve optimal partition, a drug must have a molecular structure which has a balanced lipophilic and hydrophilic nature. Un-ionized nonprotein-bound balanced molecules like alcohol will achieve milk levels equal to their serum levels. Protein binding will decrease the partition of drugs. There is some active transport of drugs but because of lack of knowledge, the importance of this factor is unknown. Finally, there seems to be a rough correlation between the dialyzability of drugs and their excretion in milk. Generally speaking, the more easily a drug can be dialyzed the greater the concentration it will achieve in milk.

Pharmacological factors may also play a significant role in altering the concentration of a drug. Drugs dependent on renal clearance will achieve higher serum and milk levels in a mother with renal insufficiency. Those medications dependent on liver metabolism may have altered half-lives if there is severe hepatic impairment in the mother. Severe impairment of other organs such as the gastrointestinal tract, heart, circulation or lungs may also alter drug absorption, distribution or excretion. Any of these factors which results in increased plasma levels of drugs as compared to normal will also produce elevated drug concentrations in breast milk.

MEDICATIONS IN BREAST MILK

It is extremely important for the breast feeding mother, the pharmacist and the physician to be aware of and avoid those substances which are toxic to the infant (Table 4.4). A lactating mother, fortunately, does not consume many medications. The most likely consumed are analgesics, barbiturates, diuretics, antimicrobials, laxatives, antinauseants and antacids. There are only a few medications within these pharmacological groups that when taken in

therapeutic doses by the mother will cause adverse effects in the infant. Infant sedation can be expected with excessive doses of narcotics, hypnotic doses of some barbiturates and large doses of alcohol, chloral hydrate, bromides, diazepam and methyprylon. Large doses of reserpine will cause nasal stuffiness. Tetracyclines will cause tooth staining and decreased bone growth. Cascara and danthron will increase bowel activity and possibly cause diarrhea. Medications with strong anticholinergic properties such as antihistamines, phenothiazines and atropine-like compounds may decrease lactation without having any appreciable effect on the infant. There are other less frequently used drugs that also cause problems.

Drugs affecting thyroid function such as iodide salts, radioactive I^{131} and propylthiouracil have had adverse effects on infant thyroids. Heavy metals such as mercury, lead and arsenicals have caused toxicities. Ergotrate maleate, given postpartum to enhance uterine contraction, has caused ergotism in a high percentage of infants. Finally, potential risks would seem to exist if antimetabolites or oral anticoagulants were taken.

There is very little data regarding the risks of using social drugs such as alcohol, tobacco or any of the abuse drugs. Excessive quantities of alcohol have produced infant sedation and smoking of more than 20 cigaretts a day has caused nicotine effects in the infant. Stimulants, depressants, narcotics and psychedelics when taken in high doses as abuse drugs would be expected to achieve high milk concentrations. Although no studies have been undertaken to measure abuse drug levels, it seems prudent for the mother to avoid them.

DISCUSSION

In general, with the exception of the preceding drugs, the infant will be unlikely to encounter adverse effects from maternally ingested drugs unless taken in excessive quantities. If a mother must consume a medication and is able to safely continue breast feeding, she should consume the drug about 15 minutes after nursing or 3 - 4 hr before the next feeding. This allows enough time for most medications to clear maternal serum and achieve a relatively low milk concentration. Conversely, medica-

TABLE 4.4
Examples of Medications in Breast Milk[a]

Drug	Explanation of Effects on Infant	Ref.
Analgesics		
Alphaprodine	Sedative effect with analgetic doses	94
Codeine	Insignificant with therapeutic doses (60 mg. P.O., S.C., I.M.)	95
Heroin	Sufficient concentration in habituated mothers to prevent withdrawals in habituated infant	96
Meperidine	Insignificant in therapeutic doses (100 mg I.M.)	94
Morphine	Sufficient concentration in habituated mothers to prevent withdrawals in habituated infant; insignificant levels with therapeutic dose (10 mg. S.C., I.M.)	95,96
Phenylbutazone	Excreted in insignificant quantities with I.M. 750-mg dose	93
Propoxyphene	Insignificant with therapeutic dose (65-130 mg P.O.) probably significant effect when used I.V. but not studied	93,94
Sodium salicylate	1-3 mg% serum level with 4-g dose (equivalent to 4 g ASA) which is insignificant; may be a problem with rheumatics with continual high dose	93,95
Antacids	Rarely absorbed to an appreciable extent — no problem unless mother develops an electrolyte imbalance	94
Antiemetics		
Antihistamines	Cause decreased lactation with large doses even though they may not be appreciably excreted	82,93
Atropine	Same as above	82,93
Chlorpromazine	Excreted but no infant effects with 1,200-mg oral dose	97
Antimicrobials	May lead to microbial resistance	
Ampicillin	Excreted, safe to use but may cause diarrhea and "allergic" sensitization	98,99
Chloramphenicol	Excreted to 50% of serum levels and possible but remote chance of "Gray syndrome" with neonate	82,93
Erythromycin	Excreted but safe to use	93
INH	Excreted but safe to use	82,93
Nitrofurantoin	Excreted but safe to use	94,98
Novobiocin	Achieves 25% of serum level and could cause possible kernicterus with neonate	82,93
Oxacillin	Excreted but safe to use	82,93

TABLE 4.4
Examples of Medications in Breast Milk[a]

Drug	Explanation of Effects on Infant	Ref.
Penicillin	Excreted but safe to use, possible allergic sensitization	98,99
Streptomycin	Excreted but safe to use	82,93
Sulfonamides	Excreted with possible occurrences of kernicterus in neonates	93,99
Tetracyclines	Excreted to 20-90% of serum levles and may cause decreased bone growth and tooth staining	82,93
Depressants **Barbiturates** Long acting	Barbital—insignificant effects with hypnotic doses (650 mg). Phenobarbital—sedative effects with hypnotic doses (100 mg). No effect with sedative doses (30 mg t.i.d.). Phenobarbital and diphenylhydantoin (390 and 300 mg) — methemoglobinemia reported in one infant; no effect on infant with 300-600 mg of diphenylhydantoin alone	93,95, 97,98, 100
Medium acting	Amobarbital—not studied adequately probably no effect with sedative doses	98
Short acting	Secobarbital, pentobarbital—no effect with sedative doses; possible effect with hypnotic doses	97,98
Ultra short	Pentothal—found in breast milk, probably insignificant	93,97
Others Alcohol	Small amounts have no effect; large doses (*e.g.,* 750 cc of wine over 24 hr or equivalent) cause sedation	93,98, 101
Bromides	Rashes and sedation with hypnotic doses	95,100,101
Chloral hydrate	1.33 g per rectum (approximately 2 g orally) have caused sedation	93
Diazepam	Large oral doses cause sedation	94
Methyprylon	Sedation with hypnotic doses	94
Reserpine	Nasal stuffiness with doses greater than 0.5 mg	82
Diuretics Hydrochlorthiazide, chlorothiazide	Excreted with remote possibility of causing problems	94,98
Hormonal Compounds Iodides	Therapeutic doses will cause goiters	93,95,101
Radioactive I[131]	Higher levels in milk than serum and will cause significant thyroid suppression	82,93

TABLE 4.4
Examples of Medications in Breast Milk[a]

Drug	Explanation of Effects on Infant	Ref.
Oral contraceptives	Decreased lactation in a minority of women, most can take low dose preparations from the 1st day postpartum without decreasing lactation; possibility of causing idiopathic jaundice	87,88, 90,97, 102
Pregnane beta-diol	Abnormal progesterone metabolite produced and excreted in some mothers and leads to jaundice	98, 103
Propylthiouracil	Excreted and will cause thyroid suppression	82,101
Thiouracil	Same as above	82,101
Thyroid	Excreted and will also cause increased milk production	93
Laxatives and fecal softeners	Bulk formers, castor oil, Dulcolax, mineral oil, DOSS, saline, phenopthalein, and other nonabsorbed types cause no problems and are safe to use	93,95, 99, 104
Anthraquinone derivatives Aloe	Small doses no effect but large doses will cause an increase in bowel activity	93,104
Cascara	Increased bowel activity with usual doses	93,104
Danthron	Increased bowel activity with usual doses	82,93
Rhubarb	Small doses no effect but large doses will cause an increase in bowel activity	93,104
Senna	Same as above	93,104
Social drugs – legal Alcohol	See under Depressants	93,98,101
Caffeine	1% of ingested dose of coffee or tea secreted, no effect on infant with moderate intake	82,93
Tobacco	More than 20 cigarettes per day has caused nicotine effects in infant, *i.e.,* restlessness, diarrhea, vomiting, and rapid pulse	82,93
Social drugs – illegal Abuse drugs	Stimulants, depressants, narcotics, psychedelics and others used in high doses have not been studied or reported and probably are excreted in high concentrations and should not be used	82
Miscellaneous Anticoagulants, oral	Not adequately studied and should be avoided	82
Antimetabolites, *e.g,* amethopterin, mercaptopurine, etc.	Possible excretion and should be avoided	82

TABLE 4.4
Examples of Medications in Breast Milk[a]

Drug	Explanation of Effects on Infant	Ref.
Arsenicals	Oral ingestion has caused infant toxicities	93
DDT	Excreted in milk at 4 times the level of cows milk but less than maximal permissible amount; death has occurred in infant whose mother inhaled a large amount	82,92
Ergotrate maleate	Excreted and causes ergotism, *i.e.,* decreased circulation, vomiting, diarrhea, tremors	82,93, 101
Fluorides	Levels of 1.13 ppm in drinking water achieve milk concentrations of 0.25 ppm	105
Foods	White navy beans, corn, egg white, chocolate, unripe fruit, pickles, peanuts, cottonseed, wheat, all reported to cause allergic reactions, *i.e.,* colic and rash, should be used sparingly or avoided	93
Lead	Topical application to nipples has caused infant toxicities	93
Mercury	Oral ingestion has caused infant toxicities	93
Poliovirus vaccine	Antibody in breast milk will neutralize some of oral poliovaccine (OPV) virus; try to avoid breast feeding 2 hr before and after immunization	106
Quinine	P.O. 300-600 mg dose excreted in insignificant quantities	93

[a]Modified from Ref. 107.

tions taken 30 to 60 min prior to a feeding usually achieve peak serum and milk concentrations during nursing. If a mother must consume a new or untested medication, breast feeding should be temporarily stopped. Fortunately, very few mothers have to discontinue breast feeding because of the consumption of medication.

Women breast feeding should avoid the use of abuse drugs, tetracyclines, cascara, danthron, antithyroid medication, anticoagulants, antimetabolites and ergot alkaloids. Excessive doses of any drug or new and untested drugs should be avoided. Finally, a pregnant or lactating woman with decreased renal or hepatic function is likely to predispose herself and the fetus or infant to drug toxicity.

SUMMARY

Both teratogenesis and maternogenesis are largely unknown fields of scientific research. Therefore, pharmacists, physicians and other members of the health care team should instruct pregnant women to avoid all medications especially during the first trimester. Drug treatment of any disease or illness in a pregnant woman must be balanced against the drug's toxicity to the fetus.

CONCLUSION

All medications, whether approved or about to be approved, should be thoroughly investigated for teratogenicity and maternogenicity. In addition to testing in animal models, drugs must be tested in humans whenever feasible. Human testing, however, is generally not desirable or feasible. Good, low cost and accurate animal model must be identified, if we are to gain the capability to test for and predict both teratogenic and maternogenic drug effects.

REFERENCES

1. Warkany, J., and Kalter, H.: Congenital malformations. N. Engl. J. Med., 265: 1047, 1961.
2. Warkany, J., and Kalter, H.: Congenital malformations. N. Engl. J. Med., 265: 993, 1961.
3. Cohlan, S. Q.: The teratogenicity of drugs in man. Pharmacol Physicians, 3: 1, 1969.
4. Underwood, T., Iturrion, W. B., and Cadwallader, D. E.: Some aspects of chemical teratogenesis. Am. J. Hosp. Pharm., 27: 115, 1970.
5. Gustafson, S. R.: Pediatric pharmacology. In The Pediatric Patient, p. 112, edited by S. R. Gustafson. J. B. Lippincott Co., Philadelphia, 1969.
6. Mirkin, B. L.: Maternal and fetal distribution of drugs in pregnancy. Clin. Pharmacol. Ther., 14: 643, 1973.
7. Warkany, J: Development of experimental mammalian teratology. In Teratology: Principles and Techniques, p. 2, edited by J. G. Wilson and J. Warkany. The University of Chicago Press, Chicago, 1965.
8. Jaffe, S. J., and Bach, N.: Neonatal pharmacology. Pediatr. Clin. North Am., 13: 527, 1966.
9. Fraser, F. C.: Some genetic aspects of Teratology. In Teratology: Principles and Techniques, p. 21, edited by J. G. Wilson and J. Warkany. University of Chicago Press, Chicago, 1965.
10. Wollman, D. H. M.: Principles of teratogenesis, mode of action of thalidomide. Proc. R. Soc. Med., 58: 497, 1965.
11. Young, J. B.: Mechanisms of teratogenesis. Part I. Bulletin of the Hospital Pharmacy and Drug Information Analysis Service, University of California, San Francisco, 17: 1, 1969.
12. Anon.: Chemical teratogenesis. In Principles of Drug Action, The Basis of Pharmacology, p. 711, edited by A. Goldstein, L. Aronson, and L. Kalman, Harper and Row, New York, 1968.
13. Lenz, W.: Epidemiology of congenital malformations. Ann. N. Y. Acad. Sci., 123: 228, 1965.
14. Anon.: Drugs in pregnancy. Med. Lett. Drugs Ther., 14: 93, 1972.
15. Cohlan, S. Q.: Fetal and neonatal hazards from drugs administered during pregnancy. N. Y. State J. Med., 64: 493, 1964.
16. Karnofsky, D. A.: Mechanisms of action of certain growth inhibiting drugs. In Teratology: Principles and Techniques, p. 185, edited by J. G. Wilson and J. Warkany. University of Chicago Press, Chicago, 1965.
17. Nelson, M. M., and Forfar, J. O.: Associations between drugs administered during pregnancy and congenital abnormalities of the fetus. Br. Med. J., 1: 523, 1971.
18. Peckham, C. H., and King, R. W.: A study of intercurrent conditions observed during pregnancy. Am. J. Obstet. Gynecol., 87: 609, 1963.
19. Nora, J. J., Trasler, D. G., and Fraser, F. C.: Malformations in mice induced by dexamphetamine sulfate. Lancet, 2: 1021, 1965.
20. Levin, J. N.: Amphetamine ingestion with biliary atresia. J. Pediatr., 79: 130, 1971.
21. Stuart, D. M.: Teratogenicity and teratogenic drugs. Pharm. Index, 8: 12, 1966.
22. Grumbach, M. M., and Ducharne, J. R.: The effects of androgens on fetal sexual development. Fertil. Steril., 2: 157, 1960.
23. Shirkey, H. C.: Adverse reactions to drugs – their relation to growth and development. In Pediatric Therapy, Ed. 4, p. 138, edited by H. C. Shirkey. C. V. Mosby Co., St. Louis, 1972.
24. Pochedly, C., and Ente, G.: Adverse hematologic effects of drugs. Pediatr. Clin. North Amer., 19: 1095, 1972.
25. Apgar, V.: Drugs in pregnancy. J. A. M. A., 190: 840, 1964.
26. Zelson, C., Rubio, E., and Wasserman, E.: Neonatal narcotic addiction, 10 year observation. Pediatrics, 48: 178, 1971.
27. Asling, J. and Way, E. L.: Placental transfer of drugs. In Fundamentals of Drug Metabolism and Drug Disposition, p. 100, edited by B. N. LaDu, H. G. Mandel and E. L. Way. Williams and Wilkins Co., Baltimore, 1971.
28. Rajegowda, B. K., Glass, L., Evans, H. E., Maso, G., Swartz, D. P., and Leblanc, W.: Methadone withdrawal in newborn infants, J. Pediatr., 81: 532, 1972.
29. Gordon, H. R.: Fetal bradycardia after paracervical block. N. Engl. J. Med., 279: 910, 1968.
30. Adamson, K., and Joelsson, I.: The effects of pharmacological agents upon the fetus and newborn. Am. J. Obstet. Gynecol., 96: 437, 1966.
31. Done, A. K.: Perinatal pharmacology (a research grant supported study). Department of Pediatrics, University of Utah, 1965.
32. Anon.: Drugs in the developing fetus. In Dilemmas in Drug Therapy, p. 140, edited by H. Beckman. W. B. Saunders Co., Philadelphia, 1967.
33. Zucker, P., and Simon, G.: prolonged symptomatic neonatal hypoglycemia associated with maternal chlorpropamide therapy. Pediatrics, 42: 824, 1968.
34. Larsson, Y., and Sterky, G.: Possible teratogenic effect of tolbutamide in a pregnant prediabetic. Lancet, 2: 1424, 1960.
35. Meadows, S. R.: Anticonvulsant drugs and congenital abnormalities. Lancet, 2: 1296, 1968.
36. Mirkin, B. L.: Diphenylhydantoin: placental transport, fetal localization, neonatal metabolism, and possible teratogenic effects. J. Pediatr., 78: 329, 1971.
37. Monson, R. R., Rosenberg, L. Hartz, S. C.,

Shapiro, S., Heinonen, O. P., and Stone, D.: Diphenylhydantoin and selected congenital malformations. N. Engl. J. Med., 289: 1049, 1973.

38. Loughnan, P. M., Gold, H., and Vance, J. C.: Phenytoin teratogenicity in man. Lancet, 1: 70, 1973.

39. Speidel, B. D., and Meadow, S. R.: Maternal epilepsy and abnormalities of the fetus and newborn. Lancet, 2: 839, 1972.

40. Sutherland, J. M., and Light, I. J.: The effect of drugs upon the developing fetus. Pediatr. Clin. North Am., 12: 781, 1965.

41. Lenz, W.: Malformations caused by drugs in pregnancy. Am. J. Dis. Child., 112: 99, 1966.

42. Weinstein, L., and Dalton, C.: Host determinants of response to antimicrobial agents. N. Engl. J. Med., 279: 467, 1968.

43. Shirkey, H. C.: The innocent child. J. A. M. A., 196: 132, 1966.

44. Sutherland, J. M.: Fatal cardiovascular collapse of infants receiving large amounts of chloramphenicol. Am. J. Dis. Child., 97: 761, 1959.

45. Weinstein, L., and Dalton, C.: Host determinants of response to antimicrobial agents. N. Engl. J. Med., 279: 526, 1968.

46. Monnet, P., Kalb, J. C., and Pujol, M.: Toxic influence of isoniazid on the fetus. Lyon Med., 218: 431, 1967.

47. Sutherland, J. M., and Mohlman, Y. M.: Antimicrobial therapy in newborn infants—major area of ignorance. Pediatr. Clin. North Am., 8: 1143, 1961.

48. Moser, R. H.: Diseases of Medical Progess, A Study of Iatrogenic Disease, Ed. 3, p. 163. Charles C. Thomas, Springfield, Ill., 1969.

49. Milunsky, A., Graef, J. W., and Gaynor, M. F.: Methotrexate-induced congenital malformations – with a review of the literature. J. Pediatr., 72: 790, 1968.

50. Shaw, E. B., and Steinbach, H. L.: Aminopterin-induced fetal malformation – survival of an infant after attempted abortion. Am. J. Dis. Child., 115: 477, 1968.

51. Shaw, E. B.: Fetal damage due to maternal aminopterin ingestion – follow-up at age 9 years. Am. J. Dis. Child., 124: 93, 1972.

52. Galina, M. P., Avnet, M. L., and Einhorn, A.: Iodides during pregnancy: apparent cause of neonatal death. N. Engl. J. Med., 267: 1124, 1962.

53. Aaron, H. H., Schneierson, S. J., and Siegel, E.: Goiter in newborn infant due to mother's ingestion of propylthiouracil. J. A. M. A., 159: 848, 1955.

54. Lopez, R., and Montoya, M. F.: Abnormal bone marrow morphology in the premature infant associated with maternal alcohol infusion. J. Pediatr., 79: 1008, 1971.

55. Dentkos, M. C.: Passage of drugs across the placenta. J. Am. Soc. Hosp. Pharm., 23: 139, 1966.

56. Yaffe, S. J.: Fetal and neonatal toxicity of drugs. Can. Med. Assoc. J., 98: 301, 1968.

57. Mellin, G. W., and Katzenstein, M.: The saga of thalidomide. Neuropathy to embryopathy, with case reports of congenital anomalies. N. Engl. J. Med., 267: 1184, 1962.

58. Rodriguez, S. U., Leikin, S. L., and Hiller, M. C.: Neonatal thrombocytopenia associated with ante-partum administration of thiazide drugs. N. Engl. J. Med., 270: 881, 1964.

59. Wilkins, L.: Masculinization of female fetus due to orally given progestins. J. A. M. A., 172: 1028, 1960.

60. Herbst, A. L., Ulfelder, H., and Poskanzer, D. C.: Adeno-carcinoma of the vagina – association of maternal stilbestrol therapy with tumor appearance in young women. N. Engl. J. Med., 284: 878, 1971.

61. Anon.: Safety of immunizing agents in pregnancy. Med. Lett., 12: 23, 1970.

62. Phillips, C. A., Maeck, J. V., Rogers, W. A., and Savel, H.: Intrauterine rubella infection following immunization with rubella vaccine. J. A. M. A., 213: 624, 1970.

63. Vaheri, A., Vesikari, T., Oker-Blom, N., Seppala, M., Parkman, P. D., Veronelli, J., and Robbins, F. C.: Isolation of attenuated rubella-vaccine virus from human products of conception and uterine cervix. N. Engl. J. Med., 286: 1071, 1972.

64. Anon.: Supplement – Collected Recommendations of the Public Health Service Advisory Committee on Immunization Practices, Morbidity and Mortality Weekly Report, 21: 27, 1972.

65. Smart, R. G., and Bateman, K.: The chromosomal and teratogenic effects of lysergic acid diethylamide. Can. Med. Assoc. J., 99: 805, 1968.

66. Dishotsky, N. I., Loughman, W. D., Mogar, R. E., and Lipscomb, W. R.: LSD and genetic damage. Science, 172: 431, 1971.

67. Eller, J. L., and Morton, J. M.: Bizarre deformities in offspring of user of lysergic acid diethylamide. N. Engl. J. Med., 283: 395, 1970.

68. Assemany, S. R., Neu, R. L., and Gardner, L. I.: Deformities in a child whose mother took LSD (letter). Lancet, 1: 1290, 1970.

69. Shearer, W. T., Schreiner, R. L., and Marshall, R. E.: Urinary retention in a neonate secondary to maternal ingestion of nortriptyline. J. Pediatr., 81: 570, 1972.

70. Palmisano, P. A., and Palhill, R. B.: Fetal pharmacology. Pediatr. Clin. North Am., 19: 3, 1972.

71. Tamer, A., McKey, R., Arias, D., Worley, L., and Fogel, B. J.: Phenothiazine-induced extrapyramidal dysfunction in the neonate. J. Pediatr., 75: 479, 1969.

72. Sobel, D. E.: Fetal damage to ECT, insulin, coma, chlorpromazine or reserpine. Arch. Gen. Psychiat., 2: 606, 1960.

73. Anon.: Drug-induced goiters in the fetus and in children and adults. Med. Lett., 12: 61, 1970.

74. Budnick, I. S., Leikin, S., and Hoeck, L. E.:

Effect in newborn infant of reserpine administered ante partum. Am. J. Dis. Child., 90: 286, 1955.

75. Desmond, M. M., Rogers, S. F., Lindley, J. E., and Moyer, J. H.: Management of Toxemia of pregnancy with reserpine. II. The newborn infant. Obstet. Gynecol., 10: 140, 1957.

76. Feldman, M. H., and Schlezinger, G.: Benign intracranial hypertension associated with hypervitaminosis A. Arch. Neurol., 22: 1, 1970.

77. Pease, C. N.: Focal retardation and arrestment of growth of bones due to vitamin A intoxication. J. A. M. A., 182: 980, 1962.

78. Lucey, J. F., and Dolan, R. C.: Hyperbilirubinemia of newborn infants associated with parenteral administration of vitamin K analogues to mothers. Pediatrics, 23: 553, 1959.

79. Woody, J. N., London, W. L., and Wilbanks, G. D.: Lithium toxicity in a newborn. Pediatrics, 47: 94, 1971.

80. Takata, A.: Adverse effects of drugs on the fetus. Drug Information Service Newsletter, Alta Bates Community Hospital, 1: 1, 1969.

81. Wickes, I. G.: Foetal defects following insulin coma therapy in early pregnancy. Br. Med. J., 2: 1029, 1954.

82. Arena, J.: Contamination of the ideal food. Nutrition Today, 5: 2, 1970.

83. Holt, L. E.: Feeding techniques and diets. In Pediatrics, Ed. 15, p. 148, edited by H. L. Barnett. Meredith Corporation, New York, 1972.

84. Catz, C. S., and Giacoia, G. P.: Drugs and breast milk. Pediatr. Clin. North Am., 19: 151, 1972.

85. Sherwood, L. M.: Current concepts — human prolactin. N. Engl. J. Med., 284: 774, 1971.

86. Tyson, J. E., Friesen, H. G., and Anderson, M. J.: Human lactational and ovarian response to endogenous prolactin release. Science, 177: 897, 1972.

87. Vorherr, H.: To breast feed or not to breast feed. Postgrad. Med. J., 51: 127, 1972.

88. Gambrell, R.: Immediate postpartum oral contraception. Obstet. Gynecol., 36: 101, 1970.

89. Jelliffe, D. B., and Jelliffe, E. F. P.: Lactation, conception, and the nutrition of the nursing mother and child. J. Pediatr., 81: 829, 1972.

90. Wong, Y. K., and Wood, B. S. B.: Breast-milk jaundice and oral contraceptives. Br. Med. J., 4: 403, 1971.

91. Werthmann, M. W., and Krees, S. V.: Excretion of chlorothiazide in human breast milk. J. Pediatr., 81: 781, 1972.

92. Kroger, M.: Insecticide residues in human milk. J. Pediatr., 80: 401, 1972.

93. Knowles, J. A.: Excretion of drugs in milk — a review. J. Pediatr., 66: 1068, 1965.

94. Shore, M. F.: Drugs can be dangerous during pregnancy and lactation. Can. Pharm. J., 8: 358, 1970.

95. Kwit, N. T., and Hatcher, R. A.: Excretion of drugs in milk. Am. J. Dis. Child., 49: 900, 1935.

96. Cobrinik, R. W., Hood, R. T., and Chusid, E.: The effect of maternal narcotic addiction on the newborn infant; a review of the literature and report of 22 cases. Pediatrics, 24: 288, 1959.

97. Matranga, A.: Drugs excreted in breast milk. Drug Information Service Newsletter, Alta Bates Community Hospital, 2: 22, 1970.

98. Knowles, J. A.: Drugs excreted into breast milk. In Pediatric Therapy, Ed. 4, p. 179, edited by H. C. Shirkey. C. V. Mosby, St. Louis, 1972.

99. Sapeika, N.: Excretion of drugs in human milk — a review. J. Obstet. Gynecol. Br. Emp., 54: 426, 1947.

100. Tyson, R., Schrader, E. A., and Perlman, H. H.: Drugs transmitted through breast milk. Part II: Barbiturates. J. Pediatr., 13: 86, 1938.

101. Illingworth, R. S.: Abnormal substances excreted in human milk. Practitioner, 171: 533, 1953.

102. Arena, J. M.: Drugs and breast feeding. J. Clin. Pediatr., 5: 472, 1966.

103. Gartner, L. M., and Arias, I. M.: Studies of prolonged neonatal jaundice in the breast-fed infant. J. Pediatr., 68: 54, 1966.

104. Tyson, R., Schrader, E. A., and Perlman, H. H.: Drugs transmitted through breast milk. Part I: Laxatives. J. Pediatr., 11: 824, 1937.

105. Bercovici, B., Gedalia, I., and Brzezinski, A.: Fluorine in human milk. Obstet. Gynecol., 16: 319, 1960.

106. Top, F. (editor): Report of the Committee on Infectious Diseases 1970, revised 1971. American Academy of Pediatrics.

107. Levin, R. H.: Drugs excreted in breast milk. Bull. Peninsula Pharmaceutical Soc., 12: 4, 1972.

chapter 5

CLINICAL TOXICOLOGY

Gary Oderda, Pharm.D.

INTRODUCTION

A great need exists today for pharmacists to be trained in the retrieval of poisoning information and be exposed to basic principles of the treatment of poisoning. Analysis of poisoning information can be traumatic but rewarding to the pharmacist equipped to handle such a medical emergency. Poisoning calls are frequently received by poison control centers, community pharmacies and hospital pharmacies. Many pharmacists who receive these calls are not equipped to handle them. It is the purpose of this chapter to provide an introduction to the retrieval of poisoning information and the treatment of poisoning.

GENERAL INFORMATION

The ingestion of a drug or chemical, be it suicidal, homicidal or accidental, is a serious problem in the United States today. In 1973 the National Clearinghouse for Poison Control Centers processed 163,500 reports of ingestions throughout the United States.[1] It is estimated that each year more than 1 million cases of poisoning occur in the United States accounting for over 3 thousand deaths.[2] About half of these deaths are accidental, and one-third occur in children under 5 years of age.[2] The figures stated above are probably lower than the actual number that exists. Both the failure of individual physicians to report poisonings and the misdiagnosis of poisoning contribute to this inaccuracy.

A child's natural curiosity can at times have disastrous consequences. He is exposed to thousands of drugs and hundreds of thousands of chemicals and household products. Fortunately, most children learn by their past poisoning experiences and thus the percentage of repeat "accidental" ingestions is low. In pediatrics, poisoning is the most common medical emergency.[2] Aspirin is still the leading ingested agent in those under 5 years old. It is interesting to note, however, that the percentage of ingestions due to aspirin in those under 5 years of age has decreased steadily from around 25% in 1966 to 6.5% in 1973.[1,3] Many factors are responsible for this decrease, and among them is an increased awareness on the part of the lay public of the dangers of aspirin. The limiting of 36 75-mg tablets per bottle of childrens' aspirin is another. The recent safety closure requirements for all products containing aspirin and all liquid preparations containing methyl salicylate will hopefully further decrease the number of salicylate intoxications. Working toward preventing poisoning is the most logical approach to this problem. The old cliche "an ounce of prevention is worth a pound of cure" obviously applies here.

ROLE AND STATUS OF POISON CONTROL CENTERS

There are 580 "official" poison control centers in the United States. Official centers are those recognized by the National Clearinghouse for Poison Control Centers, a division of the Department of Health, Education and Welfare. Official centers exist in most major metropolitan areas of the United States and are most commonly staffed by physicians, nurses and pharmacists. Phone numbers of these centers are available in a directory published by the National Clearinghouse, and they are usually available through telephone operators. Various unofficial centers also exist, and these are more difficult to locate. Most drug information centers also provide poisoning information. It is important to note, however, that these two types of centers (drug information versus poison control) do differ. Poison control centers provide services both to professionals and more commonly to the lay public, whereas drug information centers usually provide information only to professionals. It is essential that pharmacists acquaint themselves with available centers in their area so they can refer those problems that are beyond either their ability or their reference sources.

ROLE OF THE PHARMACIST IN THE TREATMENT OF POISONING

Pharmacists, because of their unique background in biopharmaceutics, drug interactions, chemistry and, of course, pharmacy, can become valuable resources in poison control centers. Many pharmacists are now officially participating in poison control and drug information centers and, of course, many more participate via their involvement in community and hospital pharmacies. It has been suggested that hospital pharmacists be trained to be able to conduct at least routine qualitative screening tests on blood and/or urine. Because of the pharmacist's background in chemistry and constant availability (both in hospitals and on call), (s)he might be the best person to perform emergency toxicology screening.[4] Pharmacists can and should try to expand their role in this area and become more involved in poison control centers.

TREATMENT — GENERAL

The treatment of poisoning is a complicated area and one that requires a background of information as well as an ability to analyze various situations quickly and carefully and apply and modify basic principles to each individual case. One must also consider all the ramifications of an ingestion. If the intent was suicidal, psychiatric counseling is also essential. If the incident was, in fact, accidental, care must be taken to avoid a recurrence. Julyan and Kuzemko[5] have suggested that accidental poisoning in small children results from four factors: an inexperienced child, a dangerous agent, an unsafe environment and a sick family. After the first ingestion, a child is no longer inexperienced and thus the likelihood of another "accidental" ingestion is low. Education of the parents can eliminate the second and third factors mentioned above (a dangerous agent and an unsafe environment) and thus further reduce the incidence of another ingestion. It is the sick family that proves to be the most difficult problem to alleviate. For reasons of poor health, low intelligence and mental instability, some families are not receptive to preventive education, and it is these families that must be followed up very closely with psychiatric and social counseling.

In general, there are two major classes of therapy for drug intoxication. They are: supportive measures, and specific measures to counteract drug effects or hasten removal of the poison from the body. Supportive measures are undoubtedly the cornerstone of therapy. Treatment for the acute poisoning is largely symptomatic and supportive. Many fatalities that are seen today are not due to the direct toxicity of the pharmacological agent; rather they are due to complications. Many complications may be seen, but the most common are respiratory or metabolic acid-base abnormalities, inadequately or improperly treated hypotension or the direct effect of prolonged coma without adequate nursing care. Respiratory nursing care is vital in the comatose patient. Care must be taken to assure the presence of an adequate airway. Since pneumonia is a frequent complication, antibiotic therapy should be initiated at the first sign of an impending infection.

Local Exposure

Various chemicals are quite toxic to the skin, eyes or mucous membranes, e.g., acids and bases. In the majority of instances, damage is caused by a direct irritation of the affected area. There are a number of compounds, however, that are capable of producing systemic toxicity via transcutaneous absorption. Examples of these agents include the chlorinated and organic phosphate insecticides and the halogenated hydrocarbons.

The clinician treating a topical or inhalation exposure must consider and treat all body areas exposed to the chemical agent. If, for example, a patient is in an enclosed area and exposed to a toxic gas, either the gas must be removed from the area or the patient must be removed from the gas. Artificial respiration is often necessary following prolonged exposure to toxic gases. Additionally, care must be taken to decontaminate all exposed areas such as the nose, mouth, eyes, respiratory tract and skin.

Materials spilled on the skin are best removed with water. Time should not be wasted looking for a specific agent that will neutralize the chemical. Large amounts of water are appropriate. Methods differ in delivering these amounts, but it can be done most conveniently using a faucet, hose or shower. Vinegar or baking soda may be used for neutralization of base or acid exposure, respectively. Combinations of the above agents and the spilled chemicals may cause tissue damage related to heat released from exothermic reactions. Other liquids that have been used in emergency situations when water has not been available include soft drinks, beer or even urine.[6]

Exposure of the eye to caustic chemicals can cause chemical burns of the cornea and conjunctiva. Instillation of a specific neutralizing agent into the eye is generally considered detrimental.[7] Two exceptions to this rule are treatment of lewisite burns with British anti-lewisite (BAL) and cocaine for iodide exposure.[8] The basic treatment of eye exposure is flooding with copious amounts of water for at least 5 to 10 min. Industrial areas where exposure is likely to take place are commonly provided with foot-operated eye baths. If this is not the case, usually the most efficient washing procedure is to place the patient's head directly underneath a faucet. The eyelids should be held open throughout the washing procedure. Any exposure of the eye to chemicals must be considered quite serious. Except in very minor cases, the eye should be seen by an ophthalmologist, preferably within 2 hr after exposure.

Exposure to agents that may not be damaging to the skin but may be absorbed and cause a systemic toxicity, *e.g.*, chlorinated and organophosphate insecticides, requires both topical and systemic therapy. Mechanical washing as described previously will reduce any irritation that might be caused by the agent as well as reduce the amount available for further absorption. Treatment must also be aimed toward the systemic sequellae of this percutaneous absorption.

REMOVAL FROM THE GASTROINTESTINAL TRACT

Emetics

Since most poisonings occur by ingestion, when applicable the most immediate and important need in acute poisoning is to empty the stomach. The trend in management has favored induced emesis with either syrup of ipecac or apomorphine over gastric lavage.[9] Lavage can be slow, traumatic and relatively inefficient (Table 5.1). Recent studies have indicated a more efficient removal from the stomach through the induction of emesis (Table 5.2).[7,10,11] The greater efficacy of induced emesis is attributable in part to some emptying of the upper small intestine (duodenum) as well as the stomach and in part to the fact that lavage often forces material past the pyloric sphincter where it can no longer be recovered. Emesis, which is more convenient, can also recover materials too large to pass through the lavage tube.

Vomiting can only be produced if medullary centers are still responsive. If the patient is comatose or unconscious, emetic agents may be ineffective as well as dangerous because of the possibility of aspiration of the vomitus. Induction of vomiting will not be successful if the stomach is empty. It is recommended that the patient be given 1 to 2 glasses of water when an emetic is given. Emetics share all of the contraindications of gastric lavage. In addition, the use of emetics is contraindicated if cardiac action is impaired because of danger of collapse or if sclerotic or other pathological changes of the blood vessels exist, as the rise of blood pressure during the act of vomiting may lead to hemorrhage. If pulmonary edema or emphysema exists, the same hypertensive mechanism may lead to complications. Vomiting should also not be induced late in pregnancy as this strain may cause a spontaneous abortion.

To produce mechanical stimulation, the patient is given either milk or water and then is gagged by gently stroking the pharynx with either a blunt object or a finger. Care must be taken to ensure that the patient does not bite the clinician's finger. The patient's body should be inverted with the head down but supported and the feet elevated. Although this method is universally available, the percentage of people who vomit after this procedure is quite low, and the mean volume of vomitus is low as compared with other methods. This was probably best illustrated by Dabbous[12]. Thirty children were studied at the emergency room of Childrens' Hospital in Seattle, Washington. Of 15 children who were gagged at home by their parents only 2 vomited with an average volume of vomitus of 50 to 60 ml. All 30 patients were gagged in the emergency room by a physician. Two of these vomited with a mean volume of vomitus of 90 ml. All 30 were then given syrup of ipecac. All vomited with an average volume of 380 ml with a range of 30 to 1000 ml.

Ipecac syrup, the emetic of first choice, is a local and centrally active emetic. Care must be taken to use syrup of ipecac instead of the much stronger (14 times) fluid extract. The Food and Drug Administration (FDA) now approves the over-the-counter (OTC) sale of appropriately labeled 1-ounce quantities of ipecac syrup. The value of ipecac as a emetic has been known for hundreds of years, but its use diminished as gastric lavage gained popularity. During the 1950's, the dosage of ipecac was increased, and it was shown to be more effective than previously believed. Analysis of reports from various sources suggest that syrup of ipecac is 90% effective in producing emesis within 30 min. Unfortunately, very little work has been done to analyze the efficacy of the ipecac-induced expulsion. Only a few individ-

TABLE 5.1
Commonly Used Specialized Gastric Lavage Fluids

Name	Mechanism of Action	Type of Poisoning	Dosage	Comments
Tannic acid	Precipitant	Apomorphine, strychnine, veratrine, cinchona alkaloids, salts of Al, Pb, and Ag	30-50 g in 1000 ml of water	Hepatotoxic; use with caution and in recommended concentration
Potassium permangenate	Oxidizing agent	Organic compounds, strychnine, nicotine, physostigmine, quinine	Usually 1:10,000 solution; NEVER greater than 1:5000	Strong irritant; use well diluted, make sure particles are well dissolved
Milk (dairy or evaporated)	Demulcent	Copper sulfate, croton oil, chlorates, thioglycollic acid	May be given straight or diluted with 50% water	
Sodium bicarbonate	Forms less corrosive and more insoluble ferrous carbonate	Ferrous sulfate	5% solution	Effective alkalinizing agent; not recommended for neutralization of acids as large amounts of carbon dioxide are released and may cause perforation
Magnesium oxide or hydroxide	Neutralizing agent	Aspirin, sulfuric, and other mineral acids, oxalic acid	25 mg/1000 ml	Does not release carbon dioxide
Normal saline	Forms insoluble and noncorrosive silver chloride	Silver nitrate	0.9% solution, approx. 1 tsp. of salt per pint of water	

TABLE 5.2
Comparison of Emetics (Arbitrary Values 0 to 4)[a]

	Ipecac Syrup (30-Ml., Limit)	Apomorphine Hydrochloride	Copper Sulfate	Zinc Sulfate	Antimony and Potassium Tartrate	Salt Water	Mustard Powder	Mechanical
Effectiveness	4	4	3	2	2	1	1	1
Speed of action								
Home	3	0	0	0	0	2	2	2
Hospital	3	4	1	1	1	1	1	4
Safety	4	3	1	1	1	4	4	4
Lack of need for antidote	4	2	1	1	1	4	4	4
Ready availability								
Home	4	1	1	1	1	4	2	4
Hospital	4	3	1	1	1	3	1	4
Low cost	4	1	4	4	4	4	4	4
Acceptance by patient	4	1	1	1	1	1	1	1

[a]Reproduced with permission from Cashman, T. M., and Shirkey, H. C.: Emergency management of poisoning. Pediatr. Clin. North Am., Vol. 17, No. 3, 1970.

uals have measured the amount of return from ipecac emesis. It is common knowledge, however, that emesis induced with ipecac is more forceful (and presumably more efficient) than mechanically induced emesis but less forceful than apomorphine. Probably the most descriptive analysis of the efficacy of ipecac syrup was reported by Boxer *et.al.*, in 1969.[11] They examined 20 patients between 12 and 20 months of age who have presumably ingested salicylates. Lavage was performed and emesis induced on each patient, and the amount of salicylates returned was measured by each method. Approximately one-half of the patients were lavaged first, and the other half were given syrup of ipecac first. In conclusion they stated that "ipecac-induced emesis is superior to gastric lavage for emptying the stomach per os of unwanted contents...and ipecac induced emesis leaves little or no salicylate which could potentially be removed by lavage."

As the average time between ingestion and delivery of the patient to the hospital is somewhat greater than 1 hr, the long onset time for ipecac (around 18 min) as compared with apomorphine (3 to 5 min) becomes less important.[12] When used according to the clearly stated directions included in the package, many lives may be saved. Pharmacists can be very influential in distributing syrup of ipecac. Local pharmaceutical organizations have provided ipecac free of charge to families with young children via community pharmacies. If this service is not available, pharmacists can display ipecac and provide information and urge that families purchase a 1-ounce container of ipecac. Parents should be cautioned to contact their physician, pharmacist or poison control center before giving the child the ipecac. In this way, a professional person can evaluate the situation and determine the appropriateness for administering an emetic and, if needed, call an ambulance service, a pediatrician or an emergency room. The combination of ipecac, water and an automobile ride will likely produce effective emesis. Obviously, a container to collect the emesis should accompany the patient so that the vomitus may be saved for later analysis.

A variety of toxic reactions to ipecac have been reported with the most frequent complications being cardiovascular. Ipecac is a specific cardiotoxin and has been shown to cause reversible depression of T waves, bradycardia, atrial fibrillation and hypotention. Toxicity is rarely seen with therapeutic doses. Clinical experience has shown that if a 1-year-old child ingests 1-ounce of the syrup (the largest amount available OTC), no real danger exists. Prudence does indicate, however, that if emesis does not occur and the dose remains in the patient, it should be removed because of possible gastric irritation. Deaths have been reported following ingestion of as little as 10 ml of the fluid extract in a 4-year-old child. The use of ipecac in a patient 1 hr after the ingestion of antiemetics such as the phenothiazines is not recommended because of its relative ineffectiveness in this circumstance.

In children over 1 year of age, the recommended dose of ipecac is 15 ml followed by water. This dose may be repeated in 15 min if emesis has not occurred. Smaller doses have been successful in children less than 1 year old. Conservative clinicians recommend the use of 8 ml in children less than 2 years old and 15 ml in those over 2. This degree of conservatism commonly leads to delay of emesis or no emesis at all.

Apomorphine is a morphine derivative that produces emesis through a central action. It acts very quickly, usually within 3 to 5 min when given subcutaneously. Apomorphine is successful in producing evacuation of large particles of food, enteric-coated tablets and a reflux of contents from the upper intestinal tract. Animal and human studies have shown apomorphine to cause a more violent emesis and a more efficient evacuation than ipecac. Apomorphine is, however, only available in a hospital setting, and thus its use is more limited than the readily available ipecac.[13]

Since apomorphine is a respiratory depressant, it should not be given to a comatose patient, if respiration is low and labored or if the ingested poison is also a respiratory depressant. The drug is centrally active and not effective in deep narcosis or shock. Apomorphine may produce protracted vomiting; this and some of its narcotic effects can be reversed by the administration of naloxone, levallorphan or nalorphine. Most practitioners who routinely use apomorphine advocate comcomitant use of one of the antagonists. The antagonist is administered at the cessation of productive vomiting. Apomorphine is unstable at room temperature and thus must be refrigerated. A green color indicates the compound has decomposed and should not be used. The normal adult dose of apomorphine is 5 mg or 0.1 mg per kg or 3.0 mg per m^2.[6] The children's dose can also be calculated using these formulas.

Copper and zinc sulfate work by direct irritation of the gastric walls and hopefully cause emesis before there is more severe irritation and injury to the gastric mucosa. Vomiting usually occurs quickly: within 5 to 10 min. If vomiting fails to occur, gradual absorption from the bowel may occur and cause systemic poisoning. The toxicity of these compounds includes widespread capillary damage and kidney and liver injury. Because of their toxicity these drugs are not generally recommended. If they are given and emesis does not occur, they must be removed by gastric lavage or successful emesis caused by another agent: 0.25 g of copper sulfate is administered as a 1% solution. If vomiting does not occur in 15 min, 0.15 g of potassium ferrocyanide in a 1% solution should be given, and then gastric lavage should be performed. Copper sulfate and potassium ferrocyanide form insoluble cooper ferocyanide and thus decrease toxicity. A dose of 0.6 to 2.0 g of zinc sulfate is given every 15 min until emesis occurs. The lethal adult dose of zinc sulfate is around 15g. If emesis does not occur, this substance must also be removed by gastric lavage.

Potassium and antimony tartrate (tartar emetic), once considered an outstanding emetic, has fallen into disfavor because of its slow action and also, in contrast to others, because it is fairly easily absorbed, and doses of 200 mg have been fatal. The ordinary emetic dose is 30 mg; if this is not effective within 30 min, it is advisable to remove the emetic by gastric lavage or to neutralize it by the administration of 1 teaspoonful of tannin in water.

Salt water and mustard water (made from dry mustard powder) are both unreliable emetics. Since they are both so unpalatable, much time is wasted in coaxing a child to drink these solutions. As a consequence, the question whether any clinical justification exists for their use is a matter of controversy.

Gastric Lavage

Gastric lavage is a procedure that is used to remove unabsorbed poison from the upper gastrointestinal tract. Lavage has been especially useful in hysterical, comatose or otherwise uncooperative patients.[14] Lavage may be lifesaving and is clearly indicated within 2 to 4 hr after ingestion of most poisons. Lavage may be effective even after 4 hr, if large amounts of milk or cream were given soon after ingestion, if the ingested poison was in the form of enteric-coated or sustained-release preparations or if the patient has been in shock.[2,8] One reason for the success of lavage so long after ingestion is the development of gastric "concretions."[8] These concretions may develop after ingestion of a large amount of a compound that normally readily dissolves in the gastrointestinal (GI) tract. In order for these concretions to develop, it is necessary that a large amount of the compound be ingested, and that this ingestion take place over a short period of time. Examples of drugs whose ingestion has caused concretions include glutethimide, barbiturates, aspirin and meprobamate.[8,15]

Lavage should obviously be begun as soon as possible. It is the delay from time of ingestion to the time lavage is begun that most limits its efficacy. Lavage is effective following moderate emesis in some situations.

Following the ingestion of toxic amounts of acids and alkali, it is generally recommended that a large bore tube should not be passed more than 30 min after the ingestion. Arena claims that lavage can be safely performed within 1 hr after a mineral acid ingestion.[2] The danger of lavage in these situations involves the possibility of perforation. The passing of a gastric tube may cause severe retching and vomiting. This is expecially true in children. In petroleum distillate poisoning (kerosene, mineral oil, mineral seal oil etc.), the vomitus readily enters the trachea because it is oily and does not stimulate the cough reflex. Aspiration can be eliminated by intubating the trachea with a tube having an inflatable cuff. Gastric lavage thus is contraindicated following petroleum distillate poisoning unless a cuffed endotracheal tube is used. Aspiration can also occur in the comatose patient during lavage, and thus it is wise to use a cuffed endotracheal tube in this situation also. With the presence of convulsions, passing a stomach tube increases both the severity and frequency of the convulsions. Following the ingestion of strychnine, the manipulation involved in intubation may precipitate convulsions, and thus in this situation, gastric lavage is contraindicated. Following ingestion (except with strychnine) after convulsions have subsided and there is reason to believe that unabsorbed poison is still present in the GI tract, gastric lavage may be carefully performed.

Gastric lavage procedure is relatively simple and one with which the pharmacist should be familiar. As large a tube as possible is generally used. This ensures that the procedure may be carried out quickly. For adults the tube should be 5/16 inch (a number 24 French tube) or larger. For children a common urethral catheter (a number 8 to 12 French tube) is satisfactory. The patient is instructed to drink a glass of water prior to passing the tube. This both lubricates the esophagus and ensures the presence of an adequate amount of fluid for insertion. The distance from the bridge of the nose to the tip of the xiphoid process is marked on the tube as this approximates the proper length of insertion. Dentures or other foreign objects are removed from the mouth. The patient is positioned on his left side with his head face down, hanging over the end of the examining table. If possible, the foot of the table should be elevated. If the patient is struggling, he should be immobilized with a sheet or blanket. This procedures is commonly required in children. The tube is immersed in water or a water-soluble jelly and is passed very gently. No great force is necessary. In older children and adults the nasal route is preferred, whereas oral passage is easier and less traumatic in infants and younger children. Care must be taken to ensure that the tube has entered the esophagus and not the trachea prior to instillation of fluid. In every case, before lavage fluid or an antidote is instilled, the stomach must first be aspirated.

In most cases the composition of the lavage fluid is less important than the amount of fluid that has been instilled. Tap water is often as good as any vehicle. In children, however, it is safer to use normal or one-half normal saline instead of water because of the child's limited tolerance to electrolyte-free solutions. Water intoxication, tonic and clonic seizures and coma can result from an increase of 5% of body water from electrolyte-free solutions.

In some cases, solutions which chemically inactivate or detoxify the unabsorbed poison can be used (Table 5.1). If these special reagents are not immediately available, lavage with water should be immediately started without them. With the exception of phenol poisoning, alcohol should never be used as lavage fluid. As well as possibly increasing central nervous system (CNS) depression, alcohol can increase absorption of certain ingested agents. Recently, castor oil emulsion lavage has been used, both because of the relative water insolubility of certain drugs and because a bolus of tablets or capsules that has been refractory to water at times responds to oil. Castor oil lavage usually follows copious water lavage. When using castor oil, the trachea must be intubated with a cuffed tube to decrease the risk of aspiration. This procedure has been shown to remove from 5 to 15 g of glutethimide several hours after ingestion and is commonly followed by an activated charcoal slurry lavage solution.

With small bore tubing (in children) 1 to 3 ounces of fluid are introduced into and aspirated from the stomach using the same syringe. The first washing is separated from the rest and all are saved for possible later analysis. This process is repeated 10 to 15 times or until all washings are clear. With large bore tubing (in adults) the stomach is filled by gravity. A funnel is introduced into the free end of the tubing. The funnel is then raised above the patient's head and 10 to 12 ounces (never more than 16 ounces) are introduced. Introduction of too much fluid can distend the stomach and force gastric contents into the duodenum. As soon as the fluid reaches the stomach, turning the patient promotes mixing within the stomach and washes all mucosal surfaces. The washings are promptly removed by a stomach pump or by gravity siphoning. This procedure is repeated 10 to 15 times (at least 3 liters of fluid) or until all returns are clear. All recovered fluid should be saved for analysis.

Cathartics

Theoretical justification does exist for the use of cathartics in poisonings. Clinical justification is more difficult to demonstrate. Most authors, however, agree that: irritant cathartics such as aloes and cascara should not be used in any kind of poisoning; cathartics should not be used in patients with disturbed electrolyte balance; and if cathartics are used after ingestion of a corrosive substance, excessive intestinal injury can be produced. Cathartics are generally used after emesis or lavage to hasten removal of the poison from the stomach and the intestinal tract. No attempt should be made to cause a severe catharsis as the consequent irritation of the bowel and loss of water and electrolytes might precipitate or aggravate shock.

Magnesium sulfate (Epsom salts) should never be used. The absorbed magnesium is rapidly excreted by normal kidneys; but if renal function is impaired by the poison, magnesium may be retained, causing depression of medullary centers.

Cathartic oils (*e.g.,* castor oil) are also normally contraindicated in poisoning. They may facilitate the absorption of some oil-soluble poisons, *e.g.,* chlorinated insecticides. An exception to this is the use of castor oil in phenol poisoning. Castor oil is normally bland until hydrolyzed to an irritant in the intestine. Phenols are highly soluble in castor oil, and for this reason, the latter facilitates its removal from the GI tract. Following castor oil with a saline cathartic is also advisable.

Sodium sulfate (Glauber's salts) is the safest of the cathartic agents. Problems with fluid balance and hypernatremia exist, but the toxicity is much less than with magnesium sulfate. This compound is the only saline cathartic that should be generally used in poisonings. Thirty grams of sodium sulfate are dissolved in 250 cc of water and given after gastric lavage or emesis. Catharsis should start in 30 min to 1 hr.

LOCAL ANTIDOTES

Local antidotes are used to neutralize any poison remaining in the GI tract. These agents can delay but not prevent absorption; thus, not too much reliance should be placed on neutralization without removal by lavage or emesis. Most neutralizing agents react chemically with the poison. They either combine with it to form a poorly soluble and therefore less toxic compound or alter it so radically that toxicity is lost. Some act solely by adsorbing the poison. Certain local antidotes can be given orally through the lavage tube along with the lavage fluid, depending on their inherent toxicity and palatability. Representative examples of commonly used specific agents are listed below.

Potassium permangenate is useful in oxidizing and precipitating certain alkaloids even though it acts somewhat slowly. No effect is seen on inorganic poisons. Potassium permangenate solutions should not exceed 1:10,000. The solution is especially effective with strychnine, nicotine, physostigmine, coniine and quinine. Care must be taken to ensure that no solid particles of potassium permangenate remain in the solution. Undissolved particles can be corrosive to the stomach. Any remaining solution must be removed from the stomach by additional washings with water.

Egg white proteins react with many poisons to form insoluble compounds. This agent is especially useful in arsenic poisoning. It is thought to adsorb or precipitate the poison and offer some protection to the gastric mucosa. Water is mixed with raw egg whites until the solution flows readily. This neutralization is often only temporary and thus the use of egg whites should serve only as an adjunct to lavage or emesis.

The protein in milk reacts with some poisons to form insoluble compounds. The calcium in milk converts fluorides, oxalic acid and oxalates to highly insoluble salts. Milk also decreases gastric irritation and thus is somewhat useful with corrosives. Milk may increase the absorption of fat-soluble compounds and thus should not be given if the poison is thought to be fat-soluble. This neutralization is also temporary, and its use is best combined with lavage or emesis.

The universal antidote is essentially universally useless. This preparation consists of activated charcoal, an antacid (usually magnesium oxide) and a supposed precipitator of alkaloids (usually tannic acid). The last two agents not only fail in large part to serve their avowed functions but instead inactivate the single useful ingredient—activated charcoal. Also important is the fact that tannic acid is a hepatotoxin. Activated charcoal alone should be used in place of the universal antidote.

Activated charcoal is an odorless, tasteless, fine black powder that is an effective nonspecific adsorbent of a wide variety of drugs and chemicals. Two characteristics are necessary for activated charcoal to be effective: first, small particle size and thus large surface area and second, low mineral content (vegetable origin). For these reasons neither burnt toast nor charcoal tablets are effective. Activated charcoal should be stored in tightly sealed glass or metal containers. Prolonged exposure to vapors of the atmosphere will decrease adsorptive capability.

When given in adequate dosage, activated charcoal is highly effective. Some say it is an effective antidote for virtually all organic and inorganic compounds and cite cyanide as the only exception. Recent evidence, however, does not support this.[16] Activated charcoal has also been shown to be relatively ineffective with ethanol, methanol, caustic alkalis and mineral acids.[16] If used, the dose should be at least 5 times by weight the amount of ingested poison. Some have suggested as high as 10 times the amount of poison be given,[16] although this may be difficult owing to the large volume that must be administered to the patient. Activated charcoal adsorbs syrup of ipecac. By this action the ipecac becomes ineffective, and the adsorptive capacity of the activated charcoal is also reduced. If both of these compounds are to be given, it is imperative that vomiting be induced with ipecac before the activated charcoal is given.

Activated charcoal has recently been compared to several other adsorbents—attapulgite, Arizona montmorillonite and evaporated milk. All four of these compounds are effective in certain situations. Activated charcoal has, however, been shown to have the broadest spectrum of adsorptive activity.[17,18] Arizona montmorillonite suffers from a poor affinity for anions and organic acids. In its favor, however, is a large surface area and greater esthetic appeal than activated charcoal. Attapulgite is much less effective than activated charcoal in limiting absorption of sodium salicylate. Evaporated milk is not as effective an adsorbent as activated charcoal. It does have the advantage, however, of universal availability. At this time this author recommends continued use of activated charcoal until the shortcomings of other agents listed above are overcome.

Acids are used occasionally to neutralize bases remaining in the oropharynx or esophagus, and bases are used occasionally to neutralize acids that may be remaining in the oropharynx, esophagus and stomach. In order for weak acids and bases to be effective they must be administered immediately after ingestion, *i.e.*, within 5 to 10 min. Generally speaking, when using a base, care must be taken not to choose one that will release carbon dioxide (*e.g.*, sodium bicarbonate or chalk), as the gas released can cause bloating and perforation and peritonitis. Specific examples of acids and bases, as well as local antidotes are summarized in Table 5.3.

DILUTION

Simple dilution is sometimes useful in retarding absorption. This decrease in absorption

TABLE 5.3
Locally Acting Antidotes Against Unabsorbed Poisons[a]

Poison	Antidote	
	Substance and dose or Concentration	Mechanism of action
Acids, corrosive	Weak alkali (magnesium oxide or hydroxide)	Neutralization
Alkali, caustic (*e.g.,* lye)	Weak acid (1:4 vinegar, 1% acetic acid, or lemon juice)	Neutralization
Alkaloids		
Coniine	Potassium permanganate, 1:10,000 (lavage)	Oxidation
Quinine		
Physostigmine[b]		
Strychnine		
Arsenic[b]	Protein (milk, egg white, etc.)	Adsorption
Barium salts	Sodium sulfate 0.3 g/kg.	Precipitation
Chlorine gas	Sodium bicarbonate aerosol	Neutralizes HCl
Detergents, cationic	Soap	Inactivation
Fluoride[b]	Calcium (milk, lime water, calcium lactate or gluconate)	Precipitation
Formaldehyde	Ammonia water, 0.2%, or ammonium acetate or carbonate, 1% (lavage)	Form methenamine
Iodine	Starch, 1-10%	Inactivation
Iron[b]	Sodium bicarbonate, 5% deferoxamine 5-10 g	Form ferrous carbonate; chelates
Mercury[b]	Sodium formaldehyde sulfoxylate, 5% (lavage), or protein (*e.g.,* milk)	Precipitation
Oxalic acid[b]	Calcium (see fluoride)	Precipitation
Phenol	A vegetable oil (olive, etc.)	Retards absorption
Phosphorus	Copper sulfate, 0.2% (lavage)	Precipitation
Silver nitrate	Normal saline (lavage)	Precipitation
Unknown and miscellaneous	Activated charcoal (5-50 g as slurry in water)	Adsorbs many poisons

[a]Reproduced from Done, A. K.: Pharmacologic principles in the treatment of poisoning Pharmacol. Physicians, Vol. 3, No. 7, 1969.

[b]Systemic antidotes also available (see Table 5.4).

is caused solely by a decrease in poison concentration and thus a subsequent decrease in concentration gradient. It is important to limit the amount of fluid to be given; 50 ml/10g is generally recognized as an appropriate amount.[9] If too much fluid is given, gastric contents (containing the poison) can be forced through the pylorus into the small intestine. For simple dilution, water is satisfactory and is universally available. Much valuable time can be lost searching for an appropriate diluent.

SYSTEMIC ANTIDOTES

A systemic antidote is an agent that specifically neutralizes or counteracts the systemic effects of a poison. Table 5.4 lists examples of specific antidotes. Most poisons do not have a specific systemic antidote. In these cases, as well as cases where a specific antidote is available, good supportive care is essential. The best antidote is of little value without good supportive care.

HASTENING ELIMINATION

In cases where a specific systemic antidote is not available, other methods of enhancing metabolism and detoxification must be considered. If a poison has been absorbed in potentially lethal quantities, it becomes necessary to examine other possible mechanisms of minimizing the toxic effects. Hastening elimination is one of these possible pathways. Drugs and chemicals are excreted through both the biliary tract and the urinary tract. At this time not enough is known about biliary excretion to utilize it for hastening elimination of poisons. Renal excretion offers much more of an opportunity. The composition of urine is determined by a combination of ultrafiltration, active tubular secretion and tubular resorption. Tubular resorption can be either an active or a passive process. Essential compounds such as glucose and sodium are actively reabsorbed, whereas foreign substances such as poisons are passively reabsorbed. No way is known to increase tubular secretion. The most one can hope to accomplish is to decrease reabsorption. Only the un-ionized form of weak acids and bases is capable of crossing membranes. For a compound with a given dissociation constant (pKa or pKb), the amount of a compound in the un-ionized form is determined by the pH. By using the Henderson-Hasselbach equation (pH = pK + log [A-]/[HA]), one can determine the amount of drug in the un-ionized form at any given pH. Examine the hypothetical example of a weak acid with a pKa of 4.4 and pay particular attention to absorption from the GI tract. In a buffer system this hypothetical weak acid HA, the un-ionized form, will be in equilibrium with H+ and A- ions. In the gastric juice (pH 1.4) HA (the un-ionized form) will be favored, and its concentration will be 1 thousand times as high as A- (the ionized form). In the plasma (pH 7.4) just the opposite will be true. Here A- will be favored, and its concentration will be 1 thousand times higher than HA. Thus in plasma the ratio of nonionized to ionized is 1:1000, and in the gastric juices, the ratio of nonionized to ionized is 1000:1. If the pH of the urine is adjusted in such a manner that a high percentage of the poison in the urine is ionized, it will not be reabsorbed and thus will be excreted. The pH of dialysis fluids can be manipulated in the same way.

The range of urinary pH that can be exogenously produced is usually 4.5 to 8.0. Unfortunately, this amount of variation is not available where it is most necessary—at the reabsorptive sites. At these sites the pH may be altered from about 6.5 to 7.5. For example, if a weak acid has a pKa of 6.5, one-half will be ionized and one-half will be un-ionized at a pH of 6.5. If the pH is raised to 7.5, approximately 90% will be ionized and 10% un-ionized, and thus reabsorption should decrease and elimination increase. Unfortunately, pH is not the only determinant of success, and the ability to accelerate removal by these means may be influenced also by the diffusibility of ionized species, the presence of specialized transport systems, degree of protein binding and the extent to which tubular reabsorption and excretion affects urinary excretion. Examples where pH manipulations are thought to be effective include long acting barbiturates, e.g., phenobarbital, and salicylates (alkalinization) and amphetamines and strychnine (acidification).

Drinking or administering intravenously large quantities of fluid and thus causing a water diuresis may increase some clearance values, but its effect on the excretion rates is minimal in most cases. The process would, of course, follow emesis or lavage if these are to be performed. If dilution fluid has been administered, additional fluid may not be necessary. The main effect of a water diuresis is to increase volume and flow in the distal renal tubules and the collecting ducts. Passive solute resorption, however, must occur to a considerable extent in the proximal tubules where it can be prevented only if water resorption can be minimized at this site.

An osmotic diuresis is far more efficient in removing a poison than a water diuresis. Osmotic diuretics such as mannitol and urea are particularly suited for this purpose. These compounds will increase the excretion of any compound that is passively reabsorbed. Probably the most useful regimen combines the use of an osmotic diuretic and an agent that alters the pH of the urine. For example, this combination is effective with salicylates, phenobarbital, amphetamines, strychnine and quinine. Osmotic diuretics are also useful in treating cerebral edema from lead poisoning. The combination of urea and sodium lactate I.V. is an example of such a combination useful for barbiturate poisoning. Also, tromethamine (THAM) appears to be a desirable drug for barbiturates as it causes both an osmotic diuresis and an alkalinization of the urine. Apnea as well as other toxicities have been reported with THAM and thus it must be used with caution.

DIALYSIS

Dialysis refers to the therapeutic procedure whereby unwanted solutes in the blood plasma

TABLE 5.4
Systemic Antidotes[a]

Poison	Antidote	Mechanism
Amphetamines	Chlorpromazine, 1 mg per kg I.M. or I.V. (0.5 mg/kg if barbiturate also taken)	Blocks excitation
Anticholinesterases (organophosphates; also the carbamates: demecardium neostigmine, physostigmine, pyridostiomine, ambenonium, but NOT carbaryl, dimetilan or carbamoyloximes)	Atropine, 1-4 mg I.M. or I.V., repeated half-hourly until atropinization is apparent	Blocks muscarinic effects
	Pralidoxime chloride, 25-50 mg/kg I.V.; repeat in 12 hr prn	Regenerates cholinesterase
Botulinus toxin	Botulinus antitoxin (type specific or polyvalent) 50,000 U I.V. then 20,000 U/day	Inactivates toxin
Bromides	Sodium or ammonium chloride, 4-6 g/day	Hastens excretion
Carbon monoxide	Oxygen (inhalation)	Hastens carboxyhemoglobin dissociation
Carboxyphen	(see Amphetamines)	
Cholinergic compounds: choline esters, pilocarpine, arecoline, muscarine; also carbaryl, dimetilan and carbamate anticholinesterases other than those listed under latter above	Atropine (as above); cholinesterase regenerators should NOT be used	Blocks muscarinic effects
Cyanide	Amyl nitrite inhalation pending sodium nitrite, 6-8 ml. 3%/m² I.V. Slowly; follow with sodium thiosulfate 12.5 g I.V. slowly	Forms methemoglobin; its iron competes with cytochromes for cyanide; forms thiocyanate
Ethylene glycol	Ethanol (as for methanol; see below)	Retards metabolism to oxalate
Fluoride	Calcium gluconate, 2-10 ml of 10% I.V.	Combats hypocalcemia and binds fluoride
Iron salts	Deferoxamine, 5 g P.O. or by tube, then 20 mg/kg I.M. 2-4 hr, (if in shock 40 mg/kg IV drip over 4 hr; may repeat in 6 hr; then 20 mg/kg drip q 12 hr	Chelation

Lead (symptomatic)	Dimercaprol (BAL), 4 mg/kg I.M.; in 4 hr, edathamil 12.5 mg/kg; repeat both q 4 hr	Chelation
Metals:		
Antimony, arsenic, bismuth, gold, mercury, nickel	Dimercaprol, 3-5 mg/kg I.M. q 4 hr on days 1-2; q 6 hr on day 3; then q 12 hr for 10 days or more	Complexation[b]
Cadmium, chromium, cobalt, copper manganese, radium, selenium, uranium, vanadium	Edathamil calcium disodium, 15-25 mg/kg q 12 hr I.V. for 5 days; interrupt for 2 days then additional courses as dictated by severity	Chelation
Methanol	Ethanol 0.75 mg/kg I.V.; then 0.5 mg/kg I.V. for 4 days; sodium bicarbonate, 4 mg/kg I.V. q 4hr pm	Retard formation of toxic metabolites; prevent or correct acidosis
Methemoglobinemic agents: nitrites, anilines, chlorates, phenacetin, etc.	Methylene blue 1-2 mg/kg I.V. as solution if cyanosis severe	Reduce methemoglobin
Narcotics (and substitutes)	Levallorphan 0.02 mg/kg or nalorphine 0.1 mg/kg I.V. as needed	Specific antagonism
Oxalate	Fluoride	Precipitation; corrects hypocalcemia
Phenmetrazine	(See Amphetamine)	
Phenothiazines (neuromuscular reactions only)	Diphenhydramine (1.5 mg/kg) or biperiden (0.04 mg/kg) HCl I.M.	Antiparkinsonian
Thallium	Sodium diethyldithiocarbamate (dithiocarb)[c] 30 mg/kg/day p.p. in divided doses, or diphenylthiocarbazone (dithizone)[c] 10 mg/kg q 12 hr P.O.	Hasten elimination
Warfarin, etc.	Vitamin K_1 or K_1 oxide, 0.5-1.0 mg/kg I.V. or I.M.	Corrects hypoprothrombinemia

[a]Adapted from Done, A. R.: Pharmacologic principles in the treatment of poisoning, Pharmacol. Physicians, 3: No. 7, 1, 1969.

[b]Many metals, especially those reacting with dimercaprol, can also be complexed by penicillamine and its derivatives (which can be given orally), but efficiency is less.

[c]Experimental, Clinical efficacy not yet established.

are allowed to diffuse across a dialysis membrane into a solution. This solution, the dialysate, is replaced continuously or intermittently with a fresh solution of carefully defined composition, so that diffusional transport is allowed to continue. In preparing solutions suitable for dialysis, all diffusible solutes should, in theory, be present in concentrations approximating those in an ultrafiltrate of normal blood plasma. Two basic types of dialysis are used. They are extracorporeal hemodialysis (the "artificial kidney") and peritoneal dialysis.

Extracorporeal hemodialysis is an effective but rather elaborate procedure. Several designs of artificial kidneys are now being used. In all types, coils of cellulose dialysis tubing are bathed on the outside by a large volume of a wash solution that is oxygenated, warmed and stirred continuously. Blood is removed continuously from one of the patient's peripheral arteries (usually the brachial). It is pumped through the dialysis tubing and back into a peripheral vein. To prevent coagulation, heparin is added and, to ensure against emboli, the blood is filtered before it is returned to the patient. Many artificial kidneys require more blood than can be safely furnished by the patient, and thus the machine must be primed with donor blood before it is connected to the patient. Contraindications for its use include inexperience of the operator and inadequate knowledge of the problem to which the apparatus is to be applied. Since heparinization is necessary to prevent coagulation of the blood in the extracorporeal circulation (it is possible, however, by "regional heparinization" to heparinize blood entering the machine and to neutralize it with protamine sulfate as it returns to the patient's venous circulation), bleeding, particularly from the gastrointestinal tract, also is a contraindication. The use of this procedure in a patient with low platelets and/or a low white cell count is not advised. Destruction of platelets and white cells by the cellophane membrane does occur during the course of hemodialysis.

Peritoneal dialysis will remove the same material as extracorporeal hemodialysis but with less efficiency. On the other hand, peritoneal dialysis offers the advantages of being adaptable to any hospital setting, requiring less experience and training, eliminating the need for elaborate equipment and avoiding the dangerous blood volume fluctuations that are often encountered when hemodialysis is used in small children. Peritoneal dialysis is much more efficient than the natural kidney for ridding the body of overdoses of barbiturates and other drugs. Contraindications for its use are infections of the peritoneal cavity and recent or extensive abdominal surgery. A small laparotomy incision is made in the right section of the mesogastric region (the umbilical area of the abdomen), and a catheter is inserted with its distal tip extending about 3 cm into the peritoneal cavity. This is used as an inflow tract. A slightly larger incision is made in the left hypogastrium (the lower middle region of the abdomen), and two catheters, each with several openings near the tip, are inserted. The tip of one catheter is advanced to about 3 cm beyond the tip of the other. This enables later movement of the catheters against each other to free any fibrin or clots from occluding the openings and thus obstructing the outlfow. A flow of about 1 liter per hr is recommended for adults and a proportionally slower flow would be used for children. Frequent checks of the outflow catheters are required to make sure that the lumens are not obstructed. A list of commonly dialyzable poisons by either the peritoneal or extracorporeal route is shown in Table 5.5.

The following sections will discuss indications for dialysis in general as well as relating these indications to two fairly commonly ingested drugs—barbiturates and glutethimide.

Conservative measures are not adequate for every patient. Dialysis is indicated in certain situations, but it must be considered an adjunct to and not a substitute for conservative therapy. Schreiner[19] suggested criteria that must be met in judging the applicability for dialysis. These criteria have been accepted as the standard, and they are:

1. Molecules should diffuse through the dialyzing membrane, be it cellophane or peritoneum, from plasma water and have a reasonable dialysance. Dialysance relates to the efficiency of transfer of a particular solute from blood to dialysate. Dialysance can be computed by the following equation:

$$D = a\left(1 - e^{\,ps/a}\right)$$

where D is the dialysance, a is the blood flow, p the membrane permeability and s the surface area. Dialysance is expressed in ml per min.

2. The drug must be distributed in plasma

TABLE 5.5
Currently Known Dialyzable Poisons[a]

Barbiturate[b]	Alcohols	Metals	Miscellaneous substances
Barbital	Ethanol[b]	Arsenic	Thiocyanate[b]
Phenobarbital	Methanol[b]	Copper	Aniline
Amobarbital	Isopropanol	Calcium	Sodium chlorate
Pentobarbital	Ethylene glycol	Iron	Potassium chlorate
Butabarbital		Lead	Eucalyptus oil
Secobarbital		Lithium	Boric acid
Cyclobarbital		Magnesium	Potassium dichromate
	Analgesics	Mercury	Chromic acid
Glutethimide[b]	Acetylsalicylic acid[b]	Potassium	Digoxin
	Methylsalicylate	Sodium	Sodium citrate
Depressants, sedatives and	Acetophenetidin	Strontium	Dinitro-ortho-cresol
tranquilizers	Dextropropoxyphene		Amanita phalloides
Diphenylhydantoin	Paracetamol	Halides	Carbon tetrachloride
Primidone		Bromide[b]	Ergotamine
Meprobamate		Chloride[b]	Cyclophosphamide
Ethchlorvynol[b]		Iodide	5-Fluorouracil
Ethinamate	Antibiotics	Fluoride	Methotrexate
Methyprylon	Streptomycin		Camphor
Diphenhydramine	Kanamycin	Endogenous toxins	Trichlorethylene
Methaqualone	Neomycin	Ammonia	Carbon monoxide
Heroin	Vancomycin	Uric acid[b]	Chlorpropamide
Gallamine triethiodide	Penicillin	Tritium[b]	Quinine
Paraldehyde	Ampicillin	Bilirubin	
Chloral hydrate	Sulfonamides	Lactic acid	
Chlordiazepoxide	Cephalothin	Schizophrenia	
	Cephaloridine	Myasthenia gravis	
Antidepressants	Chloramphenicol	Porphyria	
Amphetamine	Tetracycline	Cystine	
Methamphetamine	Nitrofurantoin	Endotoxin	
Tricyclic secondary amines	Polymyxin	Hyperosmolar state[b]	
Tricyclic tertiary amines	Isoniazid	Water intoxication	
Monoamine oxidase inhibitors	Cycloserine		
Tranylcypromine			
Pargyline			
Phenelzine			
Isocarboxazid			

[a]Reproduced with permission of Schreiner, G. E.: Dialysis of poisons and drugs, In Perspectives in Clinical Pharmacy, Ed. 1, p. 456. 1972.

[b]Kinetics of dialysis thoroughly studied and/or clinical experience extensive.

water or readily equilibrate with it. Tight protein or tissue binding limits dialysis.

3. Clinical toxicity should be related to length of exposure to the chemical and its blood concentration. This relationship is referred to as the "time-dose-cytotoxic relationship."

4. The amount of drug dialyzed should significantly add to normal body mechanisms in eliminating the drug under existing clinical conditions. For example, shock, oliguria and poor liver perfusion may decrease the body's ability

to eliminate the drug and increase the need for dialysis.

When should the practitioner turn to dialysis? Considerable controversy surrounds this topic. It is this author's feeling that the abuse of dialysis is in part responsible for this contraversy. Instances of relying on dialysis and ignoring common principles of supportive care have been seen. Dialysis has, without a doubt, been shown to be an efficient method for rapidly clearing the body of both drugs and chemicals from endogenous and exogenous sources.

Henderson and Merrill reviewed the literature in 1966 and concluded that extensive use of extracorporeal hemodialysis of barbiturates has been accompanied by a higher mortality rate than conservative management alone.[20] The highest mortality figure (12.7%) was seen in the series with the highest percentage of extracorporeal dialysis. They felt that these data suggested that possibly extracorporeal hemodialysis imposes problems not ordinarily encountered in barbiturate intoxication treated conservatively; the conservative measures are not being adequately carried out in conjunction with dialysis; or the patient populations were not comparable. These figures can be largely explained by the last two above, neglecting supportive measures and differing patient populations. Presumably, sicker patients are selected for dialysis. Dialysis is, however, a somewhat heroic measure, and it is a process that may well be responsible for an increased mortality. George Schreiner[21] has said, "We do not believe that dialysis is a substitute for an airway or nursing care. . .Our. . . experience tells us, however, that there will always be one group of patients whose intoxication is so severe that the maintenance of a good airway and support of the circulation, however effective, will not suffice. There will always be another group of patients for whom the morbidity and danger of prolonged coma or the intoxication of specific organ systems presents a risk that is no longer necessary to take. For these two groups. . .remove the poison."

Dialysis then should be used when

1. The poison meets the criteria for dialyzability.

2. A lethal amount has been ingested and conservative measures, no matter how effective, will not be sufficient.

3. Metabolism of the ingested compound yields a more toxic substance and rapid removal is necessary (two examples are methanol being metabolized to formaldehyde and ethylene glycol to oxalic acid).

4. There is underlying disease that would significantly hamper removal of the drug.

5. There is a possibility of prolonged coma.

Assuming that the decision to dialyze has been made, one now faces the choice of extracorporeal hemodialysis versus peritoneal dialysis. The main advantages of peritoneal dialysis revolve around its simplicity, availability in all centers for use by individuals with compara-

tively little special training and a decreased incidence of adverse reactions. Peritoneal dialysis is hampered, however, as the relative rate of clearance is only one-fifth to one-tenth that of hemodialysis. Also, lipid dialysate can be used more easily with hemodialysis for fat-soluble products. Peritoneal dialysis is much less efficient in patients with hypotension or vasoconstriction. If dialysis is indicated and extracorporeal hemodialysis is available, it should definitely be used. If a patient's therapy must be delayed several hours for transport to a dialysis center, and dialysis is indicated, it may be best to use peritoneal dialysis.

Barbiturate overdose is a relatively common problem in the United States today. The pKa's for the short acting barbiturates differ from those for the longer acting. For example, phenobarbital has a pKa of 7.24 whereas pentobarbital's is 7.96 and secobarbital's is 7.90. Alkalinization of the urine is effective only with phenobarbital and not the shorter acting barbiturates. Alkalinization to a high enough pH to be effective with a drug in the pKa range of 7.90 to 7.96 is not practical. Phenobarbital is metabolized slowly in the liver and excreted to a large degree unchanged in the urine. The short acting compounds rely more heavily on detoxification by metabolism and less via urinary excretion. Forced diuresis may increase the clearance of short acting barbiturates to 5.0 ml per min and phenobarbital to 17.0 ml per min.

Schreiner[21] has suggested the following specific indications for dialysis in barbiturate poisoning.

1. Known ingestion and probably absorption of a potentially fatal dose (3.0 g for short acting and 5.0 g for long acting).

2. A potentially fatal blood barbiturate level (3.5 mg% short, and 8.0% mg% long).

3. Progessive deepening of anesthesia or clinical deterioration.

4. Coexistance of a medical complication delaying elimination of drug or increasing the hazards of coma.

5. Development of a severe complication such as hyperpyrexia or aspiration pneumonia.

Hemodialysis removes barbiturates from 10 to 30 times more rapidly then diuresis. Maximal dialysance ranges from 65 ml per min for secobarbital to 100 ml per min for phenobarbital. Peritoneal dialysis is considerably less efficient.

Manipulating peritoneal dialysate solutions has shown some promising results, however. Berman and Vogelsang[22] compared ordinary dialysate with a 5% albumin solution. The albumin solution extracted approximately 50% more secobarbital and approximately 230% more pentobarbital than the ordinary solution. Kudla et.al.[23] compared normal peritoneal dialysis fluid with the same fluid plus 1% anthranilic acid and 0.25% N-mycristylbeta-aminopropionic acid. The second fluid (Ml fluid) caused an increased recovery of greater than 100% of all the following drugs: pentobarbital, amobarbital, salicylates, butabarbital, phenobarbital and diphenylhydantoin. The proposed mechanism involves displacement from binding sites occurring in the vessels of the mesentery where the agent is chiefly absorbed and where dialysis is taking place.

Glutethimide poisonings tend to be rarer and more severe than barbiturate overdosages. The mortality rate in patients taking 20 or more 0.5-g tablets is approximately 45%, yet in 1966 almost 3 million glutethimide prescriptions for patients over 65 years old were written.[24]

Glutethimide is a weakly polar, almost water-insoluble compound with a lipid-water solubility coefficient of approximately 100. Virtually no drug appears unchanged in the urine and thus forced diuresis has not proven to be very useful. Early reports showed a poor correlation of blood levels and toxicity. Schreiner,[21] however, claimed that a direct relationship between dose and toxicity does, in fact, exist. Decker et.al.[25] reported two young women who ingested glutethimide, underwent dialysis and awakened 24 hr after ingestion. Twelve hours later they returned to a comatose state and again awoke 40 hr later. At blood levels above 2.2 mg% the patients slept, and below 2.0 mg% the patients awoke.

The following are specific indications for dialysis in a patient who has ingested glutethimide:

1. After ingestion of a large dose (6.0 g or more).

2. When blood levels are high (3.0—8.0 mg%) and when patients are unresponsive and have severe hypotension and shock, cerebral or pulmonary edema or neurological signs such as fixed pupils.

Clearance values are frequently disappointing, but in vitro dialysance rates with aqueous dialysate have been reported as high as 90 ml per min. Aqueous dialysis usually can remove about 10% of the ingested dose. In severe poisoning an extended dialysis or the use of machines in a series may be desired. The rate of removal by hemodialysis is about 20 times faster than with diuresis and 12 times faster than with peritoneal dialysis.

Several interesting things have been done with glutethimide. Shinaberger[26] did work in dogs comparing a standard solution with a solution of 15% cottonseed oil and 5% glucose in water. For hemodialysis the cd/cb (concentration dialysate/concentration blood) with the standard solution was 0.32 at 3 hr. For lipid dialysate cd/cb of 1.10 at 3 hr and 2.30 at 6 hr were seen. Lipid dialysate recovered 3.43 times as much as aqueous dialysate in 3 hr. The same comparison was made with peritoneal dialysis. The cd/cb with the aqueous dialysate was 0.37 at 45 min. The ratio with lipid dialysate was 1.88 after the first exchange, 1.43 after the second, and 1.67 in the third. No adverse effects were noted.

One of the most interesting procedures beginning to be used now does not really qualify as dialysis but is actually a hemoperfusion through activated charcoal. In 1964 Yatzidis et.al.[27] performed in vitro studies and found that activated charcoal would adsorb creatinine, urea, uric acid, guanidine and other organic acids when placed in direct contact with the blood. In 1965 he reported using his method on two patients severely intoxicated with barbiturates. Both patients survived. Yatzidis et.al.[27] claimed that the only ill effects of the procedure are likely to ba a slight fall in arterial pressure and certain transitory effects which are probably caused by the release of sulfur. In this country, DeMyttenaere[28] has done some work with hemoperfusion through activated charcoal with respect to glutethimide. Severely intoxicated dogs (8.8 to 12.0 mg%) were hemoperfused. At doses of 400 mg per Kg or less, all hemoperfused dogs survived and all controls died. Clearance ranged from 84 to 150 ml per min and usually approached the flow rate indicating nearly complete estraction. The only adverse effect noted was a decreased amount of platelets. Hemoglobin levels and leukocyte levels were unchanged.

Hagstam et.al.[29] did some activated charcoal hemoperfusion work in rabbits in Sweden comparing three different particle sizes with an appropriate filter. Despite careful rinsing of the columns, microscopic charcoal particles were invariably found in the blood. Necropsy of all perfused rabbits showed no macroscopic abnormalities, but microscopic examination revealed charcoal particles in the lungs of all the hemoperfused animals, in the spleen of 66% and in the kidneys of 25% of treated animals.

Some recent work with resin hemoperfusion has been especially promising. Many of the problems associated with charcoal hemoperfusion, *i.e.*, particles distributed throughout the lungs, spleen, etc. are not seen with the use of resins. The potential range for effective resin adsorption of toxins has not been fully explored, but it promises to be broader than for hemodialysis because of the use of combinations of lipophilic, hydrophilic, anionic and cationic resins.

Recent evidence has show that aqueous dialysis with glutethimide is not very effective at increasing clearance rates. Hopefully some of the newer methods described above will prove useful.

POISONING INFORMATION AND RETRIEVAL

Introduction

The following section concerns how one answers a poisoning question, what questions are asked, how one finds and analyzes the information, and what constitutes a good answer.

Types of Questions Asked

Unfortunately, many poisoning calls do not volunteer to the pharmacist enough information to answer adequately all pertinent questions. This is especially true when the patient is discovered in a coma from an unknown cause, a child ingests an unknown amount of tablets or capsules from an unmarked container or a poisonous plant has been ingested. In addition, the incidence of multiple ingestions is also increasing. The most common question asked involves the lethality of an ingested toxic substance. Some examples: A mother calls and says, "Johnny took four of my birth control pills; should I take him to the emergency room?" A suicide prevention worker calls and says, "Mr. X took 100 Seconal; should I call an ambulance for him?"

More and more frequently, calls from physicians in emergency rooms ask, "Mr. Y took 100 Talwin; what is the lethal dose in this patient and what treatment is appropriate?"

A family physician will call and ask, "Mrs. Smith's 4-year-old son took four or five green and white capsules with Lilly H69 on them; what are they and what should I do?"

Most of the above questions can be answered with relative ease. Examples of questions more difficult to answer include a physician calling and saying, "Mrs. Jones was found comatose at her home with an empty bottle of amitriptyline, pargyline and diazepam lying next to her. How should I treat her?"

And more of a challenge, "Mrs. Doe was brought into the emergency room by friends who claim she took an unknown number of tablets of an unidentified drug and is showing the following symptoms. . .; do you know what it might be and what I should do about it?"

Often only incomplete information is available, and the pharmacist working in poison control must be ready to ask appropriate questions to uncover all of the facts from the caller. Occasionally, poisoning questions can only be extracted by clever questioning. For example, questions such as "What is a small yellow tablet with 'Roche 5' on it?" can be easily answered; "Valium® 5 mg." By asking the question, "Why do you need this information?" one might find that an ingestion has occurred and (s)he could be of further assistance in describing proper treatment.

What questions must the pharmacist ask? Standard forms placed by the telephone assure expediency and that vital information is not overlooked. An example is reproduced in Figure 5.1. It is simple to use and is self-explanatory. It is important, however, to familiarize oneself with the form before it has to be used. Caller's name, location and phone number are vital. Nothing could be more frustrating than completing the information search and realizing one neglected to ask how to reach the caller. The information about the victim is also important. Data such as age and weight are used to determine the seriousness of the amount of the ingested drug as well as the doses for any drugs used in the treatment. The name of the drug, chemical or cosmetic is usually volunteered if known. However, the amount ingested is just as important. Often this piece of information is difficult to pin down. Examination of the time

Caller's Name _____   Date _____

    Address_____   Time_____

    Phone No._____

Patient   Sex _____ Weight _____   Age _____

Drug or Chemical:

Amount:

Time of Ingestion:

Route of Administration:

Other Drugs:

Other Disease States:

Symptoms:

Previous Treatment:

FIG. 5.1
Standard poisoning telephone form.

sequence can be quite revealing. When was it taken? When was the victim found? When was treatment begun? Utilization of a pharmacist's pharmacokinetic expertise in evaluating the half-life, distribution, protein binding and other characteristics of the ingested compound can save lives as well as avoid unnecessary discomfort from such procedures as gastric lavage and forced emesis when they are not really indicated.

"Possible other intoxicants coadministered" includes others that may have been ingested at the same time as the one in question or chronic medications the patient has been taking. Questions about underlying disease states may also be useful. For example, a patient with myasthenia gravis would be expected to be unusually sensitive to anticholinergics, neuromuscular blocking agents and similar pharmacological agents. In the same vein, patients with myasthenia gravis or any other chronic disease reuqiring medication should be suspected of taking medications for that disease even it not mentioned under chronic medications. Two of the most important questions a pharmacist can ask and that he often does not are, "What symptoms is the patient exhibiting?" and, "For how long?" Obviously, treatment of an ingestion is primarily dependent on symptomatology. "Has the patient vomited?" This is important, as the patient may have already eliminated most of the toxic chemical. With a little luck and some skill at asking the appropriate questions at the right time, all of this information can be obtained quickly. Remember, time is extremely important! Treatment information is useless postmortem.

Once we have all of the available information, where do we go from here?

ANALYSIS OF A POISONING SITUATION

Perhaps a pharmacist's judgment and the ability to think on one's feet is more adequately tested in the acute poisoning circumstance than anywhere else in drug information. Information retrieval is important, but a trained lay person can gather this information as efficiently as a pharmacist. It is in the utilization of the data and arriving at a therapeutic decision that the professional judgement of the pharmacist is needed. Handling one's first poisoning call can be compared to one's first date. No matter how many times one goes over the situation in one's head, nothing seems to work out as planned. Some of the anxiety can be relieved, however, if a complete understanding of the location of various reference sources, as well as knowing how to use them, is acquired before one is thrust into the real thing. Below you will find the steps to follow in finding information for handling poison inquiries.

I. Identification of the toxic agent.
   A. What is the chemical?
   B. Which ingredients are toxic, and how toxic?
   C. How much has been ingested?
II. Analyze the symptoms.
   A. Do the symptoms the patient is experiencing match the suspected ingested agent? If not, how can this be pharmacologically explained?
   B. May any other agents be involved?
III. Evaluate previous therapy.
   A. What has been the effect of emesis or lavage?
   B. How much drug remains in the body, available to produce further toxicity?
   C. Can blood levels be easily and quickly determined to help make a rational therapy decision?
   C. How does previous therapy affect the treatment plan?
IV. Determine lethality.
   A. What are the consequences of not treating with anything but support?
   B. Are heroics in order?
   C. Should you vigorously treat a situation that is obviously nonlethal?
V. Determine the proper treatment.
   A. Is there a specific antidote?
   B. What therapy is indicated?
   C. What therapy is definitely contraindicated?

Once one is aware of what type of information to look for, how does one find it? Below is a list of references that are used in handling poisoning calls. These are of a general nature. Specifics, such as dialyzability of a certain drug can be best found in current journal articles. The following references are listed in the order that one would generally use them in retrieving poisoning information.

1. Gleason, M.N., Gosselin, R.E., Hodge, H.C., and Smith, R.P.: Clinical Toxicology of Commercial Products, 3. Ed. The Williams and Wilkins Co., Baltimore, 1969.
   This is a classical first line toxicology reference book. Although very simply laid out, in a

crisis situation with no experience with this volume, using it can be a nightmare. It is highly recommended that one carefully examine each section and practice its use. The bulk of this volume is:
   a. Trade Name Index. From this section, commercial products from A.A.A. Paste No. 1 to Zynamine Lotion are listed. If the trade name of the product is known, but not the ingredients, this is the proper section to consult first. The information provided in this section includes the names of the ingredients and probably most important, a toxicity rating for each ingredient. Also included is the amount of each ingredient, if this information is made available by the manufacturer. With this information each toxic ingredient is investigated in
   b. Ingredients Index. If the ingredients are known at the onset of the investigation, this is the first section that one would consult. One would either be given the toxicological data, be referred to another chemical in the ingredients index or be referred to
   c. The Therapeutics Index. It is here that parent compounds and drug classes are extensively discussed. Examples are acid, antihistamines, morphine, warfarin and chlorpromazine. Information such as toxicity, symptomatology, treatment, expected laboratory findings and references are listed. If the trade name is unknown, consult
   d. The General Formulations Index. Under general categories (for example, cosmetics) one would find a specific generic product such as eye makeup, foundation creams and nail polish. Listings of ingredients, amounts and toxicity are included for each product. Again, after you have this information you would proceed to the ingredients index. Also included in Clinical Toxicology of Commercial Products are a first aid and general emergency treatment section, a general supportive treatment section and a list of manufacturers' names and addresses. This volume is the primary poison reference tool and must be included in any collection of toxicology references.

2. Poison Control Cards
   These cards are published by the National Clearinghouse for Poison Control Centers, Health, Education and Welfare — Public Health Service (Fig. 5.2). Here many products are listed by trade name, and some generically. For each particular product the manufacturer, ingredients, amounts, toxicity information, symptoms and findings, recommended treatment and a list of sources of information are listed on one card. The main disadvantage of this system is unavailability, as the National

Name: Psilocybin   Type of Product: Hallucinogen

INGREDIENTS:
O-Phosphoryl-4-hydroxy-*N*-dimethyltryptamine

TOXICITY: As little as 20 mg may produce effects of 5 to 6 hr duration.

SYMPTOMS AND FINDINGS: This produces mydriasis, sweating, anxiety, hypertension and hyperactivity of tendon reflexes. Sensory perception is often clear but can be distorted with vivid, multicolored hallucinations, delusions.

TREATMENT: With an hallucinogen, basing a diagnosis of acute intoxication on the patient's statements is risky. When possible, control patient by "talking the patient down." Phenothiazines such as chlorpromazine administered I.M. have been effective. However, their hypotensive effects can be hazardous if anticholinergic drugs have been abused. Barbiturates, chlordiazepoxide (Librium) and diazepam (Valium) should be considered as alternatives in the presence of hypotension. Symptomatic and supportive procedures.

SOURCE OF INFORMATION:
The Medical Letter, Vol. 12, No. 16, Aug. 7, 1970
P.B.T., 3R*D* ED., Goodman & Gilman.
A.P.H.A. Journal, Jan. 1968.
Clearinghouse Card on LSD.

National Clearinghouse for Poison Control Centers DHEW-PHS
Name: Psilocybin   Sixty-Eighth Supplement November 1970

FIG. 5.2. *Poison control card*

Clearinghouse for Poison Control Centers carefully selects to whom they distribute these cards. Securing a complete set of all poison control cards is extremely difficult as previously printed cards are hard to obtain. The inadequacy of only having a partial set of cards is obvious. This is one reason *Clinical Toxicology of Commercial Products* has to be considered the primary source. Although the latter is still somewhat more difficult and time-consuming to use, it is definitely complete.

3. Arena, J. M.: *Poisoning: Toxicology, Symptomatology, and Treatment,* Ed. 2. Charles C Thomas, Springfield, Ill., 1970.

This volume is an excellent "all around" reference book. Its major weakness is the lack of a "trade name" index. However, general formulations are listed for the specific products and over-all listing of drugs is excellent. Arena covers the general considerations of poisoning completely and accurately. Other highlights include a broad section on insecticides, rodenticides, fungicides, herbicides and industrial chemicals. Arena also includes an excellent analysis of "street drugs," a well organized, quick and easy-to-use index and a discussion of public safety education with a list of available pamphlets, films and similar paraphernalia, as well as a list of available laboratory methods for identifying certain products.

4. von Oettingen, W. F.: *Poisoning: A Guide to Clinical Diagnosis and Treatment,* Ed. 2. W. B. Saunders Co., Philadelphia, 1963.

This volume covers general treatment principles as well as listing of individual drugs and the treatment of their overdosage. This source is especially useful in diagnostics. Its highlight is a classification by symptoms, *i.e.,* "tremors, paralysis, photophobia" and drugs known to cause that particular symptom. This section is particularly helpful in identifying the unknown poison. Unfortunately, this volume has not been recently updated and thus its utility is diminishing.

5. Other useful general poisoning information sources:

a. Manufacturer's Information. Several manufacturers provide toxicological information for their products. Examples are Geigy, Upjohn, Roche, Winthrop, William S. Merrell, Avon, Parke-Davis, and Bristol. These materials are readily available from the manufacturer. In emergency situations most pharmaceutical manufacturers will accept phone calls (collect or otherwise) and provide you with toxicology information on their products. This is sometimes true of manufacturers of household products for which ingredients are not normally released.

b. Dreisbach, R. H.: *Handbook of Poisoning.* Lange Medical Publications, Los Altos, 1971.

c. Flint, T., Jr.: *Emergency Treatment and Management*. W. B. Saunders Co., Philadelphia, 1964.

d. Deichmann, W. B., and Gerarde, H. W.: *Toxicology of Drugs and Chemicals*. Academic Press, New York, 1969.

e. Matthew, H., and Lawson, A. A. H.: *Treatment of Common Acute Poisoning*. E. and S. Livingstone, London, 1970.

CONCLUSION

The reader's introduction to the treatment of poisoning and the retrieval of poisoning information must continue. Pharmacists can become directly involved in providing first aid in the treatment of poisoning. Pharmacists in community practice can become a valuable asset to the community by providing this type of information. At least minimal involvement is seen by most practicing community pharmacists. This service may be as mundane in the beginning as distributing education materials and syrup of ipecac to patients coming into the pharmacy and coordinating emergency services (ambulance, emergency room, etc.) after an ingestion. It is from this somewhat humble beginning that one can grow and become more directly involved in providing primary care as well as serving as an available consultant for local physicians.

From here the reader should puruse in-depth treatment information. The best source of this information is, of course, from the current literature. From this type of commitment one may become more knowledgeable regarding the treatment of poisoning. With some practical experience, techniques such as retrieving information from literature sources, extracting pertinent patient information, analyzing all the data and applying it to the treatment of a patient will become more familiar to the practicing pharmacist. The pharmacist will then receive the satisfaction of knowing he is helping others, and the community will be provided with a valuable resource—a poisoning consultant.

REFERENCES

1. Anon.: Tabulation of 1973 reports. National Clearinghouse for Poison Control Centers Bulletin, p. 7, (May-June), 1974.

2. Arena, J.: General principles of treatment and specific antidotes. Mod. Treat. 8: 461, 1971.

3. Anon.: Poison prevention week. Calif. Pharm. 20: 45, 1973.

4. Winek, C. L.: A role for hospital pharmacists in toxicology and blood level information. Am. J. Hosp. Pharm., 28: 351, 1971.

5. Julyan, M., and Kuzemko, J. A.: Parents and their children in accidental poisoning. Practitioner. 208: 252, 1972.

6. Cashman, T. M., and Shirkey, H. C.: Emergency management of poisoning. Pediat. Clin. N. Am., 17: 525, 1970.

7. Abdallah, A. H., and Tye, A.: A comparison of the efficacy of emetics and stomach lavage. Am. J. Dis. Chiid., 113: 571, 1967.

8. Arena, J. M.: Poisoning, Ed. 2. Charles C. Thomas, Springfield, Ill., 1970.

9. Yaffe, S. J., Sjöquist, F., and Alván, G.: Pharmacologic principles in the management of accidental poisoning. Pediatr. Clin. North Am., 17: 495, 1970.

10. Arnold, F. J., Jr., Hodges, J. B., Jr., and Barta, R. A., Jr.: Evaluation of the efficacy of lavage and induced emesis in treatment of salicylate poisoning. Pediatrics, 23: 286, 1959.

11. Boxer, L., Anderson, F. P., and Rowe, D. S.: Comparison of ipecac-induced emesis with gastric lavage in the treatment of acute salicylate ingestion. J. Pediatr., 74: 800, 1969.

12. Dabbous, I. A., Bergman, A. B., and Robertson, W. D.: The ineffectiveness of mechanically induced vomiting. J. Pediatr., 66: 952, 1965.

13. Corby, D. G., Decker, W. J., Moran, M. J., and Payne, C. E.: Clinical comparison of pharmacologic emetics in children. Pediatrics, 42: 361, 1968.

14. Dreisbach, R. H.: Handbook of Poisoning, Ed. 7. Lange Medical Publications, Los Altos, CA., 1971.

15. Jenis, E. H., Payne, R. J., and Boldbaum, L. R.: Acute meprobamate poisoning. J. A. M. A., 207: 361, 1969.

16. Picchioni, A. L.: Activated charcoal—a neglected antidote. Pediatr. Clin. North Am., 17: 535, 1970.

17. Chin, L., Picchioni, A. L., and Duplisse, B. R.: Comparative antidotal effectiveness of activated charcoal, Arizona montmorillonite and evaporated milk. J. Pharm. Sci., 58: 1353, 1969.

18. Atkinson, J. P., and Azarnoff, D. L.: Comparisons of charcoal and attapulgite as gastrointestinal sequestrants in acute drug ingestions. Clin. Toxicol., 4: 31, 1971.

19. Schreiner, G. E.: The role of hemodialysis (artifical kidney) in acute poisoning. Arch. Intern. Med., 102: 896, 1958.

20. Henderson, L. W., and Merrill, J. P.: Treatment of barbiturate intoxification. Ann. Intern. Med., 64: 876, 1966.

21. Schreiner, G. E.: Dialysis, of poisons and drugs: annual review. Drug Intell. Clin. Pharmacy, 5: 322, 1971.

22. Berman, L. B., and Vogelsang, P.: Removal rates

for barbiturates using two types of peritoneal dialysis. N. Engl. J. Med., 270: 77, 1964.

23. Kudla, R. M., El-Bassiouni, E. A., and Mattocks, A. M.: Accelerated peritoneal dialysis of barbiturates, diphenylhydantoins and salicylates. J. Pharm. Sci., 60: 1065, 1971.

24. Melmon, K. L., and Morelli, H. F.: Clinical Pharmacology, Ed. 1, p. 607. MacMillan Co., New York, 1972.

25. Decker, W. J., Thompson, H. L., and Arneson, L. A.: Glutethimide rebound. Lancet., No. 7650, p. 778, 1970.

26. Shinaberger, J. H., Shear, L., Clayton, L. E., Barry, K. G., Knowlton, M., and Goldbaum, L. R.: Dialysis for intoxication with lipid soluble drugs: enhancement of glutethimide extraction with lipid dialysate. Am. Soc. Artif. Int. Organs, Trans., 11: 173, 1965.

27. Yatzidis, H., Oreopoulos, D., Triantaphyllidis, D., Stavroulaki, A., Voudiclari, S., Tsaparas, N., and Gavras, C.: Treatment of severe barbiturate poisoning. Lancet, No. 7405, p. 216, 1965.

28. DeMyttenaere, M. H., Maher, J. F., and Schreiner, G. E.: Hemoperfusion through a charcoal column for glutethimide poisoning. Am. Soc. Artif. Int. Organs, Trans., 13: 190, 1967.

29. Hagstam, K. E., Larsson, L. E., and Thysell, H.: Experimental studies on charcoal hemoperfusion in phenobarbital intoxication and uremia, including histopathological findings. Acta. Med. Scand., 180: 593, 1966.

section 2
Renal diseases

chapter 6

RENAL FUNCTION

Donald L. Giusti, Pharm.D.

If one were to construct a list of important diseases which alter the actions of drugs through altered pharmacokinetics, renal disease along with hepatic disease would undoubtedly be high on the list. Since most drugs are eliminated through renal or hepatic mechanisms, renal disease or hepatic disease, or both existing simultaneously, pose some very complex problems for the clinician in terms of dosage regimens and enhanced drug toxicities due to excess accumulation. It is not uncommon for a pharmacist, especially in a clinical setting, to be directly involved in solving these problems. One can state that it has almost become second nature for a competent practicing clinical pharmacist to inquire about a patient's renal status before giving a consultation on such drugs as the antibiotics or the digitalis glycosides. A pharmacist, therefore, must be well versed on the subjects of renal and hepatic disease and the laboratory tests used in their diagnosis. This section will deal primarily with renal diseases and renal function studies.

RENAL PHYSIOLOGY

Before discussing the various renal function tests, some physiological considerations are presented so that the reader may better understand the physiological basis for performing such laboratory procedures in renal disease.

The kidneys can be looked upon as complex filtering structures which maintain a constant internal environment for the optimal functioning of cells throughout the body. The biochemical nature of our internal environment is such that the slightest deviation from normal limits in such characteristics as pH, osmotic pressure, electrolyte and colloid concentration and total volume may be detrimental to health. For example, the normal pH range of plasma is relatively stabilized between 7.35 and 7.45. Variations from these values to below 6.8 or above 7.8 are incompatible with life. By ridding the body of various useless substances such as end products of metabolism, excess electrolytes, and toxic materials, the kidneys maintain, within narrow limits of normality, a homeostatic internal environment. Although the liver, lungs, sweat glands and intestines aid in the process of excretion, the kidneys are primarily responsible for this function. The process of elimination or excretion is accomplished by filtration at the glomerulus, selective reabsorption by tubular cells and the secretion of waste material by tubular cells into the tubular lumen.

The primary unit of the kidney is the nephron. Each human kidney is comprised of about 1 million nephrons. The structure of the nephron is highly adapted to perform the three functions of filtration, reabsorption and secretion. Filtration occurs at the glomerulus which is formed by the blind dilated end of the nephron invaginated by a tuft of arterial capillaries. These capillaries, which are fed by an afferent arteriole and drained by an efferent arteriole, possess some unique characteristics. The glomerular capillaries maintain a hydrostatic pressure of 60 mm Hg, which is almost twice that of other capillary beds elsewhere. This pressure is presumably due to the structure of the afferent arterioles themselves and to the relatively high resistance of the efferent arterioles. There are two opposing pressures to the hydrostatic pressure maintained within the glomerular capillaries. First is the hydrostatic pressure in Bowman's capsule ($\approx$10 mm Hg), and second is the oncotic pressure exerted by plasma proteins ($\approx$25 mm Hg). Thus, the net driving force for glomerular filtration is a pressure of about 25 mm Hg. Glomerular filtration is purely a physical process requiring no energy expenditure. Another unique property of the glomerular capillaries is that they possess autoregulation of filtration rate even when the mean arterial pressure varies from 80 to 180 mm Hg. Although this is extraordinary, any variation lower than 80 mm Hg for mean arterial pressure, such as in septicemic shock, may lead to a decrease in glomerular filtration rate (GFR) and ultimately acute renal shutdown if the pressure is not elevated. Finally, glomerular capillaries are very permeable when compared to other capillary beds. The porosity of the glomerular filter is very critical and is indicated by what is able to pass through. For example, it permits the passage of hemoglobin (molecular weight of 68,000), but it permits only minute traces of albumin (molecular weight of 69,000) to pass through. By the process of pinocytosis, most of the small quantity of albumin which is found in the glomerular filtrate is ultimately reabsorbed in the proximal tubules. Thus, if normal renal function is present, the urine should contain only minute traces of albumin or other proteins. In the presence of renal disease such as the nephrotic syndrome the permeability of the glomerular capillaries is greatly increased, and the finding of gross proteinuria is common.

Although the kidneys are small when compared to other organs, they receive 1200 cc of blood per min., which is approximately 25% of the cardiac output. This figure, the renal blood flow (RBF), corresponds to a renal plasma flow (RPF) of 650 ml per min. By filtration, 130 ml of an essentially protein-free filtrate are processed by the Bowman capsule every minute. As the filtrate passes through the tubules, the useful constituents of plasma are conserved. The proximal convoluted tubules reabsorb glucose and bicarbonate ion almost entirely. At this point also, about 80% of sodium and water are reabsorbed. Sodium is also reabsorbed further in the loop of Henle and in the distal tubules. Some water reabsorption takes place in the distal tubules and collecting ducts where antidiuretic hormone (ADH) and the countercurrent system of the loop of Henle control the process. Active secretion of substances by tubular cells occurs throughout the kidney tubules. Hydrogen and potassium ions are actively secreted in exchange for Na+ by the cells of the distal tubules. Various drugs, dyes and iodinated diagnostic compounds such as penicil-

lin G. probenecid, phenol red and iodopyracet are also actively secreted by the kidney tubules.[1-3]

Renal disease adversely affects the many functions of the kidney, and changes in renal function can be fairly accurately measured by an assortment of laboratory procedures.

MEASUREMENT OF GLOMERULAR FILTRATION RATE

The measurement of GFR is extremely important to the clinical pharmacist. Not only is this measurement an indication of glomerular function, but it is also the basis for drug dosage regimen adjustments in patients with renal impairment. Clinically, the GFR is measured by measuring the plasma clearance of certain substances removed exclusively by the kidneys. Renal clearance (RC) is an appraisal of the extent to which glomerular filtration (GF), tubular reabsorption (TR) and secretion (TS) participate in the handling of any given substance. Thus, renal clearance can be expressed by the following equation:

$$RC = GF + TR + TS \qquad (1)$$

If a substance were chosen which is neither reabsorbed nor secreted, then from Equation 1, renal clearance would equal glomerular filtration rate. The rate of clearance for any substance (x) can be expressed by the following equation[4]:

$$C_x = \frac{U_x V}{P_x} \qquad (2)$$

where U_x = concentration of x in the urine in mg%; P_x = concentration of x in the plasma in mg%; V = urine flow rate in ml per min. From Equation 2, it follows that any substance found in the plasma and urine will have a renal clearance. It also follows that the units used to express clearance are ml per min. The substances chosen to measure GFR are inulin, creatinine and urea.

The most convenient method for the clinical measurement of GFR is the endogenous creatinine clearance determination. Creatine, a creatinine precursor, is synthesized in the liver and pancreas and transported to muscle tissue via the plasma. There, it exists as either creatine or creatine phosphate. By dehydration and dephosphorylation, creatine and creatine phosphate, respectively, are converted to creatinine. Creatinine formation is therefore directly related to the total body stores of creatine and creatine phosphate. During a 24-hr. period, creatinine formation represents 1 to 2% of the body stores. Thus, creatinine is an end product of muscle metabolism, and its plasma concentration is directly related to its formation. Theoretically, creatinine production and, hence, serum creatinine concentrations could be altered by a shift in the equilibrium between creatine and creatine phosphate. However, creatinine production is very rarely altered by either endogenous or exogenous factors; therefore, plasma concentrations are usually constant. Moderate exercise, urinary flow rate or volume and diet do not influence the production of creatinine. The amount produced, however, is dependent upon lean body surface, muscle mass and a slight diurnal variation.[5] Diseases such as the muscular dystrophies or excess muscle catabolism could alter the creatinine clearance determination.[6-9]

Creatinine is freely filtered at the glomerulus; however, a small portion is also secreted by the kidney tubules. Because of this fact, the creatinine clearance may overestimate the true GFR as measured by inulin. This is especially true when the GFR falls below 30 ml per min. For this reason, patients having a creatinine clearance of 10 ml per min or less are generally considered as having negligible filtration rates.

There are many analytical methods available for the measurement of creatinine in both plasma and urine. Because of its simplicity and low cost, the most popular methods are based on the Jaffé reaction: the combination of alkaline picrate with creatinine to produce a red color. The Jaffé reaction, however, is not specific for creatinine, and the presence of other chromogens in the plasma may alter the value of the creatinine clearance determination and give false low values. Not all noncreatinine chromogens which are present in the plasma have been identified. However, important nonspecific reactants include ketone bodies, glucose, ascorbic acid, some proteins and glycocyamidine.[10,11] The more specific methods for measuring creatinine include the method described by Van Pilsum, Kito, and Hess[12,13] in which creatinine is oxidized to methylguanidine, and the method described by Benedict and Behre[14] in which 3,5-dinitrobenzoic acid is used for direct measurement of creatinine. Ionexchange procedures are also available for the separation of creatinine from interfering substances.[15] Autoanalyzer determination of serum and urine creatinine utilizes the Jaffé reaction and, hence, retains many of its inherent disadvantages such as chromogen interference. Tables 6.1 and 6.2 list factors which may alter a creatinine clearance determination by interfering with urine and plasma creatinine measurements. In renal failure, the percentage of noncreatinine chromogens is lower and not as significant as in normal patients. In general, it can be stated that the creatinine clearance will approximate the GFR within ±10%.

The length of time required for a creatinine clearance determination is over 24 hr., since an accurate determination includes a 24-hr. urine collection. Six-, 4- and 1-hr creatinine clearances can be determined, but these are generally less accurate.[16] Since the patient need not be catheterized, errors in urine collection may also be introduced into the determination. Normal values for a creatinine clearance determination range from 100 to 140 ml per min in males and from 85 to 125 ml per min in females.

The endogenous urea clearance determination is a less popular method for measuring GFR because it is less accurate than creatinine clearance. Urea, the principle product of protein metabolism, is a readily diffusible compound which is freely filtered at the glomerulus. About 40 to 60% of the filtered urea escapes into the urine, and the rest is reabsorbed by the tubules through passive diffusion. As a result, the clearance of urea varies with urine flow rates. Therefore, a high urine flow rate is needed so that the amount of urea reabsorbed is relatively constant. When the urine flow rate is 2 ml per min or greater, the portion of reabsorbed urea is fairly constant at 40%. Clearances taken at this rate are called "maximal" urea clearances and represent approximately 60% of the GFR.

When the urine flow is less than 2 ml per min, a larger portion of the filtered urea is reabsorbed, up to 70%. Attempts have been made to correct for this variability by substituting the term $\sqrt{V}$ for V in Equation 2. The square root formula should be avoided, however, since it

TABLE 6.1

Factors Which May Alter Urine
Creatinine Determinations[27]

Factors	Effect
Pathological or physiological	
Excess catabolism	I[a]
Excess exercise	I
Hyperpyrexia	I
Hyperthyroidism	I
Hypothyroidism	D[b]
Muscular dystrophies	I
Myasthenia gravis	I
Renal disease	D
Starvation	I
Agents	
Androgens	I
Corticosteroids	I
Nitrofuran derivatives	I
Thiazide diuretics	D
Nephrotoxins	D

[a]Increased.
[b]Decreased.

gives erroneously low estimates of the GFR. Generally, urea clearances taken at urine flow rates of less than 2 ml per min are of little value.

Besides the variable reabsorption of urea by the kidney tubules, additional errors are introduced into the urea clearance determination by numerous exogenous factors which affect the plasma level of urea. Serum urea will be high in patients with a large dietary protein load, gastrointestinal hemorrhage, prolonged vomiting and dehydration. Conversely, the serum urea will be low in patients during starvation, pregnancy and low protein diets. All of the above factors which may introduce errors in the urea clearance determination make it a much less accurate measurement of GFR than the creatinine clearance.

The inulin clearance determination is the most accurate approximation of GFR. Inulin is a polysaccharide which is filtered by the glomerulus, but it is neither reabsorbed nor secreted by the tubular cells. The calculations used to determine inulin clearance are identical to those used for creatinine clearance. Both the inulin and creatinine clearance determinations are standardized to 1.73 m^2 of body surface.

Although inulin clearance is extremely accurate, it is not used routinely because, in comparison with creatinine clearance, it is a complex procedure. Inulin must be injected intravenously by venoclysis, and blood levels must be maintained between 20 and 40 mg%. To insure complete emptying of the bladder, the patient is catheterized and the bladder is washed with two 20-ml portions of sterile physiological saline. At the end of three 15 to 20 min intervals, the bladder is emptied in a

TABLE 6.2

Factors Which May Alter Serum Creatinine
Determinations[27]

Factors	Effect
Pathological or physiological	
Dehydration	I[a]
Excess catabolism	I
Excess Exercise	I
Hyperpyrexia	I
Hyperthyroidism	I
Hypothyroidism	D[b]
Muscular dystrophies	I
Myasthenia gravis	I
Renal disease	D
Starvation	I
Agents	
p-Aminohippirate	I
Arginine	I
Ascorbic acid	I
Barbiturates	I
Bromsulphalein	I
Clofibrate	I
Diacetic acid	I
Glucose	I
Glycocyamidine	I
Hydroxyurea	I
Ketone bodies	I
Lipomul (oil injections)	I
Lithium carbonate	I
Mannitol	I
Methyldopa	I
Mithramycin	I
Nephrotoxins	I
Phenolsulfonphthalein	I
Proteins	I
Pyruvate	I
Triamterene	I

[a]Increased.
[b]Decreased.

similar fashion and the urine samples are saved. Ten milliliters of blood are drawn midway between urine collections.

Although inulin clearance determinations are somewhat complex, some authorities feel that the accuracy of this method justifies its routine use.[17] Table 6.3 compares creatinine clearance and inulin clearance determinations in the same patients.

MEASUREMENT OF RENAL CIRCULATION RATES

When studying renal function, it is important to know the total mass of functioning renal tissue and the rate of blood flow to these tissues. This information can be found by applying the clearance concept for certain agents with favorable characteristics.

The kidneys cannot excrete a substance faster than the arterial blood brings it to them. If the entire amount of a substance present in the plasma entering the renal artery were excreted into the urine, the rate of excretion would equual the rate at which the substance was brought to the kidneys to be excreted. Thus, RPF is equal to the clearance of a substance which is completely extracted from the blood in one circulatory pass through the kidneys. para-Aminohippurate (PAH) and Diodrast at low plasma concentrations are almost completely extracted from the plasma in one circulatory pass through the kidneys. Their clearance is approximately 90% of the renal plasma flow.

In normal adults, the clearance of PAH or Diodrast averages a little over 600 ml per min, which corresponds to a RPF of about 700 ml per min. By knowing the hematocrit, the RBF can be calculated. The clearance of PAH or Diodrast is sometimes referred to as the effective renal plasma flow (ERPF). The RBF and RPF may be grossly diminished in shock, severe hemorrhage, congestive heart failure and, of course, renal diseases.

The measurement of the total mass of functioning renal tissue is predicated upon the fact that a given mass of renal tissue can only clear from the blood a fixed maximal quantity of PAH or Diodrast per unit time. Thus, the measurement of the maximal excretion of PAH or

TABLE 6.3
Creatinine Clearance versus Inulin Clearance in the Same Patient[17]

Patient	C_{in}	C_{cr}
G. S.	113	175
D. P.	100	116
R. R.	99	111
J. H.	69	76
C. M.	86	81
J. V.	102	97
T. H.	81	71

Diodrast constitutes the measurement of tubular excretory mass of the kidney.

The ratio of GFR to RPF is referred to as the filtration fraction. Under normal conditions, its value is approximately 0.2. The filtration fraction indicates that approximately one-fifth of the plasma entering the kidneys constitutes the glomerular filtrate. Since some renal diseases cause an increase in glomerular permeability or a destruction of the glomeruli, the filtration fraction is sometimes a useful index of kidney function.

MEASUREMENT OF TUBULAR FUNCTION

The renal tubular epithelial cells are involved with the processes of active reabsorption and secretion. These functions are compromised in various renal diseases.

The extent of active reabsorption can be measured by studying the renal handling of glucose. Glucose is freely filtered at the glomeruli and almost totally reabsorbed by an active transport mechanism in the proximal convoluted tubules. In healthy individuals, only minute traces of glucose will appear in the urine within a 24-hr period. The glucose reabsorption test is predicated upon the fact that the active transport mechanism responsible for glucose reabsorption can be saturated. At normal renal function, GFR $\approx$ 120 ml per min, glucose reabsorption begins to be saturated when approximately 230 mg of glucose is filtered every minute. Once the active transport mechanism has been saturated, glucose will appear in the urine. The plasma concentration needed to affect the saturation of the glucose active transport mechanism is called the "plasma threshold." In healthy individuals the plasma threshold is approximately 190 mg%. It must be emphasized that the plasma threshold concentration varies inversely with the GFR. For example, a patient in diabetic coma with a GFR of 30 ml per min needs a plasma concentration of 760 mg% in order to filter 230 mg of glucose per min. If the active transport mechanism were intact, such a patient might not show any glycosuria despite a blood sugar of 700 mg%. When the plasma threshold is reached, the rate of active glucose reabsorption becomes constant and maximal. This rate is referred to as T_{mG} which varies from 300 to 450 mg per min in the healthy adult male and from 250 to 350 mg per min in the healthy adult female. The maximal glucose reabsorptive capacity (T_{mG}) is dependent upon the amount of healthy epithelium in the renal tubules which have functioning glomeruli.

The renal tubular epithelium is also involved in the process of secretion. Certain endogenous substances such as H^+, NH_3 and drugs such as some penicillin derivatives are actively secreted by the tubular epithelium into the tubular lumen. If the clearance of a substance is greater than GFR (creatinine or inulin clearance), then active tubular secretion must have occurred. If the clearance of a substance is less than the GFR, then reabsorption must have occurred.

The substances used to test the secretory capacity of the renal tubular epithelium are phenolsulphonphthalein (PSP, phenol red), Diodrast and PAH.

PSP is excreted into the urine at a greater rate than can be accounted for by GFR at low plasma concentrations. Only 6% of the dye is added to the urine by filtration, while 94% is added to the urine by the active transport mechanism of the renal tubular epithelium. Hence, the PSP test is a measure of renal blood flow and the secretory capabilities of the renal tubular epithelium. It only indirectly reflects changes in the GFR. The usual dose of PSP is 6 mg given intravenously. The plasma levels achieved after such a dose are not sufficiently high to saturate the tubular capacity for PSP excretion. This test, then, is not a measure of the maximal secretory capacity of the renal tubules (T_m). Also, the PSP test is not a clearance procedure. Renal function is assessed by measuring the amount of dye recovered in the urine at successive intervals. The test is based

on the observation that normal adults excrete from 28 to 35% of the dye 15 min after its administration; 13 to 17% 30 min after the injection; 9 to 12% 60 min after the injection and 3 to 6% 2 hr after the injection. At 2 hr, the total excretion of PSP should range between 53 and 70% of the injected dose.

The most accurate and reliable results are the measurements taken at the end of the first 15-min period. At the 2-hr interval, normal results may be obtained despite impaired renal function because of the repeated recirculation of the dye through the kidneys.

Urine sampling may introduce errors in the interpretation of the PSP excretion test. The patient is not catheterized, but he must void at the specified time interval. In order to facilitate voiding, many authorities feel that water loading prior to testing is necessary. Other authorities feel that water loading increases the excretion of PSP in patients with normal renal function and in patients in the diuretic phase of acute renal failure. In order to circumvent this problem, the dye may be injected only after the patient feels the urge to void. If renal impairment is severe, however, the urge to void may be nonexistent.

Residual bladder urine resulting from incomplete voiding may completely invalidate the PSP excretion test. Therefore, patients with prostatic obstruction or atonic bladders due to drug therapy or pathological conditions are not good candidates for this test.

Twenty percent of an injected dose of PSP is excreted by the liver in bile. Hence patients with liver disease may have increased urinary excretion of PSP. The position of the patient also may affect the excretion of PSP. Patients in the supine position excrete 10 to 13% greater amounts of PSP than when in the erect position. Finally, the active transport mechanism responsible for the secretory function of the renal tubular epithelium can be completely inhibited by both endogenous and exogenous agents. For example, some penicillin derivatives, sulfonamides, salicylates, diuretics, probenecid and increased uric acid will competitively antagonize the excretion of PSP. Table 6.4 lists factors which may interfere with a PSP excretion study.

The active transport mechanism responsible for the function of secretion has a limited capacity and can be saturated. The upper limit

TABLE 6.4
Factors Which May Interfere With a
Phenolsulfonphthalein Excretion Study[27,28]

Factors	Effect
Pathological or physiological	
Multiple myeloma	D[a]
Hypoalbuminuria	D
Alkalosis	D
Agents	
Anthraquinones	I[b]
Bromsulphalein	I
Carinamide	D
Cascara	I
Danthron	I
Diodrast	D
Diuretics	D
Ethoxazene	I
Formaldehyde	I
Formaldehyde- producing agents	I
Novobiocin	I
Penicillin	D
Phenazopyridine	I
Phenolphthalein	I
Probenecid	D
Radiopaque contrast media	I
Rhubarb extracts	I
Salicylates	D
Sulfinpyrazone	D
Sulfonamides	I or D
Thiazide diuretics	D

[a]Decreased.
[b]Increased.

is known as the maximal tubular secretory capacity (T_m). The substances used to measure T_m are Diodrast and PAH. If the transport mechanism is not saturated, the excretion rate of PAH and Diodrast into the urine (a function of glomerular filtration and active secretion) increases as the plasma concentration increases. The clearance at this point is constant and maximal with respect to the plasma concentration. As the plasma concentrations of PAH or Diodrast increase, a point will be reached where the renal tubules are maximally secreting either substance $(T_mD$ or $T_mPAH)$. If plasma concentrations are further increased, then only filtration continues to rise in proportion to the concentration in the plasma. At this point, the clearance of PAH or Diodrast falls. The plasma

concentration at which this occurs is called the "self-depression limit." The normal range for maximal Diodrast excretory capacity (T_mD) is 43 to 59 mg per min in the adult male and 33 to 51 mg per min in the adult female. The normal range for maximal PAH excretory capacity (T_mPAH) is 80 to 90 mg per min in both adult males and females.

MEASUREMENT OF ACCUMULATING SUBSTANCES IN THE PLASMA

As renal function decreases, there will be a proportional increase in the plasma concentration of certain endogenous substances which are normally eliminated by the kidneys. Elevated serum concentration of urea nitrogen and creatinine usually reflect impaired renal function.

The most widely used test for the evaluation of renal function is the blood urea nitrogen determination (BUN). However, the BUN must be looked upon only as a crude index of renal function. The BUN determination may often indicate only severe renal impairment. Very often a BUN determination will be within normal limits despite a 50% reduction in the GFR. Thus a BUN is not a good indicator of impaired renal function in the early stages of renal diseases. Numerous exogenous and endogenous factors may also alter a BUN. For example, the states of hydration and circulation; the urine flow rate; high and low protein intake; protein catabolism associated with trauma, infections, fever, steroids, and tetracycline; gastrointestinal bleeding; pregnancy and, finally, liver disease may affect the BUN. These error-introducing factors constitute major disadvantages of the BUN. Table 6.5 is a listing of substances and factors which may alter a BUN determination. A BUN determination may be helpful clinically only if interpreted in the proper perspective. Normal BUN values range from 10 to 20 mg%.

The serum creatinine is not appreciably altered by various exogenous factors and therefore is a more accurate measure of renal function than the BUN. Factors which may alter a serum creatinine determination are discussed under the section on creatinine clearance, and the reader is referred to Table 6.1.

The simultaneous measurement of serum

TABLE 6.5
Factors Which May Alter a BUN Determination[27]

Factors	Effect
Pathological or physiological	
Adrenal insufficiency	O or I
Congestive heart failure	O or I
Dehydration	I
Gastrointestinal bleeding	I
Hepatic failure	D
High protein intake	I
Increased nitrogen metabolism	I
Renal disease	I
Agents	
Acetohexamide	I
Acetone	I
Alkaline antacids	I
Antimony compounds	I
Arginine	I
Arsenicals	I
Blood (whole)	I
Chloral hydrate	I
Chlorobutanol	I
Chlorthalidone	I
Creatinine	I
Dextrose infusions	I
Doxapram	I
Ethacrynic acid	I
Fluid therapy, prolonged	I
Fluorides	I
Furosemide	I
Guanethidine	I
Guanochlor	I
Hydroxyurea	I
Indomethacin	I
Lipomul (oil injection)	I
Lithium carbonate	I
Methyldopa	I
Methysergide	I
Mithramycin	I
Nalidixic acid	I
Nitrofurantoin	I
Pargyline	I
Phenothiazines	O or D
Propranolol	I
Salicylates	I
Spectinomycin	I
Tetracycline	I
Thiazide diuretics	I
Thymol	D
Triamterene	I
Vancomycin	I

I = increased; D = decreased; O = no effect.

creatinine and BUN may offer more information than either test alone. Normally, the ratio of BUN to creatinine is approximately 10 : 1. A lower ratio may be associated with severe renal disease or a low protein intake. Higher ratios may be due to high protein intake, excess catabolism, gastrointestinal hemorrhages or acute renal failure.

Table 6.6 is a summary of the various renal function tests discussed in this paper. Additional information concerning the specific renal function being studied and normal values is also included.

APPLICATION OF RENAL FUNCTION TESTS TO DOSAGE REGIMEN ADJUSTMENTS

One approach to drug dosage regimen adjustments in renal impairment involves the use of nephropathically induced alterations in either drug half-lives ($t_{1/2}$) or over-all elimination rate constants (K_e) in calculating adjustments. Various schemes based on creatinine clearance or serum creatinine involving such calculations have been reported in the literature.

Orme and Cutler,[18] in their method for dosage regimen adjustments for kanamycin, use alterations in kanamycin half-life produced by renal impairment. In patients with normal renal function, 7 mg per kg of kanamycin administered every 3rd half-life (every 12 hr) will result in a peak-trough serum level curve. If a steady serum level is desired, 7 mg per kg of kanamycin may be administered initially followed by 3.5 mg per kg every half-life (every 4 hr). The same protocol may be followed in patients with varying degrees of renal impairment. However, in such patients, kanamycin half-life may be greatly prolonged. In order to calculate the new kanamycin half-life, the following equation which utilizes the creatinine clearance determination was proposed:

$$t_{1/2} = \frac{(3.5)\,(\text{body weight in kg})}{(\text{creatinine clearance})} \qquad (3)$$

According to equation 3, a 70-kg patient with a creatinine clearance of 10 ml per min would exhibit a kanamycin serum half-life of 24.5 hr. If a peak-trough serum level curve is desired, then a dose of 7 mg per kg of kanamycin can be administered every 3rd half-life (every 73.5 hr). If a steady serum level curve is desired, then a dose of 7 mg per kg of kanamy-

TABLE 6.6
Renal Function Tests[a]

Renal Function Test	Function Studied	Normal Values
Creatinine clearance (C_{cr})	Glomerular filtration rate (GFR)	Male: 100-140 ml/min Female: 85-125 ml/min
Inulin clearance (C_{in})		Male: 124 ± 26 ml/min Female: 109 ± 14 ml/min
Urea clearance (C_u)		Standard (C_{us}):54 ml/min Maximum (C_{um}):75 ml/min
p-Aminohippurate clearance (C_{PAH}) Diodrast clearance (C_D)	Effective renal plasma flow (ERPF) Renal plasma flow (RPF) Renal blood flow (RBF) Tubular excretory mass (TEM)	ERPF: 424-754 ml/min RPF: 473-840 ml/min RBF: 790-1400 ml/min TEM: 25-47 mg/min
Filtration fraction (FF)	Ratio of $\dfrac{GFR}{RPF}$	Male: 0.17-0.21 Female: 0.17-0.23
Maximal glucose Reabsorption capacity (T_{mG})	Maximal active reabsorptive capacity of the renal tubles	Male: 300-450 mg/min Female: 250-350 mg/min
PSP excretion	Renal blood flow and gives some idea of the secretory capabilities of the renal tubules	15 min 28-35% 30 min 13-17% 60 min 9-12% } 53-70% 120 min 3- 5%
Maximal Diodrast excretory capacity (T_{mD})	Maximal active secretory capacity of the renal tubules	Male: 43-59 mg/min Female: 33-51 mg/min
Maximal PAH excretory capacity (T_{mPAH})	Maximal active secretory capacity of the renal tubules	80-90 mg/min
Blood urea nitrogen (BUN)	Accumulation of urea nitrogen in the blood which gives a gross index of renal function	10-20 mg%
Serum creatinine	Accumulation of creatinine in the blood which gives a fairly accurate evaluation of renal function	0.7-1.5 mg%

[a]Adapted from Ref. 29.

cin may be administered initially, followed by 3.5 mg per kg every half-life (every 24.5 hr).

Cutler *et al.*[19] have also recommended dosage regimen adjustments for gentamicin based on serum creatinine concentrations. They recommended the initial administration of 2 mg per kg of body weight, followed by repeated injections of the same dose every 3rd half-life.

Gentamicin serum half-life in varying degrees of renal impairment can be estimated by multiplying the serum creatinine concentration (mg/100ml) by a factor of four. Thus, a patient with a serum creatinine of 5 mg/100 ml would exhibit a gentamicin serum half-life of 20 hr. According to Cutler, the new dosage regimen for gentamicin would be 2 mg per kg injected initially, followed by 2 mg per kg administered every 60 hr. Chan and associates[20] have also made recommendations for gentamicin dosage regimen adjustments. They, however, utilized the changes produced in the over-all elimination rate constant (K_e^*) by progressive renal impairment. Such alterations were calculated by using the following equation:

$$K_e^* = \frac{\log_n 2}{t_{1/2}} \qquad (4)$$

The results were plotted against the creatinine clearance determinations and the new dose was calculated using the following equation:

$$\text{New dose} = \frac{(\text{normal dose}) \, (K_e^*)}{K_e} \qquad (5)$$

where K_e is the over-all eliminations rate constant at normal renal functions. Dettli,[21] using an identical method, calculated dosage regimen adjustments for approximately 30 drugs. Finally, Jelliffe[22,23] has utilized both the creatinine clearance and the BUN for calculating dosage regimen adjustments for digoxin and digitoxin in patients with renal impairment.

The schemes described above, however, are not universally applicable to all drugs and, hence, the multiplicity of techniques becomes cumbersome in the clinical situation. In a review of the literature,[24] it was found that dosage regimen adjustments in patients with renal disease are lacking for most drugs. Further, many of the techniques available require knowledge of the variations in K_e or serum $t_{1/2}$ produced by decreasing renal function. A pharmacokinetic model based on creatinine clearance has been described which will enable the practitioner to calculate an approximate drug maintenance regimen in clinical situations where time does not permit a comprehensive literature search or when sufficient information does not exist.[24] It must be emphasized, however, that if this approach is used the subsequent dosage regimen adjustments must be looked upon as estimations to be individualized for each patient. This can be accomplished by the monitoring of serum levels as suggested by Koch-Weser[25] and Vessell[26], or by close clinical observation of the patient. The model can be described by the following equations:

$$C_\infty = \frac{D \cdot F_a}{K_e \cdot V_d \cdot \tau} \qquad (6)$$

where C_∞ = average Equilibrium state plasma concentration of drug; D = maintenance dose of drug given every τ; F_a = fraction of the dose absorbed; K_e = apparent first order rate constant for the over-all loss of drug

$$K_e = \frac{0.693}{t_{1/2}}$$

V_d = the apparent volume of distribution of the drug; τ = the dosing interval. Since

$$A = \overline{C}_\infty \cdot V_d \qquad (7)$$

where A = amount in the body at average equilibrium state and

$$1/K_e = 1.44 \cdot t_{1/2} \qquad (8)$$

substituting Equations 7 and 8 into Equation 6 gives:

$$A = \frac{(1.44) \, (t_{1/2}) \, (D) \, (F_a)}{\tau} \qquad (9)$$

where $t_{1/2}$ = the half-life for loss of drug from plasma at normal renal function. A new half-life based upon decreased renal function can be calculated as follows:

$$Nt_{1/2} = \frac{t_{1/2}}{F_e \left(\dfrac{C_{cr \; obs}}{C_{cr \; nor}} - 1 \right) + 1} \qquad (10)$$

where F_e = fraction excreted by the kidneys; $C_{cr \; obs}$ = observed creatinine clearance of the patient; $C_{cr \; nor}$ = normal creatinine clearance; $Nt_{1/2}$ = new $t_{1/2}$. The new dose based upon $Nt_{1/2}$ can be calculated as follows:

$$ND = \frac{(\tau) \, (A)}{(1.44) \, (Nt_{1/2}) \, (F_a)} \qquad (11)$$

where ND = the new dose.

CONCLUSION

Renal function studies are used not only in the differential diagnosis of renal diseases but also in monitoring the progression or regression of such diseases. Of prime importance to the clinical pharmacist is the dramatic effect which renal diseases produce on drug pharmacokinetics and subsequent drug action. Since most drugs are eliminated through a combination of renal and hepatic mechanisms, renal diseases greatly distort pharmacokinetic parameters such as serum half-lives and elimination rate constants. Proper dosage regimen adjustments must be made in order to prevent dose-related drug toxicities. Many methods have been reported which incorporate the results of renal function studies in the calculation of proper dosage regimen adjustments. In order to use such methods, the pharmacist must be well versed on renal function testing. Finally, since many drugs are known to be nephrotoxic, the pharmacist must have a working knowledge of renal function studies in order to monitor patients for such drug reactions.

REFERENCES

1. Ganong, W. F.: Review of Medical Physiology, Ed. 2, p. 548. Lange Medical Publications, Los Altos, (1965).
2. Tuttle, W. W., and Schottelius, B. A.: Textbook of Physiology, Ed. 5, p. 401, The C. V. Mosby Co., St. Louis, (1965).
3. Metcoff, J., and Yoshida, T.; Renal function and renal metabolism. Pediatr. Clin. North Am., 18: 639, (1971).
4. Levinson, S. A., and MacFate, R. P.. Clinical Laboratory Diagnosis, Ed. 7, p. 451. Lea & Febiger, Philadelphia, (1969).
5. Sirota, J. A., Baldwin, D. S., and Villarreal, H.: Diurnal variations of renal function in man, Clin. Invest., 29: 187, 1950.
6. Camara, A. A., Arn, K. D., Reimer, A., and Newburgh, L. H.: The twenty-four hourly endogenous creatinine clearance as a clinical measure of the functional state of the kidneys. Lab. Clin. Med., 37: 743, 1951.
7. Haugen, H. N., and Blegen, E. M.: Plasma creatinine concentration and creatinine clearance in clinical work. Ann. Intern. Med., 43: 731, 1955.
8. Wesson, L. G., and Lavler, D. P.: Diurnal cycle of glomerular filtration rate and sodium and chloride excretion during response to altered salt and water balance in man. Clin. Med., 40: 1967, 1961.
9. Doolan, P. D., Alpen, E. L., and Theil, G. B.: A clinical appraisal of the plasma concentration and endogenous clearance of creatinine. Am. J. Med., 32: 65, 1962.
10. Bennett, W. M., and Porter, G. A.: Endogenous creatinine clearance as a clinical measure of glomerular filtration rate. Br. Med. J., 4: 84, 1969.
11. Dunea, G., and Freedman, P.: Serum creatinine. J. A.M.A., 204: 163, 1968.
12. Newman, G. H.: Clinical significance of creatinine measurements. Postgrad. Med. J., 50: 236, 1971.
13. Van Pilsum, J. F., Kito, M. E., and Hess, J.: Determination of creatine, creatinine, arginine, guanidoacetic acid, guanidine and methylguanidine in biological fluids. J. Biol. Chem., 222: 225, 1956.
14. Benedict, S. R., and Behre, J. A.: Some application of a new color reaction for creatinine. J. Biol. Chem., 114: 515, 1936.
15. Rockerbie, R. A., and Rasmussen, K. L.: Rapid determination of serum creatinine by an ion-exchange technique. Clin. Chim. Acta, 15: 475, 1967.
16. Richardson, J. A., and Philbin, P. E.: The one-hour creatinine clearance rate in healthy men. J. A. M. A., 216: 987, 1971.
17. Price, M.: Comparison of creatinine clearance to inulin clearance in the determination of glomerular filtration rate. J. Urol., 107: 339, 1972.
18. Orme, B. M. and Cutler, R. E.: The relationship between kanamycin pharmacokinetics: distribution and renal function. Clin. Pharmacol. Ther., 10: 543, 1969.
19. Cutler, R. E., Gyselynck, A. M., Fleet, W. P., and Forrey, W.: Correlation of serum creatinine concentration and gentamicin half-life. J. A. M. A., 219: 1037, 1972.
20. Chan, R. A., Benner, E. J., and Hoeprich, P. D.: Gentamicin therapy in renal failure: a nomogram for dosage. Ann. Intern. Med., 76: 773, 1972.
21. Dettli, L., Spring, P., and Ryter, S.: Multiple dose kinetics and drug dosage in patients with kidney disease. Acta Pharmacol. Toxicol., 29: Suppl. 3, 211, 1971.
22. Jelliffe, R. W.: An improved method of digoxin therapy. Ann. Intern. Med., 69: 703, 1968.
23. Jelliffee, R. W., Buell, J., and Kalaba, R.: An improved method of digitoxin therapy. Ann. Intern. Med., 72: 453, 1970.
24. Giusti, D. L.: A review of the clinical use of antimicrobial agents in patients with renal and hepatic insufficiency. I. The penicillins. Drug Intell. Clin. Pharm., 7: 62, 1973.
25. Koch-Weser, J.: Drug therapy. Serum drug concentrations as therapeutic guides. N. Engl. J. Med., 287: 227, 1972.
26. Vessell, E. S., and Passananti, G. T.: Utility of clinical chemical determinations of drug concentrations in biological fluids. Clin. Chem., 17: 851, 1971.
27. Constantino, N. V., and Kabat, H. F.: Drug-induced modifications of laboratory test values − revised 1973. Am. J. Hosp. Pharm., 30: 24, 1973.
28. Hansten, P. D.: Drug Interactions, p. 374. Lea & Febiger, Philadelphia, 1971.
29. Krupp, M. A., Sweet, N. J., Jawetz, E., and Biglieri, E. G.: Physician's Handbook, Ed. 16, p. 141. Lange Medical Publications, Los Altos, 1970.

chapter 7

ACUTE RENAL FAILURE

Donald L. Giusti, Pharm.D.

Not long ago the diagnosis of acute renal failure was almost invariably associated with a fatal prognosis. Statistics from World War II indicate that acute renal failure secondary to crush injuries carried a 90% mortality rate. With the advent of hemodialysis and peritoneal dialysis, the mortality rate associated with acute renal failure fell to 60%. Although this mortality rate has not changed since the early 1950's, the incidence of acute renal failure has been dramatically reduced. Statistics from the Viet Nam War indicate that 1 in every 2000 wounded patients developed acute renal failure. In contrast, the statistics from the Korean War and World War II are 1 in 200 and 1 in 10, respectively.[1] These statistics emphasize the importance of prompt prophylactic measures in the prevention of acute renal failure.

DEFINITIONS

The term "renal failure" describes a level of organ function rather than a specific pathological condition such as acute tubular necrosis. Renal failure can be viewed as a later stage of renal insufficiency marked by the inability of the kidneys to maintain the volume and composition of the internal environment, *i.e.*, homeostasis. If the initiating process extends over days or weeks, the renal failure is termed *acute.* Renal failure associated with a slow deterioration of renal function, over months or years, is termed *chronic.* With today's knowledge of renal failure, prophylactic measures and sophisticated dialysis machinery, acute renal failure is usually reversible while chronic renal failure is

not. *Oliguria,* a daily urine output of less than 400 ml per day, may frequently accompany acute renal failure. However, it is quite possible to be in severe renal failure with normal daily urinary outputs.[2] In such instances, the failure is termed *high output renal failure* and is caused by the inability of the kidneys to concentrate urine. *Anuria,* a daily urinary output of 0 to 100 ml, may also accompany acute renal failure.

CLASSIFICATION AND ETIOLOGY

Acute oliguric states have been classified into three categories.[3] The first category, *prerenal*, is used to describe renal failure caused by conditions which decrease renal perfusion or renal plasma flow. The second category, *intrarenal,* is used to describe renal failure caused by functional and organic defects within the structure of the kidneys. These two classifications are very arbitrary since in actuality there is a rapid progression from prerenal to intrarenal failure. The third category, *postrenal,* is used to describe acute renal failure caused by urinary obstruction.

The prerenal causes of acute renal failure consist of circulatory disorders which impair proper perfusion of blood through the kidneys. This type of renal failure may be experienced by patients who have a negative history for renal disease. Acute renal failure caused by prerenal factors may be looked upon as a complication of the primary disease, *i.e.,* the prerenal causes. Circulatory disorders are most commonly associated with myocardial infarction, acute congestive heart failure, hypovolemic shock, excess ganglionic or adrenergic blockade, postural hypotension, massive hemorrhages, dehydration and plasma loss such as in burns. Internal fluid shifts such as in pulmonary edema or ascites can also cause a decreased circulating volume and therefore decreased renal plasma flow. No matter what the cause, when renal blood perfusion is greatly reduced, the urine output falls owing to release of antidiuretic hormone and aldosterone and increased proximal tubular reabsorption of sodium.[4,5] Although prerenal factors may be present without overt oliguria, the recognition of the existence of prerenal states is of great importance to the diagnosis, treatment and prophylaxis of acute renal failure. Prerenal causes of renal failure are summarized in Table 7.1.

The most common intrarenal cause of acute renal failure is acute tubular necrosis (ATN).[6] It must be emphasized that ATN is a histological diagnosis while acute renal failure is a clinical diagnosis. The two terms should not be used interchangeably since there may be very little correlation between the presence of ATN and the clinical diagnosis of acute renal failure. In most cases of acute renal failure the tubules are dilated owing to edematous processes and the

TABLE 7.1
Prerenal Causes of Acute Renal Failure[1,3,6]

A. Hypovolemia
  1. Loss of whole blood or plasma
    a. Hemorrhage
    b. Gastrointestinal losses
    c. Burns
    d. Trauma

  2. Loss of extracellular fluids
    a. Severe vomiting and diarrhea
    b. Fistulae
    c. Nasogastric suction
    d. Dehydration from other causes

  3. Extracellular fluid shifts
    a. Pulmonary edema
    b. Ascites

B. Impaired cardiac and circulatory function
  1. Myocardial infarction
  2. Cardiac arrhythmias
  3. Pericardial tamponade
  4. Acute congestive heart failure
  5. Pulmonary embolism
  6. Dissecting aneurysm

C. Peripheral vasodilation and vasospasms
  1. Bacteremia and septicemia
  2. Antihypertensive medications
  3. Allergic anaphylactic reactions

D. Increased renal vascular resistance
  1. Anesthesia
  2. Surgical procedures and postoperative states
  3. Hepatorenal syndrome

E. Renal vascular obstruction
  1. Embolism
  2. Renal vein thrombosis
  3. Renal artery stenosis or occlusion

tubular lumens contain pigmented casts. The microstructure of the tubular cells is generally normal in histological appearance. Frank histological necrosis is very rare.

Acute tubular necrosis is most often precipitated by a progression of all prerenal causes. Thus, sustained decreased renal plasma perfusion will ultimately result in acute renal shutdown with a histological appearance of tubular necrosis. Exogenous and endogenous nephrotoxins may also cause ATN with subsequent renal failure. Such kidney damage is often referred to as *toxic nephropathy*. Therapeutic agents such as the aminoglycoside and polypeptide antibiotics are included in Table 7.2 which is a partial list of nephrotoxic agents. Severe infectious diseases may produce acute renal failure. Urinary tract infections produced by instrumentation, obstruction, diabetes mellitus, analgesic abuse or exacerbation of pre-existing chronic pyelonephritis may lead to papillitis or medullary necrosis and ultimately to renal failure. Systemic infections such as malaria, leptospirosis, candidiasis, epidemic hemorrhagic fever and cholera may also produce acute renal failure. Intravascular hemolysis due to transfusion reactions, hemolytic anemia, malaria etc.; third trimester obstetrical complications such as placenta previa, toxemia, septic abortion, postpartum hemorrhages; increased extracorporeal pump time through the heart-lung bypass machine in open heart surgery; aortic clamping in the course of surgery for aneurysms have all been implicated in causing ATN with subsequent renal shutdown.[6] A summary of the intrarenal causes of renal failure is shown in Table 7.3.

Finally, when oliguria develops, the possibility of obstruction must always be considered. Postrenal causes of acute renal failure may be due to a disturbance in calcium metabolism leading to hypercalcemia and nephrocalcinosis. For example, parathyroid tumors, functional hyperparathyroidism, hypervitaminosis D, milk-alkali syndrome, multiple myeloma, metastatic carcinoma and finally idiopathic hypercalcemia may lead to nephrocalcinosis and finally obstruction. Acute renal failure due to obstruction has been seen with expanding cysts, prostatic hypertrophy, periureteral fibrosis, drug-induced retroperitoneal fibrosis, tumors urethral strictures, bladder neck deformities, uric acid stones, oxalate stones and cystine

TABLE 7.2
Partial List of Potentially Nephrotoxic Agents[a]

A. Metals: mercury (organic and inorganic), bismuth, uranium, lead, gold (including gold salts), cadium, arsine, arsenic, iron, silver, antimony, copper and thalium

B. Solvents (organic): carbon tetrachloride, tetrachlorethylene, methyl cellulose, methanol, toluene and benzene

C. Glycols: ethylene glycol, ethylene glycol dinitrate and diacetate, propylene glycol, ethylene dichloride, diethylene glycol, ethyl diethylene glycol, methyl diethylene glycol, butyl diethylene glycol, diethylene dioxide and dipropylene glycol.

D. Physical agents: radiation, heat stroke and electroshock

E. Diagnostic agents: iodenated contrast media

F. Therapeutic agents:
   1. Antibiotics: sulfonamides, penicillins, streptomycin, kanamycin, gentamicin, vancomycin bacitracin, polymyxin B, colistin, neomycin, tetracyclines, amphotericin B and cephaloridine
   2. Analgesics: salicylates, *para*-aminosalicylate, phenacetin, phenylbutazone and zoxazolamine
   3. Anticoagulants: phenindione and coumarin anticoagulants producing prerenal states
   4. Anticonvulsants: tridione and paradione
   5. Osmotic agents: sucrose, glucose, mannitol

G. Insecticides: biphenyl, chlorinated hydrocarbons

H. Miscellaneous chemicals: carbon monoxide, snake venom, mushroom poison, spider venom, nephroallergens (pollen, poison oak and ivy, insect repellent, wood allergens), cresol, beryllium, hemolysins, aniline and other methemoglobin producers

I. Altered serum concentrations of physiological substances: hypercalcemia, hyperuricemia, hypokalemia

[a]Reprinted with permission from Ref. 7.

stones.[1,3] A summary of postrenal causes of acute renal failure can be found in Table 7.4.

PATHOGENESIS

The pathogenesis of acute renal failure is still a controversial subject. Several theories have

TABLE 7.3
Intrarenal Causes of Acute Renal Failure[1,3,6]

A. Acute tubular necrosis
   1. Sequelae of prolonged prerenal failure
   2. Severe trauma
      a. Myoglobinuria secondary to crush trauma
      b. Burns
      c. Abdominal vascular occlusion
      d. Pancreatitis
      e. Perforated viscus
      f. Heat stress and exercise
      g. Electroshock

   3. Intravascular hemolysis
      a. Transfusion reaction
      b. Malaria
      c. Sickle cell disease
      d. Drug-induced
         1) Hemolytic anemia
         2) Serum sickness
         3) Anaphylaxis

   4. Obstetrical complications
      a. Placenta previa
      b. Placenta ablatio
      c. Postpartum hemorrhage
      d. Septic abortion
      e. Pre-eclampsia
      f. Eclampsia

   5. Postsurgical
      a. Open heart (bypass)
      b. Major abdominal surgery
      c. Surgery for aneurysms

   6. Toxic nephropathy (see Table 7.2)

   7. Infections:
      a. Papillitis or medullary necrosis from genitourinary tract infections
      b. Malaria
      c. Leptospirosis
      d. Systemic candidiasis
      e. Epidemic hemorrhagic fever
      f. Cholera

B. Other functional and organic disorders
   1. Hepatorenal syndrome
   2. Glomerulonephritis
   3. Vascular disorders
      a. Renal vein thrombosis
      b. Disseminated lupus erythematosus
      c. Polyarteritis nodosa
      d. Dermatomyositis
      e. Wegener's granulomatosis
      f. Thrombotic thrombocytopenic purpura
      g. Hypersensitivity angiitis
      h. Amyloidosis

TABLE 7.3-*continued*

C. Unknown (approximately 25% of all acute renal failure)

TABLE 7.4
Postrenal Causes of Acute Renal Failure[1,3,6]

A. Urethral obstruction
  1. Blocked catheter
  2. Stricture

B. Bladder neck obstruction
  1. Prostatic hypertrophy
  2. Bladder carcinoma
  3. Bladder infection
  4. Drug-induced urinary retention and bladder atony

C. Bilateral ureteral obstruction
  1. Intraureteral
    a. Crystalluria
      1) Sulfonamides
      2) Uric acid
    b. Blood clots
    c. Pyogenic debris
    d. Stones
      1) Calcium stones
      2) Uric acid stones
      3) Oxalate stones
      4) Cystine stones
    e. Edema
    f. Necrotizing papillitis

  2. Extraureteral
    a. Tumors
      1) Cervical tumors
      2) Prostatic tumors
      3) Endometriosis
    b. Periureteral fibrosis
    c. Drug-induced retroperitoneal fibrosis (methysergide)
    d. Iatrogenic: accidental ureteral ligation during pelvic surgery

---

been advanced which may help explain the development of oliguria in acute renal failure.

The first theory is that of generalized renal ischemia produced by excessive arteriolar vasoconstriction. Much experimental evidence gained by the induction of acute renal failure in the rat suggests that arteriolar vasoconstriction under the influence of the renin-angiotensin system does indeed play an integral role in the production of acute renal failure. However, there is also good evidence which shows that reasonable levels of renal blood flow are maintained even with virtual anuria. This theory cannot explain the clinical finding of continued anuria long after adequate renal blood flow has been re-established.[6]

The second theory is that of intrarenal shunting of blood producing a maldistribution of cortical versus medullary blood. Under normal circumstances, the cortex receives almost 90% of the renal blood flow while the medulla only receives approximately 8%. Shunting of renal blood flow from the renal cortex to the medulla is believed to occur in response to endogenous substances which control renal vascular tone, *i.e.*, renin and angiotensin. The maldistribution of blood flow produced by this shunting process impairs the concentrating ability of the kidneys. This theory also helps to explain the findings of pale cortex and congested medulla in acute tubular necrosis.

A third hypothesis suggests that tubular lumen obstruction by casts, cellular swelling, desquamation and debris is responsible for acute renal failure. This theory, a simple one from a mechanical point of view, is supported in part histologically in acute renal failure caused by multiple myeloma, hemoglobinuria, myoglobinuria and amyloidosis. These causative factors increase the possibility of tubular cast formation. Diuretic agents such as mannitol, ethacrynic acid and colloid solutions have been administered to patients with acute renal failure in an attempt to "flush out" casts from the tubular lumens. These agents are often effective as prophylactic measures. However, their mechanism of action is still unclear and may not be related to their diuretic action. Ethacrynic acid does not produce a diuretic effect in rats, but it will protect them from acute renal failure when it is used as a prophylactic measure. The mechanism for this protection is probably decreased renal vascular resistance and an over-all improvement in renal hemodynamics rather than a "flushing out" phenomenon. It has been postulated that some diuretic agents such as furosemide may actually stimulate the release of renin which would tend to deteriorate renal vascular hemodynamics.[1] Although evidence for this theory is scanty at the present time, caution should be taken when furosemide is administered to patients with acute renal failure. If, in the future, this theory is proven valid, furosemide would be an inappropriate agent for use as a prophylactic measure in acute tubular necrosis.

A fourth theory states that nephron and calyx occlusion produced by interstitial edema may be responsible for acute renal failure. This hypothesis has been supported by the frequent observation of increased renal size as seen by x-ray, and the finding of large amounts of interstitial edema in patients autopsied within 5 days after the onset of acute renal failure.[6]

The last theory suggests that tubular back-diffusion through injured cells may be responsible for oliguria in acute renal failure. This theory may explain the mechanism for early oliguria, but it fails to explain the demonstration of residual tubular function in severe oliguria.

In summary, the primary factors in the pathogenesis of acute renal failure seem to be the initiating event of afferent arteriole vasoconstriction leading to a decreased filtration rate which in turn causes a slower tubular flow rate. Cast formation and their subsequent lodgement in the collecting ducts leading to obstruction may ultimately occur in the presence of decreased tubular pressure and flow rates.

THE CLINICAL COURSE OF ACUTE RENAL FAILURE

The clinical course of acute renal failure is categorized into three parts: the oliguric or anuric phase, the diuretic phase and the convalescent phase.[8]

The period of oliguria or anuria is clinically manifested by decreased daily urine output from 0 to less than 400 ml per day. Serum concentrations of metabolic waste products which are usually excreted by the kidneys such as urea, creatinine, uric acid, fixed acids etc., are usually elevated. The patient in high output failure may be excreting a normal daily urine volume; however, the serum concentrations of metabolic end products will still be elevated. The oliguric phase of acute renal failure lasts for a variable amount of time. In patients with high output failure, the oliguric phase may last for only a few hours. Generally, however, the oliguric phase of acute renal failure may persist from 7 to 21 days.

The reversibility of acute renal failure is characterized by the onset of the diuretic phase following the oliguric phase. During this time the daily urinary output may exceed 6 liters per day. The abnormal serum concentrations of metabolic waste products, however, may continue to increase for 3 to 5 days after the onset of diuresis. This phenomenon may be termed high output failure, and its management is essentially the replacement of lost fluids and electrolytes.

An extended period of convalescence follows the diuretic phase. Debilitation and malnutrition due to the underlying causes of acute renal failure may be experienced by a majority of patients. Full physical rehabilitation and complete restoration of renal function may not occur for as long as 6 to 12 months.

DIAGNOSIS

In reviewing the many etiological factors which can predispose or cause acute renal failure, it becomes apparent that the diagnosis of the "full bloom" syndrome is simple in contrast to the diagnosis of its precipitating causes. A correct diagnosis, however, must reveal the etiological factors which were responsible for the production of renal failure. Only in this way can treatment be directed not only to the functional and organic kidney defects, but also to their precipitating causes. A discussion of the diagnosis for every etiological factor which can produce acute renal failure is beyond the scope of this chapter. However, some general guidelines which will aid in the diagnosis of functional and organic kidney defects will be discussed.

The early symptoms of acute renal failure are few in number and very nonspecific. The best way to diagnose early acute renal shutdown is to suspect it constantly, especially in the presence of prerenal factors. A thorough medical and drug history and physical examination are indispensable. Only in this way can etiological factors such as drug sensitivity, exposure to heavy metals, exposure to industrial solvents, pre-existing renal disease etc. be uncovered. The physical examination can give numerous clues to etiological factors such as aortic aneurysm, dehydration, blood loss, embolism etc. A central venous pressure will support the clinical diagnosis of blood loss or dehydration if present.

Post renal factors should always be considered in a patient with acute renal insufficiency.

A plain abdominal roentgenogram should be performed on all patients so that kidney size can be measured and radiopaque stones can be detected.

An examination of the urine can be extremely useful in the differential diagnosis of renal failure. A microscopic examination of the urine sediments may reveal epithelial casts, red blood cell casts, hemoglobin casts or bacteria which would indicate acute tubular necrosis caused by glomerulitis, intravascular hemolysis or acute pyelonephritis. Crystals of various types should be searched for; if any are found, obstructive nephrolithiasis or organic solvent poisoning should be considered.

Low urine specific gravity during the oliguric phase of acute renal failure may indicate a loss of tubular function. Low urine specific gravity, however, may be seen in elderly patients in prerenal situations. High values for urine specific gravity may indicate prerenal oliguria. Urinary sodium concentrations may be extremely helpful in distinguishing between prerenal and intrarenal failure. If renal failure is due to a decrease in circulating volume and renal plasma flow, aldosterone and antidiuretic hormone secretion will increase. Maximal water and sodium reabsorption will ensue, and urinary sodium concentration will tend to be less than 10 mEq per liter. In such instances a prerenal cause of oliguria can be entertained. If the urinary sodium concentration is above 40 mEq per liter, then renal tubular reabsorption may be impaired indicating an intrarenal cause for oliguria.[3] If maximal sodium reabsorption is taking place, potassium excretion will be increased since sodium is exchanged for potassium in the renal tubules. Thus a low urine sodium accompanied by a high urine potassium will indicate prerenal failure. The ratio of urine to plasma osmolality is usually 2:1. In prerenal oliguria, this ratio may reach 4:1 because of hypertonic urine excretion. Ratios of 1:1 or less are usually seen in intrarenal oliguria.[3]

When the drug and medical history, physical examination and clinical setting indicate a strong possibility of obstruction, special studies such as retrograde or intravenous pyelograms, arteriograms, cystoscopy and radioisotope renograms may be performed. The voiding cystourethrogram should be reserved for cases where malfunctioning bladder vesicoureteral reflux is suspected. Finally, percutaneous renal biopsy should be reserved to solve persisting major questions of etiology, treatment and prognosis. This procedure is contraindicated in the presence of solitary kidney, small kidneys and bleeding diathesis.

TREATMENT

The initial treatment of acute renal failure is largely dependent upon its etiology. If prerenal factors are present, treatment should be directed toward reversing circulatory failure and renal ischemia. This can be accomplished by the administration of whole blood, plasma expanders or saline solutions. The importance of an accurate diagnosis must be emphasized at this particular point. If prerenal azotemia is an incorrect diagnosis, the administration of these agents will lead to overhydration, pulmonary edema and subsequent congestive heart failure. Conversely, if prerenal oliguria is present, then the timid replacement of blood or saline may prolong the oliguria and cause ATN. If profound shock is present, vasoconstrictor agents should not be used since further renal ischemia may result. The infusion of 25 g of mannitol over a period of 3 min has been shown to cause an increase in renal plasma flow, a decrease in intrarenal vascular resistance and a redistribution of blood to cortical ischemic areas.[6] If diuresis is established within 3 hr, then one-half of the urine volume should be replaced along with a continued infusion of mannitol. Adequate urine flow (60 to 100 ml per hr) should be maintained for 24 to 36 hr. A lack of diuresis indicates organic renal failure, and no further attempts should be made to induce diuresis.

Fluid Balance

During the oliguric phase of acute renal failure, overhydration is the major cause of complications and mortality. Precise fluid monitoring (intake and output) is of utmost importance. It is preferable to maintain the patient in a slightly dehydrated state. In general, daily fluid requirements for patients in acute renal failure will not exceed 400 ml/24 hr. All fluid losses, sensible and insensible, such as urine, stools, stomach suction, T-tube drainage and wound drainage should be replaced. Accurate daily weights will provide an adequate index of fluid balance. When properly treated, the oliguric patient should lose approximately 1 pound per day.[8] Any increase in weight reflects over-hydration and should be corrected.

During the diuretic phase of acute renal failure, loss of fluids and electrolytes represent the major hazards. There are several reasons why a diuretic phase follows an oliguric phase in acute renal failure. First, the ability of the kidneys to concentrate urine is usually the last aspect of renal function to return. Second, elevated serum urea levels act as an osmotic diuretic. Finally, during the oliguric phase, the patient may have been in positive water balance. As renal function is restored, the accumulated fluids are presented to the kidneys for excretion.[9]

Large volumes of fluid and electrolytes should be administered during the diuretic phase of acute renal failure in order to prevent dehydration and subsequent renal ischemia. It must be kept in mind that large volume administration of fluids and electrolytes may actually perpetuate diuresis. Situations may occur where it is difficult to know whether volume replacement or the diuretic phase is responsible for the diuresis. In such instances fluid administration should be curtailed for 6 to 8 hr, and the urine flow should be determined. If the urine flow remains high, then the diuretic phase is responsible for the urine losses of fluids and electrolytes. If the urine flow decreases, then iatrogenic overhydration should be suspected.

Caloric Intake

During the early stages of the oliguric phase of acute renal failure, exogenous protein intake should be completely avoided. To minimize ketosis and negative nitrogen balance, 100 to 150 g of carbohydrates should be administered to the patient every 24 hr. The oral route of administration is preferable; however, if nausea and vomiting are present, other routes must be considered. In order to decrease urea formation and catabolism, some experts feel that the administration of anabolic steroids such as norethandrolone may be of some benefit.[10,11] However, the administration of drugs to patients with renal impairment can be extremely dangerous and should be avoided if possible. The administration of drugs of questionable efficacy in patients with renal failure should always be avoided. The administration of 20 to 40 g of protein daily may be considered after 3 to 4 days of oliguria. At this time total caloric intake can be increased to 2500 cal per day. Positive nitrogen balance usually results after such an increase. Dietary potassium intake should be negligible since serum potassium tends to rise dramatically in renal failure.

Potassium Balance

One of the important problems associated with oliguric renal failure is hyperkalemia. Untreated hyperkalemia will lead to cardiac arrythmias and death. Close electrocardiographic monitoring for hyperkalemia and blood level determinations should be performed throughout the course of acute renal failure. Any changes in the electrocardiograph indicating hyperkalemia or elevations in serum potassium concentrations require immediate measures for lowering serum potassium levels. The treatment of hyperkalemia is summarized in Table 7.5. If drug treatment fails, dialysis must be instituted.

Acid-Base Balance

Acidosis in varying degrees may appear in oliguric renal failure. If symptomatic (hyper-

TABLE 7.5
Treatment of Hyperkalemia

Drug	Dose
Prevention	
Kayexalate	10-20 g orally or as a retention enema
Sorbitol	15-20 ml of 70% Sorbitol may be added to counteract the constipating effect of Kayexalate
Dietary restriction	
Treatment	
Calcium gluconate	2-10 g I.V.
Sodium bicarbonate	45-90 mEq I.V.
Hypertonic glucose	25-50 g I.V.
Regular insulin	10-40 units I.V.
Kayexalate	50-60 g in sorbitol orally or as a retention enema

ventilation) or the serum bicarbonate level falls below 15 mEq per liter, 120 to 150 mEq of sodium bicarbonate should be administered intravenously over a 6- to 8-hr period. In a 70-kg individual, this dose will elevate the serum bicarbonate level by 5 to 6 mEq per liter.[9] Hypocalcemic tetany may develop owing to the increase in bicarbonate level.[12] In such circumstances, calcium gluconate therapy must be instituted. If the acidemia is so severe that sodium bicarbonate therapy is necessary to the point of fluid overload, dialysis is indicated.

Dialysis

The indications for dialysis are the development of the uremic syndrome characterized by anorexia, nausea, vomiting, mental confusion, muscle twitching, asterixis and convulsions; severe overhydration characterized by congestive heart failure, pulmonary edema or refractory edema; uncontrolled, symptomatic acidosis; and unresponsive hyperkalemia.

The choice of either peritoneal dialysis or hemodialysis is usually a matter of available facilities. Either method, however, will be equally effective in reversing the symptoms of the uremia and correcting fluid-electrolyte and acid-base balance. Peritoneal dialysis may not be effective when very rapid dialysis is required. This procedure is less efficient than hemodialysis for the extraction of creatine, urea and other nitrogenous substances. Peritoneal dialysis may be more efficient than hemodialysis in removing excess fluids.

Elderly patients and those suffering from trauma or infection may be dialyzed sooner irrespective of indications. The blood urea nitrogen in these patients should be kept from rising above 100 mg%. When dialysis is performed, such patients may be nourished properly, including protein; they can be ambulated; their convalescence is hastened; and infections are diminished.[1]

COMPLICATIONS

Infectious processes remain the most serious complications to acute renal failure. Infections are too often the cause of death in patients suffering from this disease. In uremia the host response is seriously depressed. Rapid recognition and prompt chemotherapy are necessary for the best prognosis. Antibiotics should be reserved for evidence of infection with an identified organism, rather than used prophylactically. Dosage regimen adjustments must be made for most antibiotics in order to prevent toxicities.

Other complications seen in acute renal failure are congestive heart failure, hypertension, uremic convulsions and anemia. Table 7.6 is a

TABLE 7.6
Partial List of Drugs Commonly Used in Renal Failure[a]

Type	Drugs Requiring Dosage Regimen Modifications	Drugs Requiring No Dosage Regimen Modifications
Antibiotics	Penicillins Cephalothin Gentamicin Streptomycin Kanamycin Isoniazid Polymyxin B Colistin Vancomycin Lincomycin Amphotericin	Erythromycin Chloramphenicol
Cardiovascular	Digoxin Digitoxin Procainamide Quinidine	Lidocaine

[a]Reprinted with permission from Ref. 13.

partial list of drugs requiring dosage regimen adjustments which are commonly used in acute renal failure.

PROGNOSIS

To some extent, recovery from acute renal failure depends upon its etiological factor. The patient with extensive trauma, infection, shock, congestive heart failure and uremic convulsions has a very poor prognosis. It is believed that renal damage which does not destroy the cellular basement membrane (toxic nephropathy) provides a better prognosis than the damage produced by ischemia. Over-all mortality rates vary between 40 and 50%. However, the incidence of acute renal failure has been dramatically cut owing to the recognition of prerenal states and prophylactic measures. Patients who recover from acute renal shutdown usually revert to normal or near normal renal function. It is believed that the restoration of normal renal function is dependent upon the severity of the original insult and upon the duration of oliguria or anuria.

REFERENCES

1. Salmon, S. E., Schrier, R. W., and Smith, L. H.: Acute renal failure – diagnosis, management and pathogenesis. Calif. Med., 115: 28, 1971.
2. Vertel, R. M., and Knochel, J. P.: Nonoliguric acute renal failure. J. A. M. A., 200: 598, 1967.
3. Keller, H. I.: The approach to the oliguric patient. Milit. Med., 135: 978, 1970.
4. Hopkins, R. W., Sabga, G., Bernardo, P., Penn, I., and Simeone, F. A.: Significance of postoperative and posttraumatic oliguria. Arch. Surg., 87: 320, 1963.
5. Young, L. E.: Complications of blood transfusions. Ann. Intern. Med., 61: 136, 1964.
6. Black, D. A. K.: Renal Disease, Ed. 2, p. 309. F. A. Davis Co., Philadelphia, 1967.
7. Schreiner, G. E., and Maher, J. F.: Toxic nephropathy. Am. J. Med., 38: 409, 1965.
8. Hedger, R. W.: The conservative management of acute oliguric renal failure. Med. Clin. North Am., 55: 121, 1971.
9. Paper, S.: Renal failure. Med. Clin. North Am., 55: 335, 1971.
10. Blagg, C. R., and Parsons, F. M.: Earlier dialysis and anabolic steroids in acute renal failure. Am. Heart J., 61: 287, 1961.
11. Gjorup, S., and Thaysen, J. H.: Anabolic steroids
12. Rosenfeld, M. G.: Manual of medical therapeutics, Ed. 20., p. 50. Little, Brown and Co., Boston, 1971.
13. Bennett, W. M., Singer, I., and Coggins, C. H.: Guide to drug usage in adult patients with impaired renal function. J. A. M. A., 223: 991, 1973.
in treatment of uremia: Lancet, 2: 886, 1958.

chapter 8

CHRONIC RENAL INSUFFICIENCY

Donald L. Giusti, Pharm.D.

The term "chronic renal insufficiency" implies irreversible renal damage. Generally, this implication is correct. Chronic renal failure with a persistently raised blood urea nitrogen concentration is most often due to irreversible kidney disease. However, in some cases, even chronic renal failure may be either partially or completely reversible. If chronic renal insufficiency is caused by sustained prerenal or postrenal factors, a chance exists that the renal damage produced may be reversible. Chronic renal failure caused by such factors probably affects every nephron by decreasing filtration pressure, increasing the pressure opposing filtration or increasing intrarenal pressure. Hence, chronic renal failure caused by sustained prerenal factors, obstruction, acute glomerulonephritis, hypercalcemia, sarcoidosis, etc. can be reversible. In true chronic renal failure, the impairment of glomerular function is due to a reduction in the number of functioning nephrons. By the time chronic renal insufficiency has been established, it is extremely difficult to identify the underlying cause. Nevertheless, efforts should be made to establish such a diagnosis so that differentiation can be made between reversible and irreversible chronic renal failure. Table 8.1 is a list of reversible causes of chronic renal insufficiency.

TABLE 8.1
Reversible Causes of Chronic Renal Insufficiency

A. Obstruction
　　1. Congenital
　　　　a. Bladder neck obstruction
　　　　b. Urethral strictures
　　2. Acquired
　　　　a. Calculi
　　　　b. Retroperitoneal fibrosis
　　　　c. Ureteric fibrosis
　　　　d. Ureteric granuloma
　　　　e. Benign or malignant tumors
　　　　f. Edema
　　　　g. Prostatic enlargements
　　　　h. Urethral strictures

B. Urinary tract infections

C. Hypertension
　　1. Essential
　　2. Malignant or accelerated
　　3. Renovascular
　　4. Pheochromocytoma
　　5. Coarctation of the aorta
　　6. Metabolic

D. Subacute bacterial endocarditis

E. Metabolic
　　1. Hypercalcemia
　　2. Hypokalemia
　　3. Hyperuricemia

F. Hematological
　　1. Intravascular hemolysis
　　2. Multiple myeloma

G. Immunological
　　1. Systemic lupus erythematosus
　　2. Polyarteritis nodosa
　　3. Hypersensitivity angiitis

H. Toxic nephropathy

ETIOLOGY

Chronic renal insufficiency is a variable loss of renal function as an end result of damage to the kidneys and a subsequent loss in the number of functioning nephrons. Thus, chronic renal insufficiency represents intrinsic renal disease with renal pathology. Acute renal failure, on the other hand, can be differentiated from chronic renal failure in that the former may be caused by both intrinsic renal disease

i.e., acute tubular necrosis (ATN) and by prerenal factors such as shock. Progressive or sustained prerenal factors, if not alleviated, however, will also lead to chronic renal insufficiency. The reversibility of such an end point is dependent upon the amount and type of renal damage produced. The deterioration of renal function associated with progressive chronic renal insufficiency may span over periods of months or years. The ultimate outcome of such a progression is a clinical syndrome known as uremia. Very often, however, patients with chronic renal failure are relatively asymptomatic until gross alterations in water, electrolyte and acid-base balance and an excess accumulation of metabolic waste products occur. Azotemia may or may not be present since the glomerular filtration rate (GFR) must fall to approximately 30% of normal before blood urea concentrations increase significantly. Monitoring patients with mild to moderate renal insufficiency for deterioration of renal function by the use of blood urea nitrogen (BUN) or serum creatinine determination may pose some problems. A graphic examination of the relationship between the BUN or serum creatinine and the GFR reveals a curve described as a square hyperbola[1] (Fig. 8.1). It is evident that the GFR may be decreased to a low of 25% of normal before substantial increases in the BUN or serum creatinine concentration are evident. The symptomatology of chronic renal failure may not appear until the BUN or serum creatinine is grossly elevated. Thus, following patients for progressive deterioration of renal function by the use of the BUN or serum creatinine determination may be misleading. These measurements will reflect only severely compromised renal function. Clearance procedures should be relied upon for the measurement of diminished renal reserves in patients with mild to moderate chronic renal insufficiency. The BUN or serum creatinine concentrations may be used to follow symptomatology in patients with severe renal impairment.

It is also evident from Figure 8.1 that the introduction of factors which tend to promote decreases in renal function (dehydration, heart failure, infections etc.) in the presence of considerable renal function may have relatively minor consequences. On the other hand, the introduction of these factors during the steep

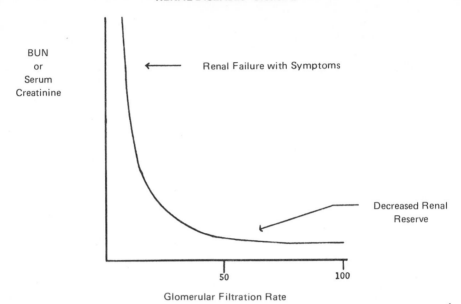

FIG. 8.1. The relationship between the GFR and the BUN or serum creatinine determination.[1]

portion of the curve may result in a significant deterioration of the clinical state of the patient.[1]

The etiological factors in chronic renal insufficiency are large in number and variety. Chronic pyelonephritis is the most frequent single cause of uremia in both children and adults, and it probably accounts for more than half of all cases.[2,3] The second most frequent cause of chronic renal insufficiency is chronic glomerulonephritis. Primary vascular diseases including hypertension are frequent causes of glomerular damage leading to renal failure. Arteriolar nephrosclerosis leading to diffuse glomerular sclerosis is a common finding in hypertensive vascular disease. Collagen diseases especially polyarteritis nodosa, systemic sclerosis and disseminated lupus erythematosis may ultimately produce severe renal damage by affecting the renal microvasculature. Indeed, the prognosis for each of these diseases is extremely poor when renal involvement is evident. Massive steroid and immunosuppresive therapy is usually employed to reverse such renal involvement. A number of metabolic diseases such as diabetes mellitus, amyloidosis, gout and hyperparathyroidism can lead to chronic renal insufficiency. In diabetes mellitus and amyloidosis, the deposition of mucopolysacchrides in the capillary walls leading to glomerular damage is the mechanism by which chronic renal failure is produced.[3] Finally, congenital kidney anomalies such as hypoplastic kidneys, polycystic kidneys; prolonged toxic nephropathy such as prolonged lead paint exposure in childhood, analgesic abuse; and chronic obstruction as seen in prostatic hypertrophy and neoplasms can all culminate in chronic renal insufficiency. Table 8.2 is a list of causative factors in chronic renal insufficiency.

PATHOPHYSIOLOGY

At the present time, there are two acceptable theories which help explain the altered physiology in chronic renal failure. The first hypothesis states that the abnormal renal function found in uremia is a composite function of all the nephrons in the kidney, each of which is diseased. The degree of malfunction and the precise histological lesions vary among each nephron. The ultimate result is an inability to excrete metabolic end products and an inability to concentrate urine.

The second and most widely accepted theory is called the "intact nephron hypothesis" or the Bricker hypothesis.[4] According to this theory, renal malfunction in chronic uremia can be explained by assuming the existence of two populations of nephrons. One population consists of nephrons which are

TABLE 8.2
Causative Factors in Chronic Renal Insufficiency

A. Glomerulonephritis

B. Primary tubular disease
　1. Fanconi syndrome
　2. Renal tubular acidosis
　3. Heavy metal poisoning
　4. Chronic kypokalemia

C. Vascular disease
　1. Hypertension
　2. Ischemic disease of the kidney

D. Collagen disease
　1. Polyarteritis nodosa
　2. Scleroderma
　3. Systemic lupus erythematosis

E. Infections
　1. Chronic pyelonephritis
　2. Tuberculosis (renal)

F. Metabolic diseases
　1. Diabetes mellitus
　2. Amyloidosis
　3. Gout
　4. Hyperparathyroidism
　5. Hypervitaminosis D
　6. Milk-alkali syndrome

G. Toxic nephropathy

H. Congenital kidney anomalies
　1. Hypoplastic kidneys
　2. Polycystic kidneys
I. Obstruction
　1. Upper
　　a. Calculi
　　b. Periureteric fibrosis
　　c. Neoplasms
　2. Lower
　　a. Prostatic enlargement
　　b. Urethral stricture
　　c. Congenital bladder and urethral anomalies

nonfunctional owing to significant destruction of any portion of the nephron. These nephrons do not measurably contribute to the production of urine. The second population consists of normally functioning nephrons. In this way, the remarkable adaptability of the kidneys can be explained. For example, sodium balance, hydrogen ion excretion and phosphate excretion are generally maintained despite marked deterioration in renal function. Deteriorated renal function, however, can be severe enough to allow eventual buildup of metabolic waste products in the blood. Owing to these products, especially urea, the intact nephrons are in a constant state of diuresis. Hence, the ability to concentrate urine is lost, and the final urine may resemble the ultrafiltrate of plasma. The ability to acidify urine is also lost. As chronic renal failure progresses, the population of intact nephrons decreases until eventually so few remain that urinary output cannot be maintained and oliguria supervenes.

DIFFERENTIAL DIAGNOSIS

The aim of differential diagnosis in chronic renal insufficiency is to distinguish between reversible and irreversible renal impairment. As in acute renal failure, the diagnosis covers a very wide field of medicine. Nevertheless, reversible prerenal and postrenal factors contributing to or causing chronic renal insufficiency must be discovered and treated. A thorough medical and drug history, physical examination, routine screening studies and urinalysis will often give clues to underlying disease processes which if alleviated may reverse the processes of chronic renal insufficiency. Thus, if any clues exist for those diseases outlined in Table 8.1, rigorous efforts in the establishment of their diagnosis and treatment should follow. Once reversible conditions have been excluded, the precise diagnosis of chronic renal failure is often immaterial to management since no specific treatment exists for this disease. The treatment of chronic renal insufficiency is aimed at maintaining the functional integrity of residual nephrons.

Many patients are unaware of the presence of chronic renal failure until renal function has seriously deteriorated. In such cases, chronic renal failure must be differentiated from acute renal failure. A plain abdominal radiograph enabling the visualization of the kidneys and their size may help in this differentiation. The presence of large kidneys accompanying symptoms of chronic renal failure may be due to diabetes mellitus, amyloidosis, multiple myeloma and myeloma kidney, systemic sclerosis, polyarteritis nodosa, systemic lupus erythematosis and accelerated or malignant hypertension. In the presence of normal sized kidneys, one of a number of reversible causes of chronic renal insufficiency outlined in Table 8.1 may be entertained. Renal biopsy may be indicated in such circumstances to determine the diagnosis. Finally, the presence of small kidneys usually indicates an irreversible process, and a renal biopsy is of no value. The radiographic abdominal film may also be useful in excluding some forms of obstructive nephropathy.

CLINICAL MANIFESTATIONS AND THEIR TREATMENT

Many patients with chronic renal insufficiency are asymptomatic especially if renal function is not seriously compromised. Symptoms, when they appear, usually can be classified into three general varieties.[1] The first class of symptoms are those directly related to fluid and electrolyte imbalance and acid-base imbalance. Thus the symptoms associated with hyponatremia, hyperkalemia and dehydration may be alleviated by correcting the underlying imbalance. The second class of symptoms are those which are not directly related to either altered excretion or accumulation of metabolic waste products. Dialysis may result in only slight improvement or no improvement of such symptoms. Thus, the symptoms associated with anemia, hypertension, renal osteodystrophy and metastatic calcification can only be relieved by specific therapy. Finally, the third class of symptoms are those which are related to uremia and are due to dialyzable substances which accumulate in the blood. Dialysis usually alleviates this class of symptoms. The composite symptomatology of a patient suffering from chronic renal insufficiency follows a somewhat logical pattern as the disease progresses. Polyuria and nocturia are usually the first signs of chronic renal failure, followed by lethargy, weakness, insomnia and slight shortness of breath. Patients generally disregard these symptoms and do not seek a physician until anorexia, nausea and vomiting appear. When acidosis and azotemia become severe, the patient becomes bedridden, increasingly lethargic and may be troubled by hiccoughs and uncontrolled twitching. Epstein and Merrill[5] eloquently described the subsequent symptomatology in the following manner:

Heart failure, progressive anemia and bleeding into the skin, mucous membranes and gastrointestinal tract herald the final illness. The skin becomes dry, with a sallow tint, the breath uriniferous. Exophthalmos may be present. Vision is impaired as hemorrhages and exudates appear in the fundi. The urinary output becomes progressively restricted. Fibrinous pericarditis or pleurisy, usually but not always painless, may appear within a few weeks of death. Disorientation and coma mercifully precede the end.

Fluid and Electrolytes

Sodium balance is retained even in the face of marked renal impairment. This observation can be explained in part by the intact nephron hypothesis. Maintenance of sodium balance is accounted for on the basis of increased sodium excretion per individual nephron. As deterioration of renal function progresses, the number of functioning nephrons decrease and excessive sodium excretion is common. The amount of sodium lost is generally a small amount, 20 to 40 mEq daily. Some patients, however, may excrete an extremely large amount of sodium. This large sodium loss is termed "salt wasting," and amounts of 200 mEq may be lost daily. Finally, in the later stages of chronic renal failure, the GFR may be so low that the residual tubules are capable of reabsorbing all filtered sodium. In this situation the hazards of salt overload are always present. Thus, depending upon the renal function, the entire range (from zero to massive losses) of sodium excretion can be seen. Quantitation of sodium loss during a 24-hr period must be done for all patients. Automatic sodium restriction solely on the basis of poor renal function may represent a significant hazard to patients with chronic renal impairment. The dietary intake of sodium should be predicated upon urinary losses. Generally patients with chronic renal insufficiency will require from 8 to 9 g of salt per day.

The agent of choice for the replacement of sodium deficit is sodium chloride. However, some patients also suffer from metabolic acidosis. In such instances, sodium bicarbonate should be used to replace part of the sodium deficit. If sodium is restricted in patients with chronic renal insufficiency, there will be a decrease in extracellular volume, decreased renal perfusion and subsequently the production of renal ischemia. The sodium intake must be titrated for each individual patient. Once this has been done, sodium should be given in the maximal tolerable amount (for that particular patient) in order to maintain the extracellular volume. Each patient must be carefully monitored for sodium intake by following his body weight, serum sodium concentration, urinary sodium concentration and GFR.

Fluids

As mentioned previously, patients with chronic renal failure may lose massive amounts of water since their intact nephrons are in a state of constant diuresis. On the other hand, if renal function is seriously impaired, oliguria predominates. It is apparent that water intake must also be individualized for every patient. Fortunately, thirst mechanisms will insure that adequate hydration is being instituted. However, hyponatremia may result if water intake is adequate but sodium intake is not. Water excess and salt wasting are major causes of hyponatremia in the azotemic patient. Also, water and salt deficiencies are major causes of reduced renal function in patients with chronic renal failure since these deficiencies produce decreased extracellular volume and renal ischemia.

During illnesses with fever, nausea, vomiting or diarrhea, supplemental fluids are very important in the maintenance of an adequate fluid volume. It is essential that proper maintenance of salt and water intake be instituted in patients with chronic renal failure. This is especially true if chronic renal insufficiency is complicated by congestive heart failure.

Potassium

Although hyperkalemia is very common in acute renal failure, it is generally not seen in chronic renal insufficiency until the end stage of the disease. This can also be explained by the intact nephron hypothesis. Intact nephrons adapt to the situation produced by chronic renal insufficiency by increasing the amount of potassium secretion per nephron. Another view is that this compensatory system is due to functional hyperaldosteronism. There may be instances, however, such as exacerbation of the underlying renal disease produced by numerous factors including dehydration, excessive potassium intake and illnesses that liberate intracellular potassium such as metabolic acidosis and catabolic states, where hyperkalemia may occur. Potassium serum levels should be monitored routinely in ambulatory patients and continuously in hospitalized patients with uremia or acute exacerbation of chronic renal insufficiency. Cardiac arrhythmias and death may be the final consequence of sustained elevated serum potassium levels. In hospitalized oliguric patients, continuous electrocardiography will give some clues to hyperkalemia. Electrocardiographic changes, however, do not usually correlate well with serum potassium levels except for the extremes of hypokalemia and hyperkalemia. In hyperkalemia, the first electrocardiographic change to appear is a tall, peaked T wave followed by S-T segment depression and decreased amplitude of the R wave with a deeper S wave. As serum potassium levels increase, the P-R interval may be prolonged followed by a disappearance of the P wave and a widening of the QRS complex. In extreme hyperkalemia, the S-T segment may be fused into the ascending limb of the T wave, and a sine wave may appear followed by cardiac arrest.[1]

Slight to moderated hyperkalemia, 4 to 5 mEq per liter, accompanied by no electrocardiographic changes or symptoms, may require no treatment. These patients, however, should be monitored closely, and potassium intake should be drastically reduced in all patients with severe renal impairment.[6] Potassium-containing foods and drugs should be avoided if possible. Elevated serum potassium levels of 6 to 8 mEq per liter accompanied by electrocardiographic changes should be vigorously treated immediately. Elevated serum potassium levels of 6 to 8 mEq per liter not accompanied by electrocardiographic changes should also be treated immediately since sudden death may occur despite a normal electrocardiogram (ECG). Immediate treatment measures consist of the intravenous administration of calcium gluconate, 5 to 10 ml of a 10% solution given over a 2-min period. Calcium will immediately antagonize the cardiac toxicity of elevated serum potassium. However, if digitalis has also been administered, digitalis toxicity may occur through a potentiation of its effects on the heart by calcium.[7,8] If ECG changes persist, another injection of calcium after 5 min have elapsed may be of benefit. A dose of 45 mEq of sodium bicarbonate may be injected intravenously over a period of 5 min. This will cause an intracellular movement of potassium, thus lowering the extracellular concentration. If ECG changes persist, more sodium bicarbonate may be administered after a 10- to 15-min delay.[7] A glucose-insulin infusion, usually containing 100 to 300 ml of a 20% solution of glucose plus 20 to 30 units of regular insulin administered I.V. over a 30- to 60-min period, will also decrease the extracellular fluid concentration of potassium by causing an intracellular shift. An alternative method is the rapid administration of 1 liter of 10% glucose containing 90 mEq of sodium bicarbonate and 40 units of regular insulin. One-half of the liter may be administered within 30 min and the remainder over a 2- to 3-hr period. The effects of these immediate measures are transient, and the repeated administration of volume may lead to hypervolemia. The use of sodium polystyrene sulfonate resin, a cation exchange resin which exchanges sodium for potassium, is generally warranted. This resin is effective in lowering serum potassium concentrations, but its effects are less rapid than the immediate measures. Thus, its administration should be instituted simultaneously with the immediate measures. It can be administered either orally if the patient does not respond to its adversities of nausea and vomiting, or rectally as a retention enema. A dose of 20 to 50 gm can be administered every 2 to 4 hr until the serum potassium is normal. Fifteen to 20 ml of 70% sorbitol are usually administered orally every 30 min until diarrhea is produced to counteract the constipating effects of the orally administered resin. The amount of sodium exchanged for potassium may be as high as 3 or 4 mEq per g of resin. Sodium overload, therefore, is a hazard in the continued use of exchange resin. If all of these measures fail to produce a response in serum potassium levels, or salt overload or hypervolemia becomes a problem, dialysis will usually be effective in restoring potassium balance.

There are a number of clinical conditions which can produce hypokalemia in the face of severe chronic renal insufficiency. These conditions include primary and secondary hyper-aldosteronism, edematous states, renal tubular acidosis, gastrointestinal loss due to vomiting or diarrhea, and finally iatrogenically by overcorrection of hyperkalemia usually by dialysis. Prolonged potassium depletion from any cause can lead to further renal damage and can also render the kidneys more liable to chronic pyelonephritis.[3] Hypokalemia, if present, should be detected early since subsequent deterioration of renal function is reversible if potassium balance is reinstituted.

Acidosis

In health, acid-base balance is normally maintained by the buffer system, CO_2 exchange in the lungs and hydrogen ion secretion by the kidneys. These three processes must compensate for acids liberated during metabolism and an average excess intake of 40 to 60 mEq of hydrogen ions daily. The kidneys eliminate hydrogen ion by forming ammonium ion (NH_4^+) from ammonia (NH_3) and by the combination of various buffers to form titratable acid which consists largely of sodium dihydrogen phosphate. In patients with chronic renal insufficiency, some degree of acidosis will be present. The development of acidosis is due to a decrease in ammonia production, a decrease in its conversion to ammonium and a decrease in its transport into the tubular lumen in response to acidosis. The residual intact nephrons are also unable to secrete enough titratable acids to keep up with daily acid loads. The plasma bicarbonate concentrations are generally stabilized at approximately 16 to 18 mEq per liter. Such low levels of bicarbonate leave little reserve for sudden acid loads. Plasma bicarbonate levels of 15 mEq per liter or lower will usually be accompanied by Kussmaul breathing. Some patients, however, will have no symptoms because of the insidious production of acidosis.

Acidosis should be treated if plasma bicarbonate levels fall below 18 mEq per liter. In ambulatory patients this can be accomplished by the oral administration of sodium bicarbonate, especially if the patient is also losing large amounts of sodium. If the patient is not losing appreciable amounts of sodium, the administration of sodium bicarbonate will lead to a salt overload. In such instances, ·5 g per day in divided doses of calcium carbonate may be used to correct the acidosis.[6] If the acidemia is severe, it should be treated with the intravenous administration of sodium bicarbonate. In a 70-kg man, 150 mEq of sodium bicarbonate can be given over a 6- to 8-hr period, and an increase in the serum bicarbonate level of 5 to 6 mEq per liter can be expected. Full correction of the acidemia is impractical, and the rapid reversal of acidosis can lead to hypokalemia and hypocalcemic tetany. For this reason, the aggressive treatment of acidosis cannot be initiated until the potassium and calcium status of the patient has been evaluated. If treatment with sodium bicarbonate represents significant potential hazards of salt and volume overload, dialysis is indicated for the correction of the acidosis.

Phosphate and Calcium

There are many factors which regulate plasma levels of ionized calcium. Such factors include plasma pH; bone dissolution and regeneration; and the equilibrium of calcium in solution, calcium bound to serum proteins and calcium in bone. The parathyroid hormone is the most potent regulator of serum calcium levels, and its secretion by the parathyroid glands is stimulated by low serum levels of ionized calcium. Serum phosphate and ionized calcium levels share a reciprocal relationship. In mild to moderate chronic renal insufficiency, serum phosphate levels usually remain normal despite a decreased filtered load. This is accomplished by a compensatory decrease in phosphate reabsorption by the renal tubules. When the GFR falls below 30 ml per min, however, serum inorganic phosphate levels rise. Ionized serum calcium levels tend to be low in chronic renal failure for reasons that are not well understood. It may be due to decreased absorption of calcium or to the high serum concentrations of phosphate (reciprocal relationship). Vitamin D resistance has been shown to occur in the early stages of chronic renal insufficiency, while the creatinine clearance is still at 70% of normal.[9-11] The reasons for vitamin D resistance are poorly understood and several theories to explain this phenomenon have been advanced. It may be due to a number of factors including defective vitamin D metabolism, the production of an antivitamin D factor, an increase in the turnover rate of the vitamin, an increased accumulation of a biologically inactive metabolite, an increased urinary excretion of an active metabolite and finally, dietary deficiently.[1,3,6,12] Whatever the reason, vitamin D resistance ultimately leads to a decreased absorption of calcium and further hypocalcemia. It can clearly be seen that the combination of hyperphosphatemia, secondary hyperparathyroidism and vitamin D resistance contributes dramatically to altered calcium metabolism leading to bone disorders. Such disorders are called azotemic osteodystrophy and are discussed under the section dealing with complications.

The treatment of hyperphosphatemia should be started early in the case of chronic renal failure. This is accomplished by reducing phosphate ingestion in the diet and by the administration of phosphate-binding antacids such as aluminum hydroxide in doses of 30 to 40 ml 3 to 4 times daily.[13] In some instances, larger doses may be needed. Magnesium-containing antacid gels should be avoided because of their potential to cause hypermagnesemia (see the following section concerning magnesium metabolism).

The hypocalcemia generally seen in chronic renal insufficiency is usually asymptomatic. However, in rare instances, frank hypocalcemic tetany may occur. The rapid reversal of systemic acidosis can also precipitate hypocalcemic tetany. Acutely, calcium gluconate infusions can be used to treat such disorders. In the ambulatory patient, serum calcium levels may be improved by increasing oral calcium intake. Calcium carbonate may be used to supply calcium and reduce acidosis, if present.[14] If calcium carbonate is overused, an alkalotic condition may ensue. For this reason, patients should be titrated carefully when calcium carbonate therapy is instituted. Calcium gluconate may be added to the regimen in cases where more calcium but less alkali is needed. Oral vitamin D supplementation can also be used in an attempt to further elevate serum calcium levels. Caution must be observed, however, since severe cases of hypercalcemia have been reported in patients on such therapy.

On rare occasions, hypercalcemia rather than hypocalcemia is seen in patients with chronic renal insufficiency. Such a finding should lead to investigations for diseases which may be existing concomitantly, which cause increased serum calcium levels. Such diseases include primary hyperparathyroidism, multiple myeloma and other cancers, sarcoidosis, milk-alkali syndrome and vitamin D intoxication. The diagnosis of these diseases is extremely important to the prognosis of chronic renal insufficiency since the hypercalcemia may be the cause rather than the result of the renal disease. In such instances, if the renal damage is not severe, the resultant chronic insufficiency may be reversible.

Magnesium

Under normal conditions, the total magnesium content of the body is approximately 2,000 mEq. Like potassium, most of the total body magnesium is intracellular, and normal serum levels range from 1.5 to 1.0 mEq per liter. Like calcium, magnesium exists in three moieties, protein-bound, complexed and ionized. These three moieties are in equilibrium with one another. The kidneys eliminate magnesium very efficiently through glomerular filtration, and some tubular reabsorption also takes place. In chronic renal insufficiency, magnesium levels tend to rise in proportion to the degree of renal impairment. Generally, the hypermagnesemia is asymptomatic until the plasma levels exceed 4 mEq per liter. Levels in excess of this amount do not occur frequently unless renal function is severely compromised or magnesium intake is increased. If plasma levels exceed 4 mEq per liter, magnesium intoxication characterized by somnolence progressing to coma, impairment of neuromuscular transmission, peripheral vasodilation and disturbance of cardiac conduction leading to cardiac arrest may occur. For this reason, patients with chronic renal insufficiency should avoid magnesium-containing compounds such as antacids and laxatives. Symptomatic hypermagnesemia may be treated by intravenous calcium infusions or dialysis.[6]

Hypomagnesemia resulting from dietary deficiency or gastrointestinal losses may also occur in chronic renal insufficiency. Most commonly, it is a result of dialysis using magnesium-free solutions. Tremors and convulsions resulting from central nervous system hyperirritability may occur as a consequence.

Carbohydrate Metabolism

Defects in carbohydrate metabolism are often found in patients with chronic renal insufficiency. Although marked hyperglycemia and ketoacidosis are rarely seen in such patients, many of them will show an abnormal glucose tolerance test (GTT). To date, the etiology for this abnormality is very poorly understood, and many investigators in the field have found contradictory and confusing results.

It has been shown that high concentrations of urea will affect enzyme systems *in vitro*, and investigators have also shown the development of an abnormal GTT in normal patients given a large urea load.[15,17] However, dialysis has a beneficial effect of returning the GTT to normal, and this can be effected without lowering the BUN.[18] These data would suggest that there is a different, dialyzable accumulating substance responsible for the alterations in carbohydrate metabolism and that urea is only a contributing factor. Other postulates which have tried to explain the alterations in carbohydrate metabolism include an abnormal plasma insulinase system which accounts for impaired peripheral utilization of glucose; a decreased sensitivity to exogenous insulin due to insensitive peripheral tissues; the presence of a circulating substance which inhibits the release of insulin or enhances its breakdown, possibly glutathione; and the inhibition of insulin by decreased plasma pH. To further complicate matters, it has been observed that insulin-dependent diabetic patients who develop uremia require less insulin for maintenance.[12] No satisfactory explanation for this phenomenon is available at present, although the increased insulin half-life seen in uremia may be partly responsible. This complication does, however, point out the difficulties encountered in uremic patients with diabetes mellitus. Continuous monitoring and individual insulin titration are extremely important in such patients.

The carbohydrate abnormalities seen in nondiabetic uremic patients rarely require treatment with exogenous insulin. However, it is important to differentiate between these abnormalities and those seen in true diabetes mellitus since diabetes is an important consideration for long term dialysis or renal transplantation therapy.

Uric Acid

Serum uric acid levels are consistently elevated in patients with chronic renal insufficiency. The hyperuricemia of renal failure, in itself, rarely leads to clinical gout; however, there are exceptions. Although hyperuricemia may generally be present, its finding should lead to investigations in the establishment of pre-existing gout since gouty nephropathy may be a reversible cause of chronic renal insufficiency.

Patients with pre-existing gout and patients with no known history of gout may experience gouty attacks especially while being maintained on dialysis. The etiology for these attacks is not clear. It is never certain whether the patient developed gout because of the hyperuricemia of renal failure or because of a predisposition to the disease. The treatment of hyperuricemia should be instituted when clinical symptoms appear. Colchicine may be used to treat the acute gouty attacks. Bennett and associates[19] have published appropriate dosage regimens for colchicine in patients with varying degrees of renal impairment.

To control serum uric acid levels, probenecid should be avoided in patients with moderate to severe renal impairment. Probenecid needs adequate renal function in order to be effective, and its excretion is dependent upon urine flow rate and pH, two variables which are difficult to control in renal failure.[19] For these reasons, allopurinol in modified dosages (100 to 300 mg per day depending upon renal function) seems to be the drug of choice for the control of hyperuricemia in patients with renal insufficiency.

UREMIA, ITS COMPLICATIONS AND THEIR TREATMENT

As renal function deteriorates, patients with chronic renal insufficiency will experience the symptoms and signs of uremia. The term "uremia" is used to describe an array of clinical findings dealing with all of the abnormalities produced by chronic impairment of renal function. The altered metabolic abnormalities, if present, may affect virtually every organ system. The clinical features of uremia and its complications may be divided into five major categories: gastrointestinal, neuromuscular, cardiorespiratory, cutaneous and miscellaneous. The gastrointestinal symptoms associated with chronic renal insufficiency include anorexia, nausea, vomiting, constipation or diarrhea, hic-

cough, coated tongue, ammoniacal breath, mouth ulcerations, parotitis, gastrointestinal bleeding and possibly pancreatitis. The neuromuscular symptoms may include drowsiness, lethargy, sleep disturbances, hallucinations, convulsions, coma, psychosis, peripheral neuropathy, muscle twitching, tetany and anxiety. The cardiorespiratory manifestations may include serofibrinous pericarditis, edema, dyspnea, acidotic respiration (Kussmaul breathing), left ventricular failure, hilar pneumonitis, "uremic lung," hypertension, normochromic normocytic anemia and polycythemia. Cutaneous manifestations may include a grayish yellow pallor, eyelid swelling, urea "frost," pruritis, purpura and skin infections. Finally, the miscellaneous category of symptoms may include epistaxis, bone disease, corneal calcification, retinal detachment, arteriosclerotic retinopathy and/or hypertensive retinopathy.

Anemia

Various anemias and coagulopathies are common findings in the uremic patient. However, there does not seem to be a good correlation between the severity of these complications and the degree of renal impairment. In early renal disease, the anemias may be mild but usually progress as renal function deteriorates. On the other hand, the anemias and coagulopathies may be stabilized even in patients with end-stage disease. An examination of peripheral blood usually reveals normochromic normocytic anemia. Hypochromia and macrocytosis have only been seen occasionally. The presence of erythrocytes with sharp, spiney, fixed projections usually termed "burr cells" are also a common finding in a peripheral blood smear of patients with chronic renal insufficiency. Hypersegmented polymorphonuclear leukocytes resembling folic acid or vitamin B_{12} deficiency are also present. This abnormality, however, is only partly reversed with the administration of vitamin B_{12} or folic acid. Although platelet number and morphology are usually normal, abnormal platelet function is common and represents the major factor in the bleeding tendency seen in uremia. Reduced availability of platelet factor III and reduced platelet aggregation and adhesiveness are the principle defects. These defects return to normal following dialysis suggesting that a circulating toxin is responsible. Thrombocytopenia may occur in the presence of microangiopathic hemolysis with intravascular coagulation. Bone marrow aspirations may look normal in early renal insufficiency, but with severe disease, hypoplasia of the erythroid elements and severe normoblastic suppression may be seen. Erythrocyte surival time may be decreased by 50% in patients with renal insufficiency. This decrease has been attributed to increased concentrations of metabolic waste products. The decreased survival time, however, is not severe enough to account for the anemia.

A plasma erythropoietin which stimulates erythropoiesis is known to exist, and it is generally accepted that the kidney is the major organ which elaborates it.[20] In renal disease, there is a deficiency in the erythrocyte-stimulating factor (ESF), and perhaps this is the cause of the anemia.

It has also been demonstrated that the red cell iron turnover rate is markedly decreased in chronic renal failure.[21] Administered iron only accumulates in the marrow for a short period of time and then moves to the liver and spleen and is stored. The end result is that very little administered iron is incorporated into the red cell. This would indicate a marrow defect not responsive to iron therapy.

Moderate intravascular hemolysis may also occur in chronic renal insufficiency. This phenomenon has been attributed to a number of causes related to abnormal metabolism in uremic subjects. Some of these abnormalities include those relating to glycolysis, glutathione metabolism and the pentose shunt pathway and sodium and potassium flux. Whatever the cause, hemolysis is often correctable by dialysis.[20]

With the exception of intravascular coagulation, many of the anemias and coagulopathies are correctable by dialysis. The normochromic normocytic anemia found in chronic renal failure, however, responds only to long term dialysis. Even then, the anemia does not revert to normal and is stabilized at a hemoglobin concentration of 7 to 10 g/100 ml. Lack of erythropoietin may be the major factor in such cases.

The treatment of anemias not responsive to dialysis is usually not warranted. Generally, these anemias are asymptomatic since many patients can tolerate considerable anemia very well. Further, the restoration of normal hematopoiesis, if it were possible, would not improve renal function, although it might restore an impaired myocardial reserve. If treatment is required, a transfusion of packed cells may be tried. Some patients may require as much as 2 units per month. The benefits versus the risks of transfusion therapy must be weighed carefully in these patients. Transfusions can not only suppress the patient's own erythropoiesis and increase the risk of siderosis and hepatitis but also introduce leukocyte antigen into the patient's circulation, stimulating antibody formation. This complication can occur despite meticulous washing of donor red cells. Such an occurrence would lead to a diminution in the number of histocompatible donors in patients awaiting renal transplantation. Hence, transfusions should be kept to a minimum.

Anabolic steroids have been shown to increase plasma erythropoietin and thus stimulate erythropoiesis in normal and anemic subjects. Clinical trials of such agents in renal anemia have been disappointing.[20] The role of such therapy cannot be clearly evaluated at this time; however, the presence of steroid-related side effects probably outweigh their doubtful advantages. Vitamin B_{12} and folic acid supplementation should be instituted only if a deficiency exists. Iron supplementation is of questionable value. However, if iron deficiency exists because of decreased dietary intake or blood loss, iron supplementation is warranted. Parenteral iron preparations are rarely indicated in the correction of iron deficiency; certainly if deficiency is not present, neither parenteral nor oral iron has any effect on hematopoiesis.

Hypertension

The mechanisms by which hypertension develops in chronic renal insufficiency are not clearly understood. Usually, however, the hypertension is volume dependent and may be controlled by achieving optimal sodium and fluid balance. On the other hand, some patients do not respond to optimal sodium and fluid balance, drastic dehydration or depressor agents. Such patients are termed "refractory." It has been shown that there is a good correlation between increased plasma renin levels and the degree of hypertension in patients who are refractory to conventional modes of therapy.

Such a correlation does not exist for nonrefractory patients.

The mechanism by which refractory, renin-dependent hypertension occurs in patients with chronic renal insufficiency has yet to be resolved. A hypothesis advanced by Merrill and Hampers[12] suggests that sodium retention followed by an elaboration of renin by damaged kidneys causes an increase in plasma volume. The inevitable increase in cardiac output causes an increased tone in the small capacitance vessels which results in an increase in peripheral resistance. Concomitantly, the renin-angiotensin mechanism is also activated, producing vasoconstriction and a further increase in peripheral resistance. The increased vascular tone causes an activation of a feedback mechanism which decreases cardiac output. At this point, the patient is hypertensive but with a normal cardiac output. In the uremic patient, the buffer mechanism within the carotid sinus is inappropriately set or triggered, resulting in an inappropriate response to changes in extracellular volume and arterial tone. The treatment for refractory renin-dependent malignant hypertension is bilateral nephrectomy.

Other explanations for the occurrence of hypertension in uremic patients have been proposed. Circulating prostaglandins with pressor and depressor properties are known to exert some influence. The exact role of prostaglandins in the production of renal hypertension, however, is not clear at this time. Hypersecretion of aldosterone has been shown to occur in patients with chronic renal insufficiency. Its contribution to renal hypertension is unclear and probably represents a secondary factor.[12] Finally, the diffuse calcification of peripheral vessels due to altered calcium metabolism is certainly a contributing cause of renal hypertension.

The treatment of asymptomatic hypertension associated with chronic renal failure is very controversial. The choice, of course, should be based on benefits versus risks, and there do exist some substantial benefits. Gradual reduction of blood pressure will prevent the further impairment of renal function and reduce the pressure load on the left ventricle, thereby improving cardiac output and renal blood flow. The treatment of borderline hypertension or symptomatic hypertension, however, will not improve pre-existing kidney lesions, and the drastic reduction of blood pressure will decrease GFR and increase the BUN. Symptomatic hypertension in the uremic patient should, of course, be treated as in other individuals.

The use of antihypertensive agents in chronic renal insufficiency warrants a few comments. There exists no safe antihypertensive agent when applied to a regimen in chronic renal insufficiency. The adversities seen with these agents in patients with normal renal function take on a more important emphasis in patients with decreased renal function. The effects of hypovolemia, hyponatremia, hypokalemia, hyperuricemia, hyperglycemia and hypercalcemia seen with diuretic agents must be meticulously monitored in patients with chronic renal failure since defects in these parameters already exist. Agents such as guanethidine and ganglionic blockers such as trimethaphan which have the capability of decreasing renal blood flow and exacerbating chronic renal insufficiency should be avoided. Depressor agents which either increase renal blood flow, such as hydralazine, or have no effect on renal blood flow, such as methyldopa and diazoxide, should be chosen preferentially. Diazoxide at a dose of 5 mg per kg administered intravenously twice daily seems to be the drug of choice in malignant hypertension associated with chronic renal insufficiency. The diabetogenic and sodium-retaining effects of diazoxide, however, must be monitored carefully.

Azotemic Osteodystrophy

As mentioned previously, abnormal calcium and phosphate metabolism associated with chronic renal insufficiency may lead to azotemic osteodystrophy. This inclusive term is used to describe three pathological bone and tissue lesions which may occur as a complication of renal insufficiency. Hyperparathyroidism secondary to initial hypocalcemia and hyperphosphatemia gives rise to osteitis fibrosa cystica with symptoms of bone pain. Radiologically, subperiosteal resorption, resorption of the ends of the clavicles and areas around fractures and loss of lamina dura are common findings in osteitis fibrosa. As hyperparathyroidism progresses, parathyroid hyperplasia increases and autonomous nodules insensitive to serum calcium and phosphate levels secrete even more parathyroid hormone. As a result, serum calcium levels increase without decreasing serum phosphate levels, and precipitation of calcium into body tissues may occur. Such a disorder is termed "metastatic calcification" and, if present, can truly complicate the course of renal insufficiency. Nephrocalcinosis may develop which would further impair renal function. Calcification of large and small vessels would certainly complicate renal hypertension and cause a variety of insufficiency disorders such as coronary, cerebral and renal insufficiency. Calcium deposits in the conduction system of the heart may lead to serious or fatal arrhythmias. Periarticular and intra-articular calcium deposits make motion extremely painful. Finally, calcium may deposit in the cornea and conjunctiva with band keratopathy which may further complicate visual nerve disturbances caused by uremia. To prevent metastatic calcification, serum levels of calcium and phosphate should be taken frequently and the calcium phosphate product, [CA] x [P], should always be kept far below 75.

Vitamin D resistance and subsequent hypocalcemia give rise to osteomalacia. Bone pain, pelvic girdle weakness, pseudofractures and widened osteoid seams in calcified bone sections are the predominant findings.

The differential diagnosis of vitamin D resistance versus hyperparathyroidism is not an easy one. The two disorders were explained separately above only for the purposes of clarity. Clinically, the two disorders occur simultaneously, and mixed osteitis fibrosa, osteomalacia and osteosclerosis generally comprise the patholigical picture. Although all patients with chronic renal insufficiency will show altered calcium and phosphate metabolism and some degree of hyperparathyroidism, fortunately, only 10% will show clinical evidence of bone disease.[12]

The treatment of azotemic osteodystrophy is very difficult. It is evident that treatment of one disorder will aggravate the other. Careful patient monitoring is essential if treatment is to be successful.

As mentioned previously, therapy with phosphate binders such as aluminum hydroxide should be started early in the course of chronic renal failure. By preventing hyperphosphatemia, it is hoped that hypocalcemia and secondary hyperparathyroidism may be averted. Vitamin D resistance and hypocalcemia leading to osteomalacia may be treated with large doses of vitamin D (50,000 to 150,000 units per day) and calcium gluconate and/or carbonate (4 to 12 g per day). The common preparations of calciferol or dihydrotachysterol may effect an increase in the gastrointestinal absorption of calcium. Some patients are extremely resistant to these preparations, and the use of 25-hydroxycholecalciferol, the active D-3 metabolite, may produce better results.[24] When calcium metabolism is near normal, vitamin D therapy should be withdrawn. Its effects may last for months since it has a long half-life.[25] If vitamin D therapy and calcium supplementation are continued, hypercalcemia and an increased calcium phosphate product sufficient to cause metastatic calcification can occur. Careful monitoring of serum calcium and phosphate levels during vitamin D therapy and calcium supplementation is essential.

The treatment for hyperparathyroidism, osteitis fibrosa cystica and metastatic calcification is total or subtotal parathyroidectomy. Many authorities have found conservative treatment to be uniformly unsuccessful.[12] Subtotal parathyroidectomy, the removal of 3 1/2 glands, or total parathyroidectomy, the removal of all 4 glands, in the experience of some has not led to severe postoperative sequelae and has alleviated hypercalcemia.[26] An important feature of parathyroidectomy is the rapid resorption of soft tissue calcification. Unfortunately, vascular calcification only improved slightly, if at all.

Gastrointestinal

Anorexia, nausea, vomiting and persistent hiccoughs are classical signs of uremia. Their etiology is still uncertain; however, the decomposition of urea by urea-splitting bacteria which results in the liberation of ammonia and subsequent irritation of the gastrointestinal mucosa may be a contributory factor. Nausea and vomiting must be controlled in order to prevent dehydration, sodium deficiency and potassium deficiency all of which can lead to further deterioration of renal function. The treatment consists of nocturnal hydration, chlorpromazine and a low protein diet. If this treatment plan fails, dialysis will almost always result in an improvement of symptoms. Ulcerations of the mucous membranes which may occur throughout the gastrointestinal tract may cause severe problems in some patients. The coagulopathy seen in chronic renal insufficiency may increase the potential for gastrointestinal hemorrhage. Mouth and tongue ulcerations occur, and *Candida* infections may result. Proper oral hygiene is imperative in such patients. Constipation may occur early in the course of renal insufficiency followed by diarrhea in the later stages. Dialysis and restoration of the imbalances associated with chronic renal failure will usually alleviate most of the gastrointestinal complications.

Neurological

Neurological manifestations in chronic renal insufficiency vary considerably. Psychological abnormalities range from mild defects of mentation to fullblown psychosis. The particular psychological manifestation presented depends upon the underlying personality. Although dialysis will improve these symptoms very often, rapid dialysis may either initiate or aggravate such symptoms, and it is termed the "disequilibrium syndrome." The etiology of this syndrome is not clear. It has been suggested that the rapid removal of extracellular urea may force water intracellularly, resulting in cerebral edema. If dialysis is not initiated, however, progressive lethargy and mental confusion leading to coma may ensue.

Peripheral motor and sensory neuropathy may be extremely debilitating. Symptoms indicating neuropathy are impaired reflexes, muscular weakness and paralysis. Dialysis may reverse some of these symptoms if the damage to the nerves is not too severe. Renal transplantation dramatically improves and invariably arrests peripheral neuropathy.

Muscle spasms are very common in chronic renal failure. They may even be present during coma. Many patients are relieved of this symptom by dialysis.

Convulsions due to uremia may also appear. These must be differentiated from convulsions due to hyponatremia, hypertensive encephalopathy and hypocalcemic tetany. Immediate measures can be taken by the administration of diazepam or diphenylhydantoin.

If diphenylhydantion is used for prolonged periods of time, interference with folate absorption may occur complicating the anemias generally seen in renal disease. The likelihood of recurrence of convulsive complications, however, is great, unless dialysis is instituted.

Cardiovascular

The cardiovascular complications of chronic renal insufficiency are generally seen late in the course of the diesease. The etiological factors in the genesis of congestive heart failure include anemia, hypertension, atherosclerosis and vascular calcification. Circulatory congestion with an increased cardiac output may also lead to congestive failure. Other factors which are not well understood but are related to altered metabolism can initiate or aggravate congestive heart failure. The treatment of choice is proper fluid and electrolyte restriction, the administration of diuretics and dialysis. This form of therapy has been successful even in the digitalis-resistant failure observed in some patients who are maintained on a low protein diet.[27] Digitalis therapy should *not* be considered unless the above mode of therapy fails. The administration of digitalis to patients with impaired renal function is highly dangerous. If such therapy, however, must be instituted, Jelliffe's[28,29] recommendations for dosage regimen adjustments in patients with renal impairment should be followed.

Uremic pericarditis may frequently complicate chronic renal insufficiency and, unlike congestive heart failure, may appear early in renal disease. It has occurred in patients on long-term hemodialysis, but, in these cases, the syndrome is probably due to inadequate dialysis. The syndrome is accompanied by pericardial tamponade, a serofibrinous exudate and sometimes hemorrhagic pericarditis. Constrictive pericarditis is a rare complication. The treatment for these complications is adequate hemodialysis or renal transplantation. In some cases, more specific therapy such as pericardiocentesis and open drainage may be necessary.

Pulmonary edema producing the "bat-wing" distribution of increased density in chest films can be seen in severe renal failure. The occurrence of this complication is due to both overhydration and increased capillary permeability. Resolution of the edema can be achieved with adequate dialysis.

Dermatological

Owing to some alterations in the immune response, uremic patients are prone to skin infections. A contributing factor to the increased incidence of skin infections is scratching because of uremic pruritis. The etiology of the "uremic itch" is not clearly understood. It may be caused by the abnormalities in calcium metabolism because some patients are relieved after parathyroidectomy. It is also thought to be an extension of the peripheral neuropathy seen in chronic renal failure.

Pallor of the skin and mucous membranes may develop because of the anemias. Dry and scaly skin is common, and fissures may occur which could contribute to skin infections. Urea frost, precipitation of urea crystals on the skin, is a rare finding. Because of the uremia-induced coagulopathies, subcutaneous hemorrhages, petechiae and ecchymoses may be seen.

Various dermatological preparations such as coal tar ointment, corticosteroid creams, dilute acetic acid solution and aquaphor ointments have been tried with varying success. The placebo effect may be the clinician's best friend when trying to relieve the uremic itch which is not responsive to parathyroidectomy. Keeping the skin moist and pliable with the use of ointments, however, is one measure which should be instituted. Fissures of the skin may thus be averted and infections reduced. Adequate maintenance dialysis will also relieve some of the dermatological manifestations.

Ophthalmological

Calcium deposition in the cornea causing irritation and hyperemia can occur in chronic renal insufficiency. Generally, this does not occur until the later stages of uremia and when hypercalcemia and the calcium-phosphate product are excessive. Calcium resorption will occur after parathyroidectomy or when proper calcium balance is maintained. Conjunctivitis without corneal calcification, retinal detachment and edema of the retina may also occur in uremia. Hypertensive and diabetic retinopathies may occur if such complications exist. A small number of patients may suffer from severe loss of vision (uremic amaurosis). The etiology of this complication is undefined, but it may be due to the neuropathies associated with uremia. Finally, neuropathies of other cranial nerves may result in nystagmus, miosis and pupil asymmetry.

Uremic Toxins

Many of the signs, symptoms and complications of uremia are etiologically well defined and understood, while others are completely confusing. Many of these etiologically undefined symptoms and complications are relieved either partially or entirely by dialysis. The theory that accumulating metabolic toxins are responsible for these conditions is rational. Finding and isolating these toxins, however, has been extremely difficult.

The signs and symptoms of uremia correlate fairly well with the accumulation of various metabolic end products such as urea. Attempts to reproduce these symptoms in normal individuals have been unsuccessful until recently. Two guanidine derivatives have been isolated from uremic patients which can reproduce the majority of symptoms associated with uremia. Anemia, decreased red cell survival time, anorexia, vomiting, ulcerations and gastrointestinal hemorrhage, decreased nerve conduction velocity, tachycardia and other arrhythmias, and generalized convulsions occur in dogs when chronically intoxicated with methylguanidine.[30] Guanidinosuccinic acid (GSA), another guanidine derivative which is found in high concentrations in uremic patients, can produce twitching, gastroenteritis, erythrocyte hemolysis and platelet defects when injected into animals. The mechanisms of GSA and methylguanidine production is not known with certainty. However, it is believed that high levels of urea may block the urea cycle, and GSA and methylguanidine may be end products of arginine metabolism through an alternate pathway.[12]

GENERAL TREATMENT

Although some forms of chronic renal insufficiency are responsive to immunosuppressive therapy, generally there is no treatment for this disorder. Therapy of any kind is aimed at preserving the functional integrity of residual nephrons, not at reversing the renal lesions. Much of the treatment discussed thus far has been either symptomatic therapy or therapy aimed at a specific defect. Three additional therapeutic measures which can be incorporated into a patient's over-all treatment program are diet, chronic hemodialysis and renal transplantation.

Diet

Chronic hemodialysis or renal transplantation is usually an inevitable end point in chronic renal failure. Prior to such measures, however, appropriate diet therapy can produce considerable alleviation of subjective complaints for prolonged periods. The purpose of diet therapy is to prevent endogenous protein catabolism which can occur because of anorexia, nausea and vomiting and to reduce the formation of urea.

It has been shown that only small amounts of protein intake are needed to establish positive nitrogen balance. Thus, protein restriction is usually started when symptoms appear or are expected to appear (generally when the BUN = 75 mg% or above). Restriction should start with 60 g per day, and, if symptoms persist, protein intake can be further decreased to 40 g per day. (These restrictions are, of course, based on a 70kg man.) The problem associated with further protein restriction is one of palatability and patient compliance. Nevertheless, highly restrictive protein diets supplying as little as 0.26 g of protein per kg of body weight per day have been established by Giordano and Giovannetti (GG diet).[31,32] Since the body can avidly manufacture nonessential amino acids, the protein component of the GG diet is made up of foods which are high in essential amino acids. Only in this way can protein intake be reduced so drastically and yet maintain positive nitrogen balance. This is accomplished by the reutilization of urea. Urea-splitting bacteria in the gut transform urea to amonia which is utilized by the body as essential building blocks for the production of nonessential amino acids. The primary caloric sources of the GG diet are fats and concentrated sugars.

A large daily allowance of fruit is incorporated into the diet, and marked increases in serum potassium have been observed in about 50% of the patients.[33] Serum potassium levels should be monitored frequently in such patients, and the addition of oral Kayexalate may be necessary.

Although the GG diet is a breakthrough in the management of patients with chronic renal insufficiency, its beneficial effects decrease as renal function decreases. When the GFR falls below 3 ml per min and the serum creatinine concentration rises above 12 mg%, the diet becomes ineffective and dialytic therapy is indicated.[33]

Chronic Intermittent Hemodialysis

Patients with end-stage chronic renal failure may live a relatively normal life while being maintained on chronic intermittent hemodialysis. However, there are some problems associated with this mode of therapy, and they are summarized in Table 8.3.

Long term intermittent hemodialysis is indicated when the following conditions exist:

1. The GFR is less than 1 or 2 ml per min.
2. The patient cannot survive on 20 g per day of protein without symptoms.
3. There are persistent symptoms of uremia.
4. A persistent BUN above 150 mg%.
5. A persistent serum creatinine above 15 mg%.
6. A persistent serum potassium above 6 mEq per liter.
7. A persistent plasma bicarbonate below 15 mEq per liter.
8. A persistent edema.
9. A persistent hyponatremia, hypertension, congestive heart failure and peripheral neuropathy.

TABLE 8.3
Problems Associated with Chronic Intermittent Hemodialysis

A. Anemia may not be alleviated
B. Peripheral neuropathy may deteriorate
C. Renal osteodystrophy may not be alleviated
D. Increased metastatic calcification may occur
E. Infections occur readily at the site of the arteriovenous cannula
F. Clots occur within the arteriovenous cannula
G. Emotional problems are frequent
H. Cost:
  1. Chronic dialysis in a center costs approximately $10,000 per year per patient.
  2. Home dialysis costs may range from $10,000 to $20,000 the 1st year; then $3,000 to $5,000 per year.

Renal Transplantation

Renal transplantation has become a recognized form of therapy for end stage renal disease over the past few years, and many more centers are now instituting this procedure. When successful, it results in almost complete restoration of renal function and health. The procedures are not, however, uniformly successful, and many problems remain in determining the proper management and immunosuppressive therapy for these patients.

By 1970, the collected experience of 3,645 transplants provided the following statistics:[34]

1. Transplants from consanguineous living donors have a 78% chance for 1-year survival and 75% chance for a 2-year survival.

2. Cadaver transplants have a 52% chance for a 1-year survival, and a 41% chance for a 2-year survival.

As immunosuppressive therapy and procedures improve, these already impressive statistics will also improve.

REFERENCES

1. Papper, S.: Renal failure. Med. Clin. North Am., 55: 335, 1971.
2. Douglas, A. P., and Kerr, D. N. S.: A Short Textbook of Kidney Disease, p. 280. J. B. Lippincott Co., Philadelphia, 1968.
3. Black, D. A. K.: Renal Disease, Ed. 2, p. 327. F. A. Davis Co., Philadelphia, 1967.
4. Bricker, N. S., Morrin, P. F., and Kine, S. W., Jr.: The pathologic physiology of chronic bright's disease; an exposition of the "intact nephron hypothesis." Am. J. Med., 28: 77, 1960.
5. Epstein, F. H., and Merrill, J. P.: Chronic renal failure, in Harrison's Principles of Internal Medicine, Ed. 6, p. 1393, edited by M. M. Wintrobe, G. W. Thorn, R. D. Adams, I. L. Bennett, Jr., E. Braunwald, K. J. Isselbacher, and R. G. Petersdorf. McGraw-Hill Book Co., New York, 1970
6. Wang, F.: Conservative management of chronic renal failure. Med. Clin. North Am., 55: 137, 1971.
7. Rosenfeld, M. G.: Manual of Medical Therapeutics, Ed. 20, p. 48. Little, Brown and Co., Boston, 1971.
8. Goodman, L. S., and Gilman, A.: The Pharmacological Basis of Therapeutics, Ed. 4, p. 805. The MacMillan Co., New York, 1970.
9. Stanbury, S. W., and Lumb, G. A.: Metabolic studies of renal osteodystrophy. I: calcium, phosphorous and nitrogen metabolism in rickets, osteomalacia and hyperparathyroidism, complicating chronic uremia. Medicine 41: 1, 1962.
10. Clarkson, E. M., McDonald, S. J., and de Wardener, H. E.: The effect of high intake of calcium carbonate in normal subjects and patients with chronic renal failure. Clin. Sci., 30: 425, 1966.
11. Kleeman, C. R., Better, O., Massry, S. G., and Maxwell, M. H.: Divalent ion metabolism and osteodystrophy in chronic renal failure. Yale J. Biol. Med., 40, 1967.
12. Merrill, J. P., and Hampers, C. L.: Uremia. In Progress in Pathophysiology and Treatment. Grune and Stratton, New York, 1971.
13. Clark, J. E., and Caedo, R. E.: Fluid and electrolyte management in renal failure. Am. Fam. Physician, 5: 125, 1972.
14. Leamon, E. J.: Metabolic acidosis – a factor in pathogenesis of azotemic osteodystrophy. Arch. Intern. Med., 124: 557, 1969.
15. Perkoff, G. T., Thomas, C. L., Newton, J. D., Soleman, J. C., and Tyler, F. H.: Mechanism of impaired glucose tolerance in uremia and experimental hyperazotemia. Diabetes, 7: 375, 1958.
16. Harris, J. L.: Effect of urea on trypsin and alpha-chymotrypsin. Nature, 177: 471, 1956.
17. Hutchings, R. H., Hegstrom, R. M., and Scribner, B. H.: Glucose intolerance in patients on long-term intermittent dialysis. Ann. Intern. Med., 65: 275, 1966.
18. Hampers, C. L., Soeldner, J. S., Doak, P. G., and Merrill, J. P.: The effect of chronic renal failure and hemodialysis on carbohydrate metabolism. J. Clin. Invest., 45: 1719, 1966.
19. Bennett, W. M., Singer, I., and Coggins, C. H.: Guide to drug usage in adult patients with impaired renal function. J. A. M. A., 223: 991, 1973.
20. Penington, D. G., and Kincaid-Smith, P.: Anemia in renal failure. Br. Med. Bull., 27: 136, 1971.
21. Chodos, P. B.: The pathogenesis of anemia in chronic renal disease. Clin. Res., 4: 141, 1956.
22. Hirschman, J. L., and Herfindal, E. T.: Essential hypertension. J. Am. Pharm. Assoc., NS11: 555, 1971.
23. Merrill, J. P.: Hypertensive vascular disease. In Harrison's Principles of Internal Medicine, Ed. 6, p. 1252, edited by M. M. Wintrobe, G. W. Thorn, R. D. Adams, I. L. Bennett, Jr., E. Braunwald, K. J. Isselbacher, and R. G. Petersdorf. McGraw-Hill Book Co., New York, 1970.
24. del Greco, F., and Krumlovsky, F. A.: Chronic renal failure, clinical and therapeutic considerations. Postgrad. Med., 52: 176, 1972.
25. Chen, P. S., Terepka, R. A., and Overslaugh, C.: Hypercalcemia and hyperphosphotemic actions of dihydrotachysterol, vitamin D^2, and hytakerol (AT-10) in rats and dogs. Endocrinology, 70: 815, 1962.
26. Katz, A. I., Hampers, C. L., and Merrill, J. P.:

Secondary hyperparathyroidism and renal osteodystrophy in chronic renal failure. Medicine, 48: 333, 1969.

27. Baily, G. L., Hampers, C. L., and Merrill, J. P.: Reversible uremic cardiomyopathy in uremia. Trans. Am. Soc. Artif. Intern. Organs, 13: 263, 1967.

28. Jelliffe, R. W.: An improved method of digoxin therapy: Ann. Intern. Med., 69: 703, 1968.

29. Jelliffe, R. W., Buell, J., and Kalaba, R.: An improved method of digitoxin therapy. Ann. Intern. Med., 72: 453, 1970.

30. Giovannetti, S., Biagini, M., Balestri, P. L., Navalesi, R., Giagnoni, P., De Matteis, A., Ferro-Milone, P., and Perfehi, C.: Proceedings of the Fourth International Conference of Nephrology, Stockholm, p. 43, June 22-27, 1969.

31. Giordano, C.: Use of exogenous and endogenous urea for protein synthesis in normal and uremic subjects. J. Lab. Clin. Med., 62: 231, 1963.

32. Giovannetti, S., and Maggiore, A.: A low nitrogen diet with proteins of high biological value for severe uremia. Lancet, 1: 1000, 1964.

33. Lange, K.: Nutritional management of kidney disorders. Med. Clin. North Am., 55: 513, 1971.

34. Rubin, A. L., Whitsell, J. C., Riggio, R. R., Schwartz, H., David, D. S., and Stenzel, K. H.: Renal transplantation: present status. Bull. N. Y. Acad. Med., 46: 869, 1970.

chapter 9

PEPTIC ULCER DISEASE

Joseph L. Hirschman, Pharm.D.
Eric T. Herfindal, Pharm.D.

If one were to prepare a list of "diseases most likely to be self-medicated before seeking the help of a physician," it is highly probable that peptic ulcer disease would head that list. This is, of course, a result of the ready accessibility of effective (or transiently effective) therapy for the symptoms of that disease—in the form of antacids. Since in most cases the pharmacist will be the first health professional contacted by the patient, who may be totally unaware that he is suffering from peptic ulcer, it is obvious that the pharmacist must have more than a layman's knowledge of the disease. Armed with a thorough understanding of the facts and folklore of the disease, he can render a service to the physician and the patient in the proper therapeutic management of this rather common disease.

ETIOLOGY

There are actually three varieties of peptic ulcer: gastric, marginal and, the most common, duodenal. An ulcer (duodenal or otherwise) can be safely defined as an acute or chronic ulceration of the digestive tract, occurring in an area which is accessible to gastric secretions. Without gastric secretions, it would be virtually impossible to develop an ulcer.

Each year, the American public spends over 1 billion dollars on the treatment of this disease. Over 75 million dollars are spent on

antacids alone.[1] Strangely, little priority has been assigned to determining the cause of this disease. Indeed, less than 5% of the money assigned to the National Institutes of Health is devoted to medical research on gastrointestinal diseases. Perhaps for this reason, little can be said with confidence about the etiology of peptic ulcers. A few things, however, can be said about its incidence and pathogenesis.

INCIDENCE

Duodenal ulcers are the most common form of the disease and thus can serve as the prototype for this discussion. Approximately 1 in 10 of us will suffer from a peptic ulcer at some time. Males will be affected more than women by a factor (depending on the source) ranging between 3 : 1 and 10 : 1. They seem to occur most commonly between the ages of 20 and 50 usually as a single ulcer, but as multiple ulcers in 20% of those affected. An ulcer is a worldwide phenomenon showing occasional but uncertain preference for certain races, cultures and seasons.[2]

PATHOGENESIS

Although the cause of peptic ulcer is unknown, there are some parameters of this disease which have been unequivocally established. A gastric ulcer never occurs in the absence of gastric acid and pepsin.[1] Thus, one can assume that for some as yet unrevealed reason the *normal* resistance of the gastric mucosa to acid and pepsin is compromised. This is by no means a simple direct process since *any* of the following factors may be involved.

1. Hormonal Factors. Since males are subject to a higher incidence than females, it is possible that the female hormones have a "protective" role.

2. Gastric Hyperacidity. While the duodenal

ulcer patient is commonly characterized as a person who generates excessive acid, this is not always the case. When hypersecretion does occur, it is frequently a result of excessive vagal stimulation.

3. Gastric Emptying Time. A number of duodenal ulcer patients show a pattern of rapid stomach emptying. If such is the case, larger than normal amounts of unbuffered stomach acid will be spilled into the duodenum. However, evidence for this as an important factor in ulcer formation is equivocal.

4. Emotions.[2] Since the peptic ulcer patient is classically characterized as a hard-driving, tense and conscientious climber, there is a great tendency to assume that this is one of the primary factors in this disease. While there is some evidence to support this point of view (e.g., emotional stress may cause complications or recurrences; anger and hostility can cause gastric mucosal engorgement, hypersecretion of acid, etc.), none of these observations has been made under controlled circumstances. The fact that ulcers cannot be healed by psychotherapy alone (and hypersecretion may continue when emotional states abate) leads one to the conclusion that some ulcers are psychosomatically induced and others are not.

5. Genetic Factors.[2] Genetic factors appear to affect the risk of peptic ulcer. Certain families reveal a long generational history of this disease. Furthermore, individuals with blood type 0 are 40% more liable to duodenal ulcers than those with blood types A, B or AB. Why blood type predisposes one to ulcers is not known, however. Racial factors have also been studied in the hopes of identifying any racial predispositions to peptic ulcer disease. However, the differences found in these studies in incidence of ulcers between various ethnic groups cannot be interpreted as being racial, as has been done. The groups studied were too genetically heterogenous to account for the variations between these ethnic groups as genetic.

It is important to stress that not one of the factors discussed above, in itself, has been *proven* to exert a powerful enough effect to result in the large variations seen between various populations in the incidence of peptic ulcers. All one can say is that these factors can be contributory to the disease—the exact significence of which is yet to be revealed.

DRUG-INDUCED PEPTIC ULCERATION

Drug-induced peptic ulcers have an etiology which is quite clear, although the mechanisms are not thoroughly understood. As pharmacists, with our drug orientation, we can be on the lookout for drug-induced disease. We can try to eliminate offending agents in those individuals who either suffer from or are predisposed to peptic ulcer disease.

In drug-induced ulcers the exact incidence and etiological relationships are difficult to determine because of differences in groups studied, concomitant and previous medications, emotional influences and other factors. However, some mechanisms of drug-induced ulceration are known. These include stimulation of gastric acidity and decreased mucosal resistance. Included in the list of drugs that can precipitate or aggravate peptic ulcers are the following.

1. Alpha-Adrenergic Blocking Agents.[3] The initial and major effect of the alpha-blocking agents and reserpine is to increase gastric secretion; any accompanying vasospasm may contribute by diminishing tissue resistance. However, the incidence of peptic ulceration with these drugs is low even when large doses are administered. In the usual dosages of reserpine used in hypertension, the incidence is almost nil.

2. Salicylates.[4,5] Aspirin and the salicylates lower mucosal resistance by producing a hemorrhagic, erosive gastritis and duodenitis. There is some evidence that aspirin does this by allowing so-called back-diffusion of hydrogen ions into the mucosal cells. This back-diffusion apparently reduces the metabolic rate of the cells, thereby making them more prone to injury and less able to regenerate when damaged. However, these effects can be minimized by the concurrent administration of an alkaline solution such as sodium bicarbonate, e.g., Alka-Seltzer. Unfortunately, this approach is not feasible for chronic administration because of the risk of systemic alkalosis secondary to the chronic use of bicarbonate. For the occasional relief of a headache, however, this approach is a reasonable one.

3. Phenylbutazone, Indomethacin and Caffeine.[5,6] Similar effects occur with phenylbutazone administration. Duration of treatment

prior to the onset of symptoms and the route of administration are unimportant because clinical evidence of an ulcer may appear a few days or several months following initiation of therapy. Indomethacin has analogous properties. The ulcerogenic action of caffeine includes both acid stimulation and mucosal effects. There are even a few reports of the precipitation of acute ulcer pain following the ingestion of a single cup of coffee.

4. Adrenocorticotropic Hormone and Corticosteroids.[4,5] The incidence of peptic ulcer occurring during the use of adrenocorticotropic hormone and corticosteroids is not known precisely, but it ranges up to 30%. Incidence is affected by dosage and duration of therapy. High dosage therapy or prolonged duration results in a much greater chance of ulcer formation. The route of administration, e.g., oral, intramuscular, makes little difference. Curiously, steroid ulcers are much more often gastric than duodenal. It has been presumed that the mechanism of steroid-induced ulcers is increased acid secretion, but recent evidence seems to implicate decreased resistance of the gastric and duodenal mucosa. There may be some interference with a hypothetical "healing factor" in the gastric mucosa. More likely, it is a combination of these factors. For this reason, patients on high doses for long periods of time should receive prophylactic antacid therapy.

5. Antineoplastics.[7] The antineoplastics also can be inducers of peptic ulcer disease. Methotrexate is probably the worst offender, but others have been implicated as well. The probable mechanism is direct damage to the mucosal epithelial cells of the gastrointestinal tract.

It is important to keep the whole subject of drug-induced ulcers in perspective. In many cases, these drugs are *not* the sole cause of a peptic ulcer. They should be considered as secondary causes of exacerbation. Ulcerogenic drugs should obviously be avoided, *but only when other reasonable alternatives are available.*

DIAGNOSIS AND CLINICAL FINDINGS

Although the diagnosis and clinical findings associated with peptic ulcers are not our primary professional concern, we should have an understanding of the essentials of diagnosis so that we can better relate to the patient and to the physician. There are several basic criteria that are essential to the diagnosis of uncomplicated peptic ulcers. The first and most prominent symptom is pain in the pit of the stomach. This epigastric distress usually occurs 45 to 60 min after meals. Most of the time, it is rapidly relieved by taking antacids or by eating. Vomiting also will produce relief, and some patients will resort to it in desperation. In the typical duodenal ulcer case, the pain is described as gnawing, burning, cramplike or aching. Some may characterize it as "heartburn." Most frequently it is mild to moderate in intensity. These symptoms are intermittent, but sometimes they may be constant. An occasional patient may also complain of nausea. Laboratory determination of free gastric acid should show increased amounts and hypersecretion. Of course, radiological evidence of an ulcer crater or deformity is usually needed for unequivocal diagnosis.

COMPLICATIONS[8]

The potential complications of peptic ulcer disease, like diagnosis, are usually not the immediate concern of the pharmacist. However, because they can be greatly influenced by drugs (usually adversely) and they can be secondary to poor medical management, which may also involve drugs, they do become our concern. The four most important complications are hemorrhage, perforation, penetration and obstruction. Hemorrhage is usually caused either by the erosion of an ulcer into an artery or a vein or by bleeding from the vascular granulation tissue at the base of the ulcer. This complication occurs in at least 25% of all ulcer patients and can be drug-induced.

Acute perforation into the peritoneal cavity is the most serious complication of peptic ulcer and the most frequent cause of death. This occurs almost exclusively in males between 25 and 40 years old with an incidence of about 1 to 2%. When it happens, it is an emergency and requires immediate surgery.

A penetrating ulcer is sometimes a difficult complication to diagnose, because ordinary ulcer symptoms may be altered. Penetration is like perforation except that the ulcer has extended into adjacent organs, rather than into the free peritoneal space. This occurs fairly frequently with duodenal ulcers and is one of the most important causes of treatment failure.

Minor degrees of pyloric obstruction are present in about 20 to 25% of patients with duodenal ulcers. However, this quite frequently is clinically insignificant. Obstruction is generally caused by edema and spasm and almost always involves some degree of pyloric constriction or stenosis.

TREATMENT

The number of treatments proposed for duodenal ulcers over the years is truly astonishing. Suggestions have ranged from gastric freezing to a wide variety of possible diets to psychotherapy. Today most clinicians rely on an elaborate group of intertwined therapeutic approaches. These include rest, diet, antacids, anticholinergics, sedatives, tranquilizers and psychotherapy. However, in terms of initiating and accelerating healing of ulcers, none of these modes of treatment has been *proven* effective. This is not to say that they are without value. Indeed they are useful in relieving symptoms and facilitating healing, but they must be chosen and applied rationally to the individual patient.

ANTACIDS

There is no question that antacids effectively relieve the pain associated with peptic ulcers and that they buffer the acid required for peptic digestion and persistence of ulceration. As a result, antacids are the mainstay of the medical management of peptic ulcer. Their use is predicated upon the fact that they neutralize hydrochloric acid, which results in an increase in gastric pH. It is known that at a pH above 3.5, 90 to 95% of peptic activity is abolished.[9] However, there is no valid evidence to indicate that antacids have any direct inhibiting effect on pepsin. Their antiulcer "activity" is due entirely to their effects on gastric acidity.

There are two groups of antacids—the absorbable and the nonabsorbable. Absorbable antacids have systemic activity and, therefore, have the potential for changing the pH of the extracellular fluid. The nonabsorbable antacids act locally in the gastrointestinal tract, and they are usually without systemic activity. From a therapeutic point of view, antacids also can be classified at a more basic level, which is divided into three groups—ineffective, possibly effective and effective.

Because clinicians over the years have observed that many patients fail to obtain satisfactory pain relief or adequate healing while taking some of the commonly used antacids, numerous attempts have been made to evaluate the theoretical potential of these agents and to categorize them on the basis of *in vitro* testing.[10,11] While these kinds of studies are useful as rough guides, they have not provided any really reliable methods of predicting with consistency the effects of any given antacid in a particular patient. This is true because no real effort was made until recently to correlate *in vitro* results with *in vivo* effects. Fordtran and his associates[12] designed and carried out a sophisticated study to compare the *in vivo* and *in vitro* properties of liquid antacids. They evolved several interpretations from their results. First, it appears likely that the degree to which acidity must be reduced to heal a peptic ulcer is variable in different patients. This may partially account for the inaccuracies associated with trying to extrapolate straightforward *in vitro* results to the *in vivo* situation. Secondly, different liquid antacids vary markedly in their *in vivo* and *in vitro* potency, and this fact should be taken into account when antacids are recommended or prescribed. Thus, antacid dosage should be based on milliequivalents of neutralizing capacity rather than by volume of the preparation. Thirdly, according to their results, the commonly recommended doses of antacids for ulcer therapy are too low, bearing out the validity of the clinical observations stated above.

SODIUM BICARBONATE[5]

The only example of a clinically useful absorbable antacid is sodium bicarbonate. It has the advantages of rapid onset and high neutralizing capacity. However, the advantages are usually outweighed by its disadvantages, which include systemic alkalosis, the milk-alkali syndrome (a hypercalcemic · condition associated with a large intake of milk and antacids) and a very short duration of action—usually less than 30 min when taken on an empty stomach. Alkalosis can be a problem with chronic use. This can result in an alkaline urine, which can lead to the formation of phosphate kidney stones.

It is generally not practical to use sodium bicarbonate in ulcer therapy except where very fast relief of pain is desired. The rest of the clinically useful antacids are of the nonabsorbable type, of which there are three major groups—the aluminum salts, the magnesium salts and calcium carbonate.

ALUMINUM SALTS[1]

The aluminum products have two distinct advantages over sodium bicarbonate: they do not cause acid rebound or systemic alkalosis. However, several disadvantages make their use questionable. They have poor neutralizing capacity, a short duration of action and they are quite constipating. Also, the aluminum preparations can inhibit the absorption of phosphate, which can become symptomatic (e.g., bone pain) if dietary intake of phosphates is low.[13] However, this ordinarily does not become clinically apparent unless the aluminum antacid therapy is prolonged.

MAGNESIUM SALTS

The magnesium salts, for example, magnesium hydroxide, magnesium oxide and magnesium carbonate, are fairly effective neutralizers and do not cause systemic alkalosis. However, they can precipitate diarrhea as a result of the osmotic effect of magnesium ion in the large bowel. One magnesium preparation, magnesium trisilicate, supposedly forms a silica gel which "coats" the ulcer crate, but it is doubtful that this "coating action" plays any role at all. Also, this compound has poor neutralizing power, and, as a consequence, doses higher than those recommended must be given.

CALCIUM CARBONATE

The last of the nonsystemic antacids is calcium carbonate, which is currently enjoying a renaissance after many years of relative disuse. It appears that this drug is the antacid of choice for many peptic ulcer patients. However, there are several disadvantages and undesirable effects associated with its use that dictate against routine selection without evaluating the possible alternatives for each patient. Among its faults are that it can cause hypercalcemia, renal calculi, constipation and acid rebound. The last certainly occurs[14,15] but should not be significant if frequent dosing is used. The so-called "milk-alkali" syndrome[1] has also been associated with the use of this drug. Although rare, it can be fatal and thus must be watched for and prevented. The constipation problem, unfortunately, is quite prevalent and is dose-related; however, this can be relieved by titrating the patient with a magnesium antacid to balance the constipating effect. Hypercalcemia secondary to calcium carbonate therapy is receiving more attention. It also appears to be dose-related, and several authorities[1,12] believe this problem to be significant enough to indicate that perhaps calcium carbonate should not be used. However, it does require relatively prolonged, high dose therapy to manifest itself in patients with normal function. This fact, along with the conflicting reports[1] on the incidence of this side effect, led these authors to believe that the prudent use of the agent is still desirable because the drug does have a number of therapeutically useful properties that outweigh some of the undesirable effects mentioned above. For example, it has a rapid onset, a fairly long duration of action and a very high neutralizing capacity as well.

There are many antacids on the market which consist of combinations of aluminum, magnesium and calcium salts in various concentrations and mixtures. The rationale behind these products is that the magnesium should override the constipating effect of aluminum and calcium and the latter should minimize the diarrheal tendencies of magnesium. Since there is no way of predicting which patients will do well on the fixed combinations, every individual should be titrated to the appropriate dose of each component. The authors emphasize the word "titration." Even though fixed combinations may be the approximate titration for some patients, they certainly will not hold for all patients. Thus, an attempt should be made to balance the calcium-magnesium ratio for each patient.

GENERAL CONCEPTS

Several points should be kept in mind when one is confronted with a selection of antacid products. The following is a brief survey of the general concepts that apply. Liquid preparations have much more surface area than tablets and so are more effective; their chemical form also differs in many cases. Unlike tablets, suspensions use hydrated chemicals. The chemicals in tablets are not rehydrated by chewing or swallowing with a glass of water. As a consequence, liquids deliver more antacid for neutralization of gastric contents. The authors believe that most tablets should not be used routinely for definitive therapy. They may be of some value if a patient finds himself in a situation where it is impractical to take a liquid preparation, in which case a calcium-containing tablet should be used; however, the tablet should be thoroughly chewed before swallowing. With any preparation, such as antacids that are to be used at frequent intervals and for prolonged periods, taste and palatability become very important as determinants of patient compliance. The pharmacist can be of great help in this aspect by selecting the most pharmaceutically "elegant" formulation of the appropriate drug. One should "taste-test" the preparations that one dispenses.

There are three important reasons for therapeutic failure with antacids. The first is a poor selection of preparations, for example, recommending milk during the acute stage of an ulcer when the rapid and potent effects of calcium carbonate are called for, or using tablet preparations instead of liquids. Secondly, failure may result from too infrequent administration of antacids. Surprisingly little attention is paid to gastric emptying time when treating gastric ulcers. The use of antacids on a "when needed" basis in active ulcer disease will usually result in therapeutic failure. Most antacids have a gastric half-life of less than 30 min and so there is very little antacid left at the end of 1 hr. Since hydrochloric acid is continuously produced, it is important to neutralize it constantly. Thus, the usual dosing frequency should be every hour or every other hour whenever possible. The third most common reason for antacid failure is the use of inadequate dosages. No antacid exceeds calcium carbonate in its acid-neutralizing ability, but differences in potency are not significant *if adequate doses of the various preparations are used.* However, for each type of antacid preparation, there is an optimal dose beyond which further increases in dose do not give more prolonged neutralization. For the aluminum preparations this is about 30 cc, which gives a mean duration of action of about 25 min. For calcium carbonate, it is 2 to 4 g, which yields a mean duration of neutralization of 40 min. Nevertheless, one should not infer from this that all antacids can be used efficaciously as long as an adequate dose is used. There are practical limitations. If the optimal dose should happen to be 60 cc or 8 tablets every hour, it is doubtful that any patient would adhere to such a regimen. Also, it should be noted that the commonly recommended doses of antacids in the literature and on the package are too low for the treatment of peptic ulcer.

To many, the suggestion of an antacid dosing schedule of one dose per hour appears to be excessive, but the majority of patients will tolerate it when advised of its importance. In most cases, this means every hour while awake, but occasionally around-the-clock therapy may be necessary, especially in duodenal peptic ulcer patients. Such patients are frequently hospitalized where this therapy can be maintained more easily. In any event, an hourly regimen (either 24 or 16 hr) is essential if antacids are to be effective during the acute phase. If this is not adhered to, prolonged healing time and recurrence may result. The hourly schedule is usually maintained for 2 to 3 weeks, when the frequency can be reduced to between meals and at bedtime. Giving antacids with meals or shortly after is not a good practice, as they will have little buffering capacity beyond the meal itself.

Ulcers probably take at least a month or longer to heal.[5] The patient should maintain the prescribed antacid regimen for this period of time even when asymptomatic, if recurrence is to be minimized. If a patient can be convinced to stay on reasonably continuous antacid therapy indefinitely, recurrence can probably be prevented altogether.

When antacids are used, there is always the possibility of incurring a drug interaction.[16] So far only one interaction has been clinically important. This is the well known interaction of di- and tri-valent cations with tetracyclines, forming a nonabsorbable chelate. A possible, but speculative, interaction is that of absorption of an active drug onto an antacid magma or gel, resulting in decreased absorption of the active drug. Drug interactions with antacids also might result from the effect of increased gastric pH on the absorption of drugs. Weakly acidic drugs, such as warfarin, the sulfonamides, penicillin G, nitrofurantoin and nalidixic acid, which would theoretically be kept in their ionized and, thus, nonabsorbable state, might be affected by such an interaction. Conversely, there would be a potential effect on weakly basic drugs, such as amphetamine, meperidine and theophylline, which would be more likely to be in the un-ionized and, thus, absorbable state which might potentiate their effects.

Although antacids are o-t-c products, they are not benign. Constipation, impaction, diarrhea, potential drug interactions and the milk-alkali syndrome are possible undesirable effects. In addition, alkalosis is possible with sodium bicarbonate. The pharmacist is in an excellent position to advise patients on the proper selection and use of antacids. Although it is true that most antacids are effective if an adequate dose is given, it is sometimes difficult for patients to adhere to an hourly schedule. As pharmacists, we are in a position to give some encouragement to these patients and to explain to them the necessity of adhering to a less than pleasant routine.

ANTICHOLINERGIC DRUGS[1,9,10]

Anticholinergic drugs are widely used in the treatment of peptic ulcer disease. However, popularity does not necessarily indicate effectiveness. The anticholinergics block the acetylcholine-mediated nerve transmissions at the neuro-effector junctions of the parasympathetic nervous system. These nerves affect the secretion of gastric juice and the motility of the intestinal tract. The use of anticholinergics in the treatment of peptic ulceration would appear to be rational—but, unfortunately, in the usual doses employed orally, they have insignificant effects on gastric secretions. In the normal dosage range, the anticholinergics may reduce the basal volume of gastric secretions, but the acid concentration remains unaltered.

At dosages that would significantly reduce gastric secretions, intolerable side effects would result. In addition, they do not abolish the response of the stomach to stimulation of food or histamine, which have a potent stimulating effect on acid secretion. Even in toxic doses, the anticholinergics cannot produce a vagal blockade such as is seen with a surgical vagotomy.

Nevertheless, these drugs provide useful adjunctive therapy in peptic ulcer patients, but not because of any effect on acid secretion. The primary therapeutic application of the anticholinergics is to delay gastric emptying time, thus facilitating the actions of the antacids. As a consequence, they are indicated for patients who are experiencing *continuing* pain—despite an adequate regimen. In addition, these drugs are often useful for the patient with nocturnal pain. In this situation, the patient should wait 1 or 2 hr after dinner (to allow the stomach to empty) before taking the anticholinergic. The anticholinergic drug should be given in 3 to 4 times the normal dose (for example, propantheline 45 mg), and the antacid dosage is doubled each hour until bedtime. The rationale for this regimen is that the basal nocturnal secretion is lowered at this dosage, even though the food-stimulated secretions are not affected.

The use of anticholinergics in the treatment of peptic ulcers is not without hazards. Because they cause paralysis of the sphincter between the stomach and the esophagus, they can cause gastric contents to reflux up into the esophagus causing some uncomfortable inflammation. The patient taking large nighttime doses and the patient with hiatus hernia should sleep with the head of the bed elevated 8 to 10 inches to prevent regurgitation of gastric contents.

Anticholinergic drugs are contraindicated in gastric ulcers because the delaying of emptying time lengthens the duration of contact between the ulcer and gastric contents. Obstruction, from the use of these drugs, is a possibility in a patient with ulcers near the pylorus. Since obstruction almost always involves some degree of pyloric constriction or stenosis, further reducing the tone of the sphincter with anticholinergics will only make things worse.

The selection of an anticholinergic agent is difficult only because of the sheer number available. All of the newer synthetic compounds are related to the belladonna alkaloids.

These alkaloids are tertiary nitrogen compounds and, as such, have greater central nervous system effects than the quaternary nitrogen compounds, such as propantheline, in equipotent doses. In some patients, this may be the determining factor in the selection of a drug (see Table 9.1).

The dose of any anticholinergic should be titrated against the appearance of side effects. If no side effects are observed at a certain dosage level, it must be assumed that no therapeutic effects are elicited. Tincture of belladonna permits very accurate titrations of dose because small variations in dose may be tried. The newer synthetic compounds are usually only available in tablet or syrup form, somewhat limiting dosage flexibility. The anticholinergics should be administered an hour before meals and at bedtime. The daytime dosage should be high enough to produce *occasional* side effects during the day and the bedtime dosage high enough to produce minor side effects *invariably* in the morning upon awakening. By giving the drug at least 1 hr before meals, maximal therapeutic effect is obtained.

SEDATION

Sedatives or tranquilizers have never been demonstrated to affect the course of peptic ulcers in controlled studies. However, there are specific patients who will benefit from sedation. These are people with a significant anxiety component to their ulcer disease. The drug of choice is phenobarbital 15 to 30 mg 1 hr before meals and at bedtime. Chlordiazepoxide and the other benzodiazepines can be used equally well but they offer no advantages, and they are more expensive. There are no indications for the use of phenothiazines, alone, or in combination in peptic ulcer disease.

REST

Rest is of value in the management of peptic ulcer. It should entail, in the ambulatory patient, reduction of social and business activities as much as practical. Adequate sleep also is important. In severe cases an initial 5- to 7-day period of bed rest at home may be tried, but if this fails or complications are present, hospitalization is necessary.

TABLE 9.1
Anticholinergic Drugs

Natural Alkaloids	Synthetic Esters (Tertiary Amines)	Synthetic Esters (Quaternary Amines)
Atropine	Dicyclomine	Anisotropine
Belladonna extract	Methixene	Diphemanil
Belladonna tincture	Oxyphencyclimine	Glycopyrrolate
Homatropine	Piperidolate	Hexocyclium
	Thiphenamil	Homatropine methylbromide
		Isopropamide
		Mepenzolate
		Methantheline
		Methscopolamine
		Oxyphenonium
		Pentapiperide
		Pipenzolate
		Poldine
		Propantheline
		Tridihexethyl
		Valethamate

DIET[17]

Diet is probably the most controversial and emotionally charged aspect of ulcer therapy. The facts are, however, that with a few exceptions, diets have no clear therapeutic effect on peptic ulcers. This conclusion is supported by a number of well designed clinical studies. By "diet," the authors mean to imply the restriction of various foods and limiting the intake of specific foods, as in a bland diet. There are some dietary principles that should be observed, however. These include nutritious diets, frequent small feedings and regularity of meals. The general diet should be determined by the patient's likes and dislikes without any unreasonable restrictions. Caffeine-containing drinks, however, should be avoided, as well as alcohol. These chemicals will stimulate excessive gastric secretions.

Milk and cream are ineffective antacids. Indeed, there are data to suggest that patients treated with milk and cream have an increased risk of myocardial infarction. It can be said that with a milk and cream regimen you may convert an ulcer patient to one who is overweight and suffering from cardiovascular disease, not to mention ulcers. Any substance, including water, put into the stomach will stimulate secretions. The reason why ulcer patients experience relief of pain after eating food or any other substance is unknown. The fact that milk and bland diets will relieve pain on a transient basis probably accounts for part of their popularity.

RESTRICTIONS

Besides coffee, tea, cola drinks and alcohol, smoking should be discouraged. Although the effect of smoking on gastric secretion is somewhat unpredictable and variable, it has been shown to delay healing. Abstinence from smoking, at least during the acute phase, is recommended.

SURGERY

Surgery becomes necessary in a minority of patients with peptic ulcers and is usually a result of complications, although it may be necessary in those refractory to medical treatment.

PROGNOSIS

If patients can be convinced to adhere to a strict antacid regimen indefinitely, the vast majority will stay well. If they are treated intensively for 5 to 6 months after complete radiological healing and all medications are stopped, the recurrence rate within 2 years is about 35%. Reducing the amount of antacids after healing does not seem to be of benefit and will lead to recurrence.

GASTRIC ULCER

Gastric ulcers are treated in the same manner as duodenal ulcers *except that anticholinergics should not be used.* About 10% of gastric ulcers prove to be due to carcinoma; thus, failure to respond to treatment in 3 to 4 weeks should be regarded as a potential cancer and appropriate measures initiated. Benign gastric ulcers have a better prognosis than duodenal ulcers. The recurrence rate is significantly less.

MARGINAL ULCER

Marginal ulcers occur following surgery for previous peptic ulcers. They usually are a result of an inappropriate choice of procedure to correct the initial ulcer, and as a result, gastric secretions were not effectively diminished. They are treated the same as a duodenal ulcer, but they are frequently more resistant to medical therapy and further surgery is often necessary.

CONCLUSION

Peptic ulcer disease continues to be an incompletely understood disease. There are many variables that contribute to the development of this common disorder. Nevertheless, peptic ulcers are *not* incurable. The authors suspect that the cure rate can be improved by the active participation of pharmacists in advising patients and physicians on the proper role of drug therapy for this disease.

REFERENCES

1. Piper, D. W., and Heap, T. R.: Medical management of peptic ulcers with reference to anti-ulcer agents in other gastro-intestinal diseases. Drugs, 3: 336, 1972.
2. Susser, M.: Causes of peptic ulcer; a selective epidemiologic review. J. Chronic Dis., 20: 435, 1967.
3. Grossman, M. I.: Physiologic approach to medical management of duodenal ulcers. Am. J. Dig. Dis., 6: 56, 1961.
4. Kirsner, J. B.: Peptic ulcer: a review of the recent literature on various clinical aspects, Part 1. Gastroenterology, 54: 611, 1968.
5. Sparberg, M.: The therapy of peptic ulcer disease. Ration. Drug Ther., 7: 1, 1973.
6. Woodbury, D. M.: Analgesic antipyretics, antiinflammatory agents and inhibitors of uric acid synthesis. In The Pharmacological Basis of Therapeutics, Ed. 4, p. 337, edited by L. Goodman and A. Gilman. The MacMillan Co., New York, 1970.
7. Salmon, S. E., and Apple, M.: Cancer chemotherapy. In Review of Medical Pharmacology, Ed. 3, p. 451, edited by F. Meyers, E. Jawetz and A. Goldfien. Lange Medical Publications, Los Altos, 1972.
8. Kirsner, J. B.: Peptic ulcer: a review of the recent literature on various clinical aspects, Part II. Gastroenterology, 54: 945, 1968.
9. Piper, D. W.: Antacid and anticholinergic drug therapy of peptic ulcers. Gastroenterology, 52: 1009, 1967.
10. Hirschman, J. L., and Herfindal, E. T.: Peptic ulcer disease. J. Am. Pharm. Assoc., NS11: 445, 1971.

11. Piper, D. W., and Fenton, B. H.: Antacid therapy of peptic ulcers, Part II: an evaluation of antacids in vitro. Gut, 5: 585, 1964.

12. Fordtran, J. S., Morawski, B. A., and Richardson, C. T.: In vivo and in vitro evaluation of liquid antacids. N. Engl. J. Med., 288: 923, 1973

13. Lotz, M., Zisman, E., and Bartter, F. C.: Evidence for a phosphorus-depletion syndrome in man. N. Engl. J. Med., 278: 409, 1968.

14. Fordtran, J. S.: Acid rebound. N. Engl. J. Med., 279: 900, 1968.

15. Barreras, R. F.: Acid secretion after calcium carbonate in patients with duodenal ulcer. N. Engl. J. Med., 282: 1402, 1970.

16. Anon.: Evaluations of Drug Interactions – 1973. American Pharmaceutical Association, Washington, D.C., p. 98, 136, 1973.

17. Buchman, E., Kanng, D. T., Dolan, K., and Knapp, R. N.: Unrestricted diet in the treatment of duodenal ulcers. Gastroenterology, 56: 1016, 1969.

chapter 10

ULCERATIVE COLITIS

Gary H. Smith, Pharm.D.
Theodore G. Tong, Pharm.D.

Ulcerative colitis is a disease of the bowel which can be characterized by the presence of diffuse inflammation and necrosis of the colonic and rectal mucosa. The clinical course of the disease is complex and unpredictable, and it can be expressed either continuously or intermittently. The duration is almost always prolonged with a wide variety of systemic and local manifestations of varying intensity. Although considered to be the most common of the "idiopathic" inflammatory bowel diseases, ulcerative colitis constitutes only a small proportion of the disorders the pharmacist encouters in his practice. However, the opportunity for a pharmacist to contribute significantly to patient care can be most rewarding since few diseases require more skill, consideration and understanding than ulcerative colitis for successful rehabilitation of those afflicted. As a consequence of pathological changes, ulcerative colitis is associated with many complex, often life-threatening, problems. Prognosis for survival can never be assured on the basis of symptom remission or absence of disease activity alone. Complex problems associated with this disease and its treatment represent a formidable therapeutic challenge for its successful management.

ETIOLOGY

Little is definitely known about the etiology of ulcerative colitis, although investigations into its pathogenesis have been extensive in number and scope. There appear to be multiple pathogenic factors involved, but their relationship to the clinical course, symptoms and response to therapy is still unclear.[1-3] It has been suggested that the etiological agent, possibly a mucolytic enzyme, within the lumen of the bowel, attacks the mucosal surface. This has not been demonstrated by the proponents of this postulate. Neither have bacteria, parasites, fungi, virus or their destructive toxins been successfully demonstrated to be etiological factors. Antibodies reacting with certain fecal anerobic bacteria have been recovered in the rectocolonic mucosa of patients with ulcerative colitis; it remains, however, to be resolved whether this is a reflection of an altered immunological status or an underlying etiological factor.[4] A great deal of emphasis and study recently has been placed on the immunological process as the cause of ulcerative colitis.[5] The pathological changes seen in colitis are compatible with an autoimmune response and frequently are associated with concurrent diseases thought to be autoimmune in nature.[6] Antibodies to colonic epithelial antigens also have been demonstrated.[7] Circulating cytotoxic lymphocytes may be involved since they are present persistently throughout the clinical course of mucosal inflammation, only to disappear soon after surgical removal of the diseased bowel. The precise significance of autoimmunity as a contributing etiological factor remains to be determined. Allergy and sensitivity to certain foods also have been suggested as possible causative factors in this disorder.[8,9]

It is widely held that ulcerative colitis patients are of a particular personality type.[10-12] They are thought to be compulsive, hostile, immature, depressed, and they frequently have difficulties expressing their aggression and sexual identity. The behavior of young patients has been described as obsessive, passive, neurotic and emotionally dependent on a parent. The mother of the child with colitis has often been characterized as being overly strict, punitive and domineering. The impression that the frequency of personality disorders among ulcerative colitis patients is greater than for patients with other medical problems has not been confirmed. Controlled studies have failed to demonstrate any relationship of personality type or psychological factors to the pathogenesis of ulcerative colitis.[13] There is greater acceptance of the association of exacerbations and remissions of colitis with changes in the emotional state once the disease has been established.[1] It appears that the most appropriate approach for the moment is to consider ulcerative colitis as a manifestation of many underlying factors and to monitor its clinical course for complications and empirically provide symptomatic treatment. In the majority of cases, therapy does not offer a permanent cure.

INCIDENCE

The incidence of ulcerative colitis varies from country to country. In the United States the incidence of the population at risk has been estimated to be from 6 to 8 per 100,000 per year.[14] On a worldwide basis the occurrence of the disease is increasing, and the available figures represent perhaps a fraction of the true incidence. Caucasians comprise a significant majority of all cases, and the condition is relatively rare among blacks. The greater frequency among the Jewish population, nearly four times more common, suggests that genetic or ethnic predisposition plays an important etiological role in ulcerative colitis.[15] Observations that the incidence of inflammatory bowel disease is higher among Israeli Jews of occidental rather than oriental extraction and the equal occurrence of the disorder in American Jews from rural or urban backgrounds support impressions that the occurrence of colitis is significantly influenced by genetics.[16,17] About 10 to 15% of patients with ulcerative colitis also have a family history of inflammatory bowel dis-

orders.[17,18] Environment does not, however, appear to be a significant factor since non-familial individuals living with families which have a predilection for ulcerative colitis have not demonstrated a greater tendency to develop this disease than the general population.[19] The disease appears to be evenly distributed between the sexes although a number of studies indicate a three to two preponderance of male children to female children with colitis.[3,20] Although it affects all ages, ulcerative colitis is considered to be a disease of adolescents and young adults. The majority of cases occur initially between the 1st and 4th decade of life, with peak rate of occurrence in the 3rd decade.[14] The relationship between age and the incidence of the disease remains unclear.

PATHOPHYSIOLOGY

Ulcerative colitis is an inflammatory and suppurative process which involves the mucosa and submucosa of the colon. Involvement at its onset is usually most active in the rectum and distal colon, progressing proximally to other portions of the colon in a continuous manner. The extent of colonic disruption varies considerably, with nearly 50% of the patients developing "universal" colitis with involvement of the entire length of the colon. The intensity of colitis varies throughout the clinical course. It may be acutely fulminant and severe or gradual with chronic recurrences of exacerbations and remissions. The morbidity and mortality risks are greatest during severe attacks where extensive total or near total colonic involvement is present. Relapses are quite common with more than half of them experienced within a year following the acute episode. About 25 to 30% of patients during their initial attack will unexpectedly present with the pathology of universal colitis similar to that encountered in patients with a history of long term colitis. A small proportion (less than 10%) of patients have ulcerative proctitis where the disease is confined to the rectum and distal sigmoid colon only. Patients with extensive colonic involvement and severe symptoms must be vigorously and rationally managed medically. Surgery must be considered where hemorrhage is acute, perforation is imminent, sepsis a complication or medical means have been unsuccessful in alleviating the acute attack.

DIAGNOSIS AND CLINICAL FINDINGS

The clinical history of patients with ulcerative colitis usually reveals the presence of bloody purulent diarrhea often of long duration. Many patients initially experience only mild rectal bleeding with either normal bowel function or mild constipation. As the bleeding gradually increases, bowel movements become greater in frequency, a characteristic of colitis. Abdominal cramping and pain are common, particularly during the early stages of the disease. The patient with advanced colitis may have as many as 30 to 40 watery, purulent and bloody bowel movements throughout the day and night. Incontinence may develop during severe episodes. When the disease is in remission or inactive, the bowel may appear to be functioning normally. Constipation is often experienced by patients with colitis limited to the rectum. In some patients, usually those with disease of greater severity and extensive colonic involvement, the symptoms are acute and occur abruptly with intense diarrhea, severe abdominal cramping, pain and rectal bleeding. Malaise, weakness, easy fatigability, mild fever, pallor, dehydration and abdominal tenderness are usually observed on physical examination in the patients with active colitis. Local and systemic manifestations involving the skin and joints are frequently encountered. Weight loss, deficiency anemias and avitaminosis are not uncommon since anorexia and malabsorption are frequently experienced during acute and chronic periods of the disease. Hematological evaluation frequently reveals a hypochromic anemia which parallels the course of the disease. During active periods of colitis, slight to moderate leukocytosis and elevated erythrocyte sedimentation rates can be seen. The clinical impression of ulcerative colitis can not be firmly established without sigmoidoscopic and radiological examination. Edema and hyperemia of the colonic mucosa are early sigmoidoscopic findings. As the disease becomes more active, ulcerations and infiltration by inflammatory cells are seen in the mucosa of the rectum and the sigmoid colon. Uniform and continuous enlargement and coalescence of ulcerations spreading to the submucosa occur as the extent and activity of the colitis progress. The bowel becomes thickened, scarred and inflexible with narrowing of the lumen as a result of continuous disease activity or episodes of exacerbation. Abdominal pain often diminishes during the later stages of the clinical course and is responsible for the erroneous impression that the disease has become less active or extensive. As a result, therapeutic management is often abated or even discontinued. Invariably the symptoms recur as a consequence. The clinical course most frequently consists of spontaneous remissions and relapses varying in severity and duration. The unpredictable and remitting pattern of this disorder may continue for years. For some patients permanent remission may be possible while for others symptoms evolve gradually into a chronic continuous course. Radiological examination establishes the extent of colonic involvement in ulcerative colitis. It can reveal significant information with respect to the degree of mucosal and luminal changes and the presence of localized complications. Rectal biopsy in mild cases of colitis may also provide more information for a definitive diagnosis. The differentiation of ulcerative colitis from a number of conditions with a similar clinical course and symptoms must always be considered during the diagnostic procedure. Serum electrolytes, proteins, liver function and other changes which diagnostically reflect the sequelae of ulcerative colitis or complications arising from its treatment must be monitored. Selection of appropriate treatment and assessment of therapeutic responsiveness must be done using the results of such tests while concurrently considering the clinical symptoms of the disease.

COMPLICATIONS

A variety of systemic and extracolonic complications can occur as a consequence of ulcerative colitis. Anemia due to occult blood loss and depletion of body iron stores is a frequent problem, especially where disease involvement is extensive.[21] Hemoglobin levels lower than 30% gm, hypochromic microcytic red cells on peripheral blood smear, low serum iron and elevated total serum iron-binding capacity characteristically are seen. Factors other than blood loss appear to be of minor significance as a source of anemia.[22] Hemolysis is rarely a primary cause of anemia in ulcerative colitis. Few cases of acquired secondary autoimmune hemolytic anemia in ulcerative colitis have been reported.[23] These patients present with fever, slight jaundice, tachycardia, hemoglobin of less than 7 g%, thrombocytopenia and marked reticulocytosis.[24] A situation which merits special attention is the occurrence of hemolytic anemia following salicylazosulfapyridine (Azulfidine, Salazopyrin) therapy in erythrocyte glucose-6-phosphate dehydrogenase (G-6-PD)-deficient individuals. Several cases have been reported in which several black patients with ulcerative colitis have developed hemolytic anemia following salicylazosulfapyridine.[25] Appropriate laboratory studies should be monitored when salicylazosulfapyridine or any other sulfonamide is used in high risk individuals such as black males or caucasians of Sardinian descent.[26] A rare condition known as Heinz-Ehrlich body anemia has been reported to occur following salicylazosulfapyridine administration but reversed subsequent to its withdrawal.[27]

Deficiencies in vitamin K and erythropoietic factors such as vitamin B_{12} and folic acid can occur after longer periods of malnutrition or when malabsorption is the result of the disease involvement extending into the terminal ileum of the small intestine. Thrombophlebitis, platelet deficiency, cardiac and thyroid abnormalities have been associated with extracolonic complications of ulcerative colitis. Severe electrolyte abnormalities, particularly with hypokalemia and acid-base imbalances, frequently complicate the clinical course of the disease.

Toxic megacolon is the most severe and acute consequence of ulcerative colitis.[28] Extreme distention or "toxic dilation" of the colon is an ominous prognostic sign deserving immediate and intensive treatment. Perforation and peritonitis are the most often feared consequences of toxic megacolon. Development of this complication is usually preceded by a rapidly deteriorating and fulminating clinical course with symptoms of severe toxicity. Patients who develop toxic megacolon most frequently have involvement of the entire colon or of the left colon. The development of this extremely severe complication is influenced by the severity of the colitis rather than its dura-

tion; therefore, it may even occur during the initial episode of colitis, or during an exacerbation of the remitting type.[28] Symptoms may suggest infarction, perforation, septicemia or partial obstruction. Appearing quite ill, the patient will have fever, leukocytosis, abdominal distention and bloody, purulent diarrhea. A decrease in the number of bowel movements without clinical improvement is not an uncommon experience. Many factors have been alleged to precipitate toxic megacolon.[3,29] However, evidence of association between its occurrence and these factors remains equivocal and circumstantial. The use of corticosteroids in acute colitis is not invariably related to the development of colonic distention or perforation.[30] Barium enemas should, however, be postponed until the disease is less acute since the further distention of an overly dilated colon could have disastrous consequences.[31,32] Table 10.1 summarizes the drugs which could complicate the diagnosis, course or treatment of ulcerative colitis.

Hepatobiliary abnormalities in the form of inflammatory liver changes are experienced by patients with ulcerative colitis. In 3 to 4% of the patients, generally those with long standing and extensive disease involvement, cirrhosis will develop.[38] This is the most serious of the hepatic complications associated with ulcerative colitis and increases the risk of morbidity and premature death. Fatty hepatic infiltrations are a frequent consequence of nutritional disturbances in the colitis patient. Resolution of relatively minor and nonspecific type hepatic changes usually occurs as the clinical course improves.[34] However, the prognosis for cirrhosis and pericholangitis is not related as clearly to the clinical course.[35]

Ulcerative colitis patients frequently experience a rheumatoid type of arthritis. Unlike the classical presentation of rheumatoid disease, the rheumatoid factor is absent from the circulation. The arthritis is usually a disorder affecting the joints of the lower limbs. Nodules are absent. The severity of symptoms will often parallel the clinical course of the colitis, although ankylosing spondylitis and sacroiliitis may progressively worsen in spite of remission of the colitis.[36]

Skin abnormalities such as erythema nodosum, erythema multiforme and purpura are common in ulcerative colitis. Lesions tend to

TABLE 10.1
Untoward Effects of Drugs on Ulcerative Colitis

Drug	Comment
A. Drugs associated with "ulcerative colitis-like" syndrome[a]	
1. Antibiotics[109-113]	
Chloromycetin Neomycin Penicillin Tetracycline Chlortetracycline Sulfonamides Ampicillin[b]	Pseudomembranous enterocolitis; a necrotizing inflammatory process affecting the mucosa of the ileum and colon; symptoms of fever, abdominal pain, oliguria, fulminating diarrhea, hypotension and collapse are experienced and appear abruptly 4-6 days following intestinal surgery, injury or antibiotic therapy; broad spectrum antibiotics are most frequently implicated; increased risk also associated with use of postoperative systemic antibiotics after preoperative courses of antibiotics; suspect resistant *Staphylococcus aureus* in postantibiotic enteritis but not always a consistent finding; combination antibiotic therapy and even penicillin alone have been associated with occurrence
Lincomycin[114,115] Clindamycin[116]	Patients receiving oral lincomycin or its congener subsequently may develop fulminant diarrhea; sigmoidoscopy reveals hyperemic and friable colonic mucosa without ulcerations; barium enema often will show mucosal changes consistent with inflammatory bowel disease; diarrhea is not uncommon following oral lincomycin; however, in cases developing protracted ulcerative colitis-like symptoms, pseudomembranous enterocolitis should be ruled out
Oral Contraceptives[117-122]	Ulcerative colitis-like symptoms and sigmoidoscopic examination following oral contraceptives suggest vascular occlusion of the distal ileum and colon in several case reports; remission of symptoms following discontinuation of drug suggests causal relationship
Chlorpropamide[123]	Edema and multiple small ulcerations of rectal and sigmoid mucosa following 500 mg for 5 days for mild hyperglycemia; concurrent exfoliative dermatitis suggests allergic disorder
5-Fluorouracil[124]	Colonic mucosal ulceration and necrosis very similar to findings of chronic ulcerative colitis have appeared in patients receiving this drug; gastrointestinal effects are commonly experienced by patients taking this drug; most of the difficulties and symptoms stop following discontinuation of drug administration
Cyclophosphamide[125]	Gastrointestinal symptoms are commonly experienced particularly with higher doses; acute hemorrhagic colitis has been reported following long term and short term cyclophosphamide administration with return to normal soon following discontinuation of therapy
6-Mercaptopurine[126]	Reports suggest intestinal ulceration is an often overlooked complication from this chemotherapeutic agent
Soap suds[127]	Colon became edematous and inflamed without ulceration following use as an enema during labor
Phenylbutazone[128,129]	Inflammatory infiltrate and ulcer of sigmoid colon following long term use reported in one patient; remission of symptoms on discontinuation and subsequent return when drug was reintroduced suggests a common etiology

TABLE 10.1–*Continued*

Drug	Comment
Gold[130]	Clinical and radiographic evidence of colitis, esophagitis, gastritis or enteritis following gold therapy should arouse suspicion of toxicity
Lithium carbonate[131]	Underlying gastrointestinal disorder may be exacerbated; one manic depressive patient reportedly developed "acute abdomen" soon after lithium therapy was begun; diagnosed as regional enteritis; diarrhea continued for several months until lithium was discontinued
Laxatives, cathartics[132-134]	Radiographic appearance of chronic inflammatory bowel has been seen in patients following excessive and chronic use of laxatives and cathartics
Digitalis[135]	Cases of enterocolitis with acute hemorrhagic necrosis of the bowel have been described in patients with congestive failure and receiving high doses of digitalis; some of these patients had definite symptoms of digitalis toxicity; whether this is a causal relationship between colitis and therapy for congestive failure remains to be established

B. Drugs associated with production of paralytic ileus
   1. Anticholinergics[29,136]

Drug	Comment
Atropine	Therapeutic doses have been demonstrated to have an inhibitory effect on colonic motility and tone; the use of anticholinergic antispasmodics for the control of diarrhea in fulminant colitis contributes little therapeutically in moderate to severe colitis since colonic tonus is already diminished; diarrhea is symptomatic of the inflammatory activity, not of hypermotility

   2. Antidepressants[137-139]

Drug	Comment
Nortriptyline Imipramine Amitriptyline[140,141]	Anticholinergic side effects have been associated with paralytic ileus in several reported cases; concomitant use of drugs with anticholinergic side effects, *i.e.,* phenothiazines, tricyclic antidepressants, antiparkinsonian drugs, should be closely monitored, particularly in the older schizophrenic or severely depressed patient or any with a concomitant disorder such as hypothyroidism

   3. Anticoagulant[142-145]

Drug	Comment
Dicumarol	Intestinal obstruction occurs secondary to intraperitoneal or intra-abdominal hemorrhage; partial or complete mechanical obstruction by an adynamic condition may be produced by intestinal hematomas; presence of echymoses, epitaxis, bloody stools with symptoms indicative of obstruction should arouse suspicion; associated with long term anticoagulant use before onset of acute abdomen
Phenidione[146]	Severe hemorrhagic colitis occurring several days after administration of drug reported in 2 patients

   4. Antihypertensives

Drug	Comment
Mecamylamine[148] Hexamethonium[149] Pentolinium tartrate[150,151] Reserpine Hydralazine	Paralytic ileus due to parasympatholytic effects of sympatholytic antihypertensives; cases reported often involve combinations of these agents used in attempts to enhance antihypertensive effects; abdominal pain is prominent feature of ileus induced by ganglionic blockade unlike "classical" paralytic ileus or acute abdomen

TABLE 10.1—*Continued*

Drug	
5. Narcotics[29,93] Meperidine Tincture of opium Tincture of paregoric Diphenoxylate	In usual therapeutic doses are potent inhibitors of gastrointestinal motility; toxic dilation of the colon has occurred in patients with mild to moderate severe ulcerative colitis; colonic motility in fulminant colitis is already impaired; diarrhea is a reflection of the generalized inflammatory activity, and treatment must be directed at managing the underlying causes; there is no therapeutic rationale for using narcotics in such situations since they can contribute to further problems such as paralytic ileus and the development of toxic dilation of the colon
6. Phenothiazines[119,136,152] Chlorpromazine Mepazine	Cases have been reported; paralytic ileus probably secondary to anticholinergic side-effects; in one report, the patient had myxedema concurrently
7. Barium enema[32]	Rapid distention of the acutely inflamed colon can induce toxic dilation and perforation
8. Others[153-155] Methocarbamol[156] Antacids[157] Diphenoxylate[158]	

[a]A patient who experiences "colitis-like" symptoms during or soon after therapy with a drug of which diarrhea is a known or suspected side effect or complication should always be evaluated for gastrointestinal disease; the reaction should not simply be considered an idiopathic or unique "sensitivity" to the agent.

[b]Schapiro, R. L., and Newman, A.: Acute enterocotitis. Radiology, 108: 263, 1972.

necrose and form chronic ulcers on the lower limbs. The severity of these dermatological disorders are greatest during periods of exacerbation of the colitis. Pyoderma gangrenosum is a rare dermatological disorder seen only in ulcerative colitis patients. Appearing usually on the limbs, these bullae-like lesions resembling "bedsores" produce chronic and severe ulcerations.[37] The onset, duration or severity of this condition, however, does not correlate well with either the extent or severity of the ulcerative colitis.[38] Aphthous ulcers of the mouth are also common. Conjunctivitis, iritis, uveitis, blepharitis and corneal ulcerations are inflammatory eye disorders which often accompany active colitis.[39] They tend to be recurrent and have been experienced during all stages of the systemic disease. The association of ulcerative colitis with many of the extracolonic disorders remains unclear; however, the suggestion that the etiology of the disease is an underlying autoimmune or hyperimmune response receives much support from their apparent relationship.

Patients with inflammatory bowel disease often have elevated concentrations of serum calcium and uric acid and appear to be predisposed to formation of renal stones.[40,41] However, the pathogenesis of nephrolithiasis in patients with colitis is poorly understood.

Prognosis for long term survival is least promising for those patients who develop ulcerative colitis during childhood or after the age of 60. Children often experience a more fulminant clinical course and respond more poorly to medical management than adults.[41] Physical growth often is severely impaired by the disease in children.[42] The risk of mortality from ulcerative colitis is greatest where the onset of symptoms is rapid, colonic involvement is extensive and severe and the patient is very young or old.[41] Carcinoma of the colon occurs more frequently among colitis patients than in the general population. This risk of malignancy increases proportionately with the duration of disease and is greatest for those patients whose disease began in childhood. It has been estimated that mortality from carcinoma increases by 20% during each decade of the disease beginning after the lst decade.[43] The survival rate of colitis patients with colonic carcinoma is significantly lower than in patients with colonic carcinoma only.[44] The predilection of carcinoma for the rectum and sigmoid colon in the general population is less well delineated for the colitis patient where malignancies in the tranverse and ascending colon are not uncommon.[39] It is quite likely that the manifestation of neoplasms in colitis patients is frequently erroneously associated with the underlying disorder, thus delaying surgery and other means for eradicating the neoplasm and quite possibly contributing to the higher mortality.[45] An awareness of the extracolonic and systemic manifestations of the disease is necessary for the early recognition and management of complications secondary to ulcerative colitis since their amelioration may significantly influence the prognosis of the high risk patients.[1,46]

TREATMENT

The goal of treatment in ulcerative colitis is to provide relief from symptoms and complications, correct deficiency states and attempt to arrest or reverse the disease process. Tailoring treatment for a disorder which is expressed by a variety of manifestations, complications and obscure etiology is a formidable task. The unpredictable clinical course, with its spontaneous remissions and exacerbations and the subjectivity by which therapeutic effectiveness is assessed, intensifies the dilemma of selecting the most appropriate and rational therapy for ulcerative colitis. Drug therapy for ulcerative colitis is nonspecific and directed against factors which have been suspected to play a role in the etiology of the disease. Agents used in the treatment of inflammatory bowel disease may be divided conveniently into those that have been found to influence the clinical course and those that correct deficiency states. Therapeutic failure with medical management and the presence of life-threatening complications are important indications for surgery.

Antimicrobials

Clinical experience with the use of antimicrobials for the treatment of ulcerative colitis has been confined primarily to the sulfon-amides.[47,48] Salicylazosulfapyridine, a diazo-linked combination of salicylic acid and sulfa-pyridine, has been the mainstay of therapy of most clinicians.[37,49] The choice of salicylazosulfapyridine is based on the widely held impression that it has been found more effective than any other sulfonamide for controlling ulcerative colitis. However, there is no clinical evidence supporting the superiority of any one of the sulfonamides, e.g., sulfasoxazole, sulfathalidine, sulfasuxidine or salicylazosulfapyridine, over another. Reliable studies have demonstrated that sulfonamides reduce the severity of colitis and the occurrence of relapses.[50] The basis for the successful use of sulfonamides in ulcerative colitis is unclear. Alteration of intestinal bacterial flora does not appear to be the mode of action.[51] It has been thought that salicylazosulfapyridine, having been demonstrated to possess an affinity for connective tissue, exerts a nonspecific anti-inflammatory effect on the surface of the colonic wall.[52,53] However, since ulcerative colitis affects primarily the colonic mucosa and submucosa, it remains equivocal whether affinity of the agent for connective tissue is the reason for its effectiveness.

The usual dosage of salicylazosulfapyridine recommended for maintenance therapy is 2 gm daily in divided doses for several weeks to months until symptoms are completely resolved. Higher doses of 4 to 8 g have been employed by some clinicians for the treatment of active and acute disease, although there is little evidence to demonstrate that this adds any real benefit to therapy or produces more effective control of the colitis. Higher doses of salicylazosulfapyridine do not reduce the occurrence of relapses and in fact usually contribute only to intensifying its side effects. Concomitant administration of corticosteroids with salicylazosulfapyridine has been successful in controlling moderate to acute symptoms.[54] Whether therapy with sulfonamides is to be continued intermittently or indefinitely should be determined by the frequency of relapses and the success of the regimen in maintaining the patient in a relatively asymptomatic state. In a few paitents with mild disease and limited colonic involvement, sulfonamides may eventually be discontinued when remission of the active disease has been present for a year or more. During acute episodes of fulminating colitis, *i.e.*, toxic megacolon, the use of oral sulfonamides including salicylazosulfapyridine appears to serve little purpose. Administration of rationally selected antibiotics parenterally is certainly an appropriate and worthwhile consideration in severe toxic dilation of the colon, threatened perforation or suspected secondary infection.

The incidence of severe untoward effects of salicylazosulfapyridine is relatively low, although minor reactions range from occasional to frequent. It can be expected that 20 to 30% of the patients receiving salicylazosulfapyridine on short term therapy will experience unpleasant side effects, usually gastrointestinal in nature. Intolerance to the gastrointestinal effects can possibly be overcome by taking the medication during meals or by gradually increasing the dose as tolerated to reach optimal therapeutic levels. Enteric-coated salicylazosulfapyridine tablets are available, however, there is no clinical evidence available to demonstrate their comparative effectiveness or toxicities with the plain tablets in ulcerative colitis patients.

Table 10.2 summarizes the untoward effects from salicylazosulfapyridine. Investigation into the absorption, metabolism and excretion of salicylazosulfapyridine and its metabolites following single dose and repeated dosage administration in man was recently reported.[55] The investigators concluded that the serum concentration of salicylazosulfapyridine is determined by highly individualized rates of absorption. About one-third of the dose absorbed is unchanged salicylazosulfapyridine while the remaining portion is reduced by the gut flora in the cecum and colon to sulfapyridine and 5-aminosalicylic acid. Further absorption then occurs in the large intestine. Only a small portion of salicylazosulfapyridine is recovered unchanged in the urine and feces.

It has been suggested recently that the capacity to metabolize salicylazosulfapyridine by acetylation may influence the onset and severity of its adverse effects. In an experimental study with healthy individuals who were given 4 gm daily on a short term basis, the slow acetylators experienced earlier and more pronounced side effects than normals or rapid acetylators. This phenomenon is not unique in therapeutics but rather reminiscent of the higher incidence of polyneuropathy in patients receiving isoniazid who were considered to be slow acetylators.[56]

Ampicillin is claimed to be as effective as the sulfonamides for the treatment of ulcerative colitis. However, clinical evaluations remain to be performed, and for the present the success of ampicillin in the treatment of colitis should be considered as preliminary observations and primarily anecdotal.

Corticosteroids

Corticosteroids are therapeutically effective in producing remission of active ulcerative colitis. Their mode of action is considered to be primarily by suppression of inflammatory activity, and their effectiveness supports the impression that an abnormally responsive immune system is significant etiological factor in ulcerative colitis.

Corticosteroids rapidly reduce the severity of acute colitis but they can not alter the basic disease process. Their use during periods of remission or in chronic continuous type colitis is controversial. Although relapses have been experienced following the discontinuation of corticosteroids, there is no evidence to justify their use as a prophylactic measure against recurrence.[57] The risk from their long term use has to be considered greater than any benefit which may be achieved by such use in ulcerative colitis.

Systemic corticosteroids should be given by the intravenous route in cases of severe colitis. The usual dose during acute episodes is 60 to 80 mg of prednisone or equivalent doses of hydrocortisone per day. Although hydrocortisone is recommended most frequently for intravenous use, it has salt- and water-retaining activity which may be undesirable where large doses are to be used and for prolonged periods. The dose of corticosteroid required to achieve the therapeutic response must be determined for every patient individually, based on the severity of symptoms and clinical course. Although the incidence of adverse effects from corticosteroids varies considerably, they are related to the amount and type administered and duration of therapy. The smallest possible dose needed to produce rapid and sustained improvement should be used. This dosage is then maintained unless symptoms are exacerbated or until the patient has improved sufficiently enough to

TABLE 10.2
Untoward Effects from Salicylazosulfapyridine[a]

Complaints	Comments
A. Minor	
Headache, nausea, gastrointestinal distress, arthralgia	These complaints comprise the majority of side effects experienced from this drug[159] ; Apparently dose-related, these complaints have been minimized by reducing the dosage; increasing the frequency of administration with smaller dose might be a worthwhile attempt
Dermatological reations[160]	Sulfonamides produce a spectrum of cutaneous reactions ranging from minor pruritus to life-threatening and even fatal toxic epidermal necrosis; dermatological reactions are not uncommon with the class of drugs having salicylazosulfapyridine as a member
Urine discoloration	Orange discoloration of alkaline urine; no color change in acid urine; should inform patient to avoid undue alarm
B. Major[b]	
Agranulocytosis[159,161,165]	The most serious of untoward effects induced by salicylazosulfapyridine; appears to be an allergic reaction; cutaneous reactions often precede the detection of agranulocytosis; complaints of sore throat, chills, fever or appearance of rash should arouse suspicion of this life-threatening reaction
Hemolytic anemia[25,166]	Particularly important in G-6-PD-deficient individuals
Heinz body anemia[27,167]	Heinz bodies occurred following salicylazopyridine administration; immediate return to normal following discontinuation of drug
Cholestatic hepatitis[168]	Bilirubin levels increased following salicylazosulfapyridine in several patients who also had cholestatic jaundice; sulfonamides have been implicated in drug-induced cholestatic hepatitis
Pancreatitis[169]	Epigastric distress and marked elevation of serum amylase occurred following administration of salicylazosulfapyridine; the association of sulfonamide derivatives with the occurrence of pancreatitis is known; pancreatitis may be overlooked since gastrointestinal side effects most frequently encountered are considered benign; in colitis, patient's symptoms may be erroneously construed as originating from underlying inflammatory disorder rather than drug-induced
Serum sickness-like syndrome[170]	A patient reported to have experienced serum sickness, skin rash, hemolytic anemia, plasmacytosis, lymphocytosis and elevation of immunoglobulins; A hypersensitivity reaction most likely cause; A patient with the allergic history of sulfonamide or salicylate sensitivity should not receive salicylazosulfapyridine
Systemic lupus erythematosus[171–173]	Several patients with chronic ulcerative colitis experienced onset or exacerbation of symptoms compatible with systemic lupus erythematosus when given sulfonamides; sulfonamides have been documented to elicit clinical manifestations of systemic lupus erythematosus in susceptible individuals
Impaired folic acid absorption[174]	Recent study demonstrated folic acid malabsorption in patients with ulcerative colitis is not an uncommon experience and can be further aggravated by Azulfidine therapy; additonal studies will be required for clinical significance and precise pharmacological mechanism of the impaired folate uptake by Azulfidine

[a]Adverse reactions to drugs of the sulfonamide class have been reported to involve all major organ systems, and the severity can range from mild discomfort to severe life-threatening reactions. The use of such agents is always accompanied by risk of complications; and an awareness of their clinical manifestations and significance and factors which contribute to their occurrence must always be exercised. Also beware of clinical significant drug-drug interactions associated with sulfonamides such as potentiation of hypoglycemic effects of sulfonylureas or increasing the anticoagulant activity of coumarin and its derivatives, etc.

[b]Incidence reported relatively infrequent to date.

have the corticosteroids decreased or withdrawn.

Oral corticosteroids can be given to the patient whose condition has improved sufficiently to allow the discontinuation of intravenous administration or who is able to tolerate oral intake. Although the goal of therapy is to improve the condition to where corticosteroids are no longer required, too rapid or premature withdrawal can result in undesirable consequences. The dosage regimen must be gradually reduced following long term use, minimizing the risk of recurrence of disease activity or adrenal-hypothalmic-pituitary insufficiency. Many of the undesirable side effects experienced following chronic therapy can be avoided if large doses of corticosteroids are given systemically over a short interval of several days to a week. Adrenal insufficiency is not seen following parenteral corticosteroids when the duration of therapy does not exceed 3 or 4 days. However, coincident diseases such as peptic ulcer, diabetes, psychological and cardiovascular disease can be exacerbated even following short term corticosteroid therapy.

When prolonged corticosteroid therapy is necessary for control of chronic severe colitis unresponsive to medical management, an alternate day single dose regimen has been suggested as a desirable method of treatment.[58] The risk of significant complications, especially adrenal insufficiency, is minimized by the intermittent administration of a cumulative single 48-hr dose every other day. The dose is given in the early morning in order to simulate the normal diurnal pattern of endogenous steroid secretion. Comparisons of the effect of giving corticosteroids in divided daily doses with alternate day therapy in ulcerative colitis patients have demonstrated less adrenal suppression during intermittent therapy; however, whether clinical effectiveness is equivalent to the daily continuous regimen of therapy is equivocal. Adrenal insufficiency and growth suppression following the long term use of corticosteroids must always be considered serious complications. Children with ulcerative colitis preferably should be treated with high doses of corticosteroids on a short term basis to induce remission, and long term therapy with these agents should be avoided if at all possible. Alternate day corticosteroid therapy has reportedly been successful in remitting symptoms without adrenal suppression in several children.[59,60] More studies of the long term effects of intermittent therapy on the clinical course of the disease in children is required.

Corticosteroids instilled intrarectally can provide beneficial relief from symptoms of colitis.[61] Extemporaneous preparations of various salts of hydrocortisone in vehicles such as safflower oil or propylene glycol or commercially available preparations for retention enema are the most popular forms of local treatment used in colitis.[52] Enemas can be given once or twice daily during active colitis or intermittently depending upon the severity of symptoms, response and clinical course. The therapeutic effect appears to be local on the colonic mucosa rather than systemic. Reports of the use of many different hydrocortisone salts in this manner show considerable variation in the amount of systemic absorption that occurs.[63,65] Studies have reported 30 to 50% absorption for hydrocortisone; the variation for systemic absorption with prednisolone is even greater. Hydrocortisone hemisuccinate is absorbed significantly, and the acetate is less readily absorbed than the alcohol. Since there is no apparent correlation between the therapeutic effects of locally instilled hydrocortisone with the degree of systemic absorption and adrenal suppression, the acetate salt, having the least capacity for absorption, would be preferred.[66-68] Patients with active colitis confined to the rectum and distal sigmoid colon respond well to this form of therapy.[69,70] There is evidence that intrarectal hydrocortisone can spread as far proximally as the midtransverse colon. Patients with extensive colonic involvement therefore may benefit from this form of treatment. If improvement is not apparent soon after intrarectal administration of corticosteroids, systemic administration should be initiated. Azulfidine and intermittent courses of topical corticosteroids may induce a reasonable state of health in children and eventual remission where colitis involvement is limited to the left and transverse colon.[62]

Ill afforded delays in the diagnosis and treatment of severe fulminant colitis may occur when corticosteroids are used because symptoms of peritonitis and perforation may unknowingly be masked by them. Opinions vary as to the contribution which corticosteroids make in increasing the operative mortality of colitis, but it appears that the complication rate reflects the severity of the disease and associated complications.[71-73] The mortality rate is increased when surgical intervention is attempted late in the course of acute, severe colitis regardless of whether corticosteroids are used. It is also important to consider that normal adrenal responsiveness will be suppressed during long term use of corticosteroids and will continue to be for many months even after complete withdrawal. Therefore, during periods of increased stress such as infection, surgery or exacerbation of colitis corticosteroids should be given in adequate amounts since pituitary and adrenal reserves may be partially or totally compromised. Judicious and rational use of corticosteroids will provide profound amelioration of the patient's symptoms, but it can never be curative. Therapy with corticosteroids is not a replacement for conventional therapy but is to be used concomitantly with rest, diet and supportive care. While corticosteroids have definitely been proven to be beneficial for the treatment of ulcerative colitis, their potential adverse effects and precautions which accompany their use should never be ignored or overlooked.[74,75]

Some clinicians prefer to use adrenal corticotropin (ACTH) alone or in combination with corticosteroids in the management of ulcerative colitis.[76,77] Although complications of adrenal and growth suppression are avoided, opinions remain divided as to the appropriateness of ACTH in the management of ulcerative colitis. There are no reliable or conclusive studies which demonstrate the superiority of ACTH over corticosteroids in the treatment of this disease. Stimulation of the adrenal gland with ACTH, either intermittently or concurrently as suggested by some clinicians, in attempts to restore or maintain adrenal cortical responsiveness is controversial. A greater suppression may be produced by such attempts than with steroids given alone. Any patient who has received corticosteroids on a long term basis should not be administered ACTH since the secretory capacity of his adrenals are very likely to be impaired and unresponsive. In acute fulminating colitis, systemic corticosteroids are preferred over ACTH since high doses of cortico-

steroids can be given rapidly with good assurance of predictable and reliable results.

Immunosuppressants

Immunosuppressive agents have been used in selected cases of ulcerative colitis.[78-81] There are reports which suggest that azathioprine (Imuran) used on a short term basis improved the condition of colitis patients who were refractory to conventional medical management.[82] The long term effects of these agents used for colitis still remains to be evaluated. Controlled evaluation of immunosuppressants is lacking. Preliminary reports of encouraging results are based on experience with patients who were concomitantly receiving corticosteroids and sulfonamides.[83] The dosage of azathioprine to produce clinical improvement remains a controversial issue. Patients in acute, toxic dilation should definitely not receive immunosuppressants.[84] A major drawback for their potential widespread use is that nearly all the patients receiving immunosuppressants reportedly developed some adverse effect. Therapy with 6-mercaptopurine for ulcerative colitis has largely been abandoned owing to the high incidence of toxic effects. Cyclophosphamide (Cytoxan) has also been utilized, but evidence suggesting it has any additional benefits over other immunosuppressants is equivocal. Until the role of autoimmunity and hyperimmune activity is better understood as an etiological factor in ulcerative colitis, the use of immunosuppressants is largely empirical.

Therapy of Anemia

The frequency with which ulcerative colitis patients experience iron deficiency anemia indicates that the body iron stores should be replenished.[21] Transfusion of whole blood is preferred for patients in acute colitis who become extremely anemic because of blood loss. Iron therapy should be reserved until the acute inflammatory activity has subsided since bone marrow utilization of iron apparently is diminished during these episodes.[85] After the acute attack, oral iron therapy can be initiated, provided there is no exacerbation of the condition. Therapy should be continued on a daily regimen until the depleted body stores of iron have completely been replenished. The course of iron therapy should be at least 3 to 6 months since the capacity for iron absorption returns to its preanemia state as the hemoglobin levels are restored and the deficiency is corrected. Continuous iron therapy should be considered for those patients who experience chronic relapses until successful remission is assured by either medical or surgical intervention.

Iron-containing products range from simple iron salts to combinations of iron, liver and vitamin B_{12} with concentrates of intrinsic factor. Ferrous sulfate tablets are the least expensive and the most efficient means of treating simple iron deficiency anemias.[86] Since many patients often complain of unpleasant side effects from such treatment, many substances have been added to iron preparations supposedly to enhance the absorption of iron while minimizing the side effects.[87] Claims that such fixed combinations are a more effective form of iron preparation should be examined very critically. There is little to choose between ferrous, lactate, carbonate, fumarate, glycine, glutamate, gluconate or sulfate in regard to absorption. Studies which have claimed the superiority of one iron preparation in many cases are based on poor experimental methods and uncritical evaluations. Iron therapy in any form will produce more side effects than placebo, and it is equivocal whether there are real differences in effectiveness and acceptability between the various forms of iron preparation. The gastrointestinal intolerance, which is the most common side effect, appears to be a function of the total amount of iron available in the preparation.[88] Nausea, vomiting, epigastric pain and other gastrointestinal discomforts can be avoided or minimized by advising that these preparations be taken with meals or that dosing be gradually increased until side effects occur or optimal dose is attained. The drawback of such recommendations is that less than optimal or desired amounts of iron may be assimilated, delaying the time for total recovery of body iron stores. However, iron deficiency is rarely a life-threatening experience, and concern for its immediate correction in the majority of ulcerative colitis patients is not warranted.

Injectable iron can be considered when the patient is unable to tolerate oral iron preparations, is unreliable or noncompliant with medications or has impaired absorption of iron. Iron dextran (Imferon) is the most commonly used parenteral preparation. Side effects experienced following intramuscular injection of iron have included local pain, skin discoloration, gastrointestinal disturbances, weakness, headache, flushing and muscle and joint pains. Systemic toxicities reportedly occur in fewer than 1% of patients receiving parenteral iron. The onset of reactions such as urticaria, rash and, rarer, bronchospasm, hypotension, tachycardia and analphylaxis is rapid, usually within 10 min following administration. Iron dextran can also be administered by the intravenous route.[89] Side effects following intravenous administration have not been shown to be of any greater severity or rate of occurrence than by the intramuscular route. The advantages of the intravenous over the intramuscular route are: the total dose can be given once; it is an acceptable route of administration for a debilitated patient with insufficient muscle mass, which is not uncommon in colitis; less local pain and discoloration is produced. Particular attention must be given to any history of eczema, asthma, hay fever or the presence of renal insufficiency, nephritis or urinary tract infection since these conditions have frequently been present in patients who develop complications following parenteral iron therapy. Patients with rheumatoid arthritis have exacerbated joint pain and swelling following intravenous administration of iron dextran. The rate of hemoglobin synthesis and erythropoiesis following parenteral iron is not significantly different from that of oral iron.[90] The average daily increase in hemoglobin is about 0.15 gm% and rarely exceeds 0.30 gm%. Therefore, the oral route of administration is indicated for these higher risk individuals. The amount of parenteral iron administered should always be calculated on the basis of body weight and the patient hemoglobin content since the body's capacity to excrete is limited. The induction of hemochromatosis should never serve as the clinical end point of therapy with parenteral iron. Experimentally, ascorbic acid has been demonstrated to act successfully as a reducing agent, converting ferric ions to ferrous ions which then can readily be assimilated.[91] However, the amount of ascorbic acid necessary to accomplish this activity is far in excess of those quantities which have been incorporated into commercially available iron preparations. Until the role of ascorbic acid in deficiency anemias can be scientifically and clinically established, its presence in iron preparations on the basis that it may offer some preventive or prophylactic measure is unacceptable. There is also at present no clinically reliable evidence to suggest that the prolonged release or enteric-coated iron preparations are more effective.[92]

Iron preparations are also available in combination with vitamin B_{12}, folic acid and dried stomach concentrates. These preparations are suitable for anemias which occur as a result of multiple deficiencies. Following gastrectomy or gastroenterostomy disorders such as gastric carcinoma or gastric ulcers, preparations containing iron and vitamin B_{12} with concentrates of intrinsic factor are appropriate choices for correcting deficiencies. The large number of iron preparations available suggest that they are often prescribed with little understanding of their proper or rational use. The patient must bear the burden of high costs of such preparations. These preparations must never serve as an excuse for poor or inadequate diagnosis or therapeutic management of any patient with symptoms of anemia.

Antispasmotics and Opiates

In mild to moderate cases of colitis, many clinicians will employ antispasmodics and opiates for purposes of diarrhea control.[3,48] However, these drugs must only be used sparingly, and long term chronic therapy with them should be discouraged. During periods of severe diarrhea, oral intake should be restricted to medications and clear fluids until the diarrhea subsides. Antidiarrheal agents containing kaolin, methylcellulose, pectin or psyllium provide minimal benefit on such occasions. Antispasmodics and opiates should be avoided in acute fulminating colitis. Therapeutic amounts of these drugs are seldom successful in controlling diarrhea in severe cases since diarrhea is symptomatic of an inflamed, hyperemic and marginally motile bowel rather than the result of hypermotility.[29,93]

Diet

Following acute attack, the patient's nutritional deficiencies should be corrected by giving small frequent feedings which are high in calories and protein but low in residue. There is

evidence that nearly 20% of patients with ulcerative colitis benefit from a milk free diet as evidenced by a decrease in their incidence of relapses.[9] It is unclear whether this is reflection of an allergic sensitivity to protein or a deficiency in the affected colon of the enzyme lactase.[94] Egg albumin, oranges, potatoes, tomatoes and wheat have been suggested as foods which can exacerbate colitis; however, substantiation of this causal relationship continues to be equivocal.[8,95] Children with ulcerative colitis who have milk products restricted from their diet should receive daily supplements of calcium and vitamin D, necessary in appropriate quantities in order to maintain biochemical function and physiological growth. Concurrent administration of corticosteroids in patients who have been restricted from milk further complicates the task of management since the effect of vitamin D on calcium absorption is antagonized. Therefore careful consideration should be given to recognizing the clinical manifestations of hypocalcemia. Adequate vitamin D as 25-hydroxycholecalciferol or dihydrotachysterol and calcium intake should be provided from sources other than milk products. Some clinicians advocate unlimited diet, while others recommend low residue diets and restricting certain foods which by patient experience and judgment have not been well tolerated. There is no universal agreement as to the benefits derived from dietary restraints for the ulcerative colitis patient. Decisions as to what constitutes a suitable dietary regimen should be individualized following an evaluation of the effect of diet on the patient's condition. The goal of dietary management for the ulcerative colitis patient is to overcome nutritional deficiencies and improve the patient's over-all sense of well-being.

Psychotherapy

Although it cannot be confirmed that there is an increased frequency of psychological or personality difficulties in patients with ulcerative colitis, an essential ingredient in the management of the disease is emotional assurance and support. The physician and pharmacist should endeavor to establish a meaningful professional relationship and rapport with the patient. It is acknowledged that emotional factors such as anxiety and stress influence the clinical course of the disease and the eventual outcome of management. Drugs such as the tricyclic antidepressants or phenothiazine tranquilizers should never be considered as appropriate substitutes for efforts at understanding and communicating with patients afflicted with ulcerative colitis. Nonspecific measures such as rest may be beneficial. Separation from emotionally stressful situation and even hospitalization for the patient may be justifiable during periods of disease activity. Medical management without conscientious, skillful and rational psychotherapy or emotional support from the physician does not meet the total needs of these patients.[96]

Surgery

Indications for surgical management of ulcerative colitis include the following: toxic megacolon, perforation, acute and severe bleeding, colonic stricture with obstruction or reasonable suspicion of malignancy.[97-99] The decision to intervene surgically in cases of intractable colitis where medical management has been unsuccessful should be made only after considering factors such as the effects of chronic invalidism, physical and developmental retardation, the drugs used, particularly corticosteroids and the risk of carcinoma.[100] There is a lack of reliable clinical information regarding the outcome of continued medical management

in these patients. In spite of maintenance therapy, the patient with near total colonic involvement or who is 60 years and older will most likely develop severe recurrent attacks eventually requiring surgery. Milder forms of colitis confined to the rectum and sigmoid colon rarely require surgery. Table 10.3 summarizes those surgical procedures which are commonly done for inflammatory diseases of the bowel. The management of toxic megacolon by medical means alone often is unsuccessful. The patient who recovers from a fulminating attack following intensive medical management usually will require surgery within a few years. The mortality rate of surgical procedures is significantly higher for emergency procudres than for elective ones.[100,101] Early surgery is encouraged in the very ill patient with severe recurrent colitis. Intensive medical treatment should be started in acute fulminant cases in order to reduce the operative risk. Careful monitoring of patient response to treatment during this period must be conducted. Although the incidence of surgical intervention has not changed appreciably in recent years, the operative mortality has decreased as has the number of emergency procedures performed. The likelihood that this is indicative of the success of intensive medical treatment prior to surgery has been suggested.

Provision for restoring and maintaining adequate electrolyte, fluid, hemoglobin levels

TABLE 10.3
Surgical Basis for Treatment of Ulcerative Colitis[175]

Procedure[a]	Comment
1. Total colectomy with ileostomy; also: panproctocolectomy	The surgical procedure of choice where colitis involvement is diffuse affecting extensive portion of colon and rectum; the entire colon is removed; an ileostomy or "artificial anus" is constructed from the ileum; this procedure does not offer opportunity for restoring the continuity of the bowel; the psychological adjustment to the impact of this procedure is important
2. Subtotal colectomy with ileorectal anastomosis	Suitable for right-sided or segmental colitis and Crohn's disease or granulomatous colitis; spares the rectum and variable amount of the distal colon; offers the opportunity for restoring continuity of the bowel; failure rate is significant where colitis is diffuse and extensive owing to continuing activity in remaining segment; risk of developing malignancies in the remaining rectal segment is considerable

[a]Twenty percent of patients with ulcerative colitis will require surgery. Prior to surgery, complete evaluation of vital signs, electrolyte levels, blood volume, hemoglobin, renal function and corticosteroid coverage must be considered. Postoperative complications (*e.g.*, fistula, serious debilitation) contraindicating oral or tube feeding may necessitate hyperalimentation by intravenous administration of protein hydrolysates, hypertonic glucose, electrolytes and vitamin solutions for prolonged periods to provide positive nitrogen balance and calories.

TABLE 10.4
Complicatons from Ileostomies

Type	Comment
1. Obstruction	Most frequent; result of high residue and high bulk foods, *e.g.,* popcorn; overeating should be avoided; scar formation and strictures can lead to obstruction; symptoms include: cramps, distention, vomiting, nonfunctioning ileostomy or diarrhea due to accumulation of pressure; contact patient's physician
2. Dehydration	Secondary to diarrhea; caution in recommending antidiarrheals since symptoms may be due to obstruction; abnormally liquefied and constant ileostomy drainage is hazardous; serious when complicated by electrolyte depletion, acid-base imbalance and hypoproteinemia
3. Electrolyte deficiency hypokalemia	Potassium deficiency; loss from ileostomy can be considerable; symptoms include muscle weakness, numbness of fingers, toes, dyspnea, irregular pulse, bradycardia, metabolic alkalosis; of particular concern in patients on digitalis glycosides and/or taking diuretics; if hypokalemia is mild and only transient, dietary replenishment often is adequate
hyponatremia	Sodium deficiency; symptoms include abdominal cramps, fatigue, oliguria, low blood pressure; should consider even in absence of diarrhea since excessive drainage and insensible loss of fluids and sodium need to be considered
4. Peri-ileostomy	Soreness around ileostoma and appliance; allergic reaction to adhesive improper fit should be ruled out; improper application or care of appliance; use of certain allergenic solvents or soaps around area should be ruled out
5. Bleeding	Contact patient's physician; cause should be determined

[a]Pharmacist considerations: enteric-coated medications are poor dosage form choices; also sustained release dosage forms; recommend liquids or soft gelatin preparations, *e.g.,* vitamins.

and corticosteroid coverage must be made prior to and after colectomy. The patient and his family should be advised of the nature of the surgery and sufficiently prepared emotionally to accept an ileostomy. The psychological adjustment required for the individual who has recently undergone an ileostomy is often facilitated by the improvement he or she experiences with respect to the quality of life. As health is restored, participation in normal activities for the patient is again possible. For most patients living with an ileostomy is invariably preferred to existing as a chronic invalid. The concerned pharmacist can often provide the ostomate patient psychological support and assurance by demonstrating an awareness and understanding of those problems which the patient might encounter. Groups have been formed in many cities and counties throughout the United States for the purpose of assisting in emotional and social rehabilitation and in dealing with those problems common to the ostomate patient.[102,103]

Especially trained individuals known as enterostomal therapists have provided valuable assistance for many ostomate patients experiencing problems, many quite complex, which required attention or simply reassurance.[104] Significant difficulties and complications have been noted to develop in many patients during the first 3 or 4 months following colectomy and ileostomy.[105,106] Obstruction is the most frequent complication.[107] It appears that proper understanding and use of judgment often are sufficient to overcome many such difficulties and complications. While servicing the ileostomy patient with the necessary appliances and supplies, the pharmacist should also make efforts to assist and inform the patient on their proper use and care.[108] Table 10.4 sum-

TABLE 10.5
Basis for the Management of Ulcerative Colitis

Area of Disease Involvement	Clinical Course	Treatment Considerations
Rectum	Acute	Local corticosteroids for short term
	Intermittent	Sulfonamides for long term; may require adjustment of dosage during exacerbations; local corticosteroids for short term during flare-ups may be useful
	Continuous	Maintenance sulfonamides, *e.g.,* salicyloazosulpyridine 2 gm daily; attempt to resolve possible etiological factors, *e.g.,* stress, anxiety, diet, allergies, cathartic abuse, etc.
Rectum/sigmoid	Acute	Local or systemic corticosteroids for short term; concomitantly sulfonamides, *i.e.,* salicyloazosulpyridine 4-6 gm may be tried; replace blood loss if anemia severe
Rectum Sigmoid colon Descending colon	Intermittent	Maintenance sulfonamides; intermittent corticosteroids locally if symptoms are successfully treated in such a manner; may need to consider systemic corticosteroids on short term basis during exacerbations; correct deficiency anemia; rule out contributing factors, *e.g.,* milk products, stress, anxiety diet
	Continuous	Maintenance sulfonamides; corticosteroids should not be used on a chronic basis, rather only when acute exacerbations occur; continuous iron therapy should be considered; rule out contributing factors; avoid long term use of opiates for diarrhea
Rectum Sigmoid colon Descending colon Transverse colon	Acute	Same as rectum/sigmoid and descending colonic involvement; sulfonamide, *i.e.,* salicylazosulpyridine, dosage may have to be adjusted upwards to 6-8 gm daily if patient can tolerate; unlikely treatment would be effective if given without corticosteroids concurrently; systemic corticosteroids may be more effective since enemas may be difficult to retain; concern for perforation, toxic megacolon and perforation; if not resolved medically within several days must consider surgery
	Intermittent	Same as for rectum/sigmoid and descending colonic involvement; if medical management is unsuccessful, surgery must be considered
	Continuous	Same as for rectum/sigmoid and descending colon; if intractable to medical management or contributing to chronic invalidism, surgery should be considered; deficiency states, *e.g.,* anemia, vitamins, especially B_{12} and K, should be restored

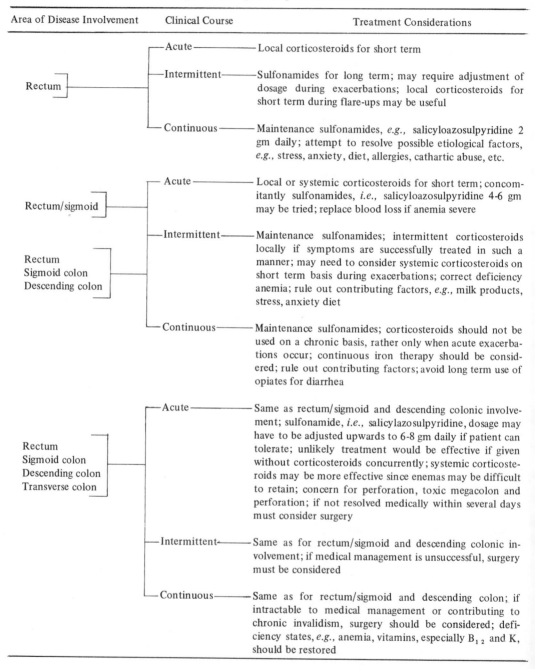

TABLE 10.5–*Continued*

Area of Disease Involvement	Clinical Course	Treatment Considerations
Entire colon	Acute	Systemic corticosteroids in sufficiently high doses for several days (4-6) during severe episodes; beware of threatened perforation and toxic megacolon; sulfonamides 4-6 gm daily subsequent to symptomatic improvement and decreasing corticosteroid dosage; repeated relapses of acute episodes almost invariably will require surgery; colonic rest, fluid electrolyte, acid-base balance important; avoid opiates and anticholinergics for diarrhea control
	Intermittent	Maintenance sulfonamides 2 gm daily; short term intermittent systemic corticosteroids during episodes of exacerbation; refractoriness to medical management for long duration, should consider surgery
	Continuous	Surgery is usually considered when medical management has been unsuccessful or has resulted in chronic invalidism; the risk of colonic malignancies is significant in children or patients with long term, extensive continuous involvement

marizes common complications from ileostomies.

PROGNOSIS

For patients with ulcerative colitis, the outlook for successful prognosis is encouraging as the quality of medical management improves. Particular attention given to intensive therapy during the onset of symptoms and a comprehensive approach to treatment with drugs, psychological support and diet have contributed to resolving the symptoms of the disease with better success. Since the therapeutic approaches to treating ulcerative colitis are largely empiric and primarily directed at providing symptomatic relief, no single approach or regimen can be recommended as universally effective. The therapy plan must be individualized with a goal of providing the patient an opportunity to resume normal activity. Mild to moderate symptoms of short duration are most likely to respond favorably to medical management. Prognosis is also improved for the patient with disease limited only to the rectum and sigmoid colon. Nearly 75% of patients with ulcerative colitis respond to medical treatment and may remain symptom-free. For some patients there may be even complete remission and reversal of the disease on clinical evaluation.

Immediate and intensive therapy is required in acute fulminating colitis since the risk of mortality from such cases is significant. Hospitalization is desirable because it facilitates efforts to assess and evaluate the clinical course of the condition and its response to management. Management of the acute attack initially should be attempted by medical means. Supportive measures such as bed rest, fluid and electrolyte replacement, colonic rest by restriction of oral intake and correction of significant anemia should be undertaken to provide relief from symptoms. Corticosteroids may be initiated at the onset of an attack depending on its severity or several days after symptomatic treatment has not produced any apparent improvement. Patients who received corticosteroids chronically prior to the acute episode or during previous attacks should be started on them immediately. One should always be aware that corticosteroids may mask symptoms of perforation. Continued evaluation for development of toxic dilation of the colon should be part of the therapy for these patients. Although not all acute attacks of colitis are terminated surgically, invariably a number of patients with recurrent severe episodes of colitis will require surgical intervention. If improvement following aggressive medical treatment is not satisfactory within several days, surgery must then be considered without further delay. Prognosis for successful recovery in such situations favors the patient whose conditions improved following medical treatment prior to surgery.

CONCLUSION

The therapeutic management of ulcerative colitis is a formidable task owing to the lack of complete understanding of its etiology, difficulty in evaluating the effectiveness of treatment and the unpredictable and chronic nature of its clinical course. The successful outcome of treatment is greatly dependent on the combined presence of psychological support, patient awareness of the limitations of the therapeutic measures employed and adherence to prescribed drug and dietary regimens (Table 10.5). The pharmacist can contribute significantly to the total management of the patient with colitis. (S)He can serve as a reliable resource of information on matters such as ostomate appliances and medications prescribed as well as being available to provide often needed emotional reassurance by virtue of accessibility to the patient. Conscientious monitoring of the patient compliance to prescribed therapeutic regimen and participation with the colitis patient's physician, therapist and nurse in evaluating the effectiveness of therapy are responsibilities which a pharmacist should assume. Success at such formidable tasks can only be achieved if the pharmacist is aware of the current concepts of the nature of the disease, problems associated with its management and the capabilities and limitations of available therapeutic approaches.

REFERENCES

1. deDombal, F. T.: Ulcerative colitis: definition, historical background, etiology, diagnosis, natural history and local complications. Postgrad. Med. J., 44: 684, 1968.
2. deDonbal, F. T., Burch, P. R. J., and Watkinson, G.: Etiology of ulcerative colitis. I. Short term prognosis. II. Long term prognosis. Gut, 4: 299, 1963.
3. Davidson, M., Bloom, A. A., and Kugler, M. M.: Chronic ulcerative colitis of childhood. J. Pediatr., 67: 471, 1965.
4. Bull, D. M., and Ignaczak, T. F.: Enterobacterial common antigen-induced lymphocyte reactivity in inflammatory bowel disease. Gastroenterology, 64: 43, 1973.
5. Lagercrantz, R., Perlman, P., and Hammarstrom, S.: Immunological studies in ulcerative colitis. V. Family studies. Gastroenterology, 60: 381, 1971.
6. Nugent, F. W., and Rudolph, N. E.: Extracolonic manifestations of chronic ulcerative colitis. Med. Clin. North Am., 50: 529, 1966.
7. Broberger, O.: Immunological studies in ulcerative colitis. Gastroenterology, 47: 229, 1964.
8. Rider, J. A., and Moeller, H. C.: Food sensitivity in ulcerative colitis. Am. J. Gastroenterol., 37: 497, 1962.
9. Truelove, S. C.: Ulcerative colitis provoked by milk. Br. Med. J., 1: 154, 1961.
10. Finch, S. M., and Hess, J.H.: Ulcerative colitis in children. Am. J. Psychiatry, 118: 819, 1962.
11. Grave, W. J.: Life stress and chronic ulcerative colitis. Ann. N.Y. Acad. Sci., 58: 389, 1954.
12. Prugh, D. G.: The influence of emotional factors in the clinical course of ulcerative colitis in children. Gastroenterology, 18: 339, 1951.
13. Meldeloff, A. I., Monk, M., Siegel, C. I., and Lilienfeld, A.: Illness experience and life stresses in patients with irriritable colon and with ulcerative colitis. N. Engl. J. Med., 282: 14, 1970.
14. Monk, M., Mendeloff, A. I., Siegel, C. I., and Lilienfeld, A.: An epidemiological study of ulcerative colitis and regional enteritis among adults in Baltimore. I. Hospital incidence and prevalence, 1960 to 1965. Gastroenterology, 53: 198, 1967.
15. Ascheson, E. D.: Distribution of ulcerative colitis and regional enteritis in United States veterans with particular reference to the Jewish religion. Gut, 1: 291, 1960.
16. Acheson, E. D., and Nefzger, M. D.: Ulcerative colitis in the United States Army in 1944. Epidemiology: comparisons between patients and controls. Gastroenterology, 44: 7, 1963.
17. Kirsner, J. B., and Spencer, J. A.: Familial occurrence of ulcerative colitis, regional enteritis and ileocolitis. An. Intern. Med., 59: 133, 1963.
18. Sherlock, P., Bell, B. M., Steinberg, H., and Almy, T. P.: Familial occurrence of regional enteritis and ulcerative colitis. Gastroenterology, 45: 413, 1963.
19. Almy, T. P., and Sherlock, P.: Genetic aspects of ulcerative colitis and regional enteritis. Gastroenterology, 51: 757, 1966.
20. Michener, W. M.: Ulcerative colitis in children, problems in management. Pediatr. Clin. North Am., 14: 159, 1967.
21. Beal, R. W., Skyring, A. P., McRae, J., and Firkin, B. G.: The anemia of ulcerative colitis. Gastroenterology, 45: 589, 1963.
22. Oremiod, T. P.: Observations on the incidence and cause of anemia in ulcerative colitis. Gut, 8: 107, 1967.
23. Fong, S., Fundenberg, H., and Perlmann, P.: Ulcerative colitis with antierythrocyte antibodies. Vox Sang., 8: 668, 1963.

24. Keene, W. R.: Uncommon abnormalities of blood associated with chronic ulcerative colitis. Med. Clin. North Am., 50: 535, 1966.

25. Cohen, S. M., Rosenthal, D. S., and Karp, P. J.: Ulcerative colitis and erythrocyte G6PD deficiency-salicylazosulfapyridine provoked hemolysis. J.A.M.A., 205: 528, 1968.

26. Carson, P. E.: Hemolysis due to inherited erythrocyte enzyme deficiencies. Ann. N.Y. Acad. Sci., 151: 765, 1968.

27. Bottiger, L. E., Engstedt, L., Lagercrantz, R., and Nyberg, A.: Occurrence of Heinz bodies during azulfidine treatment of ulcerative colitis. Gastroenterology, 100: 33, 1963.

28. Tumen, H. H.: Toxic megacolon in fulminating disease. J.A.M.A., 191: 838, 1965.

29. Smith, F. W., Law, D. H., Nickel, W. F., Jr., and Sleisenger, M. H.: Fulminant ulcerative colitis with toxic dilation of the colon: medical and surgical management of eleven cases with observations regarding etiology. Gastroenterology, 42: 233, 1962.

30. deDombal, F. T., Watts, J. M., Watkinson, G., and Goligher, J. C.: Intraperitoneal perforation of the colon in ulcerative colitis. Proc. R. Soc. Med., 58: 713, 1965.

31. Rice, R. P.: Plain abdominal film roentgenographic diagnosis of ulcerative disease of colon. Am. J. Roentgenol. Radium Ther. Nucl. Med., 104: 544, 1968.

32. Becker, M. H., Genieser, N. B., and Clark, H.: Perforation of colon during barium enema. N. Y. State J. Med., 67: 278, 1967.

33. Eade, M. N.: Liver disease in ulcerative colitis. I. Analysis of operative liver biopsy in 138 consecutive patients having colectomy. Ann. Intern. Med., 72: 475, 1970.

34. Eade, M. N.: Liver disease in ulcerative colitis. II. Long term effect of colectomy. Ann. Intern. Med., 72: 489, 1970.

35. Mistilis, S. P., Skyring, A. P., and Goulston, S. J. M.: Pericholangitis and ulcerative colitis. II. Clinical aspects. Ann. Intern. Med., 63: 17, 1965.

36. Jalan, K. N., Prescott, R. J., Walker, R. J., Sircus, W., McManus, J. P. A., and Card, W. I.: Arthropathy, ankylosing spondylitis, and clubbing of fingers in ulcerative colitis. Gut, 11: 748, 1970.

37. Perry, H. P., and Brunsting, L. A.: Pyoderma gangrenosum. A clinical study of 19 cases. Arch. Dermatol., 75: 380, 1957.

38. Johnson, M. L., and Wilson, H. T. H.: Skin lesions in ulcerative colitis. Gut, 10: 255, 1969.

39. Ellis, P. P., and Gentry, J. F.: Ocular complications of ulcerative colitis. Am. J. Ophthalmol., 58: 779, 1964.

40. Breuer, R. I., Gelzayd, E. A., and Kirsner, J. B.: Urinary crystalloid excretion in patients with inflammatory bowel disease. Gut, 11: 314, 1970.

41. Gelzayd, E. A., Brewer, R. I., and Kirsner, J. B.: Nephrolithiasis in inflammatory bowel disease. Am. J. Dig. Dis., 13: 1027, 1968.

42. McCaffery, T. D., Nasr, K., Lawrence, A. M., and Kirsner, J. B.: Severe growth retardation in children with inflammatory bowel disease. Pediatrics, 45: 386, 1970.

43. Devroede, G. J., Taylor, W. F., Sauer, W. G., Jackman, R. J., and Stickler, G. B.: Cancer risk and life expectancy of children with ulcerative colitis. N. Engl. J. Med., 285: 17, 1971.

44. Saegesser, F., and Waridel, D.: Does the frequency of canceration in ulcerative colitis justify a prophylactic proctocolectomy? Am. J. Proctol., 20: 33, 1969.

45. Diethelm, A. G., Nickel, W. F., Jr., and Wantz, G. E.: Ulcerative colitis in the elderly patient. Surg. Gynecol. Obstet., 126: 1223, 1968.

46. Edwards, F. C., and Truelove, S. F.: The course and prognosis of ulcerative colitis. III. Complications. Gut, 5: 1, 1964.

47. Spencer, J. A., and Kirsner, J. B.: The treatment of ulcerative colitis. Am. J. Gastroenterol., 37: 17, 1962.

48. Michener, W. M., Brown, C. H., and Turnbull, R. B., Jr.: Ulcerative colitis in children. II. Medical and surgical therapy. Am. J. Dis. Child., 108: 236, 1964.

49. Anon: Azulfidine in ulcerative colitis. Med. Lett. Drugs Ther., 4: 32, 1962.

50. Misiewicz, J. J., Lennard-Jones, J. E., Connell, A. M., Baron, J. H., and Jones, F. A.: Controlled trial of sulphasalazine in maintenance therapy for ulcerative colitis. Lancet, 1: 185, 1965.

51. Gorbach, S. L., Nahas, L., Patterson, J. F., Levitan, R., and Weinstein, L.: Fecal microflora in ulcerative colitis in untreated and azulfidine-treated subjects (abstract). Clin. Res., 14: 297, 1966.

52. Hanngren, A., Hansson, E., Svartz, N., and Ullberg, S.: Distribution and metabolism of salicylazosulfapyridine. Acta Med. Scand., 173: 61, 1963.

53. Muller-Wieland, K., Berndt, W., and Hirt, O.: Investigations on the absorption of azulfidine. Am. J. Proct., 21: 337, 1970.

54. Truelove, S. C., Watkinson, G., and Draper, G.: Comparison of corticosteroid and sulphasalazine (salicylazosulfapyridine) in ulcerative colitis. Br. Med. J., 2: 1708, 1962.

55. Schroder, H., and Campbell, D. E. S.: Absorption, metabolism and excretion of salicylazosulfapyridine in man. Clin. Pharmacol. Ther., 13: 539, 1972.

56. Schroder, H., and Price-Evans, D. A.: Acetylator phenotype and adverse effects of sulfasalazine in healthy subjects. Gut, 13: 278, 1972.

57. Lennard-Jones, J. E., Misiewicz, J. J., Connell, A. M., Jones, F., and Baron, J. H.: Prednisone as maintenance treatment for ulcerative colitis and remission. Lancet, 1: 188, 1965.

58. Harter, J. G., Reddy, W. J., and Thorn, G. W.: Studies on the intermittent corticosteroid dosage regimen. N. Engl. J. Med., 269: 591, 1963.

59. Cocco, A. E., and Mendeloff, A. I.: An evaluation of intermittent corticosteroid therapy in the management of ulcerative colitis. Johns Hopkins Med. J., 120: 162, 1967.

60. Sadeghi-Nejad, A., and Senior, B.: Treatment of ulcerative colitis in children with alternate day corticosteroids. Pediatrics, 43: 840, 1969.

61. Patterson, M., McGivney, J., Ong, H., and Drake, A.: Topical steroid therapy of ulcerative colitis. Gastroenterology, 103: 141, 1965.

62. Goldberg, H. I., Carbone, J. V., and Margulis, A. R.: Roentgenographic reversibility of ulcerative colitis in children treated with steroid enemas. Am. J. Roentgenol., Radium Ther. Nucl. Med., 103: 365, 1968.

63. MacDougall, I.: Treatment of ulcerative colitis with rectal steroids. Lancet, 1: 826, 1963.

64. Sherman, L. F., Tenner, R. J., and Schlottler, J. L.: Treatment of ulcerative colitis with hydrocortisone alcohol enemas: a topical and systemic anti-inflammatory agent. Dis. Colon Rectum, 10: 43, 1967.

65. Sampson, P. A., and Brooke, B. N.: Absorption of hydrocortisone in large bowel. Lancet, 1: 701, 1963.

66. Farmer, R. G., and Schumacher, O. P.: Treatment of ulcerative colitis with hydrocortisone enemas — comparison of absorption and clinical response with hydrocortisone alcohol and hydrocortisone acetate. Am. J. Gastroenterol., 54: 229, 1970.

67. Farmer, R. G., and Schumacher, O. P.: Treatment of ulcerative colitis with hydrocortisone enemas: relationship of adrenal suppression to clinical response (abstract). Gastroenterology, 56: 1157, 1969.

68. Farmer, R. G., and Schumacher, O. P.: Treatment of ulcerative colitis with hydrocortisone enemas: relationship of hydrocortisone absorption, adrenal suppression and clinical response. Dis. Colon Rectum, 13: 355, 1970.

69. Lennard-Jones, J. E., Baron, J. H., Connell, A. M., and Jones, F. A.: A double blind controlled trial of prednisone-21-phosphate suppositories in the treatment of idiopathic colitis. Gut, 3: 207, 1962.

70. Parker, J. G., and Siegelman, S.: Retrograde spread of contrast medium released from suppositories. A partial explanation for efficacy of therapeutic suppositories. Am. J. Dig. Dis., 10: 463, 1965.

71. Jalan, K. N., Prescott, R. J., Smith, A. W., Sircus, W., McManus, J. P. A., Small, W. P., and Falconer, C. W. A.: Influence of corticosteroids on the results of surgical treatment for ulcerative colitis. N. Engl. J. Med., 282: 588, 1970.

72. Kirsner, J. B.: Ulcerative colitis: "puzzles within puzzles." N. Engl. J. Med., 282: 625, 1970.

73. Brooks, J. R., and Veith, F. J.: The timing and choice of surgery for ulcerative colitis. The influence of corticosteroids. J.A.M.A., 194: 115, 1965.

74. Goldstein, M. J., Gelzayd, E. A., and Kirsner, J. B.: Some observations on the hazards of corticosteroid therapy in patients with inflammatory bowel disease. Trans. Am. Acad. Ophthalmol. Otolaryngol., 71: 254, 1967.

75. Thorn, G. W.: Clinical considerations in the use of corticosteroids. N. Engl. J. Med., 274: 775, 1966.

76. Kirsner, J. B., Palmer, W. L., Spencer, J. A., Bicks, R. P., and Johnson, C. F.: Corticotrophin (ACTH) and the adrenal steroids in the management of ulcerative colitis; observation in 240 patients. Ann. Inter. Med., 50: 891, 1959.

77. Bean, R. H. D.: Treatment of ulcerative colitis with antimetabolites. Br. Med. J., 1: 1081, 1966.

78. Bowen, G. E., Irons, G. V., Rhodes, J. B., and Kirsner, J. B.: Early experiences with azathioprine in ulcerative colitis. J.A.M.A., 195: 460, 1966.

79. Brown, C. T., and Achkar, E.: Azathioprine therapy for inflammatory bowel disease. Am. J. Gastroenterol., 54: 363, 1970.

80. MacKay, I. R.: Response to azathioprine in ulcerative colitis: report of 7 cases. Am. J. Dig. Dis., 11: 536, 1966.

81. Wisch, N., and Korelitz, B.: Immunosuppressive therapy for ulcerative colitis, ileitis and granulomatous colitis. Surg. Clin. North Am., 52: 961, 1972.

82. Patterson, J. F., Norton, R. A., and Schwartz, R. S.: Azathioprine treatment of ulcerative colitis, granulomatous colitis and regional enteritis. Am. J. Dig. Dis., 16: 327, 1971.

83. Theodor, E., Gilon, E., and Waks, U.: Treatment of ulcerative colitis with azathioprine. Br. Med. J., 4: 741, 1968.

84. Jones, F. A., Lennard-Jones, J. E., Hinton, J. M., and Reeves, W. G.: Dangers of immunosuppressive drugs in ulcerative colitis. Br. Med. J. (Corresp.), 1: 1418, 1966.

85. Henderson, P. A., and Hillman, R. S.: Characteristics of iron dextran utilization in man. Blood, 34: 357, 1969.

86. Giorgio, A. J.: Current concepts of iron metabolism and the iron deficiency anemias. Med. Clin. North Am., 54: 1399, 1970.

87. Hallberg, L., Solvell, L., and Brise, H.: Search for substances promoting the absorption of iron. Acta Med. Scand., 180 (Suppl. 459): 11, 1966.

88. Hallberg, L., Ryttinger, L., and Solvell, L.: Side effects of oral iron therapy. Acta Med. Scand., 180 (Suppl. 459): 3, 1966.

89. Wallerstein, R. O.: Intravenous iron-dextran complex. Blood, 32: 690, 1968.

90. McCurdy, P. R.: Oral and parenteral iron therapy. J.A.M.A., 191: 859, 1965.

91. Brise, H., and Hallberg, L.: Effect of ascorbic acid on iron absorption. Acta Med. Scand., 168 (Suppl. 376): 51, 1960.

92. Middleton, E. J., Nagy, E., and Morrison, A. B.: Studies on the absorption of orally adminis-

tered iron from sustained-release preparations. N. Engl. J. Med., 274: 136, 1966.

93. Garrett, J. M., Sauer, W. G., and Moertel, C. G.: Colonic motility in ulcerative colitis after opiate administration. Gastroenterology, 53: 93, 1967.

94. Gudman-Hoyer, E., and Jarnum, S.: Incidence and significance of lactose malabsorption in ulcerative colitis and Crohn's disease. Gut, 4: 299, 1963.

95. Rowe, A. H., and Rowe, A., Jr.: Chronic ulcerative colitis: atopic allergy in its etiology. Am. J. Gastroenterol., 34: 49, 1960.

96. Lepore, M. J.: The importance of emotional disturbances in chronic ulcerative colitis. J.A.M.A., 191: 819, 1965.

97. Goligher, J. C.: The surgical treatment of ulcerative colitis. Postgrad. Med. J., 44: 708, 1968.

98. Korelitz, B. I., and Lindner, A. E.: The influence of corticotrophin and adrenal steroids on the course of ulcerative colitis: a comparison with the pre-steroid era. Gastroenterology, 46: 671, 1964.

99. Turnbull, R. B., Jr.: Instructions to ileostomy patient: management of stoma. Clevl. Clin., 28: 213, 1961.

100. Frey, C. F., and Weaver, D. K.: Colectomy in children with ulcerative and granulomatous colitis. Arch. Surg., 104: 416, 1972.

101. Watts, J. M., deDombal, F. T., and Goligher, J. C.: Early results of surgery of ulcerative colitis. Br. J. Surg., 53: 1005, 1966.

102. Druss, R. G., O'Connor, J. F., and Stern, L. O.: Psychologic response to colectomy. II. Adjustment to a permanent colostomy. Arch. Gen. Psychiatr., 20: 419, 1969.

103. United Ostomy Association: 1111 Wilshire Boulevard, Los Angeles, Calif., 90017.

104. Lennerberg, E.: Role of enterostomal therapists and stoma rehabilitation clinics. Cancer, 28: 226, 1971.

105. Prudeen, J. F.: Psychological problems following ileostomy and colostomy. Cancer, 28: 236, 1971.

106. Rowbotham, J. L.: Colostomy problems—dietary and colostomy management. Cancer, 28: 222, 1971.

107. Sitt, A.: When the problem is ileostomy. Emer. Med., 2: 107, 1970.

108. Gebhardt, M. C., Caiola, S. M., and Eckel, F. M.: A hospital pharmacy ostomy patient care program. Drug Intell. Clin. Pharmacol., 6: 374, 1972.

109. Altemeirer, W. A., Hummel, R. P. and Hill, E. O.: Staphylococcal enterocolitis following antibiotic therapy. Ann. Surg., 157: 847, 1963.

110. Azar, H., and Drapanas, T.: Relationship of antibiotics to wound infection and enterocolitis in colon surgery. Am. J. Surg., 115: 209, 1968.

111. Barrett, P. V.: Complications of antibiotic therapy—gastrointestinal complications. Calif. Med., 117: 33, 1972.

112. Ecker, J. A., Williams, R. G., McKittrick, J. E.,

and Failing, R. M.: Pseudomembranous enterocolitis—an unwelcome gastrointestinal complication of antibiotic therapy. Am. J. Gastroenterol., 54: 214, 1970.

113. Khan, M. Y., and Hall, W. H.: Staphylococcal enterocolitis—treatment with vancomycin. Ann. Intern. Med., 65: 1, 1966.

114. Pittman, F. E., and Pittman, J. C.: Lincomycin colitis (abstract). Clin. Res., 20: 626, 1972.

115. Benner, E. J., and Tellman, W. H.: Pseudomembranous colitis as a sequel to oral lincomycin therapy. Am. J. Gastroenterol., 54: 55, 1970.

116. Cohen, L. E., McNeill, C. J., and Wells, R. F.: Clindamycin-associated colitis. J.A.M.A., 223: 1379, 1973.

117. Brindle, M. J., and Henderson, I. N.: Vascular occlusion of the colon associated with contraception. Can. Med. Assoc. J., 100: 681, 1969.

118. Ward, G. W., and Stevensen, J. R.: Colonic disorder and oral contraceptives. N. Engl. J. Med., 278: 910, 1968.

119. Martel, A. J., Lillie, H. J., Jr., and Sawicki, J. E.: Hemorrhage and stenosis of the jejunum following course of progestational agent. Am. J. Gastroenterol., 57: 261, 1972.

120. Silberstein, P.: Severe diarrhea caused by the therapeutic use of progestational agents. Med. J. Aust., 57: 24, 1970.

121. Brennan, M. F., Clarke, A. M., and Macbeth, W. A.: Infarction of midgut associated with oral contraceptives. N. Engl. J. Med., 279: 1213, 1968.

122. Kilpatrick, Z. M., Silverman, J. F., Betancourt, E., Farman, J., and Lawson, J. P.: Vascular occlusion of the colon and oral contraceptives. Possible relation. N. Engl. J. Med., 278: 438, 1968.

123. Rochlin, D. B., Shiner, J., Langdon, E., and Ottoman, R.: Use of 5-fluorouracil in disseminated solid neoplasms. Ann. Surg., 156: 105, 1962.

124. Rothfield, E. L., Goldman, J., Goldberg, H. H., and Einhorn, S.: Severe chlorpropamide toxicity. J.A.M.A., 172: 54, 1960.

125. Mehrotra, T. N.: Hemorrhage colitis after cyclophosphamide. Lancet, 2: 345, 1966.

126. Clark, P. A., Hsia, Y. E., and Huntsman, R. G.: Toxic complications of treatment with 6-mercaptopurine. Br. Med. J., 1: 393, 1960.

127. Pike, B. F., Phillippi, P. J., and Lawson, E. H., Jr.: Soap colitis. N. Engl. J. Med., 285: 217, 1971.

128. Bravo, A. J., and Lowman, R. M.: Benign ulcer of the sigmoid colon. An unusual lesion that can simulate carcinoma. Radiology, 100: 681, 1969.

129. Debenham, G. P.: Ulcer of the cecum during oxphenbutazone (Tandearil®) therapy. Can. Med. Assoc. J., 94: 1182, 1966.

130. Roe, M., Sears, A. D., and Arndt, J. H.: Gold reaction panenteritis. Radiology, 104: 59, 1972.

131. Varsamis, U., and Ward, R. R.: Severe diarrhea associated with lithium-carbonate therapy in regional enteritis. Lancet, 4: 1322, 1972.

132. Lemaitre, G., L'Hermine, C., and Decoulx, M.: Radiologic appearance of chronic colitis caused by laxative abuse. Report of 4 cases. J. Belge. Radiol., 53: 339, 1970.

133. Plum, G. E., Weber, H. M., and Sauer, W. G.: Prolonged cathartic abuse resulting in roentgen evidence of enterocolitis. Am. J. Roentgenol., Radium Ther. Nucl. Med., 83: 919, 1960.

134. Ramirez, B., and Marieb, N. J.: Hypokalemic metabolic alkalosis due to Carter's Little Pills. Conn. Med., 34: 169, 1970.

135. Gazes, C. P., Holmes, C. R., Moseley, V., and Pratt-Thomas, H. R.: Acute hemorrhage and necrosis of the intestines associated with digitalization. Circulation, 23: 358, 1961.

136. Scharer, L. L., and Burhenne, H. J.: Megacolon associated with administration of an anticholinergic drug in a patient with ulcerative colitis. Am. J. Dig. Dis., 9: 268, 1964.

137. Ayd, F. J.: Hazards of polypharmacy. Int. Drug. Ther. Newsl., 2: 17, 1967.

138. Gander, D. R., and Delvin, H. B.: Ileus after amtriptyline. Br. Med. J., 1: 1160, 1963.

139. Warnes, H.: Adynamic ileus during psychoactive medication: a report of three fatal and five severe cases. Can. Med. Assoc. J., 96: 1112, 1967.

140. Milner, G., and Buckner, E. G.: Adynamic ileus and amitriptyline: three case reports. Med. J. Aust., 1: 921, 1964.

141. Clarke, I. M.: Adynamic ileus and amitriptyline. Br. Med. J., 2: 531, 1971.

142. Berman, H., and Mainella, F. S.: Toxic results of anticoagulant therapy. New York State J. Med., 52: 725, 1952.

143. Goldfarb, W. B.: Coumarin induced intestinal obstruction. Ann. Surg., 161: 27, 1965.

144. Hafner, C. D., Cranely, J. J., Krause, R. J., and Strasser, E. S.: Anticoagulant ileus. J.A.M.A., 182: 947, 1962.

145. Leatherman, L. L.: Intestinal obstruction caused by anticoagulants. Am. Heart J., 76: 534, 1968.

146. Tanser, A. R., and Keat, E. C. B.: Phenidione induced hemorrhagic ulcerative colitis. Br. Med. J., 1: 588, 1966.

147. Furste, W., Phelps, D., and Taylor, P.: Antihypertensive drugs as a cause of the acute abdomen. J.A.M.A., 166: 2111, 1958.

148. Munster, A., and Milton, G. W.: Paralytic ileus due to ganglion blocking agents. Med. J. Aust., 48: 210, 1961.

149. Ettman, I. K., Bouchillon, C. D., and Halford, H. H.: Gastrointestinal roentgen findings due to untoward effects of hexamethonium. Radiology, 68: 673, 1957.

150. Becker, K. L., and Sutnick, A. J.: Paralytic ileus stimulating acute intestinal obstruction due to pentolinium tartrate. Ann. Intern. Med., 54: 313, 1961.

151. Gibson, D. S.: A case of intestinal obstruction following administration of pentapyrrolidinium bitartrate (Ansolysen®). Med. J. Aust., 2: 860, 1957.

152. Hollister, L. E., Caffey, E. M., Jr., and Klett, C. J.: Abnormal symptoms, signs and laboratory tests during treatment with phenothiazine derivatives. Clin. Pharmacol. Ther., 1: 284, 1960.

153. McHardy, G.: Gastrointestinal hazards encountered in the use of certain therapeutic agents. J.A.M.A., 168: 1868, 1958.

154. Gibson, D. S.: A case of intestinal obstruction following administration of pentapyrrolidinium bitartrate (Ansolysen®). Med. J. Aust., 2: 860, 1957.

155. Zollinger, R. M., Davis, W. D., Jr., and Curreru, A. R.: Effect of drugs on the gastrointestinal tract. Postgrad. Med., 30: 234, 1961.

156. Denneky, J. J., and Sawyer, W. D.: Paralytic ileus due to methacarbamol. J.A.M.A., 184: 516, 1963.

157. Levinsky, L., and Urca, I.: Intestinal obstruction due to antacid treatment for duodenal ulcer. Report of a case. Dis. Colon Rectum, 15: 55, 1972.

158. Figiel, L. S., and Figiel, S. J.: Diphenoxylate hydrochloride intoxication simulating intestinal obstruction. Am. J. Gastroenterol., 59: 267, 1973.

159. Collins, J. R.: Adverse reactions to salicylazosulfapyridine (Azulfidine®) in the treatment of ulcerative colitis. South. Med. J., 61: 354, 1968.

160. Carroll, O. H., Bryan, P. A., and Robinson, R. J.: Stevens–Johnson syndrome associated with long acting sulfonamides. J.A.M.A., 195: 691, 1966.

161. Caspary, E. A.: Increased platelet adhesiveness in sulphasalazine sensitivity. Lancet, 1: 94, 1964.

162. Ritz, N. D., and Fischer, M. J.: Agranulocytosis due to administration of salicylazosulfapyridine (Azulfidine®). J.A.M.A., 172: 237, 1960.

163. Evans, R. S., and Ford, W.P., Jr.: Studies of bone marrow in immunological granulocytopenia following administration of salicylazosulfapyridine. Arch. Intern. Med., 101: 244, 1958.

164. Roth, D. A., and Lindert, M. E.: A fatal case of Azulfidine® induced agranulocytosis. Gastroenterology, 37: 787, 1959.

165. Thirkettle, J. L., Gough, K. R., and Read, A. E.: Agranulocytosis associated with sulphasalazine (Salazopyrin). Lancet, 1: 1395, 1963.

166. Gardner, M. D., and Bargen, J. A.: Hemolytic anemia secondary to salicylazosulfapyridine therapy. J.A.M.A., 190: 71, 1964.

167. Spriggs, A. I., Smith, R. S., Griffith, H., and Truelove, S. C.: Heinz-body anemia due to salicylazosulfapyridine. Lancet, 1: 1039, 1958.

168. Staliffer, M. H., Sauer, W. G., Dearing, W. H., and Baggenstoss, A. H.: The spectrum of chole-

static hepatic disease. J.A.M.A., 191: 829, 1965.

169. Block, M. B., Genant, H. K., and Kirsner, J. B.: Pancreatitis as an adverse reaction to salicylazosulfapyridine. N. Engl. J. Med., 282: 380, 1970.

170. Han, T., Chawla, P. L., and Sokal, J. E.: Sulfapyridine-induced serum-sickness-like syndrome associated with plasmacytosis, lymphocytosis and multiclonal gammaglobulinopathy. N. Engl. J. Med., 280: 547, 1969.

171. Alarcon-Segovia, D.: Drug-induced lupus syndromes. Mayo Clin. Proc., 44: 664, 1969.

172. Rallison, M. L., O'Brien, J., and Good, R. A.: Severe reactions to long acting sulfonamides: erythema multiforme exudativum and lupus erythematosus following administration of sulfamethoxypyridine and sulfadimethoxine. Pediatr., 28: 908, 1961.

173. Franklin, J. L., and Rosenberg, I. H.: Impaired folic acid absorption in inflammatory bowel disease: effects of salicylazosulfapyridine (Azulfidine). Gastroenterology, 64: 517, 1973.

174. Lehr, D.: Clinical toxicity of sulfonamides. Ann. N.Y. Acad. Sci., 69: 417, 1957.

175. Ehrenpreis, R.: Surgical treatment of ulcerative colitis in childhood. Arch. Dis. Child., 41: 137, 1966.

chapter 11

HEPATITIS and CIRRHOSIS

Wayne A. Kradjan, Pharm.D.

Hepatitis and cirrhosis are two distinctively different syndromes that are classified as subgroups under the heading of liver diseases. There are a few who contend that cirrhosis is the final manifestation of repeated attacks of acute hepatitis, but this notion is generally discounted by most people in the medical profession. Cirrhosis, however, may be a sequela of long standing chronic active hepatitis.

By definition, hepatitis means an inflammation of the liver. This inflammation is usually viral in origin, but it may also be drug-induced. The virus implicated in producing viral hepatitis has never been totally isolated, but two distinct clinical patterns have been described. The first represents a spontaneously acquired infection designated as infectious hepatitis (hepatitis A), while the other, serum hepatitis (hepatitis B), is transferred by blood, blood products or infected hypodermic syringes and needles from an infected donor to a new host.

Cirrhosis, on the other hand, is characterized by a diffuse increase in the fibrous connective tissue of the liver usually associated with necrosis and regeneration of parenchymal cells imparting a nodular or glandular texture to the liver. In its later stages cirrhosis leads to such deformity of the liver that it interferes with liver function and the circulation of blood and bile to and from the liver.

ETIOLOGY

Viral Hepatitis

It is not clear whether the etiological agent that induces the two patterns of viral hepatitis are identical strains of the same virus, different strains of the same virus or two separate although closely related viruses. Immunological evidence suggests at least antigenic differences since cross immunity is not conferred, Differences in incubation periods are also seen between the two types of viral hepatitis, with infectious hepatitis having an incubation period of 2 to 6 weeks, while serum hepatitis usually has a longer incubation period of 6 weeks to 6 months. However, individual cases may vary in their length of incubation, and considerable overlap does occur.

Drug-induced Hepatitis

Drug-induced hepatitis may be divided into several types. First is the type caused by the blood and blood products which act as the vehicle for the transmission of the serum hepatitis virus. Table 11.1 lists some of these products and the relative risk from their use. Second is the small number of hepatotoxic drugs, such as carbon tetrachloride and chloroform, that when given in sufficient quantities will cause direct hepatocellular damage in all exposed individuals. The amount of damage is directly proportional to the amount and time of exposure to the toxin. Usually only zonal regions

TABLE 11.1
Risk of Hepatitis Transmission
from Blood Products[a]

A. High risk – multiple donors, cannot be heated
  1. U-V light-exposed pooled plasma (8 donors). If stored at room temperature for 6 months, the risk may be less
  2. Platelets
  3. Anti-hemophiliac (AHF) concentrate
  4. U-V exposed fibrinogen
B. Moderate risk – single donors, cannot be heated
  1. Whole blood
  2. Packed red blood cells (2-6°C)
  3. Frozen red blood cells (may be safer than refrigerated only)
  4. Single donor plasma
  5. Platelets
  6. AHF concentrate
C. No risk
  1. Human serum albumin (sterilized at 57°C)
  2. Plasma protein fraction
  3. Immune and hyperimmune gamma globulin

[a] Drying, freezing, or U-V light will not kill the hepatitis virus. Heat at 55°C for 1 hr will kill the virus but denature plasma proteins.

of the liver are destroyed, but in severe intoxication whole lobes and even the entire liver may be destroyed. Alcohol is frequently included in this category and a special type of nonviral induced hepatitis is often considered under the title of alcoholic hepatitis.[1] In contrast, there is an even larger number of agents such as halothane[2] and isoniazid[3], which usually have no effect on the liver, but on occasion have caused hepatocellular injury in random individuals via a hypersensitivity type of reaction. Often there is a history of prior exposure to the drug, but it is impossible to predict who will develop these reactions. In some cases, isolated liver cells are destroyed, while in others focal necrosis is produced. Drugs may also injure the liver without inducing frank necrosis. In these cases there is merely swelling of the liver cells with compression of the bile ducts and sinusoids leading to a prominent bile stasis in the form of thickened bile plugs within compressed bile canaliculi and droplets of bile within cells. The latter type of liver injury is termed "cholestatic jaundice" and is representative of the type of liver injury induced by chlorpromazine and methyltestosterone. Although cholestatic changes are not really classified as a form

of hepatitis, prolonged cholestatic injury may progress to hepatocellular damage, and some agents have been known to induce both hepatocellular and cholestatic effects. Table 11.2 lists some of the drugs known to cause the various types of drug-induced liver changes.

Cirrhosis

Seven major types of cirrhosis have been described in Table 11.3, but the fatty nutritional cirrhosis or Laennec's cirrhosis is by far the most commonly described in the United States. It is usually associated with chronic alcoholism but may be secondary to any dietary derangements inducing fatty changes in the liver, *e.g.,* kwashiorkor, from protein deficiency. It is agreed that cirrhosis usually begins with severe fatty changes in the liver. In the early stages this fatty infiltration is unassociated with fibrosis and scarring, while the late stages are marked by progressive loss of fat, increase of fibrous tissue, and progressive shrinkage and nodularity of the liver. However, the following questions are open to speculation:[4]

  a. Does the fatty change lead to cirrhosis, or are there some factors underlying the fatty change operating over a longer period of time that are responsible for the subsequent development of cirrhosis?
  b. Does the fatty change merely render the liver vulnerable to other noxious influences which in turn induce cirrhosis?
  c. Does alcohol itself serve as a hepatotoxic agent or does it simply substitute for a balanced diet?

Some attempts to answer these questions have led to the following proposals:[4]

  a. Sufficient fat may accumulate in liver cells to cause rupture of cell walls with the production of fatty cysts. The resultant necrotic cells may then stimulate fibrosis and scarring.
  b. The accumulation of fat in the liver cell may interfere with the structure and function of the enzyme systems of the liver and in this way cause cell necrosis as the stimulus to fibrosis.
  c. Alcohol leads to the mobilization of fat from peripheral tissue with consequent overloading of the liver. Alcohol also stimulates increased liver synthesis of

TABLE 11.2
Drug-induced Hepatitis

| Hepatotoxic | Hypersensitivity | |
	Hepatocellular	Cholestatic
Acetone	Allupurinol??	Acetohexamide
Alcohol	Antipyrine	Butyrophenones (*e.g.,* haloperidol)
Amanita phalloides	Azothioprine	Chlorpromazine and other
(mushroom)	Chloramphenicol	phenothiazines
Antimony	Diphenylhydantoin	Chlorpropamide
Arsenicals	Halothane	Erythromycin estolate
Carbon tetrachloride	Isoniazid	Methimazole and other
Chloroform	Methoxyflurane	Antithyroids
Cincophen	Methotrexate	Methyl testosterone and other
Phosphorus	6-Mercaptopurine	C-17 substituted androgens
Toluene	Methyldopa	Oral contraceptives
	Oxyphenisatin	PAS
	PAS	Sulfonamides
	Rifampin	Tricyclic antidepressants
	Thiazide diuretics	(*e.g.,* amitriptyline)
	Tetracyclines	
	Trimethadione	

TABLE 11.3
Types of Cirrhosis and Their Etiology

1. Fatty nutritional cirrhosis (Laennec's cirrhosis)— 30-50%
   Etiology: dietary derangements inducing fatty change in the liver, especially alcohol
2. Biliary cirrhosis— 15-20%
   Etiology: obstruction to bile flow, *e.g.,* stones and carcinoma, often secondary to long standing bacterial infection
3. Postnecrotic cirrhosis— 10-30%
   Etiology: scarring following massive hepatic necrosis such as that seen in chronic viral hepatitis or hepatotoxic drugs (note: some contend that viral hepatitis can not progress into cirrhosis)
4. Pigment cirrhosis— 5-10%
   Etiology: excessive deposits of hemosiderin in hemochromatosis
5. Syphilitic cirrhosis— 1-2%
   Etiology: tertiary syphilis
6. Cardiac cirrhosis— 2-3%
   Etiology: hemorrhage within the liver
7. Intermediate cirrhosis— 15-25%
   Etiology: unclear, may be a variant of fatty nutrional cirrhosis or post necrotic cirrhosis

triglycerides. These effects may lead to fatty changes and later to cirrhosis.

d. Alcoholics genererally have a severely unbalanced diet with protein deficiency, and subsequently inadequate quantities of lipotropics. This leads to a decrease of fat mobilization out of the liver.

e. When a chronic alcoholic is hospitalized and placed on an adequate diet, if fibrosis has not already intervened, excess fat can be mobilized and the liver structure and function returned to normal. In fact, if an alcoholic is able to maintain adequate diet while drinking, he may still adequately mobilize the fat out of his liver.

This last observation indicates that alcohol alone is not a direct cause of cirrhosis. Unfortunately, most chronic alcoholics do not maintain an adequate diet.

INCIDENCE

Hepatitis

In 1961 there were 72,000 cases of viral hepatitis reported.[4] Only a small fraction of these involved serum hepatitis. However, with the increased use of blood transfusions and the epidemic of intravenous drug abuse in this country, serum hepatitis has become a more significant problem. Furthermore, many drug abusers support their habit by periodically donating blood. This creates a problem since the virus cannot be detected. The disease can thus be passed on to a patient receiving transfusions. Hopefully, new screening measures using the hepatitis-associated antigen may decrease the risk.

Infectious hepatitis occurs sporadically throughout the year and may assume epidemic proportions particularly under crowded living conditions such as in the military or in underprivileged populations. It is common in children and young adults, but an increasing number of adults are contracting the disease. Serum hepatitis is commonly seen in older individuals, probably because of a greater likelihood of requiring transfusions or injections.

Cirrhosis

Cirrhosis, although a common disease throughout the world, varies in incidence not only from country to country, but from one hospital or section of a city to another. For example, it is much more common in a county hospital or veteran's hospital than in a private community hospital. It is difficult to cite an incidence of cirrhosis since patients often do not exhibit any signs or symptoms. Autopsies at various hospitals have shown an incidence ranging from 3 to 15%.[4] It also appears that cirrhosis has increased in frequency over the past 40 years. Various explanations for this increase have been proposed, including better medical care, enabling patients to live through an initial liver disease; increased incidence of alcoholism and a greater exposure to hepatotoxic drugs and chemicals which cause diffuse liver toxicity leading to cirrhosis. Table 11.3 lists the relative incidence of the various type of cirrhosis encountered. It can be seen that the largest percentage is Laennec's cirrhosis. It occurs principally in patients between 40 and 60 years of age and is found most often in males. A history of chronic alcoholism can be obtained in 50 to 90% of these patients in the United States. In Africa and Asia, children are frequently affected owing to protein-deficient diets.

CLINICAL FINDINGS AND DIAGNOSIS

Hepatitis[4,5]

The great majority of individuals exposed to the virus of infectious hepatitis or serum hepatitis do not develop clinically overt disease or have changes in their liver structure or function. Others may have subclinical disease in the form of minor liver changes without jaundice (anicteric hepatitis).

In most patients with infectious hepatitis the onset of jaundice is preceded by nonspecific constitutional and gastrointestinal symptoms. From 2 to 14 days before the appearance of jaundice, the patient abruptly develops anorexia and fatigue, and often has nausea, fever, chills and occasionally arthralgias. Right upper quadrant or epigastric discomfort, described as either a sense of fullnes or pain, is common. In contrast, serum hepatitis usually begins insidiously, with fever and flulike symptoms being uncommon. Often the first evidence of hepatic involvement in serum hepatitis is the appearance of jaundice.

One to 4 days before the onset of jaundice the urine darkens because of bilirubinemia and often the stool color lightens. Transient pruritis may occur at this stage. Once jaundice appears, the clinical features of serum and infectious hepatitis are identical. The prodromal gastrointestinal symptoms usually decrease in severity within a few days and fever rapidly subsides. The jaundice usually reaches a maximum between the 1st and 2nd weeks and decreases steadily thereafter. In typical cases, the duration of jaundice is variable but lasts less than 6 to 8 weeks. During the icteric phase the liver is often enlarged and tender to palpation. The liver may begin to decrease in size and tenderness in 1 to 2 weeks after the onset of jaundice and returns to normal size over several weeks. Table 11.4 shows some of the differentiating features between infectious and serum hepatitis. When necessary, definitive diagnosis is made by liver biopsy. It should be noted that in both forms the infective virus can be transmitted weeks before symptoms appear. There is no correlation between the histological changes in the liver and the severity of jaundice.

Serum glutamic oxaloacetic transaminase (SGOT) and serum glutamic pyruvic transaminase (SGPT) levels may be elevated 7 to 14 days prior to the onset of jaundice reflecting hepatic cell necrosis and altered cell permeability within the liver, allowing these enzymes to leak into the blood. In general the SGPT levels are higher than SGOT levels at all stages of the disease. Serum alkaline phosphatase levels are generally normal or only slightly elevated unless

TABLE 11.4

Infectious versus Serum Hepatitis

Feature	Infectious Hepatitis	Serum Hepatitis
Incubation period	2-6 weeks	6 weeks-6 months
Route of infection	Oral or parenteral	Usually parenteral
Presence of viremia during:		
Incubation period	+	+
Acute phase	+	+
Convalescence	Rare	Rare
Virus in feces during:		
Incubation period	Last 2 weeks	Rare
Acute phase	First few days	Rare
Convalescence	Rare	??

Adapted from Harrison's Principles of Internal Medicine, 6th edition[5]

cholestasis is also present (5% of cases). Protein (albumin) remains near normal or may decrease slightly if production is impaired. Globulin levels are commonly elevated and the bilirubin levels may reach 5 to 20 mg/100 ml. In severe cases an elevated bromsulphalein (BSP) retention may also be seen.

Recently an antigenic substance designated as the hepatitis-associated antigen (HAA), or Australian antigen, has been demonstrated in the serum of patients during the incubation period and acute phase of serum hepatitis. Most investigators feel the antigen is probably the protein coat or capsid material of a small virus rather than the virus itself since the antigen alone does not transfer the disease. However, transfusion of blood products positive for HAA may transmit hepatitis since the virus is probably also present. The frequency of HAA reported has varied from 50 to 95% for parenterally acquired hepatitis, and from 25 to 47% for cases of hepatitis considered to be infectious. In control populations as incidence of 0.1 to 0.2% has been reported.[6]

The diagnosis of serum hepatitis can usually be established with certainty by the incubation period after a known parenteral exposure. If there is no history of parenteral exposure, the diagnosis is usually considered to be infectious hepatitis even if the source of infection and incubation period are uncertain. If those placed in the infectious hepatitis group are divided into long versus short incubation groups, the long incubation group demonstrates a much higher incidence of positive HAA. This suggests that many of those cases designated as infectious hepatitis may actually be a variant of serum hepatitis. This observation is further strengthened by recent reports showing the development of long incubation hepatitis in staff members of renal dialysis units, suggesting nonparenteral spread of long incubation, serum hepatitis-like, viral hepatitis.[6,7]

HAA appears, on the average, 4 weeks before clinical or laboratory evidence of liver dysfunction. However, the interval may vary from 1 day to 7 weeks in individual cases. In most cases of naturally occurring hepatitis, serum obtained in the 1st week of the acute phase is likely to be positive for HAA, but it may not develop until as late as the 2nd week of illness. Persistence of antigen in the blood has been found to range from a few days to many years. In most cases, HAA disappears before symptoms subside or liver tests return to normal. There does not seem to be any correlation as to the titer of HAA and the severity of hepatitis. In patients with chronic active hepatitis, the antigen may remain positive throughout the course of the disease. As mentioned earlier, people often have a very mild or asymptomatic disease. This may explain the 0.1 to 0.2% incidence of positive HAA in the control population.

Drug-induced Hepatitis

The diagnosis of drug-induced liver disease is usually made in the absence of known exposure to viral hepatitis and with documented exposure to a known hepatotoxic drug. The hepatotoxic drugs (Table 11.2) will produce changes in all individuals consisting of fatty infiltration and zonal necrosis of liver tissue within 24 to 48 hr after exposure. Enzymatic changes and laboratory changes resemble those of viral hepatitis. The drugs that induce hepatocellular damage of the hypersensitivity type also produce laboratory changes like those of viral hepatitis. The changes may occur anywhere from 24 hr to several weeks after exposure. Drug-induced cholestatic changes usually lead to increased serum bilirubin levels as well as an increased serum alkaline phosphatase level since intrahepatic plugging prevents normal exocrine excretion of alkaline phosphatase. The drug-induced hypersensitivity reactions may also be accompanied by a fever, rash, arthralgias and eosinophilia.

Cirrhosis

Laennec's cirrhosis is insidious in its development and often produces no clinical manifestations. About 1/3 to 1/2 of all cases are discovered only on postmortem examination. If symptoms appear, the first are quite non-specific such as weight loss, loss of appetite, nausea, vomiting and ill defined digestive disturbances, and only in the more progressive stages does the patient become symptomatic. There may be leukopenia and thrombocytopenia related to hypersplenism secondary to portal hypertension. There may be anemias secondary to gastrointestinal (GI) blood loss, folic acid deficiencies, decreased RBC survival from hypersplenism or suppressive effects of alcohol on erythropoiesis in the bone marrow. There is often marked bilirubinemia with or without increased transaminase and alkaline phosphatase levels. Albumin levels are often decreased and the prothrombin time may be markedly increased owing to decreased liver production of the vitamin K-dependent factors (prothrombin group). Diagnosis is usually based on a history of predisposing factors, e.g., chronic alcoholism, and by biopsy. The hepatitis-associated antigen is not elevated in cirrhotic patients.

COMPLICATIONS

Hepatitis

Immediately following the icteric phase of acute viral hepatitis, the patient usually feels well, but recovery is seldom complete at this stage. Fatigue, mild liver enlargement and tenderness may still be evident. The duration of the posticteric phase varies from 2 to 6 weeks but may be longer in some instances. Full clinical or biochemical recovery can be expected in 3 to 4 months in most cases. In rare cases the disease may run a prolonged course for up to 1 to 2 years or more (chronic active hepatitis). The mortality rate is quite low, 0.1 to 0.4% for infectious hepatitis and 10 to 12% for serum hepatitis. Patients with chronic active hepatitis may have low grade symptoms for years and then get better; others progress into more serious stages including postnecrotic cirrhosis.

Approximately 5% of patients have an exacerbation within 6 months. The symptoms and course are identical with the first occurrence of the disease, but may be milder. The relapse usually does not alter prognosis for the patient or increase residual liver damage unless it progresses into subacute (submassive) or massive hepatitis. The prodromal stage of submassive hepatic necrosis is similar to normal acute hepatitis, but the preicteric phase is usually longer than 2 weeks. Once jaundice is present, the course of the illness is clearly different from that of typical acute viral hepatitis. The patient continues to feel ill, and weakness and vomiting may persist. Serum bilirubin may still be increasing after 2 weeks and usually plateaus at higher than 20 mg %. Transaminase lvels also remain elevated for several weeks. A liver biopsy is essential for diagnosis. Submassive hepatitis may progress to cirrhosis, portal hypertension and death after several months or years.

In massive hepatic necrosis, one usually sees a sudden shrinkage of the liver over a period of several hours or days. The patient usually develops hepatic coma and fatality is 60-90%. The interval between the onset of illness and death is usually less than 2 weeks. Figure 11.1 summarizes the clinical course of the various stages of viral hepatitis.

Cirrhosis

Cirrhosis *per se* is a relatively benign situation, but as the degree of scarring increases, the complications increase, primarily owing to a syndrome known as portal hypertension which

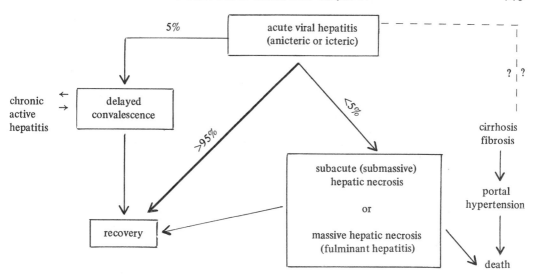

FIG. 11.1. Complications of hepatitis. (Adapted from Harrison's Principles of Internal Medicine, Ed. 6.[5])

refers to an increase in blood pressure within the portal vein from a normal of 50 to 100 mm of water up to 500 mm or higher. In simplified terms, the portal hypertension of cirrhosis is due to obstruction of the radicles of the portal vein by fibrous scarring, swelling of the liver cells and distention within the liver. Also in cirrhosis there is an increase in anastomoses between hepatic arterioles and the portal system allowing blood to be transmitted under arterial pressure into the portal system, thus increasing the portal pressure. Some of the problems arising secondary to increased portal pressure are ascites, hydrothorax, hepatomegaly, splenomegaly, gastrointestinal bleeding (ulcers and gastritis), esophagael varices, distention of abdominal vessels and hemorrhoids. With progression of the disease, the liver eventually begins to shrink in size and often is not palpable.

Endocrine disorders are also seen in far advanced cirrhosis owing to the inability of the liver to metabolize the steroid hormones of the adrenals and gonads. Commonly seen are gynecomastia, loss of body hair, impotence, spider angiomas and palmar erythema due to an increase in circulatory estrogen levels.

Ascites is one of the most striking features of cirrhosis since several liters of fluid may be accumulated within the peritoneal cavity. Although the precise mechanism of this accumulation is not known, some of the theories must be understood to appreciate the approaches to therapy.[4] Certainly a large portion of the accumulation is due to transudation of serous fluid through the serosal lining of the peritoneal cavity due to the portal hypertension. However, many other systemic and local factors may be involved. Liver disease leads to decreased albumin synthesis and thus a lowered colloid pressure in the blood, favoring transudation of fluid into the so-called third space of the peritoneal cavity. Hyperaldosteronism is well documented as well as an increase in antidiuretic hormone (ADH) activity leading to retention of sodium and water. These increases may be due to decreased metabolism of these hormones and in response to decreased effective renal blood flow. It is also felt that a large portion of the accumulation is due to direct leakage of fluid into the peritoneal cavity from the liver secondary to intrahepatic venous stasis.

Gastrointestinal hemorrhage occurs with cirrhosis in about 1/4 to 1/3 of patients, and in about 1/3 of these cases the patients die from the initial hemorrhage. Even nonfatal hemorrhages tend to be massive. Only occasionally is there an insidious leakage of blood with anemia and occult blood in the stools. Esophageal varices probably account for about 50% of the bleeding, while peptic ulcer only accounts for around 25%.

The ultimate result of far advanced cirrhosis or of severe hepatitis is liver failure and hepatic coma (hepatic encephalopathy). This is characterized by increasing personality changes and mental confusion with a characteristic flapping tremor of the fingers and hands (liver flap or asterixis), eventually followed by a deepening coma and death. The pathogenesis of these central nervous system (CNS) derangements is not well understood but is correlated by many researchers with an increased arterial and CNS ammonium level. Although a direct cause and effect relationship has not been shown to exist between encephalopathy and blood ammonium concentration, it has been shown that by decreasing factors that influence ammonium production, the patient's sensorium is often cleared. One of the most common sources of increased ammonium content of the blood is the action of bacteria in the small intestine and colon to produce ammonia from protein and urea breakdown. This ammonia is then absorbed into the blood stream and converted to ammonium ion. Normally these factors rarely lead to any CNS abnormalities since the liver converts the ammonium into urea, but when the liver is malfunctioning or the blood is being shunted away from it as in far advanced cirrhosis, encephalopathy ensues. The arterial concentration of ammonium may be accentuated by excessive dietary protein consumption, gastrointestinal hemorrhage (source of protein), overdiuresis leading to dehydration and other conditions that lead to severe electrolyte imbalances. Hepatic encephalopathy may also be induced by increased arterial pH (alkalosis) and abnormalities in various biochemical pathways.[8]

Significant azotemia sometimes occurs in patients who have liver or biliary tract disease. The concurrent impairment of renal function along with hepatic failure is often designated as the hepatorenal syndrome. The exact cause for the progression to renal failure, if a cause and effect relationship exists, is unknown. Of interest is the fact that often no structural abnormalities can be found in the kidneys at postmortem examination, and some have performed well when used as a donor for a renal transplant. It could very well be that there is simply a functional change in the kidney due to fluid and elctrolyte disturbances, shock or unmetabolized toxic substances. The use of neomycin has also been implicated as a cause of the change in renal status.

TREATMENT OF HEPATITIS

In the treatment of acute viral hepatitis,

drugs are of little value (Table 11.5). Historically, strict bed rest for several weeks or months was advocated, but now people are encouraged to maintain a certain minimal amount of exercise. They should be cautioned not to overwork but ambulate as tolerated. During the acute stages of the disease, patients are very often fatigued and cannot tolerate more than a few hours out of bed. Adequate nutrition is advocated, and if the patient is too sick to eat, parenteral feedings should be instituted. If the patient has contracted hepatitis from poor living conditions, these conditions should be ameliorated and the patient encouraged to practice good hygiene and protect himself and people with whom he has contact. If the patient is a drug user, he should be urged to discontinue the use of dirty needles. If a drug is the suspected cause of the hepatitis, its use should obviously be avoided in the future as well as structurally similar analogues.

Often the patient will complain of intense itching due to deposition of bile acids in the skin associated with biliary stasis. Cholestyramine, (Cuemid, Questran), an anion exchange resin, is occasionally given to relieve these symptoms. By forming an insoluble, nonabsorbable complex with bile acids, this drug markedly increases the fecal excretion of the bile acids. However, if the biliary obstruction is severe, the use of the drug is of little value. The usual dose is 4 g given 3 to 4 times daily for at least 2 weeks. The drug is very unpleasant to take; however, the flavor is masked when mixed with a thick juice or pulpy food such as applesauce. The main side effect of cholestyramine is constipation and GI distress. This may be relieved by taking the drug with meals and using stool softeners. Absorption of certain fat-soluble substances, e.g., vitamin, A, D or K, may be impaired by the drug. Of more im-

TABLE 11.5
Treatment of Hepatitis

Bed rest	Doubtful significance
Antiboitics	Not warranted
Cholestyramine	For pruritis
Corticosteroids	Do not alter course of disease—reserve for subacute or massive necrosis
Restrict protein	If in hepatic precoma
Neomycin (4-12 g/day)	If in hepatic precoma

portance to the pharmacist is the fact that cholestyramine will bind weakly acidic drugs such as thiazides, phenobarbital, phenyl-butazone, tetracyclines and warfarin. The pharmacist should always recommend that all other drugs be spaced as far apart from the cholestyramine as possible.

If the patient develops signs of encephalopathy or a liver flap, protein should be limited to 20 g per day and neomycin started at 2 to 4 g orally 3 to 4 times daily. By sterilizing the gut with neomycin and limiting protein intake, there is a reduction of bacterial breakdown of protein to ammonia products. Often there is a dramatic recovery in the patient's mentation with the institution of this therapy. However, hepatic failure is quite rare in hepatitis, except for very severe cases, and the treatment will be discussed more fully in the section on the treatment of cirrhosis.

Corticosteroids

Perhaps the greatest area of controversy in the treatment of hepatitis is the use of corticosteroids. It appears that the use of prednisolone or prednisone in doses of 40 to 60 mg daily brings a rapid and remarkable subjective improvement in the patient with an increase in appetite and feeling of well-being. There also appears to be a rapid initial fall of serum bilirubin which is most marked in the 1st 3 days, but becomes progressively decreased so that the serum bilirubin levels in the treated and control groups tend to be equal after the 2nd week.[9] It is important to note, however, that the subjective improvement and rapid rate of clearance of serum bilirubin are not associated with a shortened duration of the disease as evidenced by histological changes. Furthermore, not all patients respond as well and exacerbations are common if the drug is stopped abruptly or tapered to a lower maintenance level. The reduction mechanism of serum bilirubin by steroids is unknown. It is not due to increased outpouring of bile into the intestines, increased renal clearance of bilirubin or decrease in bilirubin production. Presumably, there is enhancement of the excretion of bilirubin via an additional metabolic pathway.[10,11] Routine use of steroids in acute viral hepatitis is to be discouraged since the disease is usually benign and self-limiting, and the effects are of questionable significance. Subjecting the patient to the risk of adverse effects such as GI ulceration, sodium retention, potassium loss, increased risk of infection, aggravation of diabetes and psychotic effects is usually not warranted. In addition, adverse effects would theoretically tend to be increased because of the liver's impaired ability to metabolize the corticosteroids. However, in the occasional case of chronic active hepatitis, or the cases that proceed to the more life-threatening submassive and massive necrotic hepatitis, steroids are commonly used. One study showed that in the majority of 18 cases of chronic active hepatitis, the patients not only became asymptomatic, but there was also biochemical histological evidence of improvement. Although permanent liver disease did not disappear, there was little or no progression of the disease as long as adequate doses of steroids were maintained. Those who failed to respond were found to have postnecrotic cirrhosis without active hepatitis. Carefully observed maintenance therapy for long periods was necessary in most cases to control activity of the disease. Discontinuance or rapid reduction of steroid therapy was often followed by exacerbation of the disease and in only one case was it possible to discontinue steroid therapy.[11] In two cases, this author has observed relapses with acute symptoms when the steroid dose was lowered below 20 mg of prednisone, but increasing the dose led to rapid subjective improvement.

The nature of chronic active hepatitis is obscure. It might be the result of a continuing viral infection of the liver, in which case steroid therapy would simply suppress the inflammatory reaction. It is also proposed that chronic hepatitis might be an autoimmune disease. If this were true, the effect of steroid therapy presumably would be the inhibition of antibody formation of suppression of antigen-antibody reaction. Based on the latter theory, immunosuppressive therapy with 6-mercaptopurine and azothioprene has been tried, but the results are equivocal.[8] Their use in this situation is investigational, and they should be reserved for patients with severely advanced disease as well as patients who have either not responded to or cannot tolerate corticosteroids.

Prophylactic use of gamma globulin has been suggested for persons with suspected exposure to hepatitis or who live in endemic areas. Gamma globulin in a dose of 0.1 ml per pound is given I.M. early in the incubation period after exposure to infections hepatitis. The patient still may develop a subclinical infection but will not be symptomatic. A dose of 0.05 to 0.06 ml per pound is given for protection of up to 4 months in endemic areas. Small doses of gamma globulin are ineffective against serum hepatitis. Large doses, up to 20 ml within a week of transfusion and 30 days later, give variable results. The high cost of gama globulin precludes widespread use for routine prophylaxis.[5]

TREATMENT OF CIRRHOSIS

As with hepatitis, the management of cirrhosis is largely symptomatic. In Laennec's cirrhosis, the primary treatment is to encourage the patient to abstain from alcohol. Fluid and electrolyte balance should be maintained by either parenteral administration or a good diet. If the patient is vomiting, antiemetics such as prochlorperazine may be used. For abdominal pain, analgesics may be administered, bearing in mind that aspirin-containing products may worsen gastritis or gastrointestinal bleeding. Narcotics may lead to profound CNS and respiratory depression if the patient's liver status is significantly compromised or if he is already obtunded. Sedatives and hypnotics should be avoided if there is any danger of the patient developing hepatic coma. If the patient does not exhibit signs of impending hepatic coma, he should be maintained on a 2000 to 3000 calorie diet with 1 gm of protein per kg of body weight.

Vitamin replacement is also essential in a majority of cirrhotic patients, esepcially those with a recent alcoholic history. Replacement of thiamine at 50 to 100 mg per day along with a good diet often brings about remarkable increases in mentation in chronic alcoholics as well as a decrease in peripheral neuritis and improvement in disorders in gait. Up to 1 gm per day may occasionally be required if the patient displays severe nystagmus of Wernicke's encephalopathy or oculogyric crisis. Chronic alcoholics often malabsorb folate, and their bone marrow does not adequately respond to the folate they do absorb, leading to the development of a megaloblastic anemia. Thus 1 mg of folic acid is often administered daily. Vitamin K, 10 mg daily for 3 or more days, IM or orally, is given if the prothrombin time is elevated. It should be remembered that vitamin K_1, or phytonadione, gives a more rapid response when given parenterally than the water-soluble vitamin K_3 (menadione).[12] However, if the patient is malabsorbing fats, menadione is the vitamin K of choice for oral administration since it is water-soluble. Iron therapy with ferrous sulfate or gluconate is often required if the patient is actively bleeding or if his hematocrit or hemoglobin count is depressed.

GI Bleeding

It is in the treatment of the sequela of cirrhosis that the real challenge develops. Bleeding from esophageal varices is a grave sign and is very difficult to stop; multiple transfusions are often required. Even if the bleeding is stopped, the chances of the patient hemorrhaging again are high. Placement of a Sengstaken tube and balloon in an attempt to slow the bleeding by compression is often tried, yielding varied results. Occasionally the natural hormone vasopressin (ADH)(Pitressin) is given IV in a dose of 10 to 20μ in 100 ml of 5% dextrose over 15 to 30 min. This produces a significant decrease in portal blood flow and pressure by vasoconstriction of portal arterioles. This vasoconstriction slows or stops bleeding long enough to allow thrombus formation at the site of bleeding. The dose may be repeated 3 or 4 times daily. Kinetically, it would be better to give the drug more often since it has a very short half-life (about 20 min) but, owing to its intense vasoconstrictor action, it decreases cardiac output and may cause coronary ischemia. This is especially a problem in patients with coronary heart disease or hypertension, but electrocardiograph (EKG) changes have been reported in patients with no prior evidence of heart disease.[13] It also may produce GI cramping due to stimulation of the smooth muscle contraction. Finally, it may lead to excess water retention and dilutional hyponatremia. Recently direct instillation of 0.2 units per minute of vasopressin via a catheter into the superior mesenteric artery has been tried with excellent results and fewer side effects.

Bleeding from other gastrointestinal sites, especially due to gastritis and peptic ulcer, is usually treated with nasogastric suction, iced saline and hourly antacids. Since these patients often tend to retain sodium because of a relative aldosteronism, a low sodium antacid such as Riopan should be used.

Ascites

The treatment of ascites is a frequently encountered problem in the cirrhotic patient. Ascites is often more of a cosmetic problem than a serious medical problem, but it may be a good culture medium for bacterial growth, may be painful if the abdomen becomes very tense or may cause compression of the diaphragm making respiration difficult. Often bed rest may cause a very dramatic diuresis and decrease in abdominal girth. However, after the first 1 to 2 weeks, the diuresis often slows down and drug treatment may be started. Throughout the entire treatment a 1 to 2 g low sodium diet should be maintained. Since the maximal rate at which ascitic fluid can be reabsorbed is about 700 ml per day,[4] it must be stressed that the diuresis be gentle since too rapid a diuresis can lead to volume and electrolyte depletion (*i.e.,* vascular losses occurring more rapidly than the ascitic fluid can be reabsorbed). A rising blood urea nitrogen determination (BUN) is a good sign of overdiuresis, because if the patient becomes volume depleted, his renal blood flow decreases, and he will tend to retain more fluid. This may, in turn, lead to a reaccumulation of the ascitic fluid. Treatment is usually started with a low dose of thiazides, although furosemide is often used in doses of 20 to 40 mg daily. The patient's weight is the best monitor of effectiveness of treatment with a goal of about 1 kg weight loss per day. A faster loss can often lead to the problems alluded to above, and the dose of the diuretic should be lowered. Many physicians like to use spironolactone as the diuretic because it is a relatively mild diuretic and it is a direct antagonist of the hyperaldosteronism that these patients often demonstrate. When used in combination with thiazides or furosemide it has the further advantage of an additive diuretic effect plus its potassium-sparing property. Although gentle diuresis is the rule, these patients are often refractory to normal doses of the diuretics, and it is not uncommon to see total daily doses of 120 to 180 mg or more of furosemide and 200 to 400 mg of spironolactone. Triamterene may be used as a potassium-sparing diuretic in place of spironolactone because it is a little more rapid acting. (It may take 3 to 5 days for spironolactone to induce diuresis.) However, it is not a direct aldosterone antagonist. Salt-poor albumin is used occasionally to raise the colloid pressure of the serum to draw the ascitic fluid back into the circulation. This has the disadvantage of very high cost and a possible increase of portal hypertension that may precipitate gastrointestinal bleeding. The fluid may also be tapped with a needle, but it usually reaccumulates in a matter of days, and the procedure runs the risk of introducing an infection or inducing a considerable loss of albumin. Paracentesis is usually reserved for refractory cases or in those conditions in which ascites is causing a considerable amount of pain or respiratory distress.

Hepatic Coma

If the patient should develop signs of an impending hepatic coma (*e.g.,* confusion, drowsiness, liver flap) 4 to 8 g per day of neomycin may be started and the dietary protein decreased to 20 to 30 g per day, thus decreasing ammonia production in the gut. It is also wise to back off on diuretics at this stage since hypovolemia and hypokalemia tend to aggravate the encephalopathy. If the above measures do not work and the patient slips into a coma, the dose of the neomycin should be increased to 8 to 12 g per day and the protein restriction lowered to 0 to 20 g per day. When the patient improves, the maintenance dose of neomycin may be lowered to 2 to 4 grams per day. Duration of therapy is variable and may last less than a week for some patients, months and even years in patients with very tenuous balance. The importance of protein restriction cannot be overemphasized. This author has observed a patient who was progressing nicely after recovering from hepatic coma but relapsed within 12 hr after eating a tuna fish sandwich.

If the patient is not able to take his medications orally, a retention enema of 2 to 4 g of neomycin in 200 cc of saline may be used morning and night. The addition of methylcellulose to the enema helps to thicken it and enhance retention. Neomycin is one of the "nonabsorbable" antibiotics, and thus orally it should only give local effects in the gut. However, it has been shown that from 0.1 to 0.3%[14] of a dose is absorbed and there are several reported cases of ototoxicity in patients on chronic oral neomycin therapy.[15] Most of these patients had been taking the neomycin for at least 8 months and had coexisting renal dysfunction. In any case, periodic auditory testing should be performed and the patient observed for subjective changes in hearing status if he is to be on the drug for prolonged periods.

Neomycin has also been implicated in the development of the hepatorenal syndrome since it is a known renal toxic drug when given parenterally. However, it is difficult to determine if the renal changes are due to the drug or just a progression of the disease process itself. Most people feel it is the latter mechanism that is occurring.

Another problem encountered with neomycin therapy is diarrhea due to changes in the bowel flora. However, this may not be a deleterious consequence and in fact patients are often given cathartics to cleanse the bowel and thus eliminate excess ammonia production. For this reason, orders may be written for magnesium citrate (citrate of magnesia) or for 50 g of sorbitol in 200 cc of water. However, it should be noted that these agents are not effective to any great extent when used alone and should always be accompanied by neomycin therapy and protein restriction. The danger of the cathartic procedures is that fluid and electrolyte imbalances may occur, thus worsening the encephalopathy. Therefore, it is imperative that adequate intravenous infusions of dextrose or saline with potassium supplements be maintained.

Lactulose

Another drug, lactulose, has been tried on a limited basis. It is a synthetic disaccharide, which is neither absorbed nor hydrolyzed in the small bowel. However, it is degraded by the colonic bacteria to lactic acid thus decreasing the pH of the colonic contents to about 5.5. The effects of lactulose have been attributed to replacement of proteolytic bacteria such as *Escherichia coli, Proteus,* and *Bacteroides* with organisms such as *Lactobacillus* which thrive in a more acidic medium and which are lacking in urease and other enzymes used in the production of ammonia products. However, some investigators have not been able to demonstrate a marked change in the colonic flora; they attrib-

ute the effect of lactulose solely to the pH changes that occur leading to a greater ammonium ion to ammonia concentration in the bowel lumen, and thus less absorption of the ammonia products. There may also be diffusion of ammonia from the blood to the intestinal lumen under these conditions. In any event, the final outcome of lactulose therapy is a decrease in arterial ammonium levels.[16,17]

The most common complaint of patients treated with lactulose is diarrhea due to osmotic effects of the drug in the bowel. This diarrhea may account for part of the therapeutic effects of lactulose, but when compared to sorbitol, lactulose is much more effective in overcoming the encephalopathy indicating that other mechanisms are working. In fact, the dose that is usually given (from 30 to 150 ml daily), is adjusted so that the patient has two to three soft, semiformed stools daily, avoiding watery diarrhea. The success rate at these doses has been reported to be around 85%. This includes some patients who had previously shown poor response to neomycin therapy. Unfortunately, a few patients tend to become resistant after prolonged therapy, and many patients die of other complications of the disease even though they are helped through the encephalopathy. The greatest drawback to the use of lactulose is its high cost and the fact that its use is not approved by the FDA.

One of the more exciting areas in the treatment of hepatic encephalopathy is the use of L-Dopa.[18,19] It will be recalled that L-Dopa is currently approved for use in the treatment of parkinsonism as a source of dopamine replacement. It is proposed that some of the neurological manifestations of hepatic failure, as well as the hepatorenal syndrome may be due to the accumulation of false neurotransmitters that replace normal transmitters in their peripheral and central nervous systems. The catecholamines, norepinephrine and dopamine, play important roles in normal central nervous system synaptic transmissions, while norepinephrine is the normal transmitter in the peripheral sympathetic nervous system. However, other beta-hydroxylated phenylethylamines can replace norepinephrine in the sympathetic nerve terminals and granules. One of these compounds, octopamine, has been found in higher than normal concentrations in patients in hepatic coma. These compounds can displace or coinhabit the adrenergic neuron with norepinephrine and be released in its place when sympathetic discharge is mediated. However, they are unable to elicit the normal responses that norepinephrine would mediate and may lead to some of the deficits seen in these patients.

Precursors of these false neurotransmitters, such as phenylalanine and tyrosine (Fig. 11.2), are produced from protein in the gut by the action of bacterial amino acid decarboxylases. Normally they are rapidly metabolized in the liver by monoamine oxidase (MAO) so that norepinephrine that is formed elsewhere in the body predominates. When hepatic function is impaired or when blood is shunted away from the liver, these false neurotransmitters may replace the normal transmitter. Systemically this may lead to lowered peripheral vacular resistance and shunting of blood away from the kidney. Similary, asterixis and other signs of hepatic encephalopathy might be the result of displacement of transmitters such as dopamine and norepinephrine in the basal ganglia and other areas in the brain. Finally, it should be noted that since these false neurotransmitters are amines, this theory is compatible with the idea that increased blood nitrogenous products (e.g., ammonium ions) are associated with hepatic encephalopathy.

If the displacement of normal central and peripheral transmitters by less active amines can account for hepatic coma and its cardiovascular complications, then the restoration of normal transmitter stores might restore normal function. It is impractical to use norepinephrine

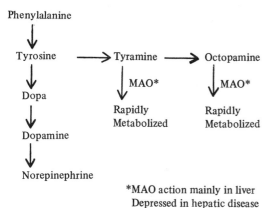

FIG. 11.2. Synthetic pathway of neurotransmitters.

itself since it is rapidly metabolized and must be given intravenously. However, L-Dopa is readily absorbed orally and converted both peripherally and centrally to dopamine, lack of which may be implicated in the encephalopathy. By referring to Figure 11.2, it can be seen that dopamine is also a precursor to norepinephrine and thus might restore natural neurotransmitter balance and lead to improvement of neurological and cerebrovascular function. L-Dopa has the added benefit that one of the effects attributed to dopamine is increased renal blood flow which may help to alleviate the renal failure of the hepatorenal syndrome.

Only a few cases are reported where L-Dopa has been used, usually as a last resort when more conventional measures failed, and the patient was near death. In one case the patient showed remarkable improvement within 1 hr after a single 250-mg dose of L-Dopa. In this author's experience the results have been varied. One case failed to respond, one case responded after several days of therapy (concurrent with neomycin which had been started 1 week earlier) and a third case showed some response after 1 day and by the 3rd day the patient was able to communicate rationally for the first time in over 1 month. Doses have usually been 500 mg 3 to 4 times daily, or in the last instance 1 g twice daily by rectal enema.

The last case was also complicated by the hepatorenal syndrome with profound hypotension and almost a total absence of urine formation. Along with L-Dopa and neomycin, the patient was given an IV infusion of metaraminol. As soon as her blood pressure increased, her urine output increased to several hundred ml daily. Other investigators have also used metaraminol in cases of the hepatorenal syndrome with very encouraging results.[18] The theory again is that sympathetic transmitter stores may be depressed and that metaraminol, by eliciting an intense alpha-adrenergic response, may increase peripheral vascular resistance, thus increasing the blood pressure and increasing the effective blood flow to the kidney. However, metaraminol does not seem to have any effect on increasing the mental status of the patient since it does not cross the blood brain barrier. For this reason, L-Dopa and metaraminol are usually given together when treating the hepatorenal syndrome.

Surgical Treatment

Surgical treatment may be required for patients who have repeated gastrointestinal bleeding, especially esophageal varices, or who have bleeding that cannot be stopped by the more conservative measures already described. The surgery performed is called a portacaval shunt and involves an anastomosis of the portal vein directly to the inferior venal cava, thus bypassing the cirrhotic liver. This serves to decrease portal hypertension and thus the back-pressure on the abdominal venous system. Unfortunately, these patients have a very poor prognosis since the only source of blood supply to carry toxins to the liver for detoxification is now the hepatic artery. Thus, if they survive the initial surgery, these patients often die of sepsis or develop hepatic failure and encephalo-pathy.[20]

PROGNOSIS

As mentioned earlier, acute viral hepatitis is not usually a life-threatening disease, although the mortality rate may be a little higher for the serum type of hepatitis than for infectious hepatitis. The rare cases that progress into chronic active hepatitis or into submassive or massive hepatic necrosis have a much poorer prognosis.

The outlook for patients with cirrhosis depends entirely upon the stage of advancement of the cirrhosis. If the liver is fatty with little fibrosis, remarkable improvement follows the initiation of a well balanced diet. The fat can be mobilized, the liver decreases in size, evidence of hepatic cell necrosis disappears and liver function is much improved. Even when there is considerable fibrosis, the forward progress of the disease can be halted by good dietary discretion although the existing fibrosis can not be reversed. If the cause of the cirrhosis is alcoholism and the patient continues to drink and neglect a proper diet, the prognosis is poor. Such patients usually die of either liver failure in hepatic coma; massive bleeding, usually from esophageal varices, or infection. About 50% die within a year of the appearance of major complications, and an additional 25% die within the next 3 to 5 years.[4] In the United States, cirrhosis has become one of the five most frequent causes of death in persons over the age of 40.

CONCLUSION

Despite the large amount of study done on the liver, and a vastly expanding understanding of its functions and pathologies, effective therapy for liver disease does not exist. At best, only symptomatic management of the complications of chronic liver disease is as yet possible. Furthermore, the etiology of viral hepatitis, probably the most frequent acute liver disease, is not established, nor do we know the initial etiology of cirrhosis or the pathways through which cirrhosis develops. One redeeming factor is that, although the lesions of advanced cirrhosis are irreversible, it is estimated that 70% or more of liver tissue must be destroyed before the body is unable to eliminate drugs and toxins via the liver. Unfortunately, it is difficult to foretell just which patients have reached this stage of involvement so that, when working with a patient with advanced liver disease, the pharmacist should always be aware of the potential inability of the patient to excrete certain drugs and see that doses are adjusted accordingly.

REFERENCES

1. Helman, R., Temko, M., Sylvanus, W., and Fallon H.: Alcoholic hepatitis. Ann. Intern. Med., 74: 311, 1971.
2. Annon.: Halothane hepatitis. Med. Lett. Drug Ther., 14: 43, 1972.
3. Goldman, A., and Braman, S.: Isoniazid: a review with emphasis on adverse effects. Chest, 62: 71, 1972.
4. Robbins, S. (editor): Pathology, Ed. 3, Chap. 12, p. 912. W. B. Saunders Co., Philadelphia, 1967.
5. Koff, R., and Isselbacher, K.: Acute hepatitis. In Harrison's Principles of Internal Medicine, Ed. 6, Chap. 326. p. 1535, edited by M. Wintrobe, G. Thorne, R. Adams, I. Bennett, E. Braunwald, K. Isselbacher and R. Petersdorf. McGraw-Hill Book Co., New York, 1970.
6. Shulmen, N.: Hepatitis associated antigen. Am. J. Med., 49: 669, 1970.
7. Rosenberg, H., Jones, D., Lipitz, L., and Kirsner, J.: Viral hepatitis: an occupational hazard to surgeons. J.A.M.A., 223: 395, 1973.
8. Melmon, K., and Morelli, H. (editors): Clinical

Pharmacology, Ed. 1, p. 91. The MacMillan Co., New York, 1971.

9. Vakil, B.: A controlled trial of prednisolone in the treatment of infectious hepatitis. J. Indian Med. Assoc., 45: 357, 1965.

10. Kern, F., Vinnik, I., Struthers, J., and Hill, R.: Treatment of chronic hepatitis with adrenocortical hormones. Am. J. Med., 35: 310, 1963.

11. Schiff, L.: The use of steroids in liver disease. Medicine, 45: 565, 1966.

12. Udall, J.: Don't use the wrong vitamin K. Calif. Med., 112: 65, 1970.

13. Beller, B., Trevino, A., and Urban, E.: Pitressin induced myocardial injury and depression in a young woman. Am. J. Med., 51: 675, 1971.

14. Breen, K., Bryand, R., Levinson, J., and Schenker, S.: Neomycin absorption in man. Ann. Intern. Med., 76: 211, 1972.

15. Berk, D., and Chalmer, T.: Deafness complicating antibiotic therapy of hepatic encephalopathy. Ann. Intern. Med., 73: 393, 1970.

16. Bircher, J., Haemmerli, U., Scollo-Lavizzari, G., and Hoffman, K.: Treatment of chronic portal-systemic encephalopathy with lactulose. Am. J. Med., 51: 148, 1971.

17. Elkington, S., Floch, M., and Conn, H.: Lactulose in the treatment of chronic portal systemic encephalopathy. N. Engl. J. Med., 281: 408, 1969.

18. Fischer, J., and Baldessarini, R.: False neurotransmitters and hepatic failure. Lancet, 2: 75, 1971.

19. Fischer, J., and James, J.: Treatment of hepatic coma and hepatorenal syndrome. Mechanism of action of L-Dopa and aramine. Am. J. Surg., 123: 222, 1972.

20. Garabedian, M., and Whitcomb, F.: Medical treatment of portal hypertension. Surg. Clin. North Am., 51: 749, 1971.

section 4

Cardiovascular diseases

chapter 12

ANGINA PECTORIS

Robert Kerr, Pharm.D.

Angina pectoris is a clinical syndrome which is most often clinically defined by the presentation of a history of substernal chest pain brought on by exertion and relieved by rest. This syndrome occurs as a result of an imbalance between the amount of oxygen delivered to the myocardium and the metabolic demands of the myocardium dictated by myocardial work (myocardial ischemia). In order to rationally approach the therapeutic management of angina pectoris, one must understand the causes of the oxygen delivery-myocardial workload imbalance, factors which precipitate the angina pectoris syndrome, the daily pattern of the syndrome in each individual patient, the relative efficacies of the drugs employed in the management regimen and the need for "total patient management."

ETIOLOGY

Coronary atherosclerosis is the identifiable pathological lesion limiting oxygen delivery to the myocardium in the vast majority of angina pectoris patients.[1,2] Atherosclerosis of the coronary arteries leads to a decrease in coronary blood flow which in turn means a decrease in oxygen delivery which leads to ischemic heart disease. One must keep in mind, however, that myocardial ischemia and, hence, angina pectoris can be caused by other factors. Some of these include systemic or pulmonary hypertension, acquired valvular disease, anemias and abnormal muscle metabolism. In addition, obstruction of the coronary arteries can be due to obstructive lesions such as arteritis or embo-

lism rather than to atherosclerosis. It is important that all possible factors be considered in a patient presenting with angina pectoris since one would obviously prefer to treat the underlying cause of the syndrome if at all possible, such as by normalizing systemic hypertension, or by valve repair if indicated, rather than only providing "symptomatic" relief, as is done in the medical management of the angina pectoris syndrome without underlying correctable etiology.

INCIDENCE

Coronary atherosclerosis begins early in life. Autopsies of 300 soldiers killed in battle showed that 77.3% of the hearts had some gross evidence of coronary atherosclerosis (the average age was 22.1 years). In 3.0% there was complete occlusion of one or more of the vessels.[1] Obviously there is not such a high percentage of young adult males who present with angina pectoris. Factors which determine whether or not patients with coronary atherosclerosis develop angina pectoris include the location of the atherosclerotic lesion, the degree of obstruction and, perhaps most important, the degree of development of collateral circulation. The tendency for coronary atherosclerosis to progress to ischemic heart disease is greater in males than in females, in diabetes, in hypertension and in certain hyperlipidemias. Of those patients presenting with angina pectoris, approximately 75% are males usually in their late 50's or early 60's.[1]

DIAGNOSIS AND CLINICAL FINDINGS

The cornerstone of the clinical diagnosis of angina pectoris is an accurate and complete patient history[3,4]; therefore, the *subjective* findings in a patient's data base will, in most instances, provide the definition of the problem: angina pectoris. *Objective* findings are usually utilized to confirm the diagnosis, to further define "atypical cases", to define exercise limitations or to provide further data on a patient who is considered to be a coronary artery bypass surgical candidate.

Subjective Findings

In establishing the diagnosis of and assessment of the problem angina pectoris, one must analyze the following features of chest discomfort[3]: quality, location, precipitating factors, factors bringing relief of distress, concurrent symptoms, duration of distress and the effect of sublingual nitroglycerin on the distress.

In assessing the quality of the discomfort of angina pectoris one should recognize that the discomfort often is not appreciated as "pain" and, therefore, the historical vocabulary should not be limited to a description of "pain." Characteristically, the discomfort may be described as being heavy, squeezing, aching, a sensation of tightness, a sense of shortness of breath or a sense of constriction around the larynx or upper trachea. The intensity of the discomfort characteristically builds up and gradually fades away. Patients rarely describe anginal pain as "stabbing like a knife" or "catching," and they usually indicate the area of discomfort with the whole hand as opposed to pointing with one finger.

The location of the discomfort of angina pectoris is usually characterized as substernal or near the sternum. However, the discomfort may occur anywhere between the epigastrium and the pharynx. The discomfort may radiate to the shoulders, arms, and/or hands. It also can appear in either shoulder or hand, the lower or upper jaw, the cervical area or the epigastrium without appearing in the chest.

Analysis of precipitating factors and relief factors is probably the most significant aspect of the history in angina pectoris, both from the standpoint of establishing the clinical diagnosis and from the standpoint of establishing a rational therapeutic regimen.[4–6] Precipitating factors are usually related to exertion or activity which would increase myocardial work and hence myocardial oxygen demand. Such exertions as climbing steps, walking a couple of blocks or sexual activity are typical precipitating factors. Anxiety-producing events or pressure will often induce anginal attacks. Eating a meal may precipitate an attack or moving from a warm to cold environment. One should also investigate the time of day anginal pain occurs: frequently, attacks are more likely to occur in the morning upon arising, or may occur at times when anxiety-producing events are present, such as driving in commuter traffic. Relief is usually obtained rapidly after cessation of the precipitating event or after the use of sublingual nitroglycerin.[7] What is obviously required in this aspect of the patient's history is a thorough analysis of the pattern of anginal distress as it relates to the patient's pattern or style of life.

The duration of stress-related anginal pain ranges between 1/2 min and 30 min.[3,7] Relief after cessation of exertion will usually occur within minutes. Relief after the use of sublingual nitroglycerin usually occurs within 45 sec to 2 min.

Two types of "atypical" angina can be identified by an accurate history. *Angina decubitus* is most often characterized by anginal attacks occurring in recumbent position, usually nocturnally. It is generally felt that angina decubitus is a form of left ventricular heart failure in which the increased venous return to the heart brought on by recumbency coupled with the increase in myocardial tension induced by left ventricular hypertrophy increases myocardial oxygen requirements, hence leading to myocardial ischemia.[2,3,7] The *intermediate syndrome,*[3] so-called because it is felt to represent an area between classical angina pectoris and myocardial infarction in the continuum of ischemic heart disease, is characterized by a history of increasing frequency and severity of anginal attacks which are "refractory" to nitroglycerin and which occur at rest as well as with exertion. Such a patient is felt to have an increased risk of sudden death secondary to ischemia-induced arrhythmias (hence the misleading terminology of "impending myocardial infarction" or "preinfarction angina") and therefore should be hospitalized and closely monitored.

Objective Findings

Objective findings in angina pectoris can be used to discover underlying causes other than coronary artery disease, to establish baseline data providing for monitoring of progression of the process, to confirm an atypical or suspected case of ischemic heart disease, to provide information in establishing exercise tolerance limits or to provide further data on a patient considered to be a candidate for coronary artery surgery. The collection of objective data revolves around the use of electrocardiography (EKG) and coronary arteriography.[3,4,7]

Typical EKG changes reflective of myocardial ischemia are T wave inversion and S-T segment displacement. However, the resting EKG is normal in 1/2 to 2/3 of patients with exertional angina without a history of myocardial infarction. Therefore, a resting EKG may prove more beneficial as a baseline to monitor progression than in providing a "diagnosis." The percentage of positive EKG changes increases when readings are taken after an exercise test and are even more revealing if taken during an exercise test. The advantages of taking EKG readings during exercise are that one can monitor the EKG changes as the ischemia occurs and, since the EKG changes usually occur prior to onset of anginal pain, the patient need not be exercised all the way up to the production of pain.

Such exercise-EKG testing may be of value in confirming the exertional character of the discomfort and also in establishing exercise tolerance limits which can then be utilized in developing a rational exercise program.

Coronary arteriography provides radiographic visualization of coronary artery lesions.[8] Such visualization can be particularly useful in the patient with an atypical case or in the patient who is considered a surgical candidate. In interpreting coronary arteriography one should keep in mind that myocardial ischemia probably does not occur until the lumen of a major coronary artery is reduced in cross section by at least 75%, and, if allowance is made for collateral circulation, it is more likely that angina occurs when there is 90 to 100% occlusion.[4,8] In addition, autopsies of persons with a history of angina pectoris show an average of 3.5 occlusions per heart. Hence, Friedberg[7] stated that "the prognosis for the patient with 1 3/4 occlusions in his coronary arteriogram is no different from the prognosis of the patient with angina pectoris without a coronary arteriogram." However, in the potential surgical candidate—that is, the patient with severely incapacitating and intractable angina, or symptoms of myocardial ischemia in early life, or the patient who is unwilling to accept restrictions on his lifestyle imposed by rational

medical management—visualization of the coronary arteries is a necessity.

MANAGEMENT

Except in cases where there is a treatable underlying cause for the ischemic heart disease, such as systemic hypertension or anemia, one should think in terms of managing angina pectoris rather than treating it. Generally, treatment aimed at reversing the atherosclerosis is not successful in ameliorating either the atherosclerosis in the vessel or the anginal syndrome itself, although frequently the management plan will involve measures aimed at slowing the progression of the atherosclerotic process. Proper rational management of an angina pectoris patient involves a firm understanding of the precipitating factors and patterns of attacks relative to the life pattern of the individual patient. The major aim of management is to reduce the frequency and severity of anginal attacks and to allow the patient to lead as normal a style of life as possible.[5,6,9] It should be pointed out that neither medical nor surgical management has been shown to alter the pathological process, alter prognosis or increase life expectancy.

General Medical Management

Once the stresses in the patient's life which precipitate anginal attacks are identified, efforts should be made to eliminate these stresses as much as possible while at the same time utilizing prophylactic drug therapy.[5,6,9] Emotional stresses in the patient's life should be approached openly with the aim of solving or eliminating them. The patient should recognize physical limitations. In some instances these may require a change in occupation, but he should be made to recognize that he has a useful life ahead of him and not be made to feel like an invalid. Reassurance is an important part of medical management since an anginal patient is almost always extremely anxious about the status of his heart and his life.

Anginal patients should be maintained at their ideal body weight. If the patient is overweight, then dietary measures should be undertaken. This usually involves caloric control along with control of fat intake, with the intention of slowing the progression of the atherosclerotic process. Some clinicians will evaluate the patient's serum lipids and attempt to correct any hyperlipidemia. However, such in-depth evaluation of hyperlipidemia in middle-aged patients with established angina pectoris is of dubious value since effective therapy for several of the hyperlipidemias is lacking and, in those cases where a hyperlipidemia may be treated, it is questionable if such treatment does anything for either the existing degree of atherosclerosis or angina or for the progression of the process. It is possible that strict dietary control, expensive and sometimes troublesome drug therapy for hyperlipidemia may place an added emotional stress on the patient.

Drug Management

Nitrites.[10-20] The nitrites have been the mainstay of drug management in angina pectoris for almost 100 years (Table 12.1). Although it is known that these drugs cause vasodilation, the exact mechanism of action by which they exert their effect in the relief of anginal pain has been the subject of controversy. For some time it was felt that the nitrites produced a vasodilation of the coronary vessels leading to a direct increase in coronary blood flow and a consequent increase in oxygen delivery to the myocardium. However, when one considers that, first, the coronary vessels of a patient with angina pectoris are diseased with atherosclerosis and, therefore, are quite possibly incapable of effectively dilating and, secondly, the coronary vessels of such a patient are probably already maximally dilated since hypoxia is a very effective physiological stimulus to vasodilation, it becomes difficult to accept coronary vasodilation as a mechanism of action for nitrites in angina pectoris. A more acceptable theory is that these drugs reduce cardiac work by creating peripheral vasodilation leading to, first, a venous pooling of blood resulting in decreased venous return to the heart and, therefore, decreased diastolic filling pressure in the left ventricle (decreased preload) and, secondly, decreased peripheral resistance against which the heart must work (decreased after-load).[2,21,6]

Many nitrites are currently available. They may be classified as being either short-acting or long acting. The short acting nitrites include amyl nitrite and nitroglycerin. While both are effective, nitroglycerin, as a sublingual tablet,

is the most commonly used medication for relief of anginal pain. Nitroglycerin is commonly used in doses of 0.16, 0.32, 0.4, and 0.6 mg sublingually. It has an onset of action of from 45 sec to 2 min and a duration not longer than 30 min. Most frequently, the drug is used to stop an attack of anginal pain, but it can be effectively utilized as a prophylactic agent if the patient is capable of anticipating events which he knows will bring on angina, such as sexual intercourse.[5] The patient can take the nitroglycerin just prior to the precipitating event and be afforded some protection. Obviously, the relationship between the patient's disease and life pattern must be well understood in order for drug prophylaxis to be effective. Patients should be educated to store their nitroglycerin tablets properly. Ideally they should be stored in the original glass or high density polyethylene container, tightly closed, with minimal amounts of filler (*e.g.*, cotton or gauze). It has been well documented that nitroglycerin vaporizes (hence the necessity of tight enclosure), is soluble in packaging materials such as plastic and fillers such as gauze or cotton, is soluble in the glue on gum labels and is unstable when stored in containers with other medicines such as aspirin.[17-20] If a sublingual nitroglycerin tablet does not produce a burning of the tongue or the characteristic sensation of fullness in the head, it is likely that the tablet has lost is potency and the supply should be replenished.[6] Initial patient responses to the drug should be monitored, especially significant postural hypotension which is particularly common in the elderly. Patients should be informed to seek medical attention if their symptoms become refractory to their usual doses of nitroglycerin.

The long acting nitrates include isosorbide dinitrate (ISDN), erythrityl tetranitrate and pentaerythritol tetranitrate (PETN). Of these only the sublingual forms of isosorbide dinitrate and erythrityl tetranitrate are effective in the prophylaxis of angina.[10]

Since these drugs are used mainly to prevent anginal attacks, rather than to treat an attack, the evaluation of their efficacy is rather difficult. There are so many physical and emotional variables in angina pectoris that there is a high degree of placebo response to prophylaxis of anginal pain. Placebo response in anginal patients is reported at 40% or higher. For ex-

TABLE 12.1
Drugs Used in the Management of Angina Pectoris

Drug	Dosage	Comments
Short acting nitrites		
Amyl nitrite	2-3 inhalations of vapor	Very short acting, usually within 30 sec but duration of action is transient; flushing and headache extremely common; generally considered obsolete for angina
Nitroglycerin	0.3 to 0.6 mg sublingually every 2-3 hr prn	Ineffective orally, despite the availability of such dosage forms
Long acting nitrates		
Erythrityl tetranitrate	10 mg qid orally or 5 mg qid sublingually	When given sublingually, the onset of effect may be as long as 10 min and usually lasts for 3-4 hr; tolerance develops with repeated use so the dose has to be gradually increased to maintain therapeutic effects
Pentaerythritol tetranitrate	10 mg orally qid	Sustained action preparations are available but are ineffective; otherwise, effects qualitatively similar to erythrityl tetranitrate above
Isosorbide dinitrate	10 mg qid orally or 5 mg qid sublingually	Similar effects to erythrityl tetranitrate
Mannitol hexanitrate	30 mg orally qid	Similar in effects to erythrityl tetranitrate
Trolnitrate phosphate	2 mg orally qid	See comment for pentaerythritol
Beta-adrenergic blockers		
Propranolol	160-400 mg a day in divided doses, for maintenance; however, lower doses should be used initially	Action enhanced by concomitant use of long acting nitrate preparations

ample, one study utilizing several placebos and several "active" drugs reported that the best response was from one of the placebos. The conclusion drawn is that the traditional "double blind controlled study" format may not be satisfactory in evaluating long acting nitrates in angina pectoris,[11] especially since most studies utilize "decreased frequency of attacks" as the success factor. The most useful studies appear to be those which utilize exercise-EKG tests after administration of drug to determine the duration of protection against exercise-induced EKG changes. Such studies indicate a definite protection induced by ISDN sublingual, as opposed to oral, with an onset of action of 5 min and a duration of action of from 1½ to 2 hr. The longer acting oral forms of ISDN, PETN and erythrityl tetranitrate are of dubious value although some clinicians do feel that they afford 4 to 5 hr of prophylaxis with an onset of action of about 1 hr. However, recent study[15] has shown that orally administered nitrites go via the portal vein directly to the liver where they are rapidly degraded so that little, if any, of the parent compound is available in the circulation. Hence, well conducted clinical and scientific work leads to the conclusion that long acting nitrites are of little more than placebo value.

There are also available sustained action formulations of most of the nitrites. These preparations have never been shown to be effective in the management of angina pectoris: however, they continue to be utilized by many clinicians. The result of the usage of these formulations, aside from the spectacular 12 hr placebo effect, is that there is a large portion of the health-care dollar expended on preparations of dubious efficacy and, more importantly, patients may be considered to have "intractable" angina when all they actually have is inadequate therapy.[5]

The FDA has classified the efficacy of coronary vasodilators as follows:

1. ISDN when administered *sublingually* is "probably" effective for treatment and prophylaxis of anginal attacks.
2. ISDN, when administered *orally* is only "possibly" effective.
3. Sustained action preparations of conventional oral dosage forms of PETN, trolnitrate phosphate, and mannitol hexanitrate, alone, or in combination with other drugs, are "possibly" effective.
4. Sustained action forms of nitroglycerin (*e.g.,* Nitrobid) are "possibly" effective.

"Probably" effective signifies that for a particular indication, the available evidence indicates that the drug probably accomplishes its proposed effect. "Possibly" effective signifies that little evidence of effectiveness for the given indication has been obtained.[16] It should be pointed out that this FDA classification was published prior to the publication of scientific evidence regarding one pass liver degradation following oral administration of nitrates.

It was once believed that chronic administration of long acting nitrates would induce development of tolerance to nitroglycerin or other nitrites or that frequent use of nitroglycerin would lead to tolerance with subsequent decrease in the efficacy of nitroglycerin. This concept of "tolerance" to nitrites is probably inaccurate. It is now generally felt that the observation of reduced efficacy of nitroglycerin tablets is more a reflection of reduced potency secondary to improper storage or of a change in the patient's life pattern or pattern of angina, rather than a reflection of the development of tolerance to the preparation.

Dipyridamole. Dipyridamole is not a nitrite, but it has been utilized as a drug which is supposed to cause marked peripheral vasodilation and increase the development of collateral vessels on the myocardium. However, since the drug also causes positive chronotropic and inotropic effects, the multiple effects apparently balance out. Dipyridamole has not been shown to be effective in the management of angina pectoris.

Beta-Adrenergic Blockade.[22-30] Beta-adrenergic blockade apparently decreases cardiac work by depressing the contractility of the myocardium leading to decreased heart rate and decreased ventricular systolic force yielding a decreased myocardial oxygen requirement. Propranolol is the beta-adrenergic blocking agent which has been used clinically.[30] Reports on propranolol's efficacy in the management of angina pectoris have been somewhat conflicting. Initial studies used low doses (60 to 120 mg) which were ineffective. Excellent results can be obtained if the dose is increased to 160 to 400 mg a day. The antianginal effect of propranolol can be further enhanced by using it in combination with a sublingual nitrate such as isosorbide dinitrate.[26] However, as with the use of any drug combination, to achieve the desired results, the dosages and regimen of each drug cannot be arrived at arbitrarily. Due consideration must be given to those parameters such as onsets of action and durations of action relative to the individual patient's pattern of anginal attacks. If properly titrated, the combination can be quite beneficial in patients who are otherwise difficult to manage. For example, if a patient's most vulnerable period is considered to be postprandial, then the patient could be instructed to take his propranolol before eating, rest for 1/2 hr after eating, and then take a sublingual ISDN 5 min before resuming activity. In this way, the drugs would come into play at the time the patient needs them. The combination works because the beta-blocking drugs and nitrates have a complementary action that results in a net reduction of myocardial oxygen consumption, thus raising the ischemic threshold. As a result, the patient will have fewer anginal attacks.[6,9,31]

One must remember when using propranolol that there is a general beta-adrenergic blockade and, therefore, complications arising from this blockade should be watched for — congestive heart failure, bronchial constriction leading to an asthma attack, bradycardia, intensification of hypoglycemic tendencies, or, more importantly, blockade of the sympathetic response to hypoglycemia thus blocking symptomatic manifestations which are important warning signs to diabetics on insulin or oral hypoglycemia agents. Propranolol is a potent myocardial depressant and should only be used in cases which do not respond to other measures such as general medical management and sublingual nitrites. Maintenance doses of propranolol for angina range from 160 to 400 mg per day. Dosing is started at lower levels and increased to maintenance levels.

Digitalis. As stated earlier, a form of angina exists in which a patient suffers from anginal attacks while in a recumbent position (angina decubitus). It is felt that part of the cause of this form of angina is left ventricular heart failure. Therefore, patients exhibiting angina decubitus frequently benefit from digitalis therapy to correct the underlying heart failure. In addition, digitalis can be used to correct propranolol-induced heart failure if it is felt that such a patient should remain on propranolol.

Tranquilizers and Sedatives. Antianxiety drugs are frequently employed in the over-all management of angina pectoris patients in an attempt to decrease the emotional and psychogenic influences on the precipitation of anginal pain. Psychogenic precipitation of anginal pain may be mediated by endogenous adrenergic humoral agents, and, with the advent of beta-adrenergic blocking agents, many clinicians do not worry about psychogenic factors. Possibly the best approach would be to deal openly with psychogenic factors so that the patient can effectively deal with them in his daily life, rather than merely utilizing drugs to cover up a problem.

Antithyroid Drugs. Antithyroid drugs and radioactive iodine have been used to decrease the frequency of anginal attacks by decreasing the rate of myocardial metabolism. This mode of therapy appears to be seldom used now and, indeed, with the current effective modes of treatment which are available, it seems unnecessary to use the antithyroid approach. However, angina may be secondary to hyperthyroidism. In this situation, antithyroid drugs are used to relieve the underlying problem.

Combination Antianginal Products. Products that contain a mixture of antianginal agents or antianginal agents and sedatives are not rational. There is no evidence that these combinations, *e.g.,* Peritrate-PB, Miltrate, Cartrax, etc., have any advantages over the individual com-

ponents. If more than one drug should be required for an individual patient, then they should be prescribed separately at the appropriate dosage regimen.

Carotid Sinus Stimulation. There are reports that electrical stimulation of the carotid sinus relieves patients with incapacitating angina. This consists of using a radiofrequency stimulator that is surgically implanted in the chest wall and connected by electrodes to the carotid sinus nerves. On the skin is a battery-powered transmitting unit that is activated by the patient at will with an off-on switch when he experiences angina. The long term value of such a procedure has yet to be evaluated, and it has been associated with a relatively high rate of immediate mortality. Therefore it cannot as yet be considered as a part of the routine mode of management in angina pectoris and should only be considered for patients extremely refractory to other therapy.

Surgery.[32–38] According to Kouchoukos and Kirklin,[32] the indication for surgery in angina pectoris patients is "disabling angina pectoris, refractory to adequate medical therapy, with angiographically demonstrated high grade obstructions in the proximal portions of the right, anterior descending, or circumflex coronary arteries, singly or in combination, and with patent vessels distally." The surgical procedures involve direct anastomosis of reversed segments of saphenous vein between the ascending aorta and the patent segments of 1 or more of the 3 major coronary arteries, or circumflex coronary arteries beyond the major obstructions. Internal mammary artery transplants (Vineberg procedure) have, for the most part, been abandoned in favor of the newer techniques.

The objectives of surgery are revascularization of the myocardium with subsequent relief of angina pectoris. Addtional objectives would be to prevent subsequent myocardial infarction and improve both the length and quality of life. Coronary artery bypass procedures have resulted in early patency rates of approximately 85 to 90%.[33] Patency rates of 1 to 2 years following operation range from 70 to 85%.[37,38] A recent study utilizing maximal graded treadmill exercise has shown that 79% of patients were free of angina 2 to 20 months after aortocoronary bypass surgery; however, only 52% could exercise for longer periods of time and 40% achieved higher heart rates.[35]

Evaluation of the results of surgical procedures in angina pectoris poses a difficult problem. Comparisons can only be made with patients who are known to have comparable symptoms and comparable degrees of atherosclerosis and left ventricular dysfunction. In addition, comparisons should be made by utilizing indices of effect which are as objective as possible. This point is illustrated by a study showing 60% of patients subjectively improving after undergoing a sham operation.[5]

Operative mortality for coronary bypass procedures seems to be related more to the preoperative degree of left ventricular dysfunction than to the number of diseased vessels or to the number of grafts inserted.[36] Early postoperative complications include myocardial infarction and serious ventricular arrhythmias.

At this point in time, increased long term survival following coronary bypass surgery has not been documented. Consequently, the procedures are still limited to a rather select group of patients until further evaluation of the accomplishment of objectives other than symptomatic relief can be obtained and correlated with both immediate and long term morbidity and mortality in matched patients, with and without surgical procedures.

CONCLUSIONS

Angina pectoris is a clinical syndrome resulting from ischemic heart disease, *i.e.*, an imbalance between myocardial work and myocardial oxygen supply. The most frequent underlying cause is atherosclerosis of the coronary vessels, but other causes such as anemia, systemic hypertension and valvular disease do exist.

Management of angina pectoris is aimed at the whole patient. Careful evaluation of the pattern of anginal episodes relative to the patient's life pattern allows for a rational approach to both general medical management and drug management. Precipitating factors in the patient's life should be eliminated as much as possible. Rational drug management involves knowledge of efficacy and pharmacokinetics of the agents available for the treatment of angina pectoris.

REFERENCES

1. Ross, R. S.: Ischemic heart disease. In Harrison's Principles of Internal Medicine, Ed. 6, p. 1208, edited by M. M. Wintrobe *et al.* McGraw-Hill Book Co., New York, 1970.
2. Epstein, S. E., *et al.*: Agnina pectoris: pathophysiology, evaluation and treatment. Ann. Int. Med., 75: 263, 1971.
3. Fowler, N. O.: Clinical diagnosis, symposium: angina pectoris. Circulation, 46: 1079, 1972.
4. Myerburg, R. J.: Diagnostic and therapeutic aspects of stable angina pectoris. Med. Clin. North Am., 55: 421, 1971.
5. Russek, H. I.: Intractable angina pectoris. Med. Clin. North Am., 54: 333, 1970.
6. Logue, R. B., and Robinson, P. H.: Medical management of angina pectoris. Circulation, 46: 1132, 1972.
7. Friedberg, C. K.: Introduction, some comments and reflections on changing interests and new developments in angina pectoris, symposium: angina pectoris. Circulation, 46: 1037, 1972.
8. Proudfit, W. L., Shirey, E. K., and Sones, F. M.: Selective cine coronary arteriography, correlation with clinical findings in 1000 patients. Circulation, 38: 901, 1966.
9. Sampson, J. J., and Hyatt, K. H.: Management of the patient with severe angina pectoris: an internists point of view. Circulation, 46: 1185, 1972.
10. Russek, H. I.: The therapeutic role of coronary vasodilators: glyceryl trinitrate, isosorbide dinitrate, and pentaerythritol tetranitrate. Am. J. Med. Sci., 252: 43, 1966.
11. Datey, K., and Dalvi, C.: Antianginal drugs: their evaluation by double blind trial. Angiology, 21: 520, 1970.
12. Goldstein, R. E., *et al.*: Clinical and circulatory effects of isosorbide dinitrate: comparison with nitroglycerin. Circulation, 43: 629, 1971.
13. Sweatman, T., *et al.*: The long acting hemodynamic effects of isosorbide dinitrate. Am. J. Cardiol., 29: 475, 1972.
14. Anon: Is peritrate life sustaining? Med. Lett. Drugs Ther., 8: 184, 1966.
15. Needleman, P., Lang, S., and Johnson, E.: Organic nitrates: relationship between biotransformation and rational anginal pectoris therapy. J. Pharmacol. Exp. Ther., 181: 489, 1972.
16. Annon: Coronary vasodilator potency. FDA Drug Bull., Feb. 1972.
17. Edelman, B. A., Contractor, A. M., and Shangraw, R. F.: The stability of nitroglycerin packaged in dispensing containers. J. Am. Pharm. Assoc., NS11: 30, 1971.
18. Shangraw, R. F., and Contractor, A. M.: New developments in the manufacture and packaging of nitroglycerin tablets. J. Am. Pharm. Assoc., NS12: 633, 1972.
19. Anon: Disintigration and storage of nitroglycerin

tablets. Med. Lett. Drugs Ther., 13: 316, 1971.

20. Anon: Nitroglycerin packaging affects potency. FDA Drug Bull., Feb. 1972.

21. Mason, D. T., *et al.*: Physiological approach to the treatment of angina pectoris. N. Engl. J. Med., 281: 1225, 1969.

22. Anon: Propranolol. Med. Lett. Drugs Ther., 10: 241, 1968.

23. Wessler, S., and Avioli, L. V.: Propranolol therapy in patients with cardiac disease. J.A.M.A., 206: 357, 1968.

24. Russek, H. I.: New dimensions in angina pectoris therapy. Geriatrics, 24: 81, 1969.

25. Zoster, T. T., and Beanlands, D. S.: Propranolol in angina pectoris. Arch. Intern. Med., 124: 584, 1969.

26. Battock, D. J., Alvarez, H., and Chidsey, C. A.: Effects of propranolol and isosorbide dinitrate on exercise performance and adrenergic activity in patients with angina pectoris. Circulation, 39: 157, 1969.

27. Zeft, H. J., Pattersen, S., and Orgain, E. S.: The effect of propranolol in the long term treatment of angina pectoris. Arch. Intern. Med., 124: 578, 1969.

28. Anon: Propranolol and other antianginal drugs. Med. Lett. Drugs and Ther., 12: 303, 1970.

29. Anon: Propranolol – new uses. Med. Lett. Drugs Ther., 15: 376, 1973.

30. Morrelli, H. F.: Drugs five years later: propranolol. Ann. Intern. Med., 78: 913, 1973.

31. Aronow, W. S.: Drug therapy: management of stable angina. N. Engl. J. Med., 289: 516, 1973.

32. Kouchoukos, N. T., and Kirklin, J. W.: Coronary bypass operations for ischemic heart disease, modern concepts of cardiovascular disease. Am. Heart Assoc. J., 41: 47, 1972.

33. Morris, G. C., *et al.*: Follow-up results of distal coronary artery bypass for ischemic heart disease. Am. J. Cardiol., 29: 180, 1972.

34. Spencer, F. C., *et al.*: Bypass grafting for occlusive disease of the coronary arteries: report of experience with 195 patients. Ann. Surg., 173: 1029, 1971.

35. Bartel, A. G., *et al.*: Changes in treadmill exercise test after aortocoronary bypass surgery (abstract). Clin. Res., 20: 24, 1972.

36. McRaven, D. R., *et al.*: Survival experience in saphenous vein bypass graft surgery (abstract). Am. J. Cardiol., 29: 277, 1972.

37. Bourassa, M. G., *et al.*: Factors influencing patency of aortocoronary vein grafts. Circulation, 46 and 46 (Suppl. I): 79, 1972.

38. Walker, J. A., *et al.*: Determinants of angiographic patency of aortocoronary vein bypass grafts. Circulation, 45 and 46 (Suppl. I): 86, 1972.

chapter 13

CONGESTIVE HEART FAILURE

Mary Anne Kimble, Pharm.D.

Robert M. Elenbaas, Pharm.D.

INTRODUCTION

The clinical syndrome of congestive heart failure (CHF) results from an inability of the heart to pump sufficient blood to meet the body's needs. Heart failure is generally considered to be a disease of the elderly, although it may occur in essentially any age group as a consequence of cardiovascular disease. The Framingham Heart Disease Epidemiology Study reported that during a 16-year period 3.5% of men and 2.1% of women in their population developed congestive heart failure.[1] This corresponded to an annual rate of 2.3 and 1.4 new cases per 1,000 males and females, respectively. These figures are in agreement with the estimated national incidence of CHF, which has been reported to vary from 0.5 to 2 per 1,000 per annum.[2] The Framingham Study clearly demonstrated a correlation between the incidence of CHF and age: by the 6th decade the incidence among men was 5 times that in the 4th decade.[1] An increase in the size of the geriatric population is making CHF one of the more commonly encountered clinical entities.

Contrary to what one might imagine, congestive heart failure appears to be a fairly rapidly fatal disease. In spite of treatment which is considered clinically effective, the long term prognosis is extremely poor. In the Framingham Study previously cited, 60% of men and 40% of women died within 5 years of the diagnosis of CHF. These figures are about 7 times the average annual death rate for persons without CHF.[3]

ETIOLOGY

Congestive heart failure has many etiologies. Most common, however, are essential hypertension, coronary heart disease and rheumatic heart disease. Pulmonary embolism, thyrotoxicosis, persistent cardiac arrhythmias and myocardiopathies, although less common, may also play an etiological role in the development of CHF. Hypertension appears to be the most important of these factors. The Framingham group, for example, found that 75% of patients who developed CHF had prior histories of hypertension.[1] It was noted that the risk of developing congestive failure in hypertensive patients was 6 times that of patients with normal blood pressures.[3] Coronary artery disease preceded the development of heart failure in 38.7% of the Framingham patients.[1] However, the majority of these had concomitant hypertension. Only 9.9% of patients had coronary artery disease alone.

An interesting study was performed by Perlman *et al.*,[4] who found a correlation between incidents of emotional upset in patients and hospital admissions for congestive heart failure. Emotional factors preceded hospitalization in 49% of patients with CHF but in only 24% of patients with diseases other than heart failure.

PATHOGENESIS

As mentioned, the clinical syndrome of congestive heart failure develops when the heart is unable to pump sufficient blood to supply oxygen needs of the tissues. Although the biochemical abnormality responsible for the myocardial failure is unknown, factors responsible for the development of the clinical manifestations of CHF are generally understood. When the heart fails and cardiac output decreases, a complex scheme of compensatory mechanisms designed to raise output is brought into play. At least in the early stages of heart failure, cardiac output is not dramatically reduced and the patient's symptoms result from the presence of these compensatory mechanisms.

In the failing myocardium, the strength with which the ventricle may contract is reduced. The reduction in stroke volume (cardiac output) which results causes an increase in residual blood volume within the ventricle at the end of the systole. If the atria continue to deliver blood to the ventricles at the same rate, the end diastolic volume will increase and the ventricles will dilate. The increased length of myocardial fibers allows an increased force of systolic contraction to be developed (Fig. 13.1). As long as the heart is on the ascending limb of the Starling curve, it will continue to compensate by progressive dilation. However, when the heart moves to the descending limb of the curve, continued dilation actually results in decreased cardiac output and no cardiac reserve exists. Fortunately, most patients seen clinically are on the ascending portion of the curve.

The failure of the heart to provide an adequate cardiac output produces several changes affecting sodium and water excretion. A reflex activation of the sympathetic nervous system and an increase in circulating catecholamines are known to exist.[5] This increase in sympathetic activity is manifest by an increase in heart rate, a redistribution of blood flow from the skin and splanchnic circulation to the brain and heart and an increase in sodium and water reabsorption by the kidney. This last effect involves a complex chain of physiological events (Fig. 13.2). Simply stated, however, sympathetic stimulation produces an increase in renal vascular resistance and a resultant decrease in glomerular filtration rate (GFR). A fall in GFR will favor sodium retention. There is also evidence that glomerular filtrate is shunted to nephrons having long loops of Henle so that reabsorption of sodium and water will be more complete.[5]

Sodium reabsorption in the proximal portion of the tubule is also increased, as is renin activity. An increase in plasma renin will lead to a corresponding increase in angiotensin formation. Angiotensin has two effects favoring

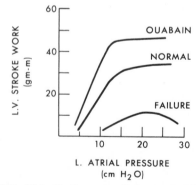

FIG. 13.1. Starling curve for normal, failing and digitalized heart.

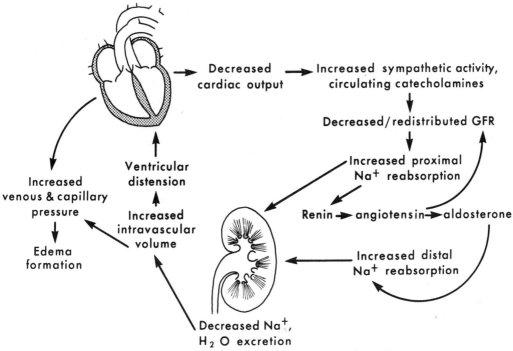

FIG. 13.2. Edema formation in CHF (after Earley[6]).

sodium and water retention: its vasoconstricting effects may further increase renal vascular resistance, and angiotensin stimulates the secretion of aldosterone, well known for its role in increasing distal tubular reabsorption of sodium.[6]

A decrease in cardiac output will also directly lower GFR and result in sodium and water retention. The net effect is an expansion of the intravascular volume in an attempt to return arterial circulation to normal.

Failure of the heart as a pump results in a congestion of blood behind the failing ventricle. Thus, if the left ventricle is functioning inadequately, the congestion is found in the systemic venous circulation. Most patients who have had left heart failure for some time, however, will present with both pulmonary and systemic congestion. A back-up of blood behind the failing ventricle results in increased venous and capillary hydrostatic pressure. The increased hydrostatic pressure causes a redistribution of fluid from intravascular to interstitial spaces resulting in the formation of edema. Because the failing heart may not be able to accept the increased sodium and water load provided by the kidneys, venous congestion, hydrostatic pressure and edema formation may increase. The patient is thus thrown into a vicious cycle.

CLINICAL FINDINGS

The clinical manifestations and physical findings of congestive heart failure are easily predicted by considering the pathogenesis of the disease. As mentioned, cardiac output is not dramatically reduced in the initial phases of heart failure, and the patient's symptoms result from the presence of compensatory mechanisms outlined above.

Table 13.1 indicates the most common symptoms and physical findings found in patients with CHF. It should be obvious that most are the result of pulmonary and systemic venous congestion as well as edema formation (Fig. 13.3). Dyspnea, orthopnea and paroxysmal nocturnal dyspnea (PND) are signs of left-sided heart failure and represent pulmonary vascular congestion. Dyspnea on exertion (DOE) is the most common symptom of heart failure. As the myocardial failure advances, dyspnea appears with less strenuous activity until eventually it is present even at rest. Orthopnea is usually taken to be an indication of more advanced heart failure and occurs when the patient assumes a recumbent position. Blood from the lower extremities and splanchnic bed redistributes to the lungs, resulting in an elevation of pulmonary venous pressure. PND (cardiac asthma) is characterized by severe shortness of breath which generally awakens the patient from sleep. PND is also the result of increased pulmonary vascular congestion which has been allowed to advance until pulmonary edema and bronchospasm develop. Pulmonary rales, pleural effusions and chest x-ray findings indicating vascular congestion in the upper lung fields are also typical of left ventricular failure.

Ankle or pretibial dependent edema, congestive hepatomegaly, jugular venous distension and hepatojugular reflux indicate systemic venous congestion and may be signs of left- or right-sided heart failure. Ankle and pretibial edema are common findings in ambulatory patients because fluid tends to localize in the dependent portions of the body secondary to gravitational forces. It should be noted, therefore, that sacral rather than ankle edema may be present in patients at bed rest. Venous congestion may also result in portal hypertension, hepatomegaly and occasional ascites. Distension of the jugular veins as a sign of systemic venous congestion may also exist.

Cardiomegaly and tachycardia have obvious causes and have been described earlier. Peripheral cyanosis resulting from compromised respiration, decreased cardiac output and shunting of blood away from the skin may be evident. Although nonspecific, fatigue and weakness are commonly found in patients with heart failure and are secondary to the reduction in cardiac output.

THERAPY — GENERAL MEASURES

The medical management of congestive heart failure includes correction of underlying disease states (*e.g.,* hypertension), bed rest, a sodium-restricted diet, digitalis glycosides and diuretics. The ultimate goal of therapy is to abolish disabling symptoms and improve the quality of the patient's life. None of the aforementioned measures are curative, and it has been dishearteningly demonstrated that despite treatment, the 5-year survival of these patients is not prolonged.[3]

Bed rest or restriction of physical activity decreases the metabolic demands of the failing heart and minimizes gravitational forces contributing to the formation of edema. Renal perfusion is also increased in the prone position resulting in diuresis and eventual mobilization of edema fluid.

A sodium-restricted diet may be instituted to offset the abnormal renal retention of sodium observed in congestive heart failure. If the ability of the kidney to excrete sodium is not severely compromised, it is possible to approach normal balance by restricting the intake of sodium to match excretion. Even though less than 1 g is required to meet physiological needs, the normal American diet contains 10 g of sodium chloride. Severe salt restriction (less than 500 mg Na or 1.3 g NaCl) is unpalatable and poorly followed. Moderate salt intake (2 to 4 g NaCl) which can be accomplished by restricting the addition of salt during cooking is much more palatable. If Na and

TABLE 13.1
Common Clinical Manifestations of Heart Failure

Cardiomegaly	Peripheral edema
Dyspnea on exertion	Pleural effusion
Fatigue	Positive hepatojugular
Jugular venous distension	reflux
Orthopnea	Rales
Paroxysmal nocturnal dyspnea	S_3 gallop rhythm

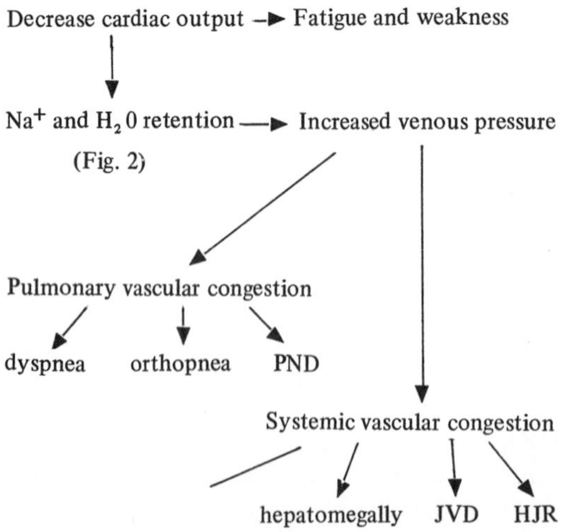

Decrease cardiac output → Fatigue and weakness

↓

Na⁺ and H₂0 retention → Increased venous pressure

(Fig. 2)

Pulmonary vascular congestion

dyspnea   orthopnea   PND

Systemic vascular congestion

hepatomegally   JVD   HJR

FIG. 13.3. Clinical manifestations of heart failure.

water retention persist despite dietary sodium restriction, diuretic therapy may be instituted. For convenience one should remember that 1 g of sodium is equivalent to 2.5 g of salt (NaCl) and that 1 level teaspoonful of salt weighs approximately 6 g.

THERAPY — DIGITALIS

Digitalis has two major pharmacological actions on the heart. Its major therapeutic effect is that of increasing the force and velocity of contraction of the normal and failing heart (inotropic effect). Although research has been extensive, the mechanisms of this effect continue to be elusive. It is currently thought that digitalis enhances excitation-contraction coupling and that this effect *may* be mediated through its inhibition of Na-K ATP-ase, an enzyme required for the active transport of sodium and potassium across cardiac cell membranes.[7] Digitalis also has electrophysiological effects on the heart which appear to be independent of its positive inotropic effects. The mechanism of these effects is also unclear but is more definitely related to an inhibition of the sodium pump which maintains intracellular electronegativity by actively transporting sodium out of the cell. The electrophysiological effects of digitalis vary in different areas of the heart and are also modified by the vagotonic actions of the drug. These effects account for the therapeutic effectiveness of digitalis in the treatment of rapid atrial rhythms associated with rapid ventricular response. Additionally, disturbances in conduction and rhythm observed with toxic doses are mediated through alteration of the myocardium's electrical function.

Although the final experimental evidence is lacking, it appears that these two effects of digitalis are independent of each other.[8] There are several important clinical implications of this fact: the practice of dosing a patient to toxicity to achieve the therapeutic benefits of inotropism is invalid since enhanced contractility may be observed before toxicity is reached; suppression of digitalis-induced arrhythmias does not simultaneously obliterate the inotropic effect of the drug; and because inotropic effects are observed at low doses of digitalis, patients who are sensitive to the toxic effect of

the drug may still benefit from doses which were previously considered subtherapeutic.[8]

Digitalis increases the force of contraction of the failing heart. As a result, cardiac output is increased and the compensatory mechanisms previously outlined begin to subside. As the end-diastolic volume is decreased, heart size is reduced; also elevated venous pressure and pulmonary congestion are eventually alleviated. As tissue perfusion improves, sympathetic tone is lowered to normal levels; subsequently, diuresis and a drop in heart rate are observed. Because it improves the primary defect responsible for the development of the syndrome, digitalis represents a rational choice in the pharmacological management of congestive heart failure.

For years, clinicians have been plagued by the fact that no sharp therapeutic end point exists for this drug. Digitalis-induced EKG changes (ST depression and T wave abnormalities) do not correlate with toxic or therapeutic effects of the drug. In general, the clinician must look for improvement of signs and symptoms of the syndrome. The patient begins to subjectively and objectively improve; he is less dyspneic and complains less of orthopnea; venous distension and signs of pulmonary congestion diminish or disappear and diuresis and diminished heart rate may also be observed. However, ankle edema does not mobilize immediately and is a poor therapeutic end point to use.

COMPARISON OF DIGITALIS PREPARATIONS

Table 13.2 compares the digitalis glycosides most frequently used. The choice of which glycoside to use in a given clinical situation will depend ideally upon the routes of administration available, the speed of onset and the duration of action required. In the vast majority of cases, however, ouabain, deslanoside, digitalis leaf and, to some extent, digitoxin offer no real advantages over digoxin, which is considered the glycoside of choice by many practitioners.

Digitalis Leaf

USP digitalis leaf is composed primarily of three glycosides: digitoxin, gitoxin, and gitalin. Digitoxin is the most important of these compounds and is responsible for the majority of

TABLE 13.2
Comparison of Digitalis Glycoside Preparations[a]

Agent	Gastrointestinal Absorption	Onset of Action min	Peak Effect hr	Average Half-life	Principal Route of Elimination	Average Digitalizing Dose Oral	Average Digitalizing Dose I.V.	Usual Daily Oral Maintenance Dose
Ouabain	unreliable	5-10	1/2-2	21 hr	Renal; some GI excretion		0.3-0.5mg	
Deslanoside	unreliable	10-30	1-2	33 hr	Renal		0.8mg	
Digoxin	50-75%	15-30	1½-5	36 hr	Renal; some GI excretion	1.25-1.5mg	0.75-1.5mg	0.25-0.5mg
Digitoxin	90-100%	25-120	4-12	4-6 days	Hepatic; renal excretion of metabolites	0.7-1.2mg	1.0mg	0.1mg
Digitalis leaf	about 40%			4-6 days	Similar to digoxin	0.8-1.2g		0.1g

[a]Reprinted with permission from Ref. 9.

the pharmacological activities of the mixture. The onset and duration of action of digitalis leaf are therefore identical to those of digitoxin (Table 13.2). The use of powdered digitalis leaf has been largely replaced by the purified crystalline preparations (digoxin; digitoxin). More accurate standardization of active drug content and an insignificant difference in cost have made these latter preparations the agents of choice.

Ouabain

Ouabain has the most rapid onset and shortest duration of action of the digitalis glycosides. It is often spoken of as having a "fast onset and short duration," which would lead one to believe that the effects of a single dose would terminate within minutes. However, as can be seen in Table 13.2, such is not the case, and the "short" duration of action is actually a relative matter.

Ouabain is absorbed very poorly from the gastrointestinal tract and is therefore only available for intravenous use. Like all the digitalis glycosides, its elimination from the body follows first order kinetics. That is, a fixed percentage of the amount of drug in the body is excreted per unit time. The elimination half-life (t ½) of ouabain is about 21 hrs in patients with normal renal function. Because the kidneys comprise the primary route of excretion for ouabain, a decrease in renal function will result in a decrease in the rate of elimination and a prolonged half-life.[10] Apparently the kinetics of ouabain in patients with varying degrees of renal dysfunction have not been extensively studied and definitive data are not available. It might be best, therefore, to avoid its use in such patients.

The clinical situations in which ouabain would be the glycoside of choice are rather limited. The time to onset of action and peak effect following an intravenous dose of ouabain is not a great deal shorter than that for digoxin. In most circumstances where prompt action is required, digoxin will suffice. Ouabain is the agent of choice in the relatively rare case where a few minutes' delay in increasing cardiac output would be life-threatening.

Deslanoside

Deslanoside is almost identical to digoxin in chemical structure. Unlike digoxin, however, it is very poorly absorbed from the gastrointestinal tract and is therefore recommended only for parenteral use. As is apparent from Table 13.2, the elimination half-life and time to onset of action and peak effect of deslanoside are not significantly different from those of digoxin. Because deslanoside offers no real advantages over digoxin, the latter agent would be the glycoside of choice if parenteral administration were desired.

Digoxin

The authors consider digoxin to be the glycoside of choice in the majority of situations encountered clinically. The availability of both intravenous and reliable oral routes of administration, relatively rapid onset of action and intermediate duration of action are the main criteria which have resulted in the predominant use of digoxin.[10]

The area of digoxin absorption and bioavailability has received a great deal of attention in recent months and has been the subject of several literature reports.[11-13] It has been reported on several occasions that digoxin administered in a well formulated tablet is rapidly absorbed and that peak serum levels are achieved within 1 hr.[11,14]

Digoxin absorption, however, is far from complete and has been reported to vary from 50 to 90%.[12,15] It is worth noting that the higher percentages of absorption were measured following administration of an alcoholic solution of the drug. Tablet administration has been reported to yield about 50 to 85% absorption.[12] A marked variation in the biological availability of digoxin from tablets produced by different manufacturers and from different lots of the same manufacturer has been reported.[11] It was noted that a 7-fold difference in serum levels resulted when two different commercial digoxin preparations were administered to the same patients. Such a pronounced variability in absorption may present an obvious hazard to the patient and could conceivably result in digitalis toxicity or underdigitalization if a patient were switched from one product to the other. It is currently recommended, therefore, that the pharmacist stock only those preparations of proven bioavailability, as for example Lanoxin.[11] Recent F.D.A. regulations regarding the certification of digoxin bioavailability and newly incorporated U.S.P. standards concerning dissolution of digoxin tablets should result in the elimination of this problem. The difference in cost between the various preparations of digoxin is insignificant when compared to the potential hazards of dispensing a poorly manufactured tablet.

Alteration of the absorption of digoxin following oral administration in patients with malabsorption syndromes has also been studied.[13] It was found that poor and erratic absorption occured in patients with malabsorption states such as sprue, short bowel syndrome and rapid intestinal transit. Bile salts and pancreatic enzymes are apparently not required for effective digoxin absorption because normal serum levels were found in patients with pancreatic insufficiency.

Digoxin is available in injectable form for both intramuscular and intravenous use. However, it is recommended that the intramuscular route be avoided and that digoxin be given intravenously if oral administration is not feasible. Digoxin is approximately 80% absorbed from an I.M. injection site;[12] however, severe pain, local muscle fasciculations and creatinine phosphokinase (CPK) elevations up to 15 times normal result when the drug is administered by this route.[16]

Caution is warranted when digoxin is given intravenously. Too rapid administration may result in acute myocardial toxicity caused by a direct effect of the drug. Additionally, the commercially available preparation contains 40% propylene glycol; rapid administration of this cardiotoxic compound may also result in acute myocardial depression. It is therefore recommended that the commercial preparation be given at a maximal rate of 1 cc per min, or preferably that it be diluted with 10 cc of normal saline for injection and then administered as a slow infusion.[16]

All digitalis glycosides are eliminated from the body following first order kinetics.[10] In the case of digoxin, approximately 35% of the total amount of drug in the body will be lost during 1 day; the kidney is the main route of elimination.[15] Glomerular filtration is primarily responsible for the renal excretion of digoxin and no significant tubular reabsorption or secretion occurs. It is worth mentioning that increased rates of urine flow caused by diuretic administration, water loading or diabetes insipidus do not increase digoxin elimination.[10] The average elimination half-life of digoxin in patients with normal renal function has been reported to be 1.6 days.[15]

Like most drugs eliminated in the urine primarily in unchanged form,[17] digoxin kinetics are altered in patients with varying degrees of renal dysfunction.[15] However, nonrenal mechanisms, principally hepatic metabolism, are also involved in digoxin elimination. It has been observed that anuric patients will eliminate approximately 14% of the total amount of drug in the body during 1 day and that the average half-life of digoxin in such patients is 4.4 days.[15,18] It is readily apparent, therefore, that the daily maintenance dose, but not the digitalizing dose, must be decreased in patients with poorly functioning kidneys. Jelliffe[15] has observed that the rate of digoxin elimination is directly proportional to creatinine clearance, and that if the creatinine clearance of a patient is known, it is possible to calculate the daily dose necessary to maintain body glycoside stores at a given level.[15] Jelliffe has reported the following relationship between creatinine clearance and percent of digoxin lost per day:

$$\% \text{ loss} = 14 + (\text{creatinine clearance})/5 \quad (1)$$

For example, a patient with a creatinine clearance of 15 ml per min will eliminate 17% of the total amount of digoxin in his body during a 24-hr period:

$$\% \text{ loss} = 14 + C_{cr}/5 = 14 + 15/5 = 17\%/\text{day} \quad (2)$$

If this patient had been digitalized with 1.0 mg of digoxin and we wished to maintain his glycoside stores at that level, the daily maintenance dose should be 0.17 mg.

Let us consider a second patient with the same creatinine clearance who has been receiving a daily maintenance dose of 0.25 mg of digoxin for the past month. We know that he will eliminate 17% of his body stores of digoxin per day and at maintenance plateau this will be equal to 0.25 mg. It is, therefore, possible to calculate that the total amount of digoxin stored by this patient is 1.47 mg immediately after taking his daily dose:

$$A_b/100\% = 0.25 \text{ mg}/17\%$$

$$A_b = 1.47 \text{ mg}$$

where A_b = the amount of drug in the body.

It should be noted that we have assumed complete availability of digoxin in performing these calculations; correcting for extent of absorption will make the results more accurate. However, because the extent of absorption of orally administered digoxin may vary and the kinetic information presented represents average data, individual patients may differ markedly from what one might calculate. It should be emphasized, therefore, that maintenance doses calculated using the principles outlined represent sophisticated estimates. Clinical evaluation of patient status and response to administered digoxin continues to be the most important method of determining dosage.[19]

The use of digoxin serum levels to monitor therapeutic response is becoming increasingly common in clinical practice and can provide the clinician with valuable information. It has been observed that digoxin steady state serum levels rise linearly with dose[19] and that there exists a direct correlation between serum level of the drug and the presence or absence of toxicity.[20] However, there is a fairly significant area of overlap in the serum levels of toxic and nontoxic patients (Table 13.3), and one must therefore interpret such data in light of the clinical situation. In general, measurement of serum levels is useful when one wishes to substantiate clinical impression with definitive data or when an unexpected response to digoxin administration is encountered.

Digitoxin

As indicated in Table 13.2, digitoxin has the slowest onset of action, peak effect and half-life of all the digitalis glycosides. Digitoxin is absorbed more completely from the gastrointestinal tract than is digoxin, and it is usually considered to be essentially 100% absorbed following oral administration.[10] However, altera-

TABLE 13.3
Digoxin Serum Levels in Toxic and Nontoxic Patients[a]

Serum Level ng/ml	Oral Dosage Given
0.8 - 1.6	Nontoxic patients, 0.25 mg/day
0.9 - 2.4	Nontoxic patients, 0.5 mg/day
2.1 - 8.7	Toxic patients

[a]From the University of California, San Francisco, Clinical Laboratories. Values at other institutions may vary.

tion of absorption in patients with malabsorption syndromes or other gastrointestinal disease has not been studied.

Digitoxin has a high affinity for plasma proteins and has been reported to be 97% bound at serum concentrations usually achieved in the clinical use of the drug.[21] This can be contrasted to digoxin which is only 20% bound to serum albumin.[10] This difference in protein binding in part explains the difference in degree of renal excretion of the two agents. Digitoxin elimination occurs primarily via hepatic metabolism and renal excretion of the metabolic by-products.[22] Digoxin has been reported to be a minor metabolite of digitoxin;[23] however, it is produced in such small amounts as to be of no significance. As far as is known, the balance of the digitoxin metabolites have little or no cardioactivity.[21] Digitoxin undergoes some degree of enterohepatic recycling,[10] a factor which may give rise to one of the few potential drug interactions for the cardiac glycosides (see below).

The elimination half-life of digitoxin has been reported to be approximately 6 days.[10,21,22] Jelliffe et al.[22] have observed that 11.4% of total body digitoxin stores will be eliminated over a 24-hr period in a patient with normal renal and hepatic function. As mentioned, the majority of digitoxin elimination occurs via hepatic metabolism. An anuric patient will eliminate approximately 7.7% of total body glycoside stores within 1 day.[22] This corresponds to an elimination half-life of approximately 9 days. It is apparent, therefore, that renal excretion accounts for approximately 1/3 of digitoxin elimination in patients with normal kidney function. On the basis of the information presented, one would not expect that any significant alteration of digitoxin maintenance dose in the presence of renal insufficiency would be necessary. Although Jelliffe has defined a mathematical relationship between the rate of digitoxin elimination and creatinine clearance similar to that of digoxin, clinical observations of patients with renal failure seem to indicate that no dose alteration is necessary.[24]

Because digitoxin relies primarily on hepatic metabolism for its elimination, liver dysfunction may conceivably reduce the rate of metabolism and prolong half-life. To date no instances of this occurrence have been reported. Nevertheless, it would be advisable to avoid the use of digitoxin in patients with liver disease and administer digoxin instead.

Digitoxin serum levels may be measured by many clinical laboratories. The discussion above with respect to digoxin serum levels in toxic and nontoxic patients applies to digitoxin as well (Table 13.3).[20]

DIGITALIZATION

The speed with which a loading dose of digitalis is administered (digitalization) depends primarily on the clinical situation. The patient may be rapidly digitalized (i.e., over a 24-hr period) or he may be digitalized slowly over a week or more. Pharmacokinetic parameters must also be considered in determining the method of digitalization.

For a given patient, the total digitalizing dose will be independent of the rapidity of administration or changes in renal function. The daily maintenance dose, however, must be altered as outlined below.

On a mg for mg basis, digoxin and digitoxin are essentially equivalent with respect to their cardiac effects. Therefore, the digitalizing dose of each will be approximately equal. When fully digitalized, most patients will have 0.75 to 1.5 mg (0.01 to 0.02 mg per kg body weight) of glycoside present in their bodies. It should be emphasized, however, that these figures represent average doses and that some patients may require much less while others much more. The initial phases of digitalis dosing are actually an exercise in titration.[15]

Rapid Digitalization

Administration of the total loading dose of digitalis within a 24-hr period is probably the method of choice for hospitalized patients. This method has several advantages: the patient is very quickly brought to maximal therapeutic effect; symptoms of toxicity are less likely to be delayed, more likely to be observed and more easily correlated to drug concentrations within the body; and diminished renal function does not affect the time required to reach maximal drug level and therapeutic effect.

Let us assume that we wish to initiate digoxin therapy rapidly in a 70-kg man with normal renal function and that we are aiming for a total dose of 1.0 mg. An initial dose of 0.5 mg should be given. Six hours later the patient should be evaluated for clinical improvement and signs of digitalis toxicity. If none exists, he should be given a dose of 0.25 mg. In another 6 hr he should again be evaluated for signs of toxicity, and if there are no contraindications, a last dose of 0.25 mg should be administered. Thus, within a 12-hr period the patient has been digitalized to a level of 1 mg. Daily losses should be replaced by adminstration of a daily maintenance dose in order to sustain this level of digitalization (1 mg). Since 35% of digoxin is eliminated per day in patients with normal renal function, the daily maintenance dose for this patient would be 0.35 mg. The above regimen could be administered either parenterally or orally. Specific details concerning routes of digoxin administration are discussed below.

If the patient presented here had developed signs and symptoms of digitalis toxicity after receiving a total dose of only 0.75 mg, further digoxin administration would of course have been discontinued. Assuming that the drug had been administered properly, we would now know that this patient becomes digitalis-toxic when the total amount in his body is 0.75 mg. In the future, it would be possible to avoid any therapeutic regimen which resulted in body glycoside stores of 0.75 mg or more.

It is important to emphasize that diminished renal function does not alter the digitalizing dose. However, because a decrease in renal function will decrease the amount of glycoside eliminated per day, an appropriate decrease in daily maintenance dose must be made. Alteration of digoxin and digitoxin dosage in renal insufficiency has been discussed in detail previously.

Because digoxin and digitoxin have essentially equal potency, a similar digitalizing regimen could be used for the rapid institution of digitoxin therapy.

Slow Digitalization

Slowly initiating digitalis therapy by placing the patient on a maintenance dose of digoxin in lieu of a loading dose is considered the method of choice for ambulatory, nonacute patients with no renal dysfunction. Its main advantage over rapid digitalization is that it does not require continuous monitoring of the patient and is thus very suitable to the ambulatory setting. The main disadvantage, however, is the length of time required to reach maximal body

glycoside stores and therapeutic effect. If the patient should develop digitalis toxicity, it is also more difficult to determine the exact amount of drug he has in his body. Additionally, changes in renal function will affect the time required to reach plateau.

The length of time required to achieve plateau concentrations of a drug administered on a routine basis at maintenance doses is dependent on the elimination half-life of that drug. It will take essentially 5 half-lives to reach plateau. Thus, a patient with normal renal function placed on a daily dose of 0.25 mg of digoxin will require 8.0 days to reach maximal glycoside concentrations (5 x 1.6 days = 8.0 days). If, however, that patient were anephric ($t_{1/2}$ = 4.4 days) it would take 22 days to reach plateau, and the maximal concentration would be approximately 2 1/2 times that of a normal patient receiving the same dose.[15] Administration of digitoxin in such a manner will require approximately 25 days to reach plateau in patients with normal kidney function and up to 45 days in patients with renal insufficiency.[22] It is therefore impractical to digitalize patients with digitoxin in this manner.

When using this method of digitalization, the pharmacist should remember to avoid increasing doses before maximal effects are observed. It would be falacious to increase a patient's maintenance dose after 3 days for example, if no clinical improvement were observed.

DIGITALIS TOXICITY

It is well recognized that digitalis has an extremely narrow therapeutic index. Studies in animals indicate that therapeutic doses are equivalent to 60% of the toxic dose which in turn is equivalent to 40% of the lethal dose. There are innumerable statistics available on the prevalence of signs and symptoms of digitalis toxicity.[20,25-27]

The incidence of digitalis toxicity has increased over the past 30 years.[25,26] This may be attributed to the greater sophistication of the clinician in recognizing digitalis toxicity and to the growing geriatric population to which digitalis is primarily administered. According to a number of prospective epidemiological studies of digitalis intoxication, approximately 20% of patients who are taking the drug eventually exhibit signs and symptoms of toxicity. Up to 18% of these patients may die from digitalis-induced arrhythmias,[20] and the over-all mortality rate of toxic patients may be twice as high as that of nontoxic patients.

Serum Levels

Recently a radioimmunoassay for serum digoxin has been developed. Prospective studies[20] show good correlation between serum digoxin levels and toxicity (see Table 13.3). Eighty-seven percent of digitalis toxic patients had levels greater than 2 ng per ml and 90% of the nontoxic patients had levels of less than 2 ng per ml.[28] However, because a significant overlap between toxic and therapeutic levels exists, serum level determinations are currently most useful as an aid in confirming suspected digitalis toxicity and in individualizing dosing regimens so that toxicity is avoided.

The pharmacist may play a role in the recognition and prevention of digitalis toxicity if he is cognizant of the signs and symptoms with which the patient may present.

Signs and Symptoms of Digitalis Toxicty

Noncardiac symptoms of digitalis toxicity are related to the central nervous system (CNS), gastrointestinal tract and endocrine effects of the drug. Allergic reactions to digitalis are extremely rare and almost unheard of. Thrombocytopenia secondary to digitoxin is also a rare phenomenon.

Recent studies[26] indicate that CNS symptoms of digitalis toxicity may be extremely common. Chronic digitalis intoxication resulting from misformulation was observed in 179 patients. Acute, extreme fatigue was a complaint in 95% of these patients. Approximately 80% experienced weakness of the arms and legs and 65% suffered from psychic disturbances occuring in the form of nightmares, agitation, listlessness and hallucinations. Visual disturbances were observed in 95% of these patients. Hazy vision, difficulty in reading and difficulty in red-green color perception were frequently present. Other complaints included glitterings, dark or moving spots, photophobia and yellow-green vision. Disturbances in color vision returned to normal 2 to 3 weeks following discontinuation of digitalis.

Gastrointestinal symptoms including anorexia, nausea, vomiting, abdominal pain (65%) and, less commonly, diarrhea were present in 80% of the patients observed.[26] Recent studies fail to support the old notion that gastrointestinal symptoms are related to impurities in digitalis products. Unilateral or bilateral gynecomastia is occasionally observed during digoxin administration and is reversible upon withdrawal of the drug.

The clinical presentation of digitalis toxicity is highly unpredictable. Unfortunately, noncardiac symptoms may precede cardiac symptoms of digitalis toxicity in up to 47% of cases. Frequently (26 to 66%) nonspecific cardiac arrhythmias may be the only manifestation of digitalis toxicity.[26,27] Vague gastrointestinal symptoms characteristic of digitalis toxicity may be difficult to evaluate since anorexia and nausea are also part of the clinical picture of congestive heart failure. Beller et al.[20] observed an equal frequency of anorexia and nausea in both toxic and nontoxic patients. Even more frustrating is the fact that digitalis toxicity may occasionally present as progressive congestive heart failure.[27]

The arrhythmogenic action of digitalis is related to its complex effects on the electrophysiological properties of the heart. Toxic doses of digitalis may simultaneously depress the automaticity of the normal pacemakers. Conduction velocity is diminished in the AV node and other specialized conducting tissues of the heart; it is increased in the atrium and ventricles.

Digitalis-induced rhythm disturbances are nonspecific but are generally characterized by decreased conduction and/or increased automaticity. It is estimated that rhythm disturbances occur in 80 to 90% of digitalis toxic patients.[27] Ventricular arrhythmias (premature ventricular contractions [PVCs], bigeminy, multifocal PVDs and tachycardia) and AV conduction disturbances (prolonged PR interval and second degree AV block) appear to be the most commonly encountered arrhythmias.

FACTORS WHICH PREDISPOSE PATIENTS TO DIGITALIS TOXICITY

A number of factors may predispose patients to digitalis toxicity. Electrolyte imbalances, including hypokalemia, hypomagnesemia and hypercalcemia, may predispose the patient to the toxic effects of digitalis.

Hypokalemia

The association between digitalis toxicity and hypokalemia is well recognized. Jelliffe[29] has observed that twice as much digitalis is required to produce toxicity in patients with a serum potassium of 5 mEq per liter than in those with a serum potassium of 3mEq per liter. Therefore, drugs, diseases and medical maneuvers which induce a hypokalemia or a drop in serum potassium from elevated to normal levels may unmask existing digitalis toxicity or allow toxicity to occur at lower doses. The mechanism of this potentiation is unclear; however, a low serum potassium has been observed to increase the uptake of digitalis by the myocardial tissue.[30]

Hypokalemia may result when excessive amounts of potassium are lost via the kidney or gastrointestinal tract or when extracellular potassium redistributes to intracellular spaces. Corticosteroids promote sodium-potassium exchange and therefore potassium excretion at the distal portion of the renal tubule. The degree of hypokalemia produced by the various glucocorticoids may be predicted on the basis of their mineralocorticoid potency. Hypokalemia is more frequently associated with hydrocortisone than with equivalent anti-inflammatory doses of prednisone. Similarly, dexamethasone which is devoid of mineralocorticoid activity would not be expected to produce hypokalemia. Diseases in which mineralocorticoid activity is high (*e.g.*, Cushing's disease, hyperaldosteronism) are also associated with low serum potassium levels.

Renal tubular acidosis is a disease characterized by an inability of the kidney to excrete acid and is associated with increased losses of urinary potassium. Drugs such as acetazolamide, amphotericin and outdated tetracycline cause a similar renal tubular defect resulting in increased urinary losses of potassium and hypokalemia.

All diuretics, with the exception of triamterene and spironolactone may cause hypokalemia through kaliuresis.

Gastrointestinal secretions contain high concentrations of potassium (8 to 10 mEq per liter). For this reason, the excessive use of cathartics or other drugs which produce diarrhea (neomycin, quinidine) increase gastrointestinal potassium loss and may eventually result in low serum potassium levels. Kayexelate, a nonabsorbable cationic exchange resin which exchanges sodium for potassium in the gastrointestinal tract, results in decreased serum potassium. Prolonged nasogastric suction and loss of fluid from ileostomies and gastrointestinal fistulas may also result in a hypokalemic state.

Potassium is required for the active transport of glucose across cell membranes and its conversion to glycogen. The administration of high concentrations of glucose without sufficient amounts of potassium (as in hyperalimentation), the correction of hyperglycemia with insulin or the simultaneous administration of glucose and insulin promotes the movement of potassium into the cells resulting in a low serum potassium.

Administration of sodium bicarbonate, correction of acidosis or the presence of alkalosis results in the redistribution of serum potassium intracellularly. Potassium moves into the cells to maintain electrical neutrality which has been altered by the presence of excess anion (HCO_3^-).

Hypomagnesemia

The observation of hypomagnesemia in the absence of hypokalemia in four digitalis-toxic patients prompted an animal study to test the effect of this electrolyte imbalance on digitalis toxicity.[31] The toxic dose of acetylstrophanthidin in dogs was reduced when the serum magnesium was reduced by hemodialysis. The long term administration of magnesium-free fluids (*e.g.*, hyperalimentation), diuretics and amphotericin B, chronic alcoholism, hemodialysis and excessive upper gastrointestinal fluid losses containing 10 to 20 mEq per liter have been associated with hypomagnesemia.

Hypercalcemia

The electrical and contractile effects of calcium on the myocardium are similar to those of digitalis.[32,33] For this reason, rapid intravenous infusions of calcium may facilitate the development of digitalis toxicity, and normal or low doses of digitalis may induce toxicity in patients with hypercalcemia (*e.g.*, hyperparathyroidism or metastatic cancer). The clinical significance of calcium-induced digitalis toxicity, however, has been questioned by Lown *et al.*[34] There have been no reports of digitalis toxicity secondary to the oral administration of calcium-containing products.

Age

Age may be an important predisposing factor in the production of digitalis toxicity. The same intravenous dose of digoxin administered to elderly and young patients produced higher serum concentrations of digoxin in the elderly. Ewy et al.[35] proposed that the higher levels and prolonged half-life observed in these patients were due to diminished renal clearance of the drug and the smaller body size of this population. It is important to emphasize that although the serum creatinine of the elderly patients (average age 77 years) was within normal limits, the mean creatinine clearance (56 ml per min) was approximately half that observed in the younger patients.

Levine et al.[36,37] have recommended the use of lower doses in premature infants and neonates (less than 1 month of age). Toxic arrhythmias were observed when infants tested during the first 72 hr of life were given doses of digoxin comparable to those recommended for children and older infants. This may be due to the decreased renal function normally observed in newborns. Their studies demonstrate that the absorption, tissue fixation and/or excretion of digoxin in infants is similar to that of adults. They point out, however, that infants excrete a smaller percentage of digoxin metabolites than do adults.

Thyroid Function

Hypothyroid (myxedematous) patients are extremely sensitive to the effects of digitalis. Although serum levels of digoxin are higher in hypothyroid patients, half-life and tissue concentrations of the drug are unchanged. Doherty and Perkins[39] postulated that the myocardium of the hypothyroid patient is more sensitive to the effects of digoxin. This observation becomes clinically important when a hyperthyroid patient managed on high doses of digoxin becomes myxedematous secondary to treatment with radioactive iodine, surgery or antithyroid drugs such as propylthiouracil.

Hepatic Function

Although never reported, diminished liver function may theoretically increase the half-life and serum levels of digitoxin because it is metabolized to a significant degree. Very little digoxin, on the other hand, is metabolized so that it is not surprising that its elimination was found to be unaltered in cirrhotic patients with normal renal function.[40]

Renal Function

As discussed previously, the half-life of digoxin may be significantly prolonged in patients with renal failure. Digitoxin is primarily metabolized to inactive products by the liver so that the half-life of this drug is only slightly altered in patients with compromised renal function. Nevertheless, the authors prefer the use of digoxin in the presence of renal failure. As can be calculated from Equations 1 and 2 above, the elimination half-life of digoxin is always less than that of digitoxin, regardless of degree of renal dysfunction. Management of toxicity would, therefore, be much easier.

An increased prevalence of digoxin toxicity has also been observed in patients with advanced cardiac disease, chronic pulmonary disease, cor pulmonale, hypoxia and atrial fibrillation.[20] Finally, the concomitant administration of several drugs has been noted to decrease the myocardial threshold to digitalis toxicity. These include cyclopropane and large doses of reserpine.

Factors which may increase dose requirements or protect against the toxicity of digitalis are listed in Table 13.4.

TREATMENT OF DIGITALIS TOXICITY

If the cardiac arrhythmia is not life-threatening, simple withdrawal of digitalis may be the only treatment required. Potassium administration should be considered in patients with digitalis-induced ectopic beats who have low or normal serum potassium levels. The oral route of administration is generally adequate and should be used unless the patient cannot take medications by mouth. The following precautions should be considered when potassium is used to treat digitalis toxicity:

Potassium should be administered with caution in patients who have conduction disturbances characterized by second degree or complete AV block.[27] Potassium also depresses conduction velocity in the AV node and its use

TABLE 13.4

Factors Which May Diminish Therapeutic Effects, Increase Dose Requirements or
Protect Against the Toxicity of Digitalis

	Reference
Poor compliance	41
Augmented metabolism of digitoxin (phenylbutazone, diphenylhydantoin, phenobarbital)	42
Diminished absorption	
Malabsorption; neomycin-induced malabsorption	13
Drug formulation	11
Cholestyramine (decreases absorption of digitoxin)	42
Increased gastrointestinal transit time (*e.g.*, cathartics)	
Hyperthyroidism	39
Age: Infants greater than 1 month to. 2 years of age are able to tolerate larger doses calculated on the basis of mg/kg or body surface area	33
Hyperkalemia: appears to protect the myocardium against toxic effects of digitalis; may occur in renal failure, acidosis, following administration of triamterene or spironolactone	43

may result in an augmentation of this cardiac arrhythmia.

Toxic doses of digitalis inhibit the uptake of potassium by myocardial, skeletal muscle and liver cells. For this reason, these patients may occasionally develop refractory hyperkalemia; large doses of potassium should be administered cautiously.[19]

Because potassium is eliminated by the kidneys, excessive potassium loads should be avoided in patients with compromised renal function.

Cardiac arrhythmias have been observed following the rapid intravenous administration of concentrated potassium solutions. If digitalis-induced arrhythmias are severe enough to warrant intravenously administered potassium, maximal recommended doses are 40 mEq per liter at a rate which does not exceed 10 mEq per hr. In no instance should the concentration of KCl exceed 80-100 mEq per liter.[33,44,45] The patient should be monitored for signs and symptoms of potassium toxicity with frequent EKG tracings (tall, peaked T waves, prolonged PR interval) and serum potassium determinations.

Virtually all of the antiarrhythmic agents have been used to treat digitalis-induced arrhythmias. Intravenous lidocaine, diphenylhydantoin and propranolol have been used with the greatest success.[33] Lidocaine and diphenylhydantoin have a theoretical advantage over propranolol and quinidine-like agents in that they probably do not further depress AV conduction.

Although lidocaine has an elimination half-life of approximately 2 hrs, an initial I.V. bolus may be lost in only 10 to 20 min because of rapid tissue distribution. Generally, the drug is administered as a constant infusion (1 to 4 mg per min) following an initial bolus dose of 50 to 100 mg (1 mg per kg). Caution should be exercised in patients with congestive heart failure since it has been demonstrated that the volume of distribution and plasma clearance of lidocaine may be decreased in these patients. Elimination half-life and time to reach plateau are therefore prolonged and symptoms of lidocaine toxicity may not be evident for several hours (2 to 3 half-lives).[46]

Reports regarding the efficacy of diphenylhydantoin (DPH) as an antiarrhythmic agent have been variable; however, the drug appears to be particularly efficacious in the suppression of digitalis-induced tachyarrhythmias with or without first or second degree AV block. A loading dose of up to 1 g (in divided doses) may be required during the first 12 to 24 hrs. Thereafter, the patient may be maintained at doses of 100 mg 3 to 4 times daily. The diluent for parenteral diphenylhydantoin contains 40% propylene glycol which is cardiotoxic; for this reason DPH should not be administered at a rate which exceeds 50 mg per min. Diphenylhydantoin is insoluble in aqueous solutions and should not be administered by intravenous infusion.

Intravenous propranolol has been useful in abolishing digitalis-induced atrial tachycardia with AV block and ventricular premature contractions. Quinidine-like actions of the drug may account for its efficacy as an antiarrhythmic agent. One to 3 mg should be given at a rate of 1 mg per min with careful EKG monitoring. A similar dose may be repeated after 2 min, but further doses should be withheld for 4 hr. Unlike diphenylhydantoin and lidocaine, propranolol depresses conduction velocity and may therefore augment AV and intraventricular block. It should not be used in asthmatic patients since it may induce bronchoconstriction, and caution should be taken when it is used in diabetics since they may experience severe protracted hypoglycemia following its administration. Should profound bradycardia occur, atropine may be used.

Procainamide and quinidine have been used less frequently because their intravenous administration is associated with hypotension and cardiotoxicity. Since conduction velocity is diminished by both of these drugs, their use should be avoided when AV or intraventricular block is present.

Other agents which are used less frequently because of unpredictable or toxic effects include EDTA (a calcium-chelating agent), magnesium and cholestyramine.

THERAPY — DIURETICS

Role of Diuretics in the Management of Congestive Heart Failure

Edema is the excessive accumulation of interstitial fluid. In congestive heart failure, it is a manifestation of the abnormal retention of sodium and water, which occurs in response to a diminished effective blood volume. Correction of the underlying disease process is most important in the removal of edema; therefore, digitalis, which improves cardiac contractility, cardiac output and tissue perfusion, should abolish the body's need to increase intravascular volume. However, a hazard of diuretic use is excessive volume depletion, diminished venous return and ultimately decreased cardiac output. It is important to re-emphasize that digitalis remains the primary therapeutic modality in the treatment of CHF.

Not infrequently, the edema of moderate to severe cases of congestive heart failure may be unresponsive to therapeutic doses of digitalis and sodium restriction. When this edema is symptomatic (e.g., pulmonary congestion, venous stasis and thrombosis of the extremities), therapy with diuretics should be initiated.

Initially, the goal of diuretic therapy is to remove the edema without causing intravascular depletion. The rate at which edema can be removed is limited by its rate of mobilization from the interstitial to the intravascular fluid compartment. Therefore, if diuresis is too vigorous, intravascular volume depletion may result. Various authors have proposed that diuretics be administered on an intermittent basis so that periods of diuresis are followed by rest periods during which diuretic-induced volume and electrolyte changes are given an opportunity to recover. Intermittent dosing may take the form of every other day therapy, single daily dose therapy, or several consecutive days of therapy followed by short rest periods.[47-49] Such regimens, of course, must be individualized to the patient's response which is measured by monitoring the improvement of signs and symptoms, weight changes as well as fluid intake and output. Once edema is removed, therapy is aimed at maintaining sodium balance in such a way that reaccumulation does not occur. A program of moderate sodium restriction coupled with diuretic and digitalis therapy generally results.

Mechanism of Action and Potency

All diuretics which are used in the management of congestive heart failure decrease the reabsorption of sodium in the renal tubules. Increased urinary sodium and water loss result.

The majority of sodium which is presented to the kidney is reabsorbed. Approximately 65% is isotonically reabsorbed with chloride ion in the proximal tubule of the kidney (see Fig. 13.4); 25% is reabsorbed without water in the loop of Henle; finally in the distal portion of the tubule 8 to 10% of the sodium is reabsorbed in exchange for potassium and hydrogen ion. This cationic exchange mechanism is stimulated by the adrenal hormone, aldosterone. In general, therefore, the potency of the various diuretics is governed by their site of action. The more proximal the site of action, the more potent the diuretic.[50,51] Therefore, diuretics acting in the loop of Henle (ethacrynic acid and furosemide) are 8 to 10 times more potent than the thiazide diuretics which act just proximally to the distal tubule. Thiazides, in turn, are more potent than those diuretics which block sodium reabsorption at the cationic exchange sites in the distal tubule (spironolactone and triamterene).

Drug Selection

Thiazide diuretics are the most commonly employed diuretic agents in the management of congestive heart failure. Aside from differences in duration of action, at maximal therapeutic doses there is essentially no difference in potency or toxicity among these compounds. The choice of agent within this class, therefore, is governed primarily by cost and bioavailability. Hydrochlorthiazide, for example, is absorbed much better than is chlorthiazide. A comparison of selected diuretics is presented in Table 13.5.

The effectiveness of diuretics is dependent upon the amount of sodium delivered to their site of action. Proximal tubular reabsorption of sodium is increased in patients with congestive heart failure, and in some instances the avidity for sodium at this site may render thiazide diuretics minimally effective. In these cases, the use of furosemide or ethacrynic acid, which work more proximally than the thiazides, should be considered. Used alone, spironolactone and triamterene are weak diuretics and are minimally effective in the treatment of symptomatic edema.

Loop diuretics (ethacrynic acid and furosemide) are the only agents which may be effective in the presence of any significant degree of renal failure (serum creatinine 3 to 8 mg%).[48] This may be due to their ability to decrease renal vascular resistance and redistribute renal blood flow. It should be pointed out, however, that in the long run these agents are also capable of inducing azotemia secondary to contraction of the vascular volume and decreased glomerular filtration rate.

Spironolactone and triamterene should be avoided in patients with renal failure (BUN>40 mg%)[48] since hyperkalemia may develop from their use.

Diuretic Escape

It is not uncommon for patients to "escape" from or become resistant to the diuretic effect of thiazides. This may be attributed to several factors,[46,47] some of which have been discussed previously.

1. A decreased delivery of sodium to the site of action secondary to the increased proximal tubular reabsorption observed in patients with congestive heart failure and/or decreased glomerular filtration rates.

2. An increased reabsorption of sodium at the distal tubule may result from increased amounts of sodium presented to this site or

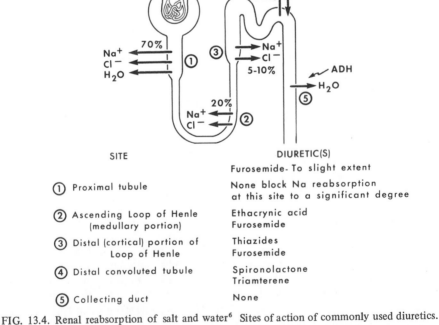

FIG. 13.4. Renal reabsorption of salt and water[6] Sites of action of commonly used diuretics.

TABLE 13.5

Selected Pharmacological Properties of Frequently Used Diuretics

Agent	Onset of Action hr	Peak Effect	Duration of Action	Usual Dosage mg/day	Commercial Availability	Relative Potency (Max Doses)	Comments
Chlorthalidone	2	18 hr	48-72 hrs.	50-100	Tablets, 100 mg	1	Long acting diuretic with thiazide-like mechanism of action and toxicity.
Ethacrynic acid	0.5-1	1-2 hr	6-8 hrs.	50 (I.V./P.O.) max: 150-200	Tablets, 25, 50 mg Injectable 50 mg vials	5	Rapidly acting, extremely potent diuretic with greater potential for toxicity; should be reserved for patients refractory to minimum doses of thiazides; works in patients with renal failure; may have more GI irritant effects than furosemide; no more than 100 mg/dose parenterally to avoid ototoxicity
Furosemide	0.5-1	1-2 hr	6-8 hrs.	40-80; may be much higher	Tablets, 40 mg Injectable, 20 mg; 10 mg/cc	8-10	Rapidly acting, extremely potent diuretic with greater potential for toxicity; should be reserved for patients refractory to minimum doses of thiazides; works in patients with renal failure; oto-toxicity with I.V. use
Hydrochlorthiazide	1-2	4 hr	4 hours	25-100	Tablets, 25, 50 mg	1	Ineffective in renal failure
Spironolactone	Delayed: 1-2 days	2-3 days	2-3 days after drug discontinued	100-200	Tablets, 25 mg	0.4	Potassium-sparing; avoid use in renal failure or in conjunction with potassium supplements
Triamterene	2	—	12-16 hr	100-200	Capsules, 100 mg	0.4	See spironolactone

from increased levels of aldosterone due to diuretic-induced sodium loss.

The latter effect may be observed by monitoring urine electrolyte levels. Initially sodium excretion is enhanced, but as diuretic therapy progresses, one may observe a drop in urine sodium and an increase in the urine potassium concentration. In such cases, the effects of thiazide or loop diuretics may be enhanced by the concomitant use of triamterene or spironolactone. The initial onset of action of these latter agents may be delayed by 3 to 7 days so that one should not be discouraged if there are no immediate results.

Problems in the Use of Diuretic Agents

Adverse affects secondary to diuretic use are common, predictable and generally preventable and treatable if recognized early.

Volume Changes. Loop diuretics, mercurials, osmotic diuretics and thiazides are all capable of producing intravascular volume depletion and hyponatremia if diuresis is too vigorous. It is important to re-emphasize that volume depletion may occur in the presence of edema if the rate of diuresis exceeds the rate of edema mobilization. A drop in blood pressure with postural changes, diminished urinary output and abnormal renal function tests may be observed. Rapid administration of osmotic diuretics such as mannitol and urea may also cause an acute volume expansion which may exacerbate congestive heart failure. The administration of these agents to patients with severe renal failure who are unable to eliminate these poorly diffusable agents would also result in a shift in body fluids to the intravascular compartment.

Hyponatremia. Hyponatremia may result when electrolyte-free fluid (water) is ingested and dietary sodium is restricted in the face of increased urinary losses of sodium. Additionally, thiazides and loop diuretics inhibit the formation of free water so that urinary sodium loss may exceed water loss. Symptoms of severe hyponatremia include lethargy, somnolence, muscle cramps and weakness which may be indistinguishable from hypokalemia without the aid of laboratory tests. Hypovolemia and hyponatremia may be minimized by dosing diuretics intermittently and by avoiding the use of long acting diuretics or severely sodium-

restricted diets (500 mg sodium or less). Hyponatremia is treated by temporary discontinuation of diuretic therapy, liberalization of sodium intake and, if severe, the administration of hypertonic saline.

Hypokalemia. All diuretics, with the exception of the potassium-sparing agents spironolactone and triamterene, are capable of producing hypokalemia. By inhibiting reabsorption of sodium in the proximal portion of the tubule, more is presented to the distal tubule for exchange with potassium and hydrogen ions. As mentioned previously, the avoidance of potassium depletion is particularly important in congestive failure patients in whom digitalis toxicity may be potentiated. When hypokalemia is accompanied by hypochloremic alkalosis, it is important to supplement potassium as the chloride salt. Low serum chloride levels perpetuate urine potassium losses so that replacement of potassium without chloride (*e.g.*, gluconate and citrate salts) will be minimally effective. Potassium supplementation (40 to 60 mEq per day) should be used with caution in patients with compromised renal function since they are frequently unable to eliminate large potassium loads. Administration of potassium with spironolactone and especially triamterene in renal failure patients should also be avoided since severe, life-threatening hyperkalemia may result.

Hyperuricemia. With the exception of spironolactone, decreased renal clearance of uric acid and secondary hyperuricemia is a complication of all diuretics frequently used in the management of congestive heart failure. In general, diuretic-induced hyperuricemia rarely induces gouty attacks and is not a contraindication to use. If uric acid levels are in excess of 9 to 10 mg% or if patients have a history of gouty arthritis, probenecid or allopurinol may be used.

Diabetes. By mechanisms which are yet unclear, diuretics may induce a diminished glucose tolerance and elevate blood glucose levels in patients with a genetic predisposition to diabetes (again, all except spironolactone). The effect is reversible upon discontinuation of the diuretics. The use of diuretics is not necessarily contraindicated in diabetic patients, and blood sugar can generally be controlled by adjusting the dose of diabetic medications. However, nonketotic, hyperosmolar coma and ketoacidosis have been induced by diuretic administration on occasion.

Miscellaneous. Transient and infrequently permanent deafness following the intravenous use of large doses of ethacrynic acid and furosemide has been reported. Patients with poor renal function and those receiving other ototoxic drugs appear to be predisposed to this adverse effect.

Painful gynecomastia secondary to spironolactone has been reported and is virtually indistinguishable from that produced by digoxin. Discontinuation of the medication results in reversal of the symptoms. Irregular menses in females and decreased libido in both sexes have also been reported as side effects of spironolactone.

MISCELLANEOUS DRUG CONSIDERATIONS IN THE MANAGEMENT OF PATIENTS WITH CONGESTIVE HEART FAILURE

Drugs which produce expansion of the intravascular volume or decrease cardiac contractility should be avoided or used with caution in patients with congestive heart failure (see Table 13.6).

Drugs may produce volume expansion by several mechanisms: They may increase retention of sodium and water by the kidney, increase the intravascular osmotic pressure causing a redistribution of interstitial and intracellular water into intravascular space and increase total body sodium and water by their high sodium content.

Agents which cause sodium retention are listed in Table 13.6. Phenylbutazone reportedly

TABLE 13.6
Drugs Which May Exacerbate CHF

Drugs Which May Cause Sodium Retention	Drugs Which Decrease Myocardial Contractility
Androgens	Daunomycin
Corticosteroids	Guanethidine
Diazoxide	Propranolol
Estrogens	
Guanethidine	
Licorice	
Lithium carbonate	
Methyldopa	
Phenylbutazone	
Salicylates	

TABLE 13.7
Sodium Content of Selected Antacids[a,b]

Drug	Sodium Content Mg Na:15 cc or Tab
Greater than 15 mg/tablespoonful or per tab	
Amphogel	15
Basal gel	27
Creamalin tabs	25
Gelusil	21
Maalox	18
Phosphagel susp.	39
Less than 15 mg/tablespoonful or per tab	
Dicarbosil, tab	
Maalox, tabs	
Mylanta, liq., tab.	
Riopan, liq., tab.	
Titralac, liq., tab.	
Tums, tab.	
Wingel, liq., tab.	

[a]Note: In general, the sodium content of antacids does not become significant unless thay are given in quantities of 15-30 cc every 1-2 hr. Please note that sodium content of liquids is that contained in 15 ml.

[b]Reprinted with permission from Ref. 52.

increases intravascular volume by 50% and has been reported to exacerbate pre-existing heart failure. The administration of diazoxide, an antihypertensive agent, is also accompanied by a significant degree of sodium retention. The drug may have a direct effect on renal tubules and/or stimulate the release of antidiuretic hormone. Significant sodium retention and edema may result from the chronic administration of androgenic substances to patients with metastatic carcinoma. Glucocorticoids cause sodium retention through the stimulation of sodium reabsorption in exchange for potassium in the distal tubules of the kidneys. High doses of salicylates have induced congestive failure in patients with rheumatic fever and heart disease presumably owing to a sodium-retaining effect.

The rapid intravenous administration of slowly diffusable substances capable of exerting osmotic activity may result in acute volume overload and the exacerbation of congestive heart disease. Such agents include mannitol, albumin, urea, hypertonic glucose and saline.

Propranolol, a beta-adrenergic blocking agent with negative inotropic effects, may induce overt congestive failure in an already damaged or compromised myocardium. Theo-

TABLE 13.8
Sodium Content of Medicinals[a,b]

Drug	Unit	Mg Na/ unit
1. Parenteral products		
Amcillin S	1 g/inj	62
Dynapen	63 mg/5 ml	67
Geopen	5 g	680
Keflin	1 g vial	62
Methicillin	1 g vial	55
Omnipen N	2 g vial	124
Penbritin-S	1 g vial	66
PenG Na (Squibb)	5 mu/vial	233
Polycillin	1 g vial	68
Principen N	1 g/inj	70
Prostaphlin	4 g vial	144
Staphcillin Buff	1 g vial	61
Unipen Inj.	1 g vial	73
2. Oral liquids		
Dristan Cough Formula	5 ml	59
Phenergan Expectorant	5 ml	51
(plain or VC)		
Phospho-Soda	5 ml	55
Vicks Cough Syrup	5 ml	54
Vicks Formula 44 Syrup	5 ml	68
3. Oral solid dosage forms		
Alkaseltzer	Tab	521
Bisodol Powder	10 g	1,540
Bromoseltzer	80 gr/capful	717
Erythrocin Filmtab	250 mg	70
Fizrin	pkt	673
Kayexelate Powder	15 g	550
Nervine Effervescent	Tab	544
Panteric Granules	Teaspoonful	161
Pasna Pak Granules	6 g pkt	600
Pasna Tri-Pak Granules	5.5 g pkt	490
Rolaids	Tab	53
Sal Hepatica	Rounded Tsp	1,000
Sodium salicylate	10 gr tab	97
4. Food supplements		
Carnation Slender	10 oz can	440
Lytren	1 oz	189
Meritene Powder	1 oz	113
Vivonex-100	6 doses	2,385
5. Miscellaneous		
Fleets enema	4.5 oz	5,000[c]

[a]Reprinted with permission from Ref. 52.
[b]Selected adult medications with an extraordinarily high sodium content (50 mg/dose).
[c]Average absorption = 250-300 mg/enema[53]

retically, sympatholytic agents such as guanethidine may further compromise the myocardium which is dependent upon increased sympathetic tone to maintain cardiac contractility and cardiac output. Furthermore, many of these agents cause mild degrees of sodium retention, perhaps by decreasing cardiac output and therefore glomerular filtration rate. Thus far, however, such agents have not been implicated in the production of overt heart failure. Finally, the direct toxicity of daunomycin on the myocardium may initially manifest itself as confestive heart failure.

Drugs which contain significant amounts of sodium are listed in Table 13.8. The amount of sodium contained in most commercial antacids is insignificant unless the diet is severely sodium-restrictive (500 mg Na per day). Examples of antacids with exceptionally low sodium contents are listed in Table 13.7.

CONCLUSION

The pharmacist may have a very significant role in the management of the patient with congestive heart failure. As has been emphasized, the incidence of toxicity in patients taking digitalis is alarmingly high. It has been shown that a good working knowledge of digitalis pharmacology, kinetics and factors affecting its use may have a marked influence on decreasing the incidence of toxicity.[54] Additionally, it has been shown that patients with CHF who understand their disease and the importance of properly taking prescribed medications have a much higher compliance rate than those that do not.[55] The pharmacist is in an ideal position to provide such patient education and should consider it his responsibility to do so.

REFERENCES

1. McKee, P. A., Castelli, W. P., McNamara, P. M., and Kannell, W. B.: The natural history of congestive heart failure: the Framingham study. N. Engl. J. Med., 285: 1441, 1971.
2. Klainer, L. M., Gibson, T. C., and White, K. L.: The epidemiology of cardiac failure. J. Chronic. Dis., 18: 797, 1965.
3. Kannel, W. B., Castelli, W. P., McNamara, P. M., McKee, P. A., and Feinleib, M.: Role of

blood pressure in the development of congestive heart failure: the Framingham study. N. Engl. J. Med., 287: 781, 1972.

4. Perlman, L. V., Ferguson, S., Bergum, K., Isenberg, E. L., and Hammarsten, J. F.: Precipitation of congestive heart failure: social and emotional factors. Ann. Intern. Med., 75: 1, 1971.

5. Brod, J.: Pathogenesis of cardiac edema. Br. Med. J., 1: 222, 1972.

6. Early, L. E.: Edema formation and the use of diuretics. Calif. Med., 114: 56, 1971.

7. Smith, T. W., and Haber, E.: Medical progress: digitalis (first of four parts). N. Engl. J. Med., 289: 945, 1973.

8. Mason, D. T., and Braunwald, E.: Symposium on congestive heart failure, II. digitalis: new facts about an old drug. Am. J. Cardiol., 22: 151, 1968.

9. Smith, T. W., and Haber, E.: Digitalis (third of four parts). N. Engl. J. Med., 289: 1063, 1973.

10. Smith, T. W.: Digitalis glycosides (first of two parts). N. Engl. J. Med., 288: 719, 1973.

11. Lindenbaum, J., Mellow, M. H., Blackstone, M. O., and Butler, V. P., Jr.: Variation in biologic availability of digoxin from four preparations. N. Engl. J. Med., 285: 1344, 1971.

12. Greenblatt, D. J., Duhme, D. W., Koch-Weser, J., and Smith, T. W.: Evaluation of digoxin bioavailability in single-dose studies. N. Engl. J. Med., 289: 651, 1973.

13. Heizer, W. D., Smith, T. W., and Goldfinger, S. E.: Absorption of digoxin in patients with malabsorption syndromes. N. Engl. J. Med., 285: 257, 1971.

14. White, R. J., Chamberlain, D. A., and Howard, M.: Plasma concentrations of digoxin after oral administration in the fasting and postprandial state. Br. Med. J., 1: 380, 1971.

15. Jelliffe, R. W.: An improved method of digoxin therapy. Ann. Intern. Med., 69: 703, 1968.

16. Greenblatt, D. J., Duhme, D. W., and Koch-Weser, J.: Pain and CPK elevation after intramuscular digoxin. N. Engl. J. Med., 288: 689, 1973.

17. Bennett, W. M., Singer, I., and Coggins, C. H.: A practical guide to drug usage in patients with impaired renal function. J.A.M.A., 214: 1468, 1970.

18. Jelliffe, R. W.: A mathematical analysis of digitalis kinetics in patients with normal and reduced renal function. Mathematical Biosci., 1: 305, 1967.

19. Smith, T. W.: Digitalis glycosides (second of two parts). N. Engl. J. Med., 288: 942, 1973.

20. Beller, G. A., Smith, T. W., Abelmann, W. H., Haber, E., and Hood, W. B.: Digitalis intoxication, a prospective clinical study with serum level correlations. N. Engl. J. Med., 284: 989, 1971.

21. Lukas, D. S.: Of toads and flowers. Circulation, 46: 1, 1972.

22. Jelliffe, R. W., Buell, J., Kalaba, R., Sridhar, R., Rockwell, R., and Wagner, J. G.: An improved method of digitoxin therapy. Ann. Intern. Med., 72: 453, 1970.

23. Doherty, J. E.: The clinical pharmacology of digitalis glycosides: a review. Am. J. Med. Sci., 255: 382, 1968.

24. Rasmussen, K., Jewell, J., Storstein, L., and Gjerdrum, K.: Digitoxin kinetics in patients with impaired renal function. J. Clin. Pharmacol. Ther., 13: 6, 1972.

25. Rodensky, P. L., and Wasserman, F.: Observations on digitalis intoxication. Arch. Intern. Med., 108: 61, 1961.

26. Lely, A. H., and van Enter, C. H. F.: Noncardiac symptoms of digitalis intoxication. Am. Heart J., 83: 149, 1972.

27. Chung, E. K.: Digitalis induced cardiac arrhythmias. Am. Heart J., 79: 845, 1970.

28. Smith, T. W., and Haber, E.: Digoxin intoxication: the relationship of clinical presentation to serum digoxin concentration. J. Clin. Invest., 49: 2377, 1970.

29. Jelliffe, R. W.: Factors to consider in planning digoxin therapy. J. Chronic. Dis., 24: 407, 1971.

30. Prindle, K. H., Jr., Skelton, C. L., Epstein, S. E., and Marcus, F. I.: Influence of extracellular potassium concentration on myocardial uptake and inotropic effect of tritiated digoxin. Circ. Res., 28: 337, 1971.

31. Seller, R. H., Cangiano, J., Kim, K. E., Mendelssohn, S., Brest, A. N., and Swartz, C.: Digitalis toxicity and hypomagnesemia. Am. Heart J., 79: 57, 1970.

32. Resnick, N.: Digitalis: a double-edged sword. Med. Sci., 4: 31, 1964.

33. Chung, E. K.: The current status of digitalis therapy. Mod. Treat., 8: 643, 1971.

34. Lown, B., Black, H., and Moore, F. D.: Digitalis, electrolytes and the surgical patient. Am. J. Cardiol., 6: 309, 1960.

35. Ewy, G. A., Kapadia, G. G., Yao, L., Lullen, M., and Marcus, F. I.: Digoxin metabolism in the elderly. Circulation, 39: 449, 1969.

36. Levine, O. R., and Somlyo, A. P.: Digitalis intoxication in premature infants. J. Pediatr., 61: 70, 1962.

37. Levine, O. R., and Blumetnal, S.: Digoxin dosage in premature infants. Pediatrics, 29: 18, 1962.

38. Hernandez, A., Burton, R. M., Pagtakham, R. D., and Goldring, D.: Pharmacodynamics of ^{3}H-Digoxin in infants. Pediatrics, 44: 418, 1969.

39. Doherty, J. E., and Perkins, W. H.: Digoxin metabolism in hypo- and hyper-thyroidism — studies with tritiated digoxin. Ann. Intern. Med., 64: 489, 1966.

40. Marcus, F. I., and Kapadia, G. G.: The metabolism of digoxin in cirrhotic patients. Gastroenterology, 47: 517, 1964.

41. Weintraub, M., Au, W. Y. W., and Lasagna, L.: Compliance as a determinant of serum digoxin concentration. J.A.M.A., 224: 481, 1973.

42. Solomon, H. M., and Abrams, W. B.: Interactions

between digitoxin and other drugs in man. Am. Heart J., 83: 277, 1972.

43. Irons, G. V., Jr., and Orgain, E. S.: Digitalis-induced arrhythmias and their management. Prog. Cardiovasc. Dis., 8: 539, 1966.

44. Seltzer, A., and Cohn, K. E.: Production, recognition and treatment of digitalis toxicity. Calif. Med., 113: 1, 1970.

45. Bigger, J. T., and Strauss, H. C.: Digitalis toxicity: drug interactions promoting toxicity and the management of toxicity. Semin. Drug Treat., 2: 147, 1972.

46. Thomson, P. D., Melmon, K. L., Richardson, J. A., Cohn, K., Steinbrunn, W., Cudihee, R., and Rowland, M.: Lidocaine pharmacokinetics in advanced heart failure, liver disease and renal failure. Am. Heart J., 82: 417, 1971.

47. Kleit, S. A., Hamburger, R. J., Martz, B. L., and Fisch, C.: Diuretic therapy: current status. Am. Heart J., 79: 700, 1970.

48. Gantt, C. L.: Diuretic therapy. Ration. Drug Ther., 6: 1, 1972.

49. Schreiner, G. E., and Lauler, D. P.: Edema and diuretics. Medcom, New York, 1969 (Riche Therapeutic Series).

50. Early, L.: Diuretics. N. Engl. J. Med., 276: 966, 1967.

51. Early, L.: Diuretics (concluded). N. Engl. J. Med., 276: 1023, 1967.

52. Diet Committee of the San Francisco Heart Association in cooperation with the U.C. Hospital Pharmacy: sodium in medicinals., San Francisco Heart Association, San Francisco, 1973.

53. Anon.: Hospital Pharmacy Notes. Veterans Hospital, Brooklyn, N.Y., May, 1972.

54. Ogilvie, R. I., and Ruedy, J.: An educational program in digitalis therapy. J.A.M.A., 222: 50, 1972.

55. Marsh, W. W., and Perlman, L. V.: Understanding congestive heart failure and self-administration of digoxin. Geriatrics, 27: 65, 1972.

chapter 14

ACUTE MYOCARDIAL INFARCTION

Robert A. Kerr, Pharm.D.

Myocardial infarction represents one extreme in the clinical spectrum of ischemic heart disease. Ischemic heart disease includes asymptomatic coronary atherosclerosis, angina pectoris, the "intermediate syndrome," myocardial infarction and sudden death. Angina pectoris and myocardial infarction represent the most usual clinical pictures; however, sudden death, presumably from an arrhythmia secondary to myocardial ischemia, can occur in patients with no apparent previous history of angina pectoris or myocardial infarction. Patients may also present with acute myocardial infarction with no previous history of angina pectoris. Patients may pass into the symptomatic phases of ischemic heart disease and then return to an asymptomatic phase, presumably because of development of collateral coronary circulation.

This mixture of clinical progression in ischemic heart disease is easier to understand when one considers that coronary atherosclerosis can progress for 40 years or longer in a preclinical form and may be asymptomatic even when the pathological disease is fairly extensive. In fact, when symptomatic disease occurs in the form of angina pectoris, it represents, in most cases, advanced and very severe occlusive atherosclerosis of the coronary arteries (angina pectoris probably occurs when there is 90 to 100% occlusion of a major coronary artery).[1] It has been demonstrated that, as a rule, angina occurs after two major coronary arteries are occluded and the remaining major branches are severely narrowed. This compromised coronary blood flow leads to the relative imbalance between oxygen delivery and myocardial work which presents the "pain on exertion" picture of the angina pectoris syndrome. Myocardial infarction, on the other hand, results from lack of coronary blood flow to an area of myocardium leading to prolonged ischemia and tissue damage. Consequently, acute myocardial infarction usually is not precipitated by exertion or relieved by rest.

Approximately 800,000 Americans die of coronary heart disease annually.[2] An estimated 600,000 of these deaths are the result of acute myocardial infarction.[3] Other statistics indicate that acute myocardial infarction is responsible for more than one-half of deaths occurring before the age of 65.[2] However, precise computation of the total mortality from all acute myocardial infarctions is difficult since some patients with mild symptoms never consult a physician and others die suddenly with the exact cause of death not apparent. The American Heart Association in its public education materials states that heart attack (*i.e.,* myocardial infarction) is the greatest threat to the life of a businessman between the ages of 35 and 64.[4]

DIAGNOSIS AND CLINICAL FINDINGS

As with angina pectoris, perhaps the most significant aspect of diagnosis in acute myocardial infarction is an accurate history of the patient's clincial presentation. The most frequent presenting complaint of the patient with myocardial infarction is a deep visceral pain involving the central portion of the chest and epigastrium. The pain is usually described as being extremely severe; "crushing" or "heavy"; relatively constant and prolonged; often occurring at rest (or, at any rate, not brought on by exertion or relieved by rest); and often accompanied by profuse sweating, nausea and vomiting, shortness of breath, and marked weakness or faintness. The pain may radiate to the shoulder, arm, neck, jaw, abdomen or back (radiation to the arms occurs in about 25% of cases). It is important to realize that many patients will not describe a pain but rather will talk of an unusual discomfort. One should, therefore, not limit the historical vocabulary to an investigation of "pain." At times difficulties may arise in those patients who have a chronic gastrointestinal disorder and chronically complain of "heartburn" (as in the patient with hiatus hernia). The significant point in such a patient is the presence of a new type of pain (example: a prolonged substernal or epigastric distress occurring during recumbency helped by sitting up which is described as a "new occurrence"). In the patient with known angina, the significant point is the change in pattern of symptomatology (example: longer duration and occurring at rest). The significance of "new pain" or "first time pain" is greater than pain which is chronically experienced.[5]

Some patients, particularly the elderly, may present with acute shortness of breath (perhaps progressing to pulmonary edema), sudden loss of consciousness, altered state of consciousness (confusion), an arrhythmia or sudden drop in blood pressure rather than with classical complaints of pain. It is estimated that at least 15 to 20% of myocardial infarcts are "painless" (this is probably a low estimate since such a patient may not seek medical attention).[2]

Physical findings in acute myocardial infarction may be present and helpful to the clinician; however, they are rarely diagnostic when taken alone. Initial observation of the patient usually shows that reaction to the chest pain is the dominant feature. Anxiousness and restlessness, often accompanied by moving about in an attempt to relieve the pain, are common. It is not uncommon for the patient to try to "walk off" the pain of myocardial infarction. Pallor accompanied by sweating and coolness of the extremities is common. The pulse is usually rapid; however, some patients exhibit profound bradycardia. Heart sounds are usually diminished but are often normal. An atrial gallop, or S_4, is the most common extra heart sound. Fewer patients exhibit a ventricular gallop, or S_3, and occasionally a paradoxical split of the second heart sound is heard. However, with the possible exception of the reaction of the patient to his chest pain, none of these findings is specific for myocardial infarction and, in fact, may not be present.

The most frequently utilized laboratory tests for the diagnosis of myocardial infarction are serial enzyme studies and electrocardiographic studies (EKG). Of course, there are several nonspecific laboratory indications of tissue necrosis and inflammation which may be helpful such as elevation of erythrocyte sedimentation rate and elevation of the white blood cell count.

With prolonged ischemia, myocardial cells are damaged, and the cell membranes become permeable to enzymes which leak into the blood. These enzymes are present in tissues other than myocardium; however, the rate of liberation following injury differs. Therefore, the time course of serum concentrations of these enzymes can be utilized to confirm diagnosis of myocardial infarction (see Fig. 14.1). The three most frequently used enzyme concentrations are creatinine phosphokinase (CPK), serum glutamic oxaloacetic transaminase (SGOT) and lactic dehydrogenase (LDH). CPK is more specific than SGOT since it is present in fewer tissues; however, its usefulness is limited for two reasons: first, its elevation may be missed unless levels are drawn early, and secondly, elevations may occur secondary to intramuscular injections of drugs; a fair number of patients receive such injections prior to blood testing. (However, it must be

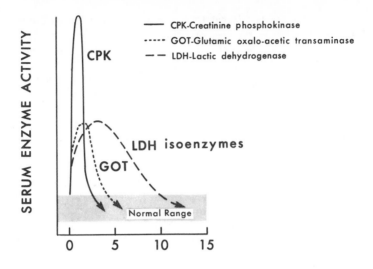

DAYS AFTER ONSET

FIG. 14 1. Time course of serum enzyme concentration changes following a typical myocardial infarction.

admitted that severe myocardial infarction elevates CPK more dramatically than a simple I.M. injection.) SGOT is the most widely used enzyme test; however, it too can be missed since it usually falls off to normal within 3 days. LDH peaks at 3 to 4 days and falls to within normal limits within 14 days. While rapidly migrating LDH isoenzyme is more specific for myocardial infarction than is total LDH, it is normally not necessary to obtain LDH isoenzyme studies since the important point of enzyme studies is the time course of the serum concentrations of the three enzymes, CPK, SGOT and LDH. Owing to the limitations of CPK studies, and since many laboratories are not equipped to measure CPK, one finds that serial SGOT and LDH studies are the most frequently used.

The electrocardiogram can be of great value in the study of ischemic heart disease since the electrophysiological processes within the heart are sensitive to alterations in perfusion of the myocardium. The three EKG changes observed in the infarcted heart are T wave inversion, ST elevation and the appearance of Q waves (see Fig. 14.2). Only Q waves are diagnostic of infarction (i.e., necrosis), however, ST and T wave changes provide suspicion and, in fact, are the only changes seen if the infarction does not involve the entire thickness of the myocardium (i.e., subendocardial infarction).[6]

Time relationships are important in EKG

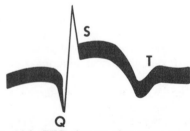

NORMAL EKG

FIG. 14.2. EKG changes after acute myocardial infarction: Three indicative changes—Q wave, ST elevation and T inversion.

tracings with myocardial infarction since changes may not occur for several days or even for 2 to 3 weeks. Some changes, however, usually do occur within the first few hours after infarction. ST segment changes appear early and progress. T waves initially become taller and then later become inverted. Evolution of EKG changes (*i.e.,* progressive changes in EKG pattern from day to day) are necessary for electrocardiographic diagnosis of *acute* myocardial infarction. These time relationships and evolutionary processes are important to consider when one is evaluating the significance or usefulness of a tracing taken within the 1st hr of the infarction. Such a tracing, for most practical purposes, would only be helpful as a baseline for further tracings (at least as it would relate to diagnosis).[5] Certainly if one suspects an early arrhythmia, an EKG tracing is needed for indentification of the arrhythmia. EKG tracings can be utilized to identify the location of the infarction, anterior or inferior (diaphragmatic or "posterior" by older terminology), and such detailed discussions of the electrocardiogram in myocardial infarction can be found in various electrocardiography textbooks.[6] However, such a dissertation is not deemed within the scope of our discussion here.

MANAGEMENT

Prehospital Phase

Approximately 70% of the 600,000 people who die annually in the United States from acute myocardial infarction die before receiving medical aid.[2,3] Approximately 50% of all deaths from acute myocardial infarction occur during the first 2 hr after the onset of symptoms.[3] The delay in seeking medical attention is usually the result of indecision by the patient. The average "decision time" to seek medical help is 3 hr after the onset of symptoms.[2,5] The patient experiencing warning symptoms[4] (see Table 14.1), especially the patient who has been unusually healthy, will frequently delay before he communicates with anyone. This delay in communication may be the result of denial that anything serious is happening ("This can't be happening to me") or the hope that the symptoms will go away and everything will be all right. Those observing the patient, such as family or friends, are more prone to recognize the potential severity of the situation and seek medical assistance than is the patient himself; however, by this time, much critical time may have been lost.

TABLE 14.1
Warning Symptoms of Myocardial Infarction

The symptoms vary, but these are the usual warnings of heart attack:
1. Prolonged, oppressive pain or unusual discomfort in the center of the chest, behind the breast bone
2. Pain may radiate to the shoulder, arm, neck or jaw
3. The pain or discomfort is often accompanied by sweating; nausea, vomiting and shortness of breath may also occur
4. Sometimes these symptoms subside and then return; do not wait; act immediately

It is obvious that all the sophistication of the coronary care unit is useless for those patients who never reach the hospital. Since recognition of symptoms and their seriousness by the patient seems to be a critical point (*i.e.,* once this recognition is made, transportation to medical assistance is usually quite rapid), the importance of better education of the public regarding the nature and significance of the early symptoms of acute myocardial infarction and what to do about them cannot be overemphasized. How to obtain medical attention is a vital part of this educational process. It is generally felt that immediate transportation to the closest emergency room is a better mode of action than going to or calling a physician's office. Calling for an ambulance (or a mobile coronary care unit, if available) to provide transportation is reasonable provided one does not have to wait any extended period of time for the arrival of the ambulance.[5]

The role of the practicing pharmacist in providing this type of public education is obvious. Not only can the pharmacist verbally educate those patients who may be at high risk (*e.g.,* patients with history of angina pectoris or previous myocardial infarction, or long standing hypertension with evidence or end organ disease), but he can also display and provide public educational materials.

First aid treatment of the patient with acute myocardial infarction may merely require making the patient as comfortable as possible, sitting him up if there is shortness of breath, or lying him down if there is marked weakness or faintness suggestive of hypotension and providing for rapid transportation to medical assistance; or, cardiopulmonary resuscitation may be required. Resuscitation efforts by untrained individuals are almost always unsuccessful. Even in the hospital setting cardiopulmonary resuscitation by trained, well motivated personnel is all too often unsuccessful; however, it is true that properly applied resuscitation techniques can save many lives.[2,5] It would behoove all allied health personnel to obtain continuing training in cardiopulmonary resuscitation. It is quite possible that adequately trained allied health personnel, and not physicians, offer the most in terms of availability, competency and economy for prehospital emergency management of myocardial infarction.[5]

The medical emergency treatment of acute myocardial infarction in the prehospital phase involves analgesia, oxygen, treating or trying to prevent cardiac arrhythmias and treating other early complications. The goal in this phase of treatment is to keep the patient as stable as possible prior to the availability of close monitoring in a hospital coronary care unit.

As mentioned earlier, the pain of myocardial infarction is severe and, in fact, is often described as the most severe pain the patient has ever experienced. Therefore, prompt treatment of this pain is in order to provide comfort and to alleviate the extreme anxiety associated with cardiac pain. However, one must use potent analgesics with extreme care in the acute myocardial infarction patient since all of these agents have effects on the hemodynamics of the cardiovascular system.[7,8] The choice of analgesic seems to boil down to selection of either morphine or pentazocine, since all of the narcotic analgesics seem to have hemodynamic effects comparable to those of morphine in equianalgesic doses. The hemodynamic effects of morphine and pentazocine postmyocardial infarction have been studied.[7,8] Morphine decreases oxygen consumption, decreases left ventricular end-diastolic pressure, decreases blood pressure via venous pooling and causes an over-all decrease in cardiac work. Pentazocine increases myocardial oxygen requirement, increases mean aortic pressure, increases left ventricular end-diastolic pressure, increases mean pulmonary artery pressure, causes a small increase in cardiac output and causes an over-all increase in cardiac work. In general, a decrease in myocardial oxygen consumption and cardiac work would seem to be beneficial in the myocardial infarction patient; therefore, morphine appears to be the analgesic of choice in most of these patients. However, in those patients exhibiting hypotension or suspected elevation of sympathetic activity in which an excessive hypotensive response to morphine may be experienced, pentazocine may offer advantages to such a patient who requires continued analgesia. (It should be remembered, however, that pentazocine will increase cardiac work and myocardial oxygen consumption, which could increase the degree of myocardial ischemia.) An important principle to remember in the use of these agents is that only an amount of drug necessary to alleviate the pain should be administered. Some patients require less analgesia than others and, therefore, minimal doses should be used initially with subsequent doses being titrated to individual patient response. Since, in effective dosage, none of the presently available potent analgesics is entirely free from circulatory effects in patients with acute myocardial infarction, knowing what to expect ahead of time increases the efficiency in monitoring these patients.

Ventricular fibrillation is the apparent cause of most sudden deaths in the prehospital phase of acute myocardial infarction.[3] Consequently, recognition and treatment of ventricular arrhythmias or cardiac rhythms which are felt to predispose to ventricular arrhythmias during the prehospital phase are currently areas of intense investigation and discussion. While there is no definite formula (since there is some degree of apparent contradictory information both clinically and experimentally), it is possible to formulate a fairly rational approach to the problem utilizing current available information.

If the patient has frequent premature ventricular contractions (PVCs), he is more prone to ventricular fibrillation, especially if the PVCs are on top of the T waves. Lidocaine hydrochloride has proven to be the most successful agent currently available to treat this problem. In prehospital management, one can use 50 to 100 mg (2.5 to 5 cc of 2% solution) as an I.V. bolus to obtain rapid therapeutic blood levels (1 to 4 μg per ml). This blood level can then be maintained during transit to the hospital by giving an I.M. injection of 200 mg (5 cc of 4% solution or 4 cc of 5% solution), which will provide serum levels above 1 μg per ml for at least 60 min.[9,10] Obviously, if the patient is in shock or hypotensive, an I.M. injection is not reasonable owing to erratic absorption from the site in injection. Currently there is some literature suggesting that all patients with acute myocardial infarction should be given a prophylactic intramuscular injection of lidocaine because EKG tracings often are not available prior to hospitalization. When one considers the mortality statistics secondary to ventricular arrhythmia during this critical time period, and also that lidocaine in normal doses usually does not impair atrioventricular conduction, this course of action may seem quite reasonable provided that the patient is not severely bradycardic, is not hypotensive and is not in decompensated heart failure. One must remember, though, that the routine use of antiarrhythmic agents, either self-administered or administered by paramedical personnel in the prehospitalized patient, has not been adequately studied. Indeed, principles of rational therapeutics tell us that each individual should be analyzed relative to the variables in hemodynamic and electrophysiological status that affect the necessity of the use of an agent prophylactically or that affect potential toxicities.[11]

Management of the patient exhibiting bradycardia during the prehospital phase is somewhat more controversial.[3,12,13] One of the reasons for the controversy over the management of this problem is that there is some uncertainty about the significance of bradycardia in acute myocardial infarction. It has been generally believed that bradycardia in these patients has certain disadvantages: it may result in decreased cardiac output with subsequent hypotension with poor tissue perfusion leading to possible aggravation of myocardial ischemia; and it is also believed by many that bradycardia may be an important cause of electrical instability leading to ventricular fibrillation. It is the latter point that has recently been challenged by some experimental and clinical data.[3] Some of these data indicate that persons with untreated sinus bradycardia have a lower incidence of development of serious ventricular tachyarrhythmias than those persons without sinus bradycardia. While some clinicians feel that decreased cardiac output secondary to bradycardia increases myocardial inschemia and that this ischemia increases the incidence of arrhythmias, others feel that bradycardia (provided it is

not too severe) will decrease myocardial oxygen consumption and hence lead to less ischemia. In addition, there is some evidence that the use of atropine in "bradycardia-induced" PVCs may abolish only the more benign arrhythmias not associated with high mortality and may be ineffective in abolishing more severe arrhythmias (e.g., close coupled PVCs).[3] Where does all this leave us with respect to the emergency use of atropine immediately after acute myocardial infarction? Certainly the evidence suggests that routine use of atropine is not warranted and in fact may be dangerous. There are an increasing number of reported cases of fatal atropine-induced tachyarrhythmias. It seems quite reasonable to administer atropine to the patient who is severely bradycardic and has marked hypotension. Atropine should be dosed carefully by using aliquot of 0.3 mg I.V. to achieve the desired response. Too high a dose can lead to abolishment of vagal tone with consequent decrease in electrical stability of the heart. Atropine is not indicated in a patient with mild to moderate bradycardia who is otherwise stable.[13]

The use of nitroglycerin during the prehospital phase of acute myocardial infarction has also been the subject of some discussion.[3] It has long been felt that the administration of nitroglycerin or other hypotensive agents should be avoided in this circumstance owing to their propensity to decrease arterial pressure causing a reflex increase in heart rate and subsequent extension of the ischemic process.[5] However, there is some clinical evidence that the administration of a vasodilator to patients with decreased left ventricular function postmyocardial infarction may result in hemodynamic improvement.[14,15] In addition, there is some experimental evidence that coadministration of nitroglycerin with an alpha-agonist (to prevent nitrate-induced hypotension and reflex tachycardia) may enhance the electrical stability of the heart during acute myocardial ischemia.[3] However, it still would seem best to avoid nitroglycerin and other vasodilators in acute myocardial infarction until more convincing clinical evidence is available concerning efficacy, safety and the variables which should be considered.

Other complications in the early phase of acute myocardial infarction are cardiogenic shock and acute left ventricular failure with subsequent pulmonary edema. The patient who presents outside the hospital with cardiogenic shock is unlikely to survive.[5] Management of this problem will be discussed later in the section on the hospital phase of management. Briefly and basically, the management of pulmonary edema is to: sit the patient up to decrease venous return; administer morphine to alleviate apprehension and to provide venous pooling; administer oxygen; provide positive pressure breathing to increase intrathoracic pressure thereby decreasing venous return; apply rotating tourniquets to decrease the relative circulating blood volume; and, if necessary, perform phlebotomy to decrease circulating blood volume.[5]

It is important that all of the procedures and drugs administered to the patient during the prehospital phase be accurately communicated to the hospital staff. This provides for total knowledge of the status of the patient and allows for continuity of care.

HOSPITAL PHASE

Monitoring

The development of coronary care units with subsequent close monitoring of patients has been a major advance in the management of acute myocardial infarction.[16,17] Continuous cardiac monitoring together with recent advances in electrophysiology and the use of antiarrhythmic agents has been shown to decrease mortality significantly during the hospital phase of acute myocardial infarction.[18] Cardiac monitoring in coronary care units provides for rapid detection of arrhythmias and allows for decisions concerning specific treatment as they appear. Of course, monitoring involves more than the utilization of a cathode ray oscilloscope, The high nurse-to-patient ratio in coronary care units allows for close monitoring with respect to heart rate, blood pressure, rate and quality of breathing, character of heart sounds, signs and symptoms of congestive heart failure and the psychological status of the patient. Certainly "eyeball monitoring" and observation of the patient can be as important as oscilloscope monitoring.

Arrhythmias

As stated previously, early detection and treatment of arrhythmias are paramount in the management of the acute myocardial infarction patient. Following acute myocardial infarction, especially during the first 48 hr after the onset of chest pain, some form of arrhythmia is exhibited by nearly 95% of patients. Lemberg et al. provided a breakdown concerning the incidence of arrhythmias encountered postmyocardial infarction (see Table 14.2).[18]

Two forms of heart block can be seen with myocardial infarction.[12] The first is a result of a diaphragmatic (inferior) infarction (DMI) with compromised blood flow to the atrioventricular (AV) node. The second results from anterior infarction (AMI) with disease affecting primarily the intraventricular conduction system. DMI usually results from right coronary disease and the resulting heart block usually is AV nodal, whereas AMI usually results from disease of the anterior descending coronary artery and, therefore, involves the bundle branch system. Mortality from AMI with heart block is higher than that seen in DMI with heart block; however, the incidence of DMI with heart block is higher.

The conduction defects seen with DMI are, for the most part, secondary to ischemia and are usually reversed within the 1st week of admission. The QRS complexes are narrow and the ventricular rate is relatively rapid (40 to 60 beats per min). The conduction defects seen

TABLE 14.2
Incidence of Arrhythmias Post-Myocardial Infarction[a]

Arrhythmia	Incidence %
Electrical instability	
Premature ventricular contraction	80
Paroxysmal ventricular tachycardia	28
Bradyarrhythmias	
Sinus bradycardia	30
Junctional rhythms	8
Slow ventricular tachycardia	16
Atrioventricular block	8
Pump failure	
Atrial arrhythmias	27.3
Premature atrial contractions	
Paroxysmal atrial tachycardia	
Atrial fibrillation	

[a]Reprinted with permission from Ref. 18.

with AMI reflect involvement of the ventricular system and can be due either to ischemia or to necrosis of the conduction tissue itself. Consequently, the associated mortality from heart failure and cardiogenic shock, reflecting extensive infarction, is rather high. With AMI and heart block there is a paroxysmal onset of AV block, wide QRS complexes and a very slow heart rate.[12]

In DMI with first degree block no specific therapy is necessary. The few patients who progress to second degree block do so slowly, allowing time for evaluation. DMI with second or third degree block is treated depending upon both ventricular rate and hemodynamic status. Increase in heart rate is indicated if the ventricular rate is less than 50 beats per min and/or there is evidence of heart failure or cardiogenic shock. One can first attempt careful administration of atropine (remembering that atropine can induce dangerous tachyarrhythmias or can paradoxically worsen AV block). If atropine is unsuccessful, then transvenous pacing is indicated.

In AMI with either second or third degree block, transvenous pacing is usually recommended even though the mortality in such patients is extremely high, with or without pacing. Atropine would not be effective since the site of the conduction defect and the escape pacemakers are not under significant parasympathetic control, and since the block in AMI is usually secondary to destruction of conduction tissues.

The use of isoproterenol in myocardial infarction with heart block has been suggested by some clinicians since it may facilitate conduction in both the AV node and the His Purkinje system. Isoproterenol, however, can also increase myocardial oxygen demands (with the potential of increasing size of the infarct) and also can increase ventricular irritability with subsequent risks of inducing premature ventricular contractions and ventricular fibrillation.

Ventricular arrhythmias, specifically premature ventricular contractions, represent the most frequently encountered rhythm disturbance in acute myocardial infarction.[18] The increased cardiac irritability seems to be due to myocardial ischemia. Since electrical death is primarily due to ventricular fibrillation, early recognition and treatment of potentially fatal ventricular arrhythmias is vital.

Patterns felt to be potentially dangerous and therefore requiring immediate treatment are: a high frequency of premature ventricular contractions (more than 6 per min), repetitive ventricular beats or ventricular tachycardia with ectopic rates greater than 100 beats per min, multiform PVC's or even 1 PVC which interrupts the T wave of a preceding sinus or ectopic beat.

Lidocaine hydrochloride is the drug of choice for immediate treatment of ventricular arrhythmias (Table 14.3). It is administered as an intravenous bolus of 50 to 100 mg followed by an infusion of 1 to 4 mg/min. Lidocaine has a distribution half-life of 20 min and a metabolic half-life of approximately 2 hr. Dosage must be reduced to one-third normal in patients with decompensated right-sided heart failure or with severe liver disease. Overdose toxicities include drowsiness, mental confusion and, rarely, convulsions.[18]

If continued antiarrhythmic therapy is required beyond 24 hr, either procainamide or quinidine can be added to the regimen. Both of these agents have been shown to be effective in both the treatment and prevention of ventricular arrhythmias postmyocardial infarction.[18,21] Both drugs can cause hypotension when administered parenterally. Quinidine should be given only I.M. and never I.V. since I.V. administration is frequently followed by profound hypotension. Procainamide can be administered both I.M. and I.V. with caution. Under most circumstances both agents are administered orally.[18] Both drugs have a half-life of approximately 3 hr. It has been demonstrated that procainamide should be administered every 3 to 4 hr, whereas current data seem to indicate that a 6-hr dosing interval is adequate for quinidine.

Propranolol may be an effective alternative drug in myocardial infarction patients with ventricular arrhythmias who do not respond to or have a sensitivity to lidocaine. Small doses of 0.5 mg every 2 min I.V. up to a total dose of 3 to 4 mg have been used successfully.[18] When using this agent, one must keep in mind that it is a potent myocardial depressant with the potential for inducing bradycardia or heart failure.

When a life-threatening ventricular tachyarrhythmic does not respond to drug therapy, electrical cardioversion is indicated. It should be pointed out that optimal efficacy of either

TABLE 14.3

Drugs Commonly Used in the Management of Myocardial Infarction

Drug	Dose	Comments
Analgesics		
Morphine	3-10 mg S.Q., I.M., I.V.	Causes an over-all decrease in cardiac work; use smallest dose possible; can induce hypotension, nausea and vomiting, constipation and respiratory depression
Pentazocine	30-60- mg I.M.	Causes an over-all increase in cardiac work; causes hallucinations and/or psychoses in some patients
Antiarrhythmics		
Atropine	Aliquots of 0.3 mg I.V.	For severe bradycardia; 0.6-0.9 mg total usually sufficient; can induce fatal tachyarrhythmias
Lidocaine	50-100 mg I.V. bolus 200 mg I.M. 1-4 mg/min. I.V. infusion	I.V. bolus necessary to obtain therapeutic levels; I.M. injection will maintain levels for about 60 min; decrease dose in liver congestion or severe liver disease; most efficacious for ventricular arrhythmias
Propranolol	0.5-4 mg I.V. in aliquots of 0.5 mg q 2 min	An alternative agent for ventricular arrhythmias; can induce a bradycardia
Digoxin	0.25 mg I.V. q 5 h x 3-4 doses then individualized maintenance dose	For control of ventricular response in atrial arrhythmias; loading dose to obtain desired response; maintenance dose based on renal function and clinical response
Quinidine	200-400 mg q 6 h po or I.M.	For control of PVCs; for conversion of atrial fibrillation *after* digitalization; never to be used I.V.
Procainamide	250-500 mg q 4 h	For ventricular arrhythmias; dosing interval of 3-4 hr necessary to maintain blood level; chronic use associated with high incidence of lupus syndrome

antiarrhythmic drug therapy or electrical cardioversion is obtained when the patient is in good acid-base and electrolyte balance. One should not assume that a patient is "refractory" to a mode of antiarrhythmic therapy when there may be an underlying physiological cause that may lead the patient to be refractory to other therapeutic efforts as well.

Supraventricular arrhythmias can occur post-myocardial infarction, and in most cases they are considered to be benign and transient. Atrial fibrillation occurs in about 10 to 15% of myocardial infarction cases, and it is usually preceded by premature atrial beats or short runs of atrial tachycardia.[18] There are two considerations in the decision to treat supraven-

tricular arrhythmias: the ventricular response and the decrease in cardiac output secondary to loss of atrial transport of blood into the ventricles. Rapid ventricular response to atrial fibrillation or flutter may aggravate left ventricular failure thereby inducing hypotension and possibly extending the area of damage or injury in the myocardium. Digoxin is particularly effective in controlling ventricular response to supraventricular tachyarrhythmias. A reasonable approach in such a situation is to select a predetermined index of effect (*i.e.*, a controlled ventricular response) and then dose the digoxin (*e.g.*, 0.25 mg every 5 hr) until the response is obtained. Once a desired index is obtained, maintenance dosing, if indicated, can be determined based upon the ability of the patient to clear the drug and the clinical response observed.

Since atrial fibrillation can decrease cardiac output by as much as 30% in some patients, it may be desirable to convert the supraventricular arrhythmia to improve atrial transport. Electrical cardioversion has been successful in terminating atrial flutter, but its success in atrial fibrillation is often transient.[18] Propranolol has been successful in the treatment of supraventricular arrhythmias postmyocardial infarction. In digitalized patients, less propranolol is used owing to synergistic effects on depression of atrioventricular transmission. Quinidine has also been effective in atrial arrhythmias. Since quinidine has an antivagal activity which acts to increase AV conduction, it is mandatory that digitalization be accomplished prior to the use of quinidine to convert an atrial tachyarrhythmia.

Shock

Approximately 15% of hospitalized patients with acute myocardial infarction exhibit cardiogenic shock, which is a serious complication usually leading to death.[22,23] Shock associated with myocardial infarction is most often the result of insufficient cardiac output to maintain adequate tissue perfusion and is usually manifest by hypotension, oliguria and signs of sympathetic vasoconstriction. While mortality in cardiogenic shock is extremely high, an agressive but rational therapeutic approach can save some patients.

First one should remember that many of the agents used in the management of other problems in acute myocardial infarction can induce profound hypotension and precipitate or aggravate the shock syndrome.[22] Potentially offending agents include narcotic analgesics, myocardial depressants, sedatives and tranquilizers and antihypertensives. Consequently, a review of the medication history, paying particular attention to dose, dosing interval and temporal relationship with the development of hypotension may uncover precipitating or aggravating agents which should be discontinued.

If there is evidence of a reduced effective plasma volume, intravenous fluids such as Lactated Ringers Injection USP, or 5% dextrose

TABLE 14.4
Risk Factors Associated with Increased
Mortality between End of First Week and Three Months[a]

1. Coronary prognostic index of 6 or more
2. Significant ventricular arrhythmias in the first 48 hr
3. Sinus tachycardia
4. Persistent S-T segment elevation
5. Recurrent ischemic pain or recurrent arrhythmias

[a]Reprinted with permission from Ref. 32.

in water or plasma expanders such as low molecular weight dextran or albumin can be used. Such fluids are best given prior to the use of sympathomimetic amines in situations of relative hypovolemia. One must remember that the frequent cause of shock in acute myocardial infarction is pump failure, and, therefore, close monitoring of the patient's volume status and the ability of the left ventricle to handle volume (*e.g.*, central venous pressure, clinical signs of circulatory overload in the lungs) is mandatory, if volume expansion is attempted.[22,23]

Sympathomimetic amines which increase arterial pressure are considered principle modes of therapy in the shock syndrome.[23] Metaraminol, which acts in part by the release of endogenous norepinephrine, is frequently used, as is levarterenol. Both agents provide peripheral vasoconstriction and some heart stimulatory effects. While such agents do indeed raise arterial pressure, they can also act to decrease peripheral perfusion via peripheral vasoconstriction which at times can lead to end organ damage (*e.g.*, renal failure). Some clinicians have counteracted this "peripheral clamping" effect by titrating doses of the beta-agonist isoproterenol. The use of isoproterenol in shock must be undertaken with considerable caution since it can worsen hypotension, especially in cases of relative hypovolemia, and it can induce arrhythmias (as can the other sympathomimetics), especially in patients with ischemic myocardium who are already prone to development of arrhythmias.

Since in many incidences this shock syndrome is associated with pump failure, some clinicians will digitalize these patients. Several points should be kept in mind if digitalization is considered. First is the differentiation between decreased output due to heart block versus left ventricular failure. Digoxin may worsen the former and may improve the latter. Secondly, there is some evidence that the myocardium is more sensitive to digitalis-induced arrhythmias in early postmyocardial infarction. Thirdly, digitalization is *not* an immediate process and takes several hours to a day to achieve, even with "rapid acting" glycosides. Obviously, if the decreased cardiac output is secondary to an arrhythmia, one should deal specifically with the arrhythmia to help correct the shock syndrome.

Heart Failure

As mentioned earlier, one of the complications of acute myocardial infarction is acute left ventricular failure leading to pulmonary edema. The basic approach to this problem was also discussed earlier. It should be pointed out that several of the therapeutic maneuvers in pulmonary edema can conceivably precipitate other problems. For example: morphine administration can lead to profound hypotension and/or respiratory depression (*e.g.*, in a patient with chronic lung disease); and potent diuretics such as furosemide, ethacrynic acid and mercurials can lead to major fluid and electrolyte imbalance which can manifest hypotension, shock and/or arrhythmias. Therefore, an understanding and recognition of the patient's current physiological status coupled with an understanding of the ways this physiological status may change are imperative for effective monitoring of therapeutic response as well as toxicity.

Some patients may manifest clinical evidence of congestive heart failure without frank pulmonary edema. It is important to remember that the patient experiencing an acute myocardial infarction is more prone to the potential toxicities associated with the use of digitalis glycosides and diuretics and therefore, definite indications with precise therapeutic objectives and accurate indices of effect are mandatory.

Anticoagulation

There is a great deal of controversy over the use of anticoagulants in association with acute myocardial infarction.[24-28] It is now generally believed that the risk-benefit ratio does not warrant long term anticoagulation of individuals with myocardial infarction. Generally, it is felt that short term anticoagulation is indicated for individuals for whom prolonged immobilization is likely or in those patients with a history of thromboembolism. This is a prophylactic measure directed at preventing deep vein thrombosis which could produce pulmonary embolism. Interestingly, it has been demonstrated that a significant number of patients develop thrombosis within the 1st 72 hr of the acute infarction and that prolonged immobilization probably favors proximal extension of the thrombus to the thigh and femoral vein leading to clinical recognition of the thrombus.[28] There is some statistical evidence that women over 55 years of age with moderately severe infarction[27] and men with a history of angina or previous infarction may benefit from anticoagulation therapy.[24] However, there is much disparity in the literature concerning benefit in a variety of subgroup classifications. At our current level of knowledge it seems reasonable that anticoagulation therapy in the form of heparin should be considered in patients felt to be at risk for the development of pulmonary embolism, *i.e.*, prolonged immobilization or those with history of thromboembolic episodes. In spite of the controversy over efficacy relative to postmyocardial infarction anticoagulation and over who should or should not receive anticoagulation, anticoagulants are used as frequently now as in 1966 by physicians treating uncomplicated myocardial infarction (71% of surveyed physicians in 1970 used anticoagulants in uncomplicated myocardial infarction).[29]

Other Complications

Anxiety. Patients experiencing an acute myocardial infarction have good reason for anxiety. Not only are they anxious because of the initial severe pain; they are also anxious about their state of health during the recovery process, about their prognosis and about the surroundings in the environment of a coronary care unit (and probably about a multitude of other real or imagined pressures). The anxiety of pain is best treated with potent analgesia as discussed earlier. Other antianxiety agents, such as diazepam or barbiturates, may be considered and should be used according to individual situations in a cautious manner. Remember that all antianxiety agents and tranquilizers can have deleterious effects on the hemodynamics of the cardiovascular system.

Nausea and Vomiting. Frequently nausea and vomiting are part of the early symptoms accompanying the initial pain of acute myocardial infarction. In addition, narcotic analgesics have, as frequently encountered side effects, nausea and vomiting.[30] The risk of vomiting in these patients relates to the possibility of aspiration leading to respiratory compromise, pneumonitis and pneumonia. One should attempt to prevent this complication by administering only as much narcotic as is needed to relieve pain, by observing the patient closely and, if possible, by positioning the patient so that aspiration is less likely to occur.

Constipation. Immobility coupled with the use of narcotic analgesics frequently produces constipation in the recuperating myocardial infarction patient. Aside from the inconvenience and potential anxiety this produces (since our society is unusually bowel conscious), the constipated patient who strains at stool is performing a Valsalva maneuver with its consequent effects on myocardial conduction. To prevent or minimize this straining, it is invariably routine to administer a stool softener such as dioctyl sodium sulfosuccinate 2 or 3 times a day.[22]

Mobilization.[30-33] Traditionally, immobilization and prolonged hospitalization have been part of the cautious management of patients with acute myocardial infarction (Table 14.5). This approach has been theoretically defended by arguing that exercise would increase both mechanical stress and tissue hypoxia resulting in increased risk or arrhythmia, reinfarction and ventricular rupture or aneurysm. On the other hand, there is increasing evidence that prolonged immobilization in the form of strict bed rest for up to 4 weeks may not be beneficial in terms of risk of thromboembolism, cardiac failure, cardiac output, pulmonary congestion, and psychological effects on the patient.[31]

Proponents of early mobilization suggest that cardiac work tends to be higher when a patient is lying in bed versus when he is seated comfortably in a chair; that the physical effort of defecation is much greater on a bedpan than on a bedside commode; and that the risk of leg vein thrombosis is increased in the immobile, recumbent patient—provided that the alternative is not a hard-edged chair that compresses the popliteal veins. It is also felt that the hypotension and faintness experienced by many coronary patients during mobilization are results of loss of postural vasomotor reflexes during prolonged immobilization rather than myocardial injury.[31] The risk of myocardial rupture, when it occurs, is encountered in the 1st week, and mainly within the 1st 4 days, after myocardial infarction.[31,34]

Up to this point in time, studies have indicated that early mobilization in uncomplicated acute myocardial infarction is not associated with adverse effects and, in fact, have demonstrated a significant benefit psychologically and in terms of return to work. It would seem reasonable, then, to recommend the following program relative to mobilization of the myocardial infarction patient.[31]

TABLE 14.5
Early Mobilization Vs. Late Mobilization:
Major Complications in the 1st 8 Months of a Controlled Trial[a]

	Early Mobilization (N=95)	Late Mobilization (N=104)
	%	%
Death from coronary heart disease	5	8
Nonfatal reinfarction	19	19
Late cardiac failure	3	8
Serious arrhythmia	1	1
Ventricular aneurysm	4	3
At work 2 months after admission	41	17[b]

[a]Reprinted with permission from Ref. 33.
[b]Statistically significant.

1. An initial period of 7 days' rest should apply to all patients, since there is currently little published evidence that a shorter period would be safe.

2. This initial period of rest should include leg exercises, a bedside commode, and comfortable positioning (flat or propped up) unless there is some contraindication such as severe pain or shock.

3. Based on the *absence* of persistent pain, cardiac failure, low output state, ventricular arrhythmias and prolonged sinus tachycardia (after the first 48 hr), a "good risk" group can be identified. In this group, myocardial function has generally returned to normal within the 1st week postmyocardial infarction, and the patient can be allowed to walk on the 8th day, and barring complications, can be discharged from the hospital a few days later and can return soon to work.

4. For the rest of the patients there should be no fixed rules. Patients with persistent cardiac failure should be kept at rest in bed or in a chair. Patients with recurrent pain or arrhythmias do not seem to have an increased risk of either reinfarction or serious rhythm disturbance with moderate physical activity; however, such patients do present a more difficult management problem. In any case, progressive mobilization after the 2nd week is probably indicated except when there has been a further ischemic episode.

5. In those patients who for one reason or another experienced unusually or unnecessarily prolonged bed rest during hospitalization, a period of convalescence following discharge is usually indicated.

POSTHOSPITAL PHASE

Aside from the period of convalescence mentioned under the discussion on mobilization, the posthospital phase of the management of myocardial infarction patients is concerned with patient education, return to work and medical management of chronic processes (such as the angina pectoris syndrome). Nearly all physicians will counsel their patients prior to discharge from the hospital concerning return to work, smoking, diet, and sexual activity, but less than half of these physicians provide educational materials to their patients.[29]

Anxiety and depression are the most common noncardiac causes of persistent invalidism, and these symptoms are more frequently seen in patients who are still at home than those who are at work. Many patients merely suffer from simple lack of instruction or reassurance, rather than any formal psychiatric disease.[35]

If cardiac damage, which may cause ill health later, is present and recognizable during the initial few days of the illness, then rehabilitation, which should begin during these early days, can be properly directed from the start with a high degree of accuracy.[35]

SUMMARY

The management of the patient with acute myocardial infarction can be divided into prehospital, hospital and posthospital phases. During the prehospital phase, the major concerns are *early* recognition of symptoms with *rapid* transportation to medical assistance while maintaining the patient in a stable condition by either providing emergency treatment of early complications or providing prophylactic therapy for potentially life-threatening complications. The hospital phase of management is basically concerned with *close monitoring* of the patient to allow for immediate recognition and treatment of complications (especially life-threatening arrhythmias). The posthospital phase concerns itself mainly with a rational program of mobilization and patient education, with a goal toward returning the patient to as normal a pattern of life as possible.

REFERENCES

1. Friedberg, C. K.: Symposium on angina pectoris: introduction. Circulation, 46: 1037, 1972.
2. Hershberg, P. I., and Alexander, S.: Prevention and treatment of sudden cardiac death. Med. Clin. N.Am., 56: 625, 1972.
3. Epstein, S. E., *et al.*: The early phase of acute myocardial infarction: pharmacologic aspects of therapy. Ann. Intern. Med., 78: 918, 1973.
4. Heart Association: What every executive should know about heart attacks.
5. Oglesby, P.: Prehospital management of acute myocardial infarction. Med. Clin. N. Amer., 57: 119, 1973.
6. Marriott, H. J. L.: Practical Electrocardiography,

Ed. 4, p. 181. The Williams and Wilkins Co., Baltimore, 1968.

7. Scott, M. E., and Adgey, A. J.: Circulatory effects of I.V. pentazocine in patients with acute myocardial infarction. Curr. Ther. Res., 13: 81, 1971.

8. Alderman, E. L., et al.: Hemodynamic effects of morphine and pentazodine differ in cardiac patients. N. Engl. J. Med., 287: 623,1972.

9. Bernstein, V., et al.: Lindocaine I.M. in acute myocardial infarction. J.A.M.A., 219: 1027, 1972.

10. Scott, D.B., et al.: Plasma levels of lidocaine after intramuscular injection. Lancet, 2: 1209, 1968.

11. Halkin, H. H., and Melmon, K. L.: Should antiarrhythmic drug prophylaxis be routine after acute myocardial infarction? Ration. Drug Ther., 7: No. 6, 1973.

12. Rose, K. M., et al.: Myocardial infarction complicated by conduction defect. Med. Clin. N. Am., 57: 155, 1973.

13. Anon.: Atropine after myocardial infarction (editorial). Lancet, 2: 1183, 1972.

14. Gold, H. K., et al.: Use of sublingual nitroglycerin in congestive heart failure following acute myocardial infarction. Circulation, 46: 836, 1972.

15. Franciosa, J. A., et al.: Improved left ventricular function during nitroprusside infusion in acute myocardial infarction. Lancet, 1: 650, 1972.

16. Day, H. W.: Acute coronary care: a five year report. Am. J. Cardiol., 21: 472, 1968.

17. Marshall, R. M., et al.: Acute myocardial infarction. Arch. Intern. Med., 122: 472, 1968.

18. Lemberg, L., et al.: The treatment of arrhythmias following acute myocardial infarction. Med. Clin. N. Am., 55: 273, 1971.

19. Bloomfield, S. S., et al.: Quinidine for prophylaxis of arrhythmias in acute myocardial infarction. N. Engl. J. Med., 281: 253, 1969.

20. Koch-Weser, J., et al.: Antiarrhythmic prophylaxis with procainamide in acute myocardial infarction. Ration. Drug Ther., 11: No. 7, 1973.

21. Koch-Weser, J.: Antiarrhythmic prophylaxis in acute myocardial infarction. N. Engl. J. Med., 285: 1024, 1971.

22. Davison, R., and Brandfonbrener, M.: Treatment of acute myocardial infarction. Ration. Drug Ther., 7(9), 1973.

23. Anon.: Treatment of shock associated with myocardial infarction. Med. Lett. Drugs Ther., 11: No. 7, 267, 1969.

24. International Anticoagulant Review Group: Collaborative analysis of long term anticoagulant administration after acute myocardial infarction. Lancet, 1: 203, 1970.

25. Handley, A. J.: Low dose heparin after myocardial infarction. Lancet, 2: 623, 1972.

26. Michaels, L.: Heparin in acute coronary insufficiency. J.A.M.A., 22: 1235, 1972.

27. Drapkin, A., and Merskey, C.: Anticoagulation therapy after infarction. J.A.M.A., 222: 541, 1972.

28. Mauerer, B. J.: Frequency of venous thrombosis after myocardial infarction. Lancet, 2: 1385, 1971.

29. Wenger, N. K., et al.: Uncomplicated myocardial infarction—current physician practice in patient management. J.A.M.A., 224: 511, 1973.

30. Gordon, B. M., et al.: Management of myocardial infarction effect of early mobilization. Scott. Med. J., 12: 435, 1967.

31. Rose, G.: Early mobilization and discharge after myocardial infarction. Mod. Concepts Cardiovasc. Dis., 46: 59, 1972.

32. Barber, J. M., et al.: Early mobilization and discharge of patients with acute myocardial infarction. Lancet, 2: 57, 1972.

33. Harpur, J. E., et al.: Controlled trial of early mobilization and discharge from hospital in uncomplicated myocardial infarction. Lancet, 2: 1331, 1971.

34. Mallory, G. K., et al.: Speed of healing of myocardial infarction: a study of the pathological anatomy in 72 cases. Am. Heart J., 18: 647, 1939.

35. Nagle, R., et al.: Factors influencing return to work after myocardial infarction. Lancet, 2: 454, 1971.

chapter 15

ESSENTIAL HYPERTENSION

Joseph L. Hirschman, Pharm.D.
Eric T. Herfindal, Pharm.D.

At least 25 million people in the United States have hypertension. Of these, perhaps 60% have developed cardiovascular disease secondary to their hypertension. About 300,000 of these patients will die this year from complications of high blood pressure.[1] However, the mortality rate among the treated patients is significantly lower than among the untreated. It is apparent, therefore, that medical and pharmacological treatment of high blood pressure is effective. Nevertheless, one wonders whether all of the patients receiving treatment are being managed in a rational fashion.

This attitude of skepticism must prevail

because of the nature of the disease and the drugs used to treat it. Hypertension is one of the few diseases that lends itself to multiple drug therapy on a rational and clinical basis. Using more than one drug, however, to treat a single disease is quite difficult. It requires a thorough understanding on the part of the clinician of the etiology, pathology and other contributing factors, if the blood pressure is to be reduced significantly without precipitating unnecessary adverse reactions.

Unfortunately, a rational approach does not always prevail, and there sometimes is a tendency to treat with fixed combinations of drugs without titrating or assessing the effects of the individual agents on the patient. Because of this, and the fact that antihypertensive medications represent a substantial proportion of the drugs that pharmacists dispense, the pharmacist should also have a thorough understanding of the factors that influence the selection of drug therapy. With a substantial knowledge of the basic principles upon which the drug therapy of hypertension is based, the pharmacist is in an excellent position to monitor the antihypertensive therapy of his patients and advise the physician on the appropriate use of these drugs.

When the terms "hypertension" and "high blood pressure" are used clinically, they mean increased systemic arterial pressure above that which is usually considered normal. The upper limits of normal blood pressure are 140 systolic over 90 diastolic, commonly expressed as 140/90. However, there are variations from this, and "normal" readings may vary. For example, blood pressure tends to rise gradually with age, and thus a blood pressure of 150/95 or so would be normal for people over 60 years of age. There are also a number of factors that can cause brief rises in blood pressure so that single readings do not necessarily indicate that a person has hypertension. Such factors include emotions, posture, smoking and digestion which all can transiently increase or decrease blood pressure measurements.

CLASSIFICATION AND ETIOLOGY

There is sometimes a tendency to make the classification of hypertension an all-inclusive, complex listing that becomes rather cumber-some to use. It is easier simply to classify hypertension into primary essential hypertension and secondary hypertension. This chapter is primarily concerned with essential hypertension, but a few comments on secondary hypertension are appropriate. High blood pressure may be a result of some other underlying disease such as chronic pyelonephritis or hyperthyroidism.[2] In such cases the high blood pressure can be cured by treating the underlying disease. Often no specific antihypertensive therapy is required because vigorous treatment of the primary problem results in a return to normal blood pressure. This is not the case with essential hypertension, which accounts for about 85% of all hypertensive patients.[2] Essential hypertension can be controlled or contained, but it is not curable. Thus, since only secondary hypertensions can be "cured," it is imperative that the clinician thoroughly rules out the possibility of other diseases before settling on a diagnosis of essential hypertension.

The term "essential" really means "I don't know." The cause or etiology of essential hypertension is still unknown. Perhaps if the cause were known, the disease could be cured. However, since the cause is not known, it cannot be removed. The only alternative, then, is to treat the disease by blocking the symptoms.

INCIDENCE[3]

High blood pressure is more common in women than in men. The average age of onset is about 35, although it is not unusual to find it in younger people. Onset after 55 years of age, however, is uncommon. Diabetics are at least twice as liable to develop high blood pressure as nondiabetics. Also, it is generally accepted that heredity is of great importance in the etiology of hypertension. There is ample evidence to indicate that hypertension tends to have a familial concentration. For example, a child whose parents both have high blood pressure has a greater chance of becoming hypertensive than he has of remaining normotensive during his lifetime. The exact mode of genetic transmission remains undetermined, but it may be a biochemical aberration or an inborn error of metabolism.

PATHOPHYSIOLOGY[4]

While the etiology of essential hypertension remains unknown, we do know that cardiac output (CO) and peripheral vascular resistance (PR) are altered, resulting in high blood pressure (BP). As can be seen in Figure 15.1, blood pressure is dependent upon the interaction of CO and PR. Also, since CO is equal to the product of stroke volume (SV) and heart rate (HR), blood pressure can also be determined by measuring these parameters as well. Thus, if there is an increase in one or a combination of CO, PR or HR, the blood pressure is also going to be elevated. Conversely, if we can reduce any one or a combination of these blood pressure determinants, we should be able to lower the blood pressure. Although all of these factors do affect blood pressure, most patients with essential hypertension show an increased peripheral resistance while the cardiac output is usually normal.

Peripheral resistance is mainly determined by the volumetric capacity of the arterioles or vessels that function to transfer blood from the arteries to the tissue capillaries and venous system. When the arterioles contract, peripheral resistance goes up, resulting in an elevation of the blood pressure. When these vessels are dilated, blood pressure will fall. Actually, blood pressure normally remains constant despite changes in posture and wide variations in demand for blood through particular organs such as the kidneys. Maintenance of blood pressure at normal levels is achieved through the functioning of homeostatic mechanisms which alternately change cardiac output and peripheral vascular resistance to meet the needs of the body at any particular time. For some inexplicable reason, these control mechanisms do not function properly in essential hypertension. It should now be apparent why most of the antihypertensive therapy described is aimed at reducing peripheral resistance.

DIAGNOSIS AND CLINICAL FINDINGS[5]

Many patients with hypertension have had transient episodes of high blood pressure in the past. Frequently these episodes of high blood pressure are related to anxiety, resentment and

Blood pressure (BP) = cardiac output (CO) X peripheral resistance (PR)

and

CO = stroke volume (SV) X heart rate (HR)

therefore

BP = SV X HR X PR

FIG. 15.1. Pathophysiology of hypertension.

other environmental stress. Since transient hypertension often becomes permanent, such early observations of increased blood pressure should not be dismissed as being purely situational. Other initial symptoms that might be encountered are headaches, dizziness, nervousness and palpitations. However, these symptoms are not peculiar to high blood pressure and are not diagnostic in themselves. Furthermore, they are not indicative of the general severity of the disease. Many patients may have no symptoms other than measurable high blood pressure, while still others may have signs of progressing disease such as nosebleeds and intermittent hematuria.

In addition to the measurements of blood pressure, the examination of the retina is very important in assessing the severity of the hypertensive process in any patient. The techniques of assessing hypertensive retinopathy are beyond the scope of this chapter, but one should be aware that no physical examination for evaluating the hypertensive patient is valid without funduscopic examination.

One other factor that is sometimes overlooked is that it is not unusual for a patient who has been diagnosed and told that he has high blood pressure to start exhibiting some of the symptoms described above, such as headaches and palpitations. When this occurs, it is most often a result of anxiety over the disease rather than being directly related to its pathology.

COMPLICATIONS

Persistent high blood pressure that is not relieved by treatment is very likely to result in serious and even fatal complications. Approximately 10% of all hypertensive patients suffer strokes or die from cerebral hemorrhages.

Another 10% of these patients will develop angina pectoris or experience myocardial infarctions. The rather predominant complication of renal vascular sclerosis develops in about 30% of all of the patients with hypertension. This results in an increased frequency of urination, nocturia, proteinuria and, as mentioned previously, occasional hematuria. In severe cases, this may result in death from uremia.[3]

So-called "malignant" hypertension may develop in about 5% of all patients with hypertension. The term "malignant" is used because the mortality is virtually 100% within several years if the disease is not treated vigorously. Malignant hypertension is manifested by diastolic pressures that are sustained above 130 mm Hg, causing widespread arterial and tissue damage along with rapidly progressing renal failure. Onset is abrupt and may not necessarily be preceded by established hypertension.[1]

TREATMENT

The primary goal of the treatment of hypertension is the prevention of morbidity and death. Experience shows that lowering the blood pressure to a normal or near normal level and keeping it there is the only successful therapeutic pathway to achieving this goal. We have already noted that reducing peripheral resistance will lower blood pressure. This approach is, in fact, the most rational mode of therapy. As peripheral resistance is really arterial resistance, effective therapeutic agents lower pressure by inducing vasodilation either directly or indirectly by decreasing adrenergic vasoconstrictor impulses to the vessel walls. Effective treatment, however, usually involves more than drugs. Diet and psychotherapy are frequently useful adjuncts to drug therapy.

DIET THERAPY[5]

Twenty years ago, diet therapy was the mainstay of the therapeutic regimen. With the advent of effective drugs, the importance of dietary control has diminished, but by no means has it been eliminated. However, one should not rely solely upon drugs for several reasons. For example, obesity is frequently found in hypertensive patients. Weight reduction in an obese hypertensive frequently will, in itself, reduce blood pressure.

While perhaps controversial in some minds, it is prudent to reduce the intake of dietary saturated fats in the hypertensive patient. Evidence for an association between hypertension and progressing atherosclerosis is sufficient enough to advise these patients to restrict intake of eggs, cheese, milk and related foods. The atherosclerotic processes contribute to the progression of hypertensive cardiovascular disease, and, since myocardial infarction and strokes are the leading causes of death in these patients, there is sufficient reason to adhere to a low saturated fat diet.[6]

Sodium restriction is a time-honored therapeutic measure utilized to treat high blood pressure and is still very important, although with the availability of oral sodium-depleting agents such as the thiazides, rigorous programs of severe dietary salt restrictions are no longer necessary. Sodium restriction results in a reduced blood pressure by causing a depletion of the extracellular fluid volume and a reduction in the circulating blood volume which subsequently results in a decreased cardiac output. In addition, it probably reduces peripheral vascular resistance by making arterioles less responsive to the vasoconstricting action of circulating catecholamines. Thus, as we see from Figure 15.1 there is a reduction in blood pressure secondary to the reduction in cardiac output. The average salt intake in a hypertensive patient should consist of 5 g or less per day. This is not difficult and can be achieved with minimal interference of the patient's normal diet.[7] However, there are many drugs which have relatively high sodium contents, for example, Alka-Seltzer, and pharmacists should advise their hypertensive patients to avoid these products.

PSYCHOTHERAPY[3]

Psychotherapy is less well established as a useful adjunct in the treatment of high blood pressure, but it seems to be worthwhile. What we mean by psychotherapy is not psychiatric care but rather emphasizing the value of good "bedside manners." Hypertensive patients are commonly emotionally labile and respond to environmental stresses by an elevation of blood pressure. In other words, they are in a sense reactive hypertensives whose blood pressure goes up as a response to an external stress. The successful clinicians will help the patient learn to deal with stress in such a way as not to aggravate hypertension.

DRUG THERAPY: PHARMACOLOGY OF ANTIHYPERTENSIVE DRUGS

All currently used antihypertensive drugs act by impairing normal homeostatic mechanisms which in turn reduce peripheral resistance. These include sedatives, diuretics, ganglionic blocking agents, alpha-blockers, catecholamine depleters, false neurotransmitters and vasodilators. Understanding the mechanisms by which these agents work will enable one to assess the efficacy and potential toxicity of any antihypertensive regimen selected for a given patient (Table 15.1).

Sedatives[8]

In tense, agitated or anxious hypertensive patients, sedatives may be effective in reducing blood pressure. They do this through their central depressant or "tranquilizing" effects which take the edge off emotional responses to environmental stresses, thus minimizing any reactive blood pressure elevation. Phenobarbital is the most useful drug for this purpose, although the benzodiazepines (chlordiazepoxide, diazepam or oxazepam) and meprobamate can also be used, albeit at more expense to the patient. Blood pressure reduction is not pronounced, but, in selected patients, such as those with systolic hypertension, the use of sedatives will make over-all control easier.

Diuretics[9]

The diuretics are a very useful class of drugs in the treatment of high blood pressure. The most important diuretics are the thiazides such as chlorothiazide and hydrochlorothiazide. These drugs lower blood pressure by volume depletion and by a direct action on the arterial wall reducing both cardiac output and peripheral resistance. The thiazides are the best diuretics, and there is no reason to use any but the

cheapest. There are no clinically significant differences between them. Although ethacrynic acid and furosemide are effective antihypertensives, their extreme diuretic potency makes them a poor initial choice. These agents should be used only in patients shown to be refractory to the thiazides. Diuretics alone are more effective therapy than the sedatives. On the average, the diuretics elicit a fall of 15 percent in both the systolic and diastolic pressures.

Ganglionic Blocking Agents[10]

The ganglionic blocking drugs were the first really effective antihypertensives to be widely used. However, because of their unpleasant side effects and the availability of more effective agents, they are now seldom used in the routine management of hypertension. Pentolinium tartrate, mecamylamine and trimethaphan are examples of this class. They act by inhibiting synaptic nerve transmission in both the sympathetic and parasympathetic ganglia. Because they also block the parasympathetic ganglion, these drugs cause a lot of annoying effects such as bladder retention, constipation, visual blurring and other symptoms associated with parasympathetic blockade. Accordingly, these drugs are used currently only in very severe or accelerated hypertension (hypertensive crisis) for short periods of time when their extremely potent hypotensive action outweighs the undesirable side effects.

Alpha-Adrenergic Blocking Agents[3]

Phenoxybenzamine and phentolamine are the two best known examples of this class of antihypertensives. Alpha-blockers specifically inhibit the vasoconstriction mediated by vascular alpha-receptors, thereby inducing vasodilation and diminution of peripheral resistance. These agents, like the ganglionic blockers, generally are not used in the routine management of hypertension because of their high incidence of side effects which include nausea, vomiting, headache and tachycardia. However, they do have specialized indications—phentolamine is useful in some patients with severe renal disease because it can lower blood pressure without further compromising renalvascular perfusion.

TABLE 15.1
Effective Antihypertensive Drugs

Drug	Pharmacology	Dosage (mg/day)	Side Effects
Hydrochlorothiazide	Sodium diuresis; direct vasodilation	100-150	Hypokalemia Hyperglycemia Hyperuricemia
Reserpine	Depletion of catecholamines	0.1-0.5	Sedation Depression Nasal congestion Bradycardia
Hydralazine	Direct vasodilation	50-250	Headache Nausea Lupus-like syndrome
Guanethidine	Depletion of catecholamines; blocks storage of catecholamines	10-400	Orthostatic hypotension Impaired ejaculation Diarrhea
Methyldopa	Blockade of catecholamine synthesis; false neurotransmitter	500-3000	Drowsiness Impotence Hemolytic anemia Drug fever Orthostatic hypotension
Mecamylamine	Blocks autonomic ganglia transmission	10-100	Dry mouth Blurred vision Urinary retention Constipation Impotence
Diazoxide	Arteriolar dilation	5 mg/kg (IV)	Hyperglycemia Sodium retention
Phenobarbital	Central sedation	45-90	Sedation

Catecholamine-Depleting Agents[11]

These drugs are the most widely used in the therapy of hypertension. This group of drugs includes reserpine, guanethidine and methyldopa. All of these drugs reduce peripheral resistance by interfering with the transmission of impulses by the postganglionic adrenergic nerve fibers. Since norepinephrine is necessary for arteriolar vasoconstriction, deficiencies of this catecholamine will result in vasodilation. However, the norepinephrine depletion is not achieved by the same mechanism with each drug, a fact that can be of great advantage when using multiple drug therapy to treat hypertension.

Reserpine. Reserpine causes norepinephrine depletion by inhibiting its storage in the intraaxonal granules of the adrenergic nerve endings. In ordinary circumstances, this stored norepinephrine is released during transmission of a nerve impulse, resulting in adrenergic stimulation and consequent powerful vasoconstriction. Obviously, if this norepinephrine is not available, there will be no vasoconstriction. However, the depletion is not an immediate reaction, as reserpine does not cause direct depletion. Instead, there is a blockade of norepinephrine uptake by the storage sites in the first place, and this results in the depletion. Before hypotensive effects can become apparent, existing stores must be used up. As a consequence, the usual onset of action for oral reserpine is anywhere from 3 to 6 days. Reserpine is not without side effects such as drowsiness and depression, but with the dosage used in hypertension, the effects are usually tolerable. However, in an occasional patient, the mental depressive effects are noticeable enough so that continued use of the drug is not warranted even though control of the blood pressure may have been attained. Since there have been a few cases of suicide by patients who became severely depressed as a result of reserpine therapy, it is wise to switch to another agent when depression becomes a problem.

Guanethidine. The qualitative effects of guanethidine are very similar to those of reserpine in that peripheral vascular resistance is reduced by impairing the transmission of adrenergic vasoconstrictor impulses. However, guanethidine does this in a more complex fashion. As with reserpine, guanethidine also prevents the uptake of norepinephrine into the storage sites. But guanethidine also has what appears to be direct depleting effects on norepinephrine from the storage sites. The onset of action of guanethidine is much faster than that of reserpine since the relative amounts of norepinephrine depletion are much greater. Because of the depleting properties of guanethidine, it is important that the initial dose be low with gradual increases to the maintenance dose. If a large dose were given initially, it is possible to get a sudden release of an excessive amount of norepinephrine and possibly precipitate a para-

doxical hypertensive reaction. The most aggravating side effect with this drug is orthostatic hypotension. Most patients become accustomed to this and tolerate it quite well. They should be instructed to get out of bed slowly to avoid fainting, particularly when they first start on the drug. Fortunately, guanethidine does not enter the central nervous system and thus does not share the depressant properties of reserpine.

Alpha-Methyldopa. Of all the hypertensive agents, methyldopa has the most fascinating pharmacology (Fig. 15.2). For one thing, there are several proposed mechanisms which in themselves are not entirely sufficient to explain the actions of the drug. The hypotensive effects of the drug probably result from the sum of all the various mechanisms. One of the actions of methyldopa which is presumed to be partially responsible for its vasodepressor activity is the inhibition of the biochemical conversion of dopa to dopamine which should result in a depletion of neuronal norepinephrine. This occurs because of a competition between dopa and methyldopa for decarboxylase, which is the enzyme responsible for converting dopa to dopamine. Since dopamine is the precursor of norepinephrine, a lack of dopamine in the neurons will result in a deficiency of norepinephrine with a consequent reduction of blood pressure. In addition, methyldopa also behaves as a false neurotransmitter. It is believed that methyldopa is taken up by sympathetic nerve endings and then becomes sequentially converted to methyldopamine, and then to methylnorepinephrine within the axonal granules. The methylnorepinephrine behaves as a false transmitter displacing norepinephrine, the true transmitter, from the axonal granules. Subsequent

a. Decarboxylase inhibition:

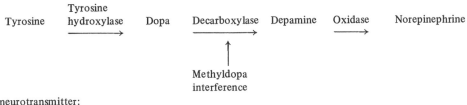

b. False neurotransmitter:

FIG. 15.2 Methyldopa—mechanism of action.

adrenergic stimulation would lead to the release of the false transmitter. Since methylnorepinephrine lacks the biological activity of norepinephrine, adrenergic inhibition results. Methyldopa can also cause orthostatic hypotension, but not as severe as that seen with guanethidine. Occasionally, serious adverse reactions such as hemolytic anemia and drug fever are seen with methyldopa.

Vasodilator Antihypertensives

Drugs in this class directly lower peripheral vascular resistance and do not affect the sympathetic reflexes, resulting in little or no postural hypertension. They act directly on the smooth muscle of the arteriolar wall, causing vasodilation and thus reducing peripheral vascular resistance. It is known that this vasodilation is not a result of adrenergic interference, but it is not completely understood just what does cause the vasodilation. The most important agent in this class is hydralazine, although the thiazide diuretics partially fall in this group. Other drugs in this class include diazoxide, a thiazide derivative, and sodium nitroprusside.

Hydralazine.[12] As mentioned above, hydralazine has a direct vasodilating effect by virtue of an unexplained interference with arteriolar contractility. However, this effect of hydralazine can produce a compensatory homeostatic stimulation of heart rate and cardiac output which could offset the decrease in peripheral resistance. For this reason, the drug is frequently used in combination with other antihypertensive agents which act to deplete the norepinephrine which mediates the homeostatic response. More recently some clinicians have begun to use propranolol in combination with hydralazine. The rationale for this mixture is that propranolol, by virtue of its beta-adrenergic blockade in cardiac tissue, results in the decrease of the hydralazine-induced chronotropic and inotropic effects on the heart. Thus, a greater over-all reduction in peripheral vascular resistance may be achieved with hydralazine when used in this manner than would ordinarily be expected at the same dosage level.[7] Hydralazine has a few mild side effects such as nausea that are usually transient. With chronic use and high doses, serious complications, such as a drug-induced lupus-like syndrome, can result. When this happens, the drug must be discontinued and should never be used in that patient again, even after resolution of the lupus. Because of the cardiac stimulatory effects, hydralazine should also be avoided in patients with existing coronary disease or angina pectoris.

Sodium Nitroprusside.[13] Until recently this drug was not commercially available, but was prepared by hospital pharmacists for use in hypertensive emergencies where conventional therapy had failed. While it is now readily available it still is confined to the treatment of hypertensive crisis. Sodium nitroprusside is a potent antihypertensive agent and appears to exert its effects by a direct peripheral vascular relaxation. Following intravenous administration, there is a prompt fall in arterial and renal blood pressure and a slight increase in heart rate. The onset of action of this agent following intravenous use is almost immediate, and dissipation of action occurs several seconds after the infusion is stopped. Adverse effects include restlessness, agitation, nausea, vomiting, muscular twitching and a reversible hypothyroidism with prolonged usage.

Diazoxide.[14] This drug is very effective in the treatment of hypertensive crisis. It is a thiazide derivative, but, interestingly enough, it is not a diuretic and in fact causes sodium retention. However, it shares the property of vasodilation seen with other thiazides, except that it is extremely potent in this regard and has a rapid onset of action with intravenous administration. Unfortunately, it has the significant side effect of being diabetogenic with chronic therapy, obviously negating long term use of the drug in the treatment of chronic hypertension.

Monoamine Oxidase Inhibitors[11]

The only monoamine oxidase inhibitor (MAOI) used clinically in the treatment of hypertension is pargyline. The mechanism of action of pargyline in hypertension is not understood, but it does produce a mild orthostatic hypotension which results in a lower blood pressure. However, the great potential for serious drug interactions with this drug should contraindicate its use. Although there are some interesting theoretical considerations with MAOIs, they have no place in the rational therapy of hypertension because of their toxicity.

Veratrum Alkaloids[10]

The veratrum compounds act to decrease both cardiac output and peripheral resistance. Their clinical application is extremely limited because of their rather low therapeutic index. The dose at which desirable lowering of the blood pressure is reached quite often results in a high incidence of severe nausea and vomiting. As a consequence, the patient tolerance is not good, and these drugs are generally not used because of the availability of safer and more effective agents.

Beta-Adrenergic Blocking Agents[15]

The only clinically available beta-adrenergic blocker is propranolol. In addition to its possible use with hydralazine to overcome the cardiac stimulatory effects of this drug, it also has an intrinsic hypotensive action of its own, especially in treating high blood pressure that is caused by excessive renin secretion by inhibiting it. In addition, the drug has a cardiac beta-adrenergic blocking action which produces a decrease in the heart rate, consequently lowering the cardiac output. The net effect is a reduction in blood pressure. This therapeutic application of propranolol is not out of the clinical investigatory stage, but it appears that it will find a permanent place in antihypertensive therapy in the very near future.

DRUG THERAPY: CLINICAL USE OF ANTIHYPERTENSIVE DRUGS[4,7,9,10]

There is still some controversy as to when treatment of hypertension should be started. Most physicians agree that advanced hypertension, whether or not there are clear signs of tissue damage, must be treated. Such a consensus, however, is not apparent when it comes to treating mild and earlier reactive hypertension. There is growing evidence to suggest that treatment of the early phase may result in a more favorable prognosis by preventing some of the irreversible vascular changes that increase the morbidity in established cardiovascular hypertensive disease. We subscribe to this school of thought and believe therapy should begin when the diagnosis of hypertension is first made, whether or not there is any evidence of tissue damage. As previously mentioned, therapy should be aimed at lowering the blood pressure to acceptable levels and keeping it there. An "acceptable" level cannot be defined arbitrarily. It depends upon the severity of the patient's hypertension and the therapeutic response to the drugs vis-a-vis their toxicity.

The severity of hypertension is usually judged by considering the degree of tissue damage and the diastolic pressure measurements. Utilizing both parameters, the severity of the disease can be broken into groups (Table 15.2). Mild hypertension is present when the diastolic pressure is consistently between 90 and 105 mm Hg in the absence of tissue damage. The patient is also asymptomatic at this stage. Moderate hypertension is diagnosed when the diastolic pressure falls within the range of 105 to 130 mm Hg whether or not there is tissue damage apparent. These patients may or may not be symptomatic. High blood pressure is rated severe when the patient is symptomatic with evidence of tissue damage with concomitant diastolic pressure measurements in the range of 130 to 140 mm Hg. The hypertension may also be considered severe, even at a lower blood pressure, if there is a moderate amount of tissue damage detected. If diastolic readings are above 140 mm Hg, this constitutes a hypertensive crisis which is a medical emergency and must be treated accordingly.

TABLE 15.2
Classification of Hypertensive Disease

Class	Diastolic Blood Pressure mm Hg	Clinical Signs
Mild hypertension	90-105	Asymptomatic; no tissue damage
Moderate hypertension	105-130	May be either asymptomatic or symptomatic with evidence of some tissue damage
Severe hypertension	130-140	Symptomatic with definite tissue damage
Hypertensive crisis	Above 140	Medical emergency; moderate to severe tissue damage

The patient with mild hypertension usually does not know he has a problem with blood pressure. It is most frequently detected on a routine physical examination. Many of these patients do not exhibit continual elevations of blood pressure but are often reactive. Early treatment of these patients is important to prevent the development of progressive cardiovascular disease. However, therapy should be handled in a manner that produces negligible side effects. Since these patients are asymptomatic, it is not conducive to patient acceptance if the drugs themselves produce undesirable symptoms.

Initial therapy consists of phenobarbital 15 to 30 mg 3 or 4 times a day. This may be enough in the reactive hypertensive because it may reduce the anxiety level sufficiently so that the blood pressure does not rise at every emotional stimulus. If this is insufficient, hydrochlorothiazide 50 mg twice a day, or its equivalent, should be added. If upon follow-up these drugs are found to be ineffective, reserpine can be added and phenobarbital discontinued. Reserpine has enough of a sedative component that the sedative itself becomes redundant. The initial dose of reserpine should be 0.25 mg twice a day for 5 days followed by a reduction to 0.25 mg once a day. Thereafter, the response to reserpine is gradual, and maximal therapeutic results might not be seen for several weeks. This is usually sufficient therapy for the mild hypertensive, but an occasional patient will be refractory. In this event, therapy should be approached in a manner similar to that outlined below for moderate hypertension. The end point of any therapy for the mild hypertensive should be a diastolic pressure below 90 mm Hg.

Patients with moderately high blood pressure will also require a thiazide diuretic as part of their therapy. However, reserpine, although it should be tried initially, will usually prove to be inadequate. If reserpine is discarded, then methyldopa becomes the primary drug of choice. It should be started at doses of 250 mg 2 or 3 times a day. Depending upon the response, the dose can gradually be increased at 3- to 5-day intervals until either the desired blood pressure reduction is achieved or total daily intake reaches 3 g. Although some patients will respond at somewhat higher dosage levels, for practical purposes the 3-g limit is valid because of the necessity of taking a large number of tablets every day and the fact that tachyphylaxis will develop in some patients with moderate hypertension. If the methyldopa proves to be ineffective, guanethidine should be substituted. In this event, a starting dose of 10 mg daily can be increased at 5- to 7-day intervals in 10-mg increments until a sufficient hypotensive response is achieved without excessive side effects. Most patients require from 10 to 50 mg per day for effective therapy, but some may require as much as 300 mg per day. These dosages need only be given once a day, in the morning.

Hydralazine can also be used effectively in patients with moderate hypertension in conjunction with 0.25 mg of reserpine daily, but because of the side effects, especially the lupus-like syndrome, it is a distant third choice of therapy. If it is used, the starting dose should be 10 mg twice a day gradually increased in increments of 25 mg per day every 3 or 4 days until the blood pressure is lowered to the desired point. Eventually most patients will require somewhere between 50 and 200 mg daily for maintenance. The incremental approach to the maintenance dosage is imperative if one is to avoid unpleasant side effects, especially headaches. In the very rare patient who is refractory to guanethidine, methyldopa or hydralazine, mecamylamine should be tried. A starting dose of 2.5 mg orally per day should be used.

In patients with severe disease there are no precise treatment regimens. Accelerated hypertension requires immediate treatment in the hospital. Severe hypertension should always be considered a life-threatening medical emergency. Therapy invariably requires parenteral administration of rapidly acting agents such as trimethaphan, diazoxide or nitroprusside. Once control of the blood pressure is achieved, maintenance therapy with an oral agent, usually guanethidine, is established. Many of these patients will, however, require combination therapy for an indefinite period.

It can be seen from the foregoing discussion that combinations of different drugs are used to treat the many varied forms of hypertensive vascular disease. This is a rational approach as long as advantage is taken of the fact that the decrease in peripheral resistance that occurs is a result of drug activity at different sites of action so that additive effects are obtained. For example, it is rational to use reserpine in combination with hydralazine because one is a sympatholytic agent while the other is a direct vasodilator. The same reasoning applies when combining a thiazide diuretic and methyldopa which results in an additive effect. However, it is not rational to combine guanethidine and reserpine as both essentially act at the same site, *i.e.,* the postganglionic adrenergic neuron. The use of fixed ratio drug combinations such as Ser-Ap-Es, Diupres and so on is generally a poor approach. Each individual drug should be specifically titrated to the individual patient. If in the end the titration matches the fixed ratio product, then the latter can be used to the economic advantage and convenience of the patient, but this method should never be used as the initial therapeutic approach.

Whether multiple therapeutic agents or single drugs are used, each drug should be titrated to a near maximal dose. This dose is determined by an end-point of either the attainment of the desired lowering of blood pressure or the development of prohibitive side effects. If this is not done, one will never know whether the maximal utility has been reached with the agent in question.

Some side effects may be encountered initially that, though unpleasant, tend to abate as the patient develops tolerance. The sedative effect of methyldopa is one such side effect. The early appearance of such side effects should not result in the premature discontinuance of the drug until it has been established that the side effect is not transient and that blood pressure cannot be controlled at a dosage at which the effect is not manifested. If side effects are a definite problem, then lower doses of several drugs, acting at different sites, provide a very rational approach to that patient's therapy.

There are a number of significant drug interactions that occur with the antihypertensive agents, and the pharmacist should be thoroughly aware of such inappropriate combinations. There are many published reviews and descriptions, in addition to product brochures, on this subject to which the pharmacist can refer.[16,17]

PROGNOSIS[18,19]

The prognosis for the patient with essential hypertension tends to be variable, and there are some factors which make the prognosis less favorable for some than for others (Table 15.3). In any event, statistically, there is a definite decrease in longevity for patients with essential hypertension because of the development of the secondary cardiovascular and cerebral vascular diseases. Nevertheless, the prognosis is more favorable in patients who have early and adequate therapy for their hypertension. Obviously, therapy must continue for the life of the patient since the disease is not curable, only controllable. With early therapy, a large number of hypertensive patients will escape secondary cardiovascular disease. Even patients with organic changes may continue their normal physical and intellectual activities for many years without noticeable incapacities. If essential hypertension is left to progress without treatment, the odds are vastly in favor of the development of complicating cardiovascular disease. In those with severe disease, lack of treatment is rapidly fatal.

CONCLUSION

There is no drug panacea for hypertension. Each patient requires individually tailored treatment and therapy is always long term. In most instances, the therapy of hypertensive patients will require judicious use of several drugs. Unfortunately, not all the people who prescribe or monitor these drugs understand them, and rational, optimal therapy is not achieved in many patients. Pharmacists, at the very least, should have an in-depth understanding of the actions and uses of the hypertensive agents. Armed with this knowledge, the pharmacist can promote the rational use of these drugs.

TABLE 15.3
Adverse Prognostic Factors

a. Young age of onset
b. Negro
c. Male
d. Diastolic pressures greater than 110 mm Hg
e. Enlarged heart
f. Abnormal kidney function
g. Retinopathy
h. Existing cardiovascular disease, *e.g.,* angina, congestive heart failure
i. Strokes
j. Uremia

REFERENCES

1. Page, L. B., and Sidd, J. J.: Medical management of primary hypertension (first of three parts). N. Engl. J. Med., 287: 960, 1972.
2. Armstrong, M. L.: Progress in the diagnosis of secondary hypertension. Med. Clin. North Am., 52: 1213, 1968.
3. Bienuenu, O. J.: Essential hypertension. Med. Clin. North Am., 51: 967, 1965.
4. Bourne, H. R., and Melmon, K. L.: Guides to the pharmacologic management of essential hypertension. Ration. Drug Ther., 5: 1, 1971.
5. Merrill, J. P.: Hypertensive vascular disease. In Harrison's Principles of Internal Medicine, Ed. 6, p. 1252, edited by M. Wintrobe. McGraw-Hill Book Co., New York, 1970.
6. Deming, Q. B.: Blood pressure: its relation to atherosclerotic disease of the coronaries. Bull. N. Y. Acad. Med., 44: 968, 1968.
7. Page, L. B., and Sidd, J. J.: Medical management of primary hypertension (second of three parts). N. Engl. J. Med., 287: 1018, 1972.
8. Merrill, J. P.: Hypertensive vascular disease. In Harrison's Principles of Internal Medicine, Ed. 6, p. 1259, edited by M. Wintrobe. McGraw-Hill Book Co., New York, 1970.
9. Moser, M.: Use and abuse of antihypertensive drugs. G. P., 35: 87, 1967.
10. Page, L. B., and Sidd, J. J.: Medical management of primary hypertension (third of three parts). N. Engl. J. Med., 287: 1074, 1973.
11. Nies, A. S., and Melmon, K. L.: Recent concepts in the clinical pharmacology of antihypertensive drugs. Calif. Med., 106: 388, 1967.
12. Brest, A. N., Onesti, G., and Swartz, C.: Mechanisms of antihypertensive drug therapy. J.A.M.A., 211: 480, 1970.
13. Cacace, L., and Thomas, T.: Treatment of hypertensive emergencies with sodium nitroprusside. Drug Intell. Clin. Pharmacy, 4: 187, 1970
14. Anon.: Diazoxide (Hyperstat). Med. Lett. Drug Ther., 15: 53, 1973.
15. Prichard, N. C.: Propranolol as an antihypertensive agent. Am. Heart J., 79: 128, 1970.
16. Hansten, P. D.: Drug Interactions, Ed. 2. Lea and Febiger, Philadelphia, 1973.
17. Anon.: Evaluations of Drug Interactions, Ed. 1. American Pharmaceutical Association, Washington, D.C., 1973.
18. Veterans Administration Cooperative Study Group on Antihypertensive Agents: Effect of treatment on morbidity in hypertension: results in patients with diastolic blood pressures averaging 115 through 129 mm Hg. J.A.M.A., 202: 1028, 1967.
19. Veterans Administration Cooperative Study Group on Antihypertensive Agents: Effects of treatment on morbidity in hypertension. II. Results in patients with diastolic blood pressures averaging 90 through 114 mm Hg. J.A.M.A., 213: 1143, 1970.

Respiratory diseases

chapter 16

ASTHMA

Peter M. Penna, Pharm.D.

Bronchial asthma is a chronic disease which many pharmacists see daily in either their community or hospital practices. The term "bronchial asthma" has been best defined by the American Thoracic Society as: ". . .a disease characterized by an increased responsiveness of the trachea and bronchi to various stimuli and manifested by a widespread narrowing of the airways that changes in severity either spontaneously or as a result of therapy."[1] The most important aspect of the disease is that there is widespread obstruction to airflow. The disease may cause a number of distressing symptoms including wheezing and dyspnea, and less commonly a cough with the production of a thick mucoid sputum. In some patients, the frequency of attacks increases until there is a state of chronic airway obstruction. This situation may be virtually indistinguishable from chronic bronchitis and emphysema, but classically, asthmatics respond more readily to bronchodilators and corticosteroids than do patients with these other diseases. As emphasized in Chapter 17, there is a great deal of overlap in these conditions, and the methods of treatment for each are very similar.

Many people believe that asthma is more of a nuisance than a serious threat to life. While this may be true in some patients, there are many deaths reported every year, and a large number of hospital beds are occupied by asthmatic patients. Acute attacks, exacerbations, and even overzealous use of drugs produce a great amount of morbidity and mortality.

ETIOLOGY

The basic problem in asthmatics is that their bronchi overreact to various specific or nonspecific stimuli. There are several systems of classifying asthma depending on the type of precipitating factors. Perhaps the most popular is a system in which the stimuli may come from either the external environment, producing "extrinsic" asthma, or from the internal environment producing "intrinsic" asthma. Table 16.1 summarizes the properties of these two types. While some patients will fit exclusively into one category or the other, many will exhibit properties from each. Some authorities believe that external causative agents can be found for all asthmatics, if a thorough search is conducted.[2]

Another more complete and meaningful way to classify the stimuli, and therefore the asthma, is to break them down into: allergic stimuli, psychological stimuli, pulmonary infections, physical exertion and pollution.

Most asthmatics will demonstrate allergy to one substance or another, particularly those whose symptoms start in later childhood and young adulthood. The types of allergens commonly found vary greatly and include such things as pollen (in patients with hay fever), fungi and mold spores, animal dander (especially cat, dog and horse), house dust (thought to be due to an allergen derived from the mite species Dermatophagoides) and orris root used in face powders.[2,3]

The reaction which takes place is thought to be the immediate, or type 1, allergic reaction. Patients may also have asthmatic attacks due to allergies to certain substances in their working environments; for example, a bakery worker may become allergic to flour. Also, some patients may have asthmatic attacks because of allergies to foods such as eggs, chocolate, fish, nuts, etc. Industrial and food allergies as a cause of asthma are somewhat rare compared to the other allergic causes of asthma.

Psychological stimuli are known to precipitate asthmatic attacks in predisposed individuals, although it is likely that there are other factors involved. The important point to remember here is that these patients have

TABLE 16.1
*Common Features of Intrinsic
and Extrinsic Asthma*[a]

	Intrinsic Asthma	Extrinsic Asthma
Other names	Nonallergic; infective Nonatopic	Allergic Atopic
IgE levels	Normal	Elevated
Skin tests	Negative	Positive
History of family allergies	Negative	Positive
Age at onset	Usually over 35 (middle age)	Usually below 5 (childhood to young adulthood)
Nasal symptoms	Polyps	Hay fever
ASA sensitivity	Strong associations	None

[a]Modified from Cecil-Loeb Textbook of Medicine, p. 887.

hyperresponsive bronchi just like other asthmatics, but their attacks may be precipitated by the nervous system rather than pollen, infections, etc.

Psychological disturbances occur in many asthmatics; however, there is some question whether these abnormalities are a cause or effect of the asthma. An extremely anxious person who suffers an emotional upset may respond by having an asthmatic attack. On the other hand, a person who suffers from severe asthma may be expected to have an altered psychological outlook due to the morbidity he has endured. In addition, there is some evidence, mainly in children, that certain people are able (often subconsciously) to precipitate an asthmatic attack when it is to their advantage.[3,4]

Pulmonary infections are commonly associated with asthmatic attacks, particularly in children under 5, and in those who have their first episode in middle age. It is thought that the infection, which often starts in the upper respiratory tract and descends to the bronchopulmonary tree, causes a buildup of antibodies in the inflamed tissue of the lung. In later infections, these antibodies elicit an asthmatic response. It is also possible that these patients have a predisposition to asthma, including hypertrophy of mucus-producing glands and increased numbers of goblet cells. If there is an increase in mucus production, infections take hold more easily, and the inflammation caused could produce bronchospasm and, therefore, asthma.[3,5]

Physical exertion may precipitate attacks in some asthmatics. The immediate effect of exercise may be bronchodilation, but if the exertion is prolonged for more than a few minutes, the dilation may give way to bronchoconstriction. Even if these patients stop the exercise before wheezing and dyspnea have started, they may go on to have a full attack. Some authorities feel that this type of attack is brought on by hyperventilation or by the release of some constricting substance. It is interesting to note that the type of exercise may determine whether or not the patient has an attack. It appears that swimming produces fewer episodes than either running or cycling.[2,3,6,7]

Atmospheric pollution and cigarette smoking have been implicated in causing asthma in some people, although the evidence is incomplete. It may be that these patients actually have chronic bronchitis or emphysema which are known to be adversely affected by pollution and smoking. In any event, many asthmatics find things like sulfur dioxide, paint fumes, smoke, cold air etc., to be irritating to their lungs. Once a person develops the hyperreactive bronchi which characterize asthma, any irritant, if present in sufficient quantities, may produce an attack.[3,4]

Regardless of the cause of asthma in a specific patient, it is important to remember that there is often a degree of overlap, and many factors may be involved in attacks. In a study by Williams *et al.*[8], it was found that out of 487 cases, allergy was a factor in 64.1%, infection in 88.1%, and psychology in 70.2%.

Thirty-eight percent were affected by all three conditions, while allergy alone was important in only 3.3%, infection alone in 11.3% and psychological factors alone in only 1.2%. It would seem that once the bronchi had conditioned themselves to an asthmatic response, a number of influences *should* be able to set the system off.

Most medical texts do not discuss the one etiological factor of asthma which is of the most interest to pharmacists—asthma induced by drugs. One of the most common pulmonary adverse effects following drugs is asthma, and the most frequently implicated drug is aspirin. Sensitivity to aspirin most often occurs in middle-aged patients who have had chronic asthma for several years. They also frequently suffer from rhinitis and nasal polyps. The reactions which occur are often severe and prolonged and may even be fatal. A reaction may start within a few minutes to several hours after ingestion of the aspirin, but it usually begins within 30 min. The patient will first notice a profuse, watery rhinorrhea followed by a scarlet flush of the head, neck, upper chest and extremities, then wheezing and cyanosis due to bronchoconstriction. Gastrointestinal upset may occur. The mechanism of the reaction is unknown, but it has been blamed on such things as acetylation of serum albumin, acetylsalicylic acid anhydride present in aspirin tablets

and direct allergy to aspirin itself. The evidence is still inconclusive. It is important to remember that most other salicylates, *e.g.*, sodium salicylate, will not produce a reaction in sensitive individuals. However, indomethacin, mefenamic acid and certain yellow food dyes such as tartrazine or F D & C yellow No. 5 may precipitate asthma in these patients.[9-13]

A number of other drugs have been reported to precipitate asthmatic attacks in sensitive individuals by a hypersensitivity reaction. Any drug which can cause an anaphylactic reaction might be considered to cause asthma because the changes which take place in asthma are among the many which take place in an anaphylactic reaction. Table 16.2 lists those drugs which have been reported to cause asthma by allergic reactions. Other than aspirin, which is associated with a relatively high incidence of asthma, the reports concerning these drugs are not very common, and many are highly questionable.

Drug-induced asthma may also be the result of the pharmacological properties of the drug. In contrast to the preceding type of reaction, these are much easier to anticipate because they are an extension of the normal pharmacology of the agent. They usually precipitate attacks in pre-existing asthmatics. The most commonly implicated drugs are the parasympathomimetics, histamine, and propranolol, and

TABLE 16.2
Drugs Which Have Been Reported to Precipitate Asthmatic
Attacks by Hypersensitivity Reactions

Drug	Reference	Drug	Reference
Acetaminophen	53	Nitrofurantoin	64, 65
Allergenic extracts	54, 17	Oral contraceptives	66, 67
Antisera	54, 55	Penicillins	54, 68, 69
Aspirin	9, 10, 12, 54	Pituitary snuff	
		(vasopressin)	9, 54
Azathioprine	56	*d*-Propoxyphene	53
Bromsulphalein	54, 57	Quinidine	70, 71
Hashish and marihuana	9, 58	Radio-opaque organic	
		iodides	54, 72
Indomethacin	13, 54, 53	Reserpine	73-75
Iron dextran	54, 59, 60	Succinylcholine	54, 76
Local anesthetics (ester		Tetracyclines	54, 77
type)	54, 61		
MAO inhibitors	62	*d*-Tubocurarine	54, 76, 78
Mefenamic acid	53	Vaccines	54
Mercurials	54, 63		

they should be used with great caution, if at all, in asthmatics.

Some of the bronchodilator aerosols, notably isoproterenol and epinephrine, have been implicated in causing a worsening of asthma in a few patients. This is thought to be due to metabolic products of the drugs, including 3-methoxyisoproterenol, which have a paradoxical beta-blocking effect. It has been observed that in an asthmatic attack, these people will begin using or overusing their aerosols, and after an initial period of relief they will have a worsening of their symptoms.[14-16]

Finally, there are drugs used by asthmatics which can precipitate attacks because of their irritating effects. N-Acetylcysteine often causes bronchospasm because it releases hydrogen sulfide. When it is used in asthmatics, they should be pretreated with a bronchodilator.[9,17] Also, the new drug, cromolyn sodium may be irritating when administered, and it has been associated with precipitation of asthma. This will be discussed further in the section on treatment.

INCIDENCE

The over-all incidence of asthma appears to be about 1 to 2% of the population. It is more common in children, occurring at the rate of 2.3 to 4.8% and it appears to be determined in part by heredity. After the age of 7, there is a decrease in the incidence, probably because the increased bronchial diameter makes the bronchi less susceptible to obstruction. In adults, the rate is 0.5 to 1%, and women are affected more commonly than men. There does not seem to be a genetic predisposition in this group. Pulmonary infections are the major precipitating cause here.[2,3]

PATHOLOGY

The bronchial obstruction of asthma is due to three processes. The first is easily reversible, while the last two processes are not readily terminated.[17,18] They are: bronchial smooth muscle contraction; thickening of the mucus membrane lining of the lung; and plugging of the bronchi and bronchioles with thick, tenacious mucus.

Examination of the lungs of asthmatics reveals large numbers of eosinophils and goblet cells in the bronchial walls as well as hypertrophied mucus glands. At autopsy, the lungs usually do not collapse when the chest cavity is opened, which indicates that there is an obstruction to the outflow of air due to mucosal edema and excess mucus.[2,3,19]

Several causes of the bronchoconstriction, mucosal edema, and mucus plugging in asthmatics have been postulated. In those persons whose asthmatic attacks are related to allergies due to pollen, bacteria, etc., it is thought that the antibody "gamma E immunoglobulin" (IgE, or reagin) is particularly important. IgE is formed in a number of areas of the body related to the site of exposure including the plasma cells of the respiratory tract. The IgE produced here usually remains in the area attached to mast cells near the surface of the lung tissue. When an antigen attaches to the cell-bound IgE antibody, a series of reactions is set up which allows the cell to release histamine, slow releasing substance (SRS), serotonin, bradykinin, chemotactic substances for eosinophils and other chemicals. The results of this are that: the histamine causes bronchoconstriction and capillary vasodilation (edema); the SRS causes prolonged bronchial smooth muscle contraction; serotonin also causes contraction of the smooth muscle; the bradykinin causes an increased capillary permeability (edema and secretions), as well as smooth muscle contraction; and eosinophils are brought into the area. The net effect, then, is bronchoconstriction, mucosal edema and increased secretions. Histamine and SRS are probably the most important mediators of the asthmatic attack. The content of cyclic adenosine 3', 5'-monophosphate (cyclic AMP) in the mast cells is important here because increased levels of this compound inhibit the release of histamine and SRS. Drugs like epinephrine, isoproterenol, prostaglandins E and E2, and the methylxanthines cause the levels of cyclic AMP in the cells to increase. It may be that this is part of the basis for the activity of these drugs in relieving bronchospasm.[2,17,18,20,21] The role of IgE in asthma is much more complex than presented here. There are two excellent reviews by Beall et al.[18] and Dockhorn[21] which discuss this aspect of asthma in more detail.

Another theory of the mechanism of the

asthmatic attack concerns beta-adrenergic blockade. The proponents of this theory believe that some asthmatics suffer either from partial beta-adrenergic blockade or a deficiency of active beta-adrenergic substances. Szentivanyi[22,23] stated that beta-receptors in lungs of asthmatics are not as responsive as they are in normal people. Therefore, when challenged by a noxious stimuli, the bronchial smooth muscle is not able to respond normally (by relaxation) to the output of beta-active substances, mainly epinephrine. There is also evidence that some asthmatics have a decreased ability to produce epinephrine in stressful, asthma-producing situations. When evaluating these theories on beta-adrenergic blockade or deficiency, it is important to remember that most asthmatics have been exposed to various sympathomimetics for long periods, and, therefore they may react abnormally to endogenous or exogenous beta-stimulators.[18,21]

The final theory of the pathogenesis of asthma deals with increased parasympathetic activity. Parasympathetic or vagal stimulation causes the bronchial smooth muscle to constrict. In normal people, the effects of this are insignificant. In some asthmatics, it is hypothesized that pre-existing damage in the pulmonary tree (*e.g.,* from chronic bronchitis) makes them overly sensitive to further stimuli, thereby causing an asthmatic attack.[18]

DIAGNOSIS AND CLINICAL FEATURES

Classically, asthmatics suffer acute attacks of dyspnea and wheezing. These attacks may vary in length from a few minutes to several days, and the patient appears physically well between episodes. The symptoms usually begin a few minutes after exposure to an allergen or other precipitating factor. The patient may first notice tightness in his chest followed by wheezing and coughing and then dyspnea. In some people, the constriction may be so great that there is no wheeze. As in chronic obstructive pulmonary disease, the patient will have more difficulty with expiration than inspiration. Other signs and symptoms which sometimes occur include orthopnea, cyanosis, tachycardia, agitation and confusion, overinflation of the chest with decreased respiratory movements, and thick viscous sputum which may contain mucus plugs called Curshmann's spirals. [2-4,20]

Skin tests may be used as an aid in the diagnosis of allergic bronchial asthma. However, it should be remembered that these patients may react to many injected allergens, but that few of these are actually the cause of asthma. Allergic asthmatics will also usually show an increased number of eosinophils in blood and sputum.

Pulmonary function studies show hyperinflation of the lung and elevated airway resistance. Hypoxia is usually present in attacks, but the carbon dioxide levels may be low, normal or increased depending on the severity of the asthma.[2-4]

When attacks first occur, the patient usually has no abnormalities between episodes, and he may be able to participate in vigorous exercise with no problem. Fortunately, some patients never progress beyond this degree, and many children even experience a diminished number of attacks as they grow into adulthood. Other patients, however, may find that although they begin having less severe, and even less frequent attacks, they begin to have chronic airflow obstruction, possibly as a result of concomitant emphysema or chronic bronchitis.

TREATMENT

At present, there is no method, procedure or drug which is curative for asthma, and there is nothing available which will permanently correct the basic abnormality of the disease. Therefore, the treatment involves various processes and drugs which are used in an effort to prevent or treat acute attacks and exacerbations. It is hoped that, if the attacks are properly handled, the patient will eventually outgrow the disease.

Hyposensitization

As in many other conditions, a search is made for a precipitating cause of the asthma, and every effort is made to remove these factors. This involves a number of things. First, the physician will search for responsible allergens, and the patient is then cautioned to avoid these if possible. This may give very good results. Skin tests can be used but often they do not give much information. The history of the occurrence of attacks can be very helpful. For example, if the patient is a child who suffers allergic asthma when taking naps or sleeping at night, a responsible allergen may be found in his room—pillow feathers, wool, house dust, etc. In this case, daily vacuuming of the room or damp mopping, replacement of wool and feathers by other materials or covering pillows with plastic containers may produce dramatic results. If there are allergens or irritants in the atmosphere which cause severe problems, it may be advisable for the patient to move to an area which does not have these agents.

In other cases, an attempt at desensitization or hyposensitization can be made, but the results of this procedure sometimes have been disappointing. It appears to be most effective in children with extrinsic asthma. The mechanism of hyposensitization is incompletely understood, but it is thought that small injections of responsible allergens (antigens) cause an increase in IgG antibodies to the antigen. Therefore, when the patient is exposed to naturally occuring antigen, the IgG will combine with it and prevent it from reacting with the "asthma-producing" IgE antibodies. There also appears to be a nonspecific desensitization of mast cells. That is, some patients who undergo desensitization for one allergen may find that they are less allergic to other allergens. While there is some controversy concerning hyposensitization, some patients do benefit from it. Many physicians however, feel that the procedure has only placebo value. The process may take several years to complete, and it is not without danger. If a small number of responsible allergens can be identified, and if the patient is not substantially helped by some of the standard forms of therapy, then hyposensitization may be a worthwile venture.[2-4,17,24-26]

Sedatives

It is well known that psychological factors greatly affect asthmatics, and for this reason, control of the emotional state is extremely important. The family of the asthmatic must be made aware of this factor so that, if possible, they can aid in avoiding stressful situations. Sometimes it is beneficial to remove the asthmatic from his family; however, this is usually an unacceptable remedy. "Tranquilization" may be of benefit but also may cause problems. Many patients have benefited from low doses of barbiturates, benzodiazepines, phenothiazines

and tricyclic antidepressants, but they must be used with extreme caution, if at all, in patients who are hypoxic. Their respiratory depressant effects may further worsen the hypoxia. Many of these agents, especially the phenothiazines and tricyclics, have antihistaminic side effects which cause drying of the mucous membranes. Since one of the problems in asthmatics is thick, tenacious mucus, it is best to avoid any drug that causes this effect.

Sympathomimetics

Symptomatic treatment of asthma involves the use of bronchodilators, hydration, expectorants and mucolytics, and for severe cases, corticosteroids. Bronchodilators are the mainstay of asthma therapy, both in acute attacks and in relieving generalized obstruction. They are most effective in milder asthma but are used in combination with other measures in even the most severe cases. A number of sympathomimetics are available, but the most widely used in the United States is isoproterenol in various inhalant preparations. This drug mainly affects the beta-adrenergic receptors, and, therefore, it works very well as a bronchodilator. However, it is nonspecific in its action on the beta system and therefore affects other structures, notably the heart, as well as the bronchial smooth muscle. The result is that some patients who overuse the drug will have undesirable side effects including tachycardia and other arrhythmias, anginal pain, tremors, headache, etc. A number of deaths have been attributed to the cardiac side effects.

The drug is well absorbed by inhalation, but sublingual and oral administration produce unreliable results. The usual dose is 0.1 mg (0.05 to 0.25 mg) by aerosol. Using the small pressurized-metered aerosols, this amount is provided in 1 to 2 inhalations. The patient should allow 1 to 2 min to pass after the 1st dose before administering it again. He should not use the device any more than 3 times for any attack, and not more often than every 3 hr. If the patient uses a hand-held bulb nebulizer, the usual dose is 5 to 15 inhalations of a 0.5% solution, repeated in 10 to 30 min if necessary. With intermittent positive pressure breathing, 0.5 to 1.0 ml of a 0.5% solution, diluted to 2 to 4 ml with water or saline may be used for a period of 5 to 10 minutes.[27,28]

Epinephrine is another popular sympathomimetic for asthmatics, especially those who are having very severe attacks. Its actions are similar to those of isoproterenol except that it does affect the alpha-receptors, thereby causing vasoconstriction in the bronchial mucosa which helps relieve edema of this tissue. It is felt that this alpha-activity is not significant in most cases. In severe cases, it has been postulated that it could even be deleterious because it may lead to thickening of the mucus. Adequate hydration of the patient should help to avoid this problem. The toxicities of the drug are essentially the same as those of isoproterenol. Ephinephrine may be given by inhalation, but it is more commonly injected subcutaneously for severe episodes. The dose is 0.1 to 0.5 ml of a 1 : 1000 solution, repeated in 5 to 10 min if needed, up to a maximum of 2.0 ml. It is wise to massage the site of injection to hasten absorption.[17,27-29]

Phenylephrine is sometimes used, but it has very little effect on bronchoconstriction because it has no beta-adrenergic activity. Its alpha-activity will help to relieve mucosal edema by its vasoconstrictive effects, and this is the basis of its use. It is most often given in combination with isoproterenol.

Some patients will appear to be refractory to either epinephrine or isoproterenol, especially if they are having a severe attack. There are several possible causes for this phenomenon, and each of them must be evaluated. The first is that the patient's bronchi may be so severely plugged with mucus that the sympathomimetic, if given by inhalation, may not be able to reach the constricted area. In this situation, removal of the mucus by hydration, suction, mucolytics, etc. should restore the effectiveness of the inhaled agents. Even if the sympathomimetic is given systemically, the patient will still experience difficulty in breathing as long as the mucus is present. Second, the particles or droplets from the aerosol may not reach or may not be retained in the bronchi and bronchioles if they are the wrong size. This is rarely a problem in the metered aerosol sprays but sometimes will occur with nebulizers. Third, a patient may continue to wheeze after aerosol administration because the mucus is moving out of the smaller bronchioles and bronchi into the larger structures where it may cause wheezing. Humidification and coughing with deep breathing should help resolve this problem. Finally, and most important, some patients have actually become unresponsive or refractory to the sympathomimetics because of either acidosis or simple overuse of the agent. Respiratory acidosis is a common complication of severe asthmatic attacks and is best relieved by improving the patient's ventilation. This should restore very rapidly the effectiveness of the bronchodilators. Patients who overuse these drugs may find that they no longer respond when they most need the agents. Withdrawal of the drug for a few days may restore responsiveness. Related to this last point is the fact, mentioned previously, that one of the metabolites of isoproterenol, 3-methoxyisoproterenol, is a weak beta-blocking agent which theoretically may reverse the effects of the sympathomimetic. In actual situations, it is doubtful that enough of this metabolite could be produced to reverse the effects of the bronchodilator.[17,15,30,31]

Recently, a controversy has arisen concerning the potential problems of overuse of the various metered bronchodilator aerosols. Briefly, it had been reported that there was an increase in the mortality rate due to asthma in England and Wales which correlated very well with the increased use of these sprays. It was also found that the aerosols used in England and Wales contained 5 times as much isoproterenol as those used in other countries. Some of these other countries, however, also demonstrated a modest rise in asthma mortality. The question of toxicity due to the propellant used in the aerosol was raised. It was found that these chemicals can cause sudden death but that the amount supplied in aerosols was probably insignificant. Then, it was pointed out that at autopsy most of these patients had evidence of severe asthma. Perhaps the bronchodilators in actuality kept these patients alive longer than normal and they ultimately died of an especially severe attack. Others feel that these sudden deaths were the result of a drug interaction with corticosteroids that the patient may have been taking concomitantly. There are many more theories and questions which have been raised by these reports, but one conclusion seems evident: metered aerosol sympathomimetics have been a great boon to the asthmatic, but misuse of these preparations (as with any drug) can cause problems. It should be tactfully yet vigorously stressed to patients that these drugs do have their limitations and toxicities. They must not be used more often than directed, and if it appears that the patient is not responding to 1, 2, or 3 doses, he should seek medical aid immediately.[17,14,16,30,32-38]

In addition to making certain that the patient understands the above cautions, the pharmacist should also be sure that the person using these aerosols understands their proper use. He should exhale fully, then inhale the aerosol slowly, hold it in for several seconds, then exhale normally.

Patients who suffer from mild chronic asthma may obtain relief with the use of oral ephedrine. It is not effective in the more severe forms of the disease. The doses used may vary from 15 to 60 mg given up to 5 times daily, but most patients get adequate relief with 25 mg 3 or 4 times per day. The last dose should be not later than 6 or 7 p.m. if the person has problems sleeping. Ephedrine has the same side effects as isoproterenol, except that some patients may also suffer from urinary retention. There are several other orally active sympathomimetics which may be used by asthmatics, including methoxamine, methoxyphenamine, phenylpropanolamine and pseudoephedrine. It has not been shown that these have any significant advantage over ephedrine.[3,17]

Salbutamol, which is not yet commercially available in the United States, is a sympathomimetic which selectively stimulates the beta-adrenergic receptors in pulmonary tissue. It has been theorized that there are two types of beta-receptors: The beta-1 receptors which are located in the cardiovascular system and the beta-2 receptors which are located in the lungs. Therefore, salbutamol, which stimulates only the beta-2 system in the lung, will cause bronchodilation, but it will have little effect on cardiac function. Up to this time, it appears that the claims for this drug are valid, and fewer cardiac side effects have been reported than with isoproterenol.[39-41]

Theophylline Derivatives

The methylxanthines are the other major class of drugs used as bronchodilators. The various theophylline salts (ethylenediamine, choline, etc.) are the most popular agents in this group because they have very pronounced peripheral effects with minimal central nervous system (CNS) effects when compared with the other xanthines. The mechanism by which they cause bronchodilation is questionable, but it is currently thought that they inhibit the enzyme phosphodiesterase which is responsible for the metabolism of cyclic AMP. It is known that cyclic AMP is involved in the bronchodilating effects of the sympathomimetics and methylxanthines and that it also may inhibit the release of the chemical mediators of bronchospasm from mast cells. The xanthines act to increase levels of cyclic AMP, like the sympathomimetics, but by a different mechanism. It is thought that this is the reason that xanthines and sympathomimetics are additive in their effects and that the xanthines will still work in sympathomimetic-resistant patients.[18]

The effectiveness of theophylline is related to its blood levels in most cases; 0.5 to 1.0 mg% is necessary for dilation, although there is some variability outside these bounds in patient responsiveness. It may be difficult to achieve these levels with oral administration because absorption is erratic. Uncoated tablets are the most rapidly absorbed, but they may produce local irritation. Alcoholic elixirs of theophylline appear to be an exception to the above. In this dosage form, the drug is rapidly absorbed and provides very good therapeutic blood levels. Because of the added alcohol, this dosage form may be particularly irritating to patients with ulcer symptoms. Rectal suppositories are popular, and they may give slightly better absorption than oral tablets, but the blood levels produced may still be erratic. Retention enemas are better, but are expensive. In emergency situations, aminophylline is best given by the I.V. route. In less acute situations, it may be injected I.M., but it is extremely painful.[42-44]

Oral and rectal doses range from 100 to 500 mg every 6 to 8 hr for adults, and 3 to 4 mg per kg in children, depending on the patient's response to the specific medication used. If the patient does not take the drug regularly (uses it only during attacks), it may be necessary to give a loading dose of 500 mg, followed by normal maintenance doses. The I.M. and I.V. doses, used mainly in acute situations, are 250 to 500 mg. Care must be taken not to administer the drug too fast by the I.V. route because hypotension and arrhythmias may occur. It is best to administer it over a 10- to 15-min period. Some physicians like to dilute it in 100 to 200 ml D5W to be administered over ½ hr to avoid toxicities. After the initial dose, if the patient has had continuous bronchospasm, 500 mg may be added to a suitable I.V. fluid and infused over 6 hr.[20,29,42]

The side effects of the xanthines include hypertension, nausea, vomiting, diarrhea, headache, arrhythmias (tachycardia and extrasystoles) and CNS excitation. The gastric side effects are fairly common and are due to the central effects of the drug (increased HC1 production and medullary stimulation) as well as local effects. Some patients take the drug orally after meals to cut down gastric irritation. Unfortunately, this method may be effective by decreasing absorption. Asthmatics who take corticosteroids may be particularly sensitive to the gastric problems of the xanthines due to an additive effect.

Hydration, Expectorants and Mucolytics

Adequate hydration is necessary if the patient is to be able to remove mucus plugs. Dehydration is often thought to be responsible for recurring attacks. Therefore, it is important that patients realize the necessity of a high fluid intake. In addition, some receive benefit by breathing in steam (hot showers, electrolytic vaporizers, etc.) or nebulized water. If the patient is receiving oxygen therapy, it must be humidified because gases can be very drying. A few patients benefit from expectorants (ammonium chloride, glyceryl guaiacolate, the iodides, etc.) but, generally, they have not been too effective N-Acetylcysteine, which is discussed in detail in Chapter 17 can be very useful in patients with extremely thick mucus. It is best applied directly to the affected areas of the lung with a catheter which will then aid in the removal of the liquefied mucus. This drug can cause bronchospasm, and therefore it should be used with extreme caution in asthmatics who should be pretreated with bronchodilators. Generally, plain water, either as an increased fluid intake, steam or mist, will help very adequately to liquefy a patient's mucus. In severe situations, N-Acetylcysteine can be very useful.[17,25,29]

Corticosteroids

If a patient has not responded to the standard forms of treatment, it may be necessary to place him on corticosteroids. While these drugs give dramatic relief, their side effects limit their usefulness, and a patient should be placed on them only after an extensive re-evaluation of previous therapy. If the patient is to be placed on continuous corticosteroids, the lowest possible dose should be used, and he should be started on alternate day therapy to lessen the incidence of side effects. This would necessitate the use of short acting agents such as prednisone, prednisolone, methylprednisolone, cortisone or hydrocortisone. The initial dose regimen should be sufficient to suppress the symptoms, and then an attempt should be made to lower the dose as much as possible. These drugs may be given by inhalation, but there is no major advantage using this route.

In acute situations, extremely high doses of parenteral or oral corticosteroids may be required for short periods in order to reverse attacks. Three hundred milligrams or more of hydrocortisone (or equivalent) per day may be required. These doses are usually continued for 3 to 5 days, then decreased over a week or so. Adrenal suppression following this type of therapy is minimal. There is some evidence that patients on chronic steroid therapy have a higher rate of cortisol metabolism. If this is true, then a large dose of corticosteroid which normally produces a response in a nonsteroid-dependent patient may have little or no effect in one who is on chronic steroids. These patients will then require even higher doses in acute exacerbations.[2-4,17,20]

Cromolyn

The newest drug to be made available for asthmatics in this country is cromolyn sodium or disodium cromoglycate (DSCG). This preparation is unique among all antiasthmatic drugs in that it is the only agent which inhibits the release of bronchoconstrictive substances from mast cells. There is some evidence that it may also inhibit the bronchospasm caused by exogenous histamine. DSCG is a prophylactic agent, and it appears that it must be used for several weeks for maximal effectiveness. It has been shown to be useful in allergic and exercise-induced asthma and therefore should be of benefit to the majority of asthma sufferers. The usual dose is 20 mg of the powder inhaled 3 or 4 times daily. The drug is ineffective when given orally since it must be applied directly to the tissues it is to protect. Some asthmatics find the powder irritating and will respond with an asthmatic attack when dosing themselves. In this case, it is advisable to have the patients premedicate themselves with a bronchodilator.[29,45-47]

Several benefits have been attributed to the drug. It obviously decreases the incidence of attacks in many of those who use it. In addition, patients who must take corticosteroids may find that they can reduce the dose of the steroid. Many children who have used the drug go through a phase of "catch up" growth. Pulmonary function tests may reveal an improvement after the patient has been on the drug, but often the amount of improvement does not equal the greater subjective improvement that the patient feels. Many people, particularly children, will go through a state of euphoria when they find that they can lead more normal lives.[48-51]

The drug seems to have few toxicities. The only major problem is that it is irritating and can induce an attack when inhaled. There has also been a report of slightly abnormal liver function tests.[45]

It should be stressed that while DSCG offers an unusual and effective approach to the therapy of asthma, it certainly is not a cure all and should not be used in place of adequate hydration, avoidance of precipitating factors, etc. In addition, its cost may make it prohibitive for some patients.

Miscellaneous Agents

Antibiotics may be used when infections are a precipitating or complicating factor of asthma. Some physicians give prophylactic antibiotics to asthmatic patients, but most authorities agree that this is an unacceptable practice. Prophylactic antibiotics not only expose the patient to potential adverse effects of the drugs, but they rarely, if ever, protect him from infection. They may stop colonization by a specific sensitive organism but, if the patient is predisposed to get an infection, he will be infected by a resistant organism.

Antihistamines, it would appear, should be beneficial in asthma since histamine is involved in the reaction. There are two basic problems, however. First, histamine is not the only mediator in asthma, and therefore antihistamines have little effect in aborting attacks. Secondly, antihistamines tend to dry the mucous membranes. In the lungs, this leads to mucus which is thicker and more difficult to remove. For this reason, these drugs are generally contraindicated in asthmatics.

Combination products are a relatively popular item prescribed for asthmatics. Most of these contain ephedrine, a methylxanthine, a sedative, and sometimes expectorants, antihistamines, other sympathomimetics, etc. Most of these preparations owe their efficacy to the ephedrine because the doses of sedative or xanthine are often subtherapeutic. While these preparations offer a simple method for a patient to dose himself with a number of drugs, it would be best if the patient were individuallly titrated with the necessary drugs so that he could obtain the best therapeutic response.

COMPLICATIONS

Status asthmaticus is an unrelenting asthmatic attack lasting more than 24 hr which does not respond to the bronchodilators. This is considered a medical emergency and requires hospitalization for the most effective treatment. Most deaths due to asthma are the result of status asthmaticus. The usual causes of death in these patients include: respiratory depression due to the overuse of either sedatives or oxygen, xanthine or sympathomimetic toxicity, extensive plugging of the bronchi with thick mucus due to dehydration and poor coughing efforts, and cardiac failure. The usual precipitating causes include pulmonary infection, dehydration, massive exposure to allergen or misuse of medications.[3,25,29]

The treatment of this condition is similar to that for milder forms of asthma except that it is more vigorous, and the corticosteroids are almost always used in high doses (*e.g.,* 300 mg or more of hydrocortisone per day) for short periods. They are rapidly tapered after a few days. The sympathomimetics, by definition, are ineffective in status asthmaticus, if the latter is due to respiratory acidosis, a refractory state or extensive plugging of the bronchi. The acidosis is best treated by improving ventilation or, if this fails, by I.V. sodium bicarbonate. This may restore responsiveness to the sympathomimetics, but care must be taken to avoid overtreatment with sodium bicarbonate. To correct dehydration, I.V.s should be started, and the patient should receive 3 to 5 liters the first 24 hr, depending on cardiac and renal function. Xanthines probably should be administered also, preferably by the I.V. route. After a loading dose of 500 mg of aminophylline in an adult, it is convenient to add the drug to the I.V. bottles.

Oxygen therapy should be considered in these patients, but it is important that blood gases be monitored before and during treatment. It is desirable to keep the pO_2 above 60 mm Hg. It may be necessary to perform a tracheostomy and use assisted ventilation and bronchial lavage. Patients who are on assisted ventilation may be given sedatives safely. Deaths have been reported in patients with compromised respiratory function who were given even low doses of depressants. However, a patient in status asthmaticus may be in a state of exhaustion and may desperately require rest. Once his ventilatory functions are being handled by an external force, it is safe to give a sedative to allow rest.

If there are signs of pulmonary infection, antibiotics should be started after material for culture and sensitivity is obtained. A Gram stain of the sputum may aid in narrowing the choice of antibiotics. Also the experience of the physician, the patient's history and consultation with the medical laboratory may give a clue to the most likely infecting organism.[2-4,20,25,29]

PROGNOSIS

The prognosis of asthmatic patients is extremely variable. In those whose symptoms begin in childhood, the outlook is very good. Fifty to 95% have a remission of symptoms when they reach adulthood. Five to 10% of this group, especially those who have associated eczema, will continue to have severe disability. In asthmatics whose symptoms started in adulthood, a study by Rackemann showed that after 15 years, 22% of patients were free of symptoms, 44% had improved, 33% remained the same and 3% had died. There is no doubt that in either group chronic asthma has a poorer prognosis than the intermittent type.[2,3,52]

SUMMARY

Asthma is the result of constriction of the bronchi, edema of the mucosal walls and production of viscous mucus. A number of factors are known to precipitate attacks, including allergens, irritants, physical exertion, emotions and infections. Adequate treatment involves, 1st, the recognition and removal, if possible, of causative factors. Next the patient should be taught to keep himself adequately hydrated and to use properly sympathomimetics and xanthines, if needed. If these things do not afford significant relief, the use of corticosteroids and DSCG should be considered. The main point to remember is that asthma rarely can be treated by a single procedure or drug. It must be approached from several different directions, using different agents and methods to gain the maximal benefit at the least therapeutic cost. Pharmacists come in contact with asthmatics daily and can be of considerable help by monitoring therapy and making sure that they understand the proper use of their drugs.

REFERENCES

1. American Thoracic Society: Chronic bronchitis, asthma, and pulmonary emphysema. Am. Rev. Respir. Dis., 85: 762, 1962.
2. Howell, J. B. L.: Airway obstruction, In Cecil-Loeb Textbook of Medicine, Ed. 13, p. 881, edited by P. B. Beeson and W. McDermott. W. B. Saunders Co., Philadelphia, 1971.
3. Crofton, J., and Douglas, A.: Respiratory Diseases, p. 394. Blackwell Scientific Publications, Oxford, England, 1969.
4. Norman, P. S.: Asthma, hayfever, and other manifestations of allergy, In Harrison's Principles of Internal Medicine, Ed. 6, p. 363, edited by M. W. Wintrobe, G. W. Thorn, R. D. Adams, I. L. Bennett, Jr., E. Braunwald, J. J. Isselbacher, and R. G. Petersdorf. McGraw-Hill Book Co., New York, 1970.
5. Coleman, W. P.: Infectious asthma. South. Med. J., 63: 800, 1970.
6. Fitch, K. D., Turner, K. J., and Morton, A. R.: The relationship between serum IgE levels and exercise-induced asthma. Ann. Allergy, 30: 497, 1972.
7. Fitch, K. D., and Morton, A. R.: Specificity of exercise in exercise-induced asthma. Br. Med. J., 4: 577, 1971.

8. Williams, D. A., Lewis-Faning, E., Rees, L., Jacobs, J., and Thomas, A.: Assessment of the relative importance of the allergic, infective, and psychological factors in asthma. Acta Allergol., 12: 376, 1958.

9. Rosenow, E. C.: The spectrum of drug-induced pulmonary disease. Ann. Intern. Med., 77: 977, 1972.

10. Samter, M., and Beers, R. F.: Intolerance to aspirin. Clinical studies and consideration of its pathogenesis. Ann. Intern. Med., 68: 975, 1968.

11. Juhlin, L., Michaelsson, G., and Zetterstrom, O.: Urticaria and asthma induced by food-and-drug additives in patients with aspirin hypersensitivity. J. Allergy Clin. Immunol., 50: 92, 1972.

12. Miller, F. F.: Aspirin-induced bronchial asthma in sisters. Ann. Allergy, 29: 263, 1971.

13. Vanselow, N. A., and Smith, J. A.: Bronchial asthma induced by indomethacin. Ann. Intern. Med., 66: 568, 1967.

14. Tothill, A.: Death from asthma. Br. Med. J., 1: 837, 1968.

15. Falliers, C. J., Garces, F., Bates, J. W., and Molk, B.: Isoproterenol aerosols for asthma. Experiences with severe chronic asthma in children. Clin. Pediatr., 9: 318, 1970.

16. Reisman, R. E.: Asthma induced by adrenergic aerosols. J. Allergy Clin. Immunol., 46: 162, 1970.

17. Thompson, P. D., and Cohen, A. B.: Respiratory disorders. In Clinical Pharmacology: Basic Principles in Therapeutics, p. 262, edited by K. L. Melmon and H. F. Morrelli. Macmillan Co., New York, 1972.

18. Beall, G. N., Heiner, D. C., and Whipp, B. J.: Asthma: new ideas about an old disease. Ann. Intern. Med., 78: 405, 1973.

19. Spencer, H.: Pathology of the Lung, Ed. 2, p. 715, Pergamon Press, Oxford, England, 1968.

20. Weiss, E. B., Faling, L. J., Brooks, S. M., Mintz, S., Chodosh, S., and Segal, M. S.: Bronchial asthma: current concepts in pathophysiology and management of status asthmaticus. Mod. Treat., 6: 278, 1969.

21. Dockhorn, R. J.: The immunologic and adrenergic aspects of asthma. Ann. Allergy, 29: 539, 1971.

22. Szentivanyi, A., Fishel, C. W., and Talmage, D. W.: Adrenaline mediation of histamine and serotonin hyperglycemia in normal mice and the absence of adrenaline-induced hyperglycemia in pertussis-sensitized mice. J. Infect. Dis., 113: 86, 1963.

23. Szentivanyi, A.: The beta adrenergic theory of the atopic abnormality in bronchial asthma. J. Allergy, 42: 203, 1968.

24. Reed, C. E.: Asthma. In Current Therapy 1973, p. 531, edited by H. F. Conn. W. B. Saunders Co., Philadelphia, 1973.

25. Fink, J. N., and Sosman, A. J.: Therapy of bronchial asthma. Med. Clin. North Am., 57: 801, 1973.

26. Levy, D. A., Lichtenstein, L. M., Goldstein, E. O.,

and Ishizaka, K.: Immunologic and cellular changes accompanying the therapy of pollen allergy. J. Clin. Invest., 50: 360, 1971.

27. Innes, I. R., and Nickerson, M.: Drugs acting on postganglionic adrenergic nerve endings and structures innervated by them (sympathomimetic drugs). In The Pharmacological Basis of Therapeutics, Ed. 4, p. 478, edited by L. S. Goodman and A. Gilman. Macmillan Co., New York, 1970.

28. Anon.: Sympathomimetic (adrenergic) agents. In American Hospital Formulary Service, Vol. 12, p. 12, edited by M. J. Reilly, J. A. Kepler, D. M. Johnson, and P. M. Douglas. American Society of Hospital Pharmacists, Washington, D.C., 1973.

29. Blumstein, C. G.: Drug treatment in bronchial asthma. Semin. Drug Treat., 2: 385, 1973.

30. Dollery, C. T.: Symposium on isoproterenol therapy in asthma. Ann. Allergy, 31: 25, 1973.

31. Ayers, S. M.: Symposium on isoproterenol therapy in asthma. Ann. Allergy, 31: 3, 1973.

32. Silverglade, A.: Isoproterenol aerosol not responsible for increased mortality from asthma. N. Engl. J. Med., 288: 738, 1973.

33. Anon.: Asthma deaths: a question answered. Br. Med. J., 4: 443, 1972.

34. Herxheimer, H.: Asthma deaths. Br. Med. J., 4: 795, 1972.

35. Harris, M. C.: Symposium on isoproterenol therapy in asthma. Ann. Allergy, 31: 19, 1973.

36. Grandevia, B.: Symposium on isoproterenol therapy in asthma. Ann. Allergy, 31: 30, 1973.

37. Lehr, D.: Isoproterenol and sudden death of asthmatic patients in ventricular fibrillation. N. Engl. J. Med., 287: 987, 1972.

38. Stolley, P. D.: Asthma mortality: why the united states was spared an epidemic of deaths due to asthma. Am. Rev. Respir. Dis., 105: 883, 1970.

39. Spitzer, S. A., Goldschmidt, Z., and Dubrawsky, C.: The bronchodilator effect of salbutamol administered by IPPB to patients with asthma. Chest, 62: 273, 1972.

40. Racoveanu, C., Stanescu, D. C., Manicatide, M., and Stroescu, V.: The bronchodilator effects of orciprenaline and salbutamol. A double blind study. Postgrad. Med. J., 47: 83, 1971.

41. Parker, S. S., Choo-Kang, Y. F. J., Cooper, E. J., Cameron, S. J., and Grant, I. W. B.: Bronchodilator effect of oral salbutamol in asthmatics treated with corticosteroids. Br. Med. J., 4: 139, 1971.

42. Tong, T. G.: Aminophylline—review of clinical use. Drug Intell. Clin. Pharmacol., 7: 156, 1973.

43. Ritchie, J. M.: The Xanthines. In The Pharmacological Basis of Therapeutics, Ed. 4, p. 358, edited by L. S. Goodman and A. Gilman. Macmillan Co., New York, 1970.

44. Segal, M. S., Weiss, E. B., and Carta, C.: Rectal aminophylline (blood levels with concentrated solutions). Ann. Allergy, 29: 135, 1971.

45. Toogood, J. H., Lefcoe, N. M., Rose, D. K., and

McCourtie, D. R.: A double blind study of disodium cromoglycate for prophylaxis of bronchial asthma. Am. Rev. Respir. Dis., 104: 323, 1971.

46. Brompton Hospital/Medical Research Council Collaborative Trial: Long-term study of disodium cromoglycate in treatment of severe extrinsic or intrinsic bronchial asthma in adults. Br. Med. J., 4: 383, 1972.

47. Hermance, W. E., and Brown, E. B.: Cromolyn sodium (disodium cromoglycate) in treatment of asthma. N. Y. State J. Med., 73: 430, 1973.

48. Gebbie, T., Harris, E. A., O'Donnell, T. V., and Spears, G. F. S.: Multicentre, short-term therapeutic trial of disodium cromoglycate, with and without prednisone, in adults with asthma. Br. Med. J., 4: 576, 1972.

49. Taylor, B., and Psiloinis, M. P.: Disodium cromoglycate in childhood asthma. N. Z. Med. J., 74: 374, 1971.

50. Mathison, D. A., Condemi, J. J., Lovejoy, F. W., and Vaughan, J. H.: Cromolyn treatment of asthma: trials in corticosteroid-dependent asthmatics. J.A.M.A., 216: 1454, 1971.

51. Glass, R. D.: Experience with disodium cromoglycate in the treatment of asthmatic children. Med. J. Aust., 1: 1382, 1971.

52. Rackemann, F. M., and Edward, M. C.: Asthma in children: a follow-up study of 688 patients after an interval of twenty years. N. Engl. J. Med., 246: 815, 1952.

53. Smith, A. P.: Response of aspirin-allergic patients to challenge by some analgesics in common use. Br. Med. J., 2: 484, 1971.

54. Anon.: Lung disease caused by drugs. Br. Med. J., 3: 729, 1969.

55. Haigné, R.: Hypersensitivity to drugs. In Drug-Induced Diseases, Vol. 4, p. 220, edited by L. Meyler and H. M. Peck. Excerpta Medica, Amsterdam, 1972.

56. Kroese, W. F. S.: Immunosuppressive drugs. In Side Effects of Drugs, Vol. 7, p. 640, edited by L. Meyler and A. Herxheimer. Excerpta Medica, Amsterdam, 1972.

57. Katz, W. A., and Scarf, M.: Bromosulphalein reactions. A. J. Med. Sci., 248: 545, 1964.

58. Tennant, F. S., Preble, M., Prendergast, T. J., and Ventry, P.: Medical manifestations associated with hashish. J.A.M.A., 216: 1965, 1971.

59. Refshauge, W. D.: Adverse effects of parenteral iron preparations. Med. J. Aust., 1: 314, 1969.

60. Herbert, V.: Drugs effective in iron-deficiency and other hypochromic anemias. In The Pharmacological Basis of Therapeutics, Ed. 4, p. 1397, edited by L. S. Goodman and A. Gilman. Macmillan Co., New York, 1970.

61. Ritchie, J. M., Cohen, P. J., and Dripps, R. D.: Cocaine; procaine and other synthetic local anesthetics. In The Pharmacological Basis of Therapeutics, Ed. 4, p. 371, edited by L. S. Goodman and A. Gilman. Macmillan Co., New York, 1970.

62. Mathov, E.: The risks of monoamine oxidase inhibitors in the treatment of bronchial asthma. J. Allergy, 34: 484, 1963.

63. Mathews, K. P., and Pan, P. M.: Immediate type hypersensitivity to phenylmercuric compounds. Am. J. Med., 44: 310, 1968.

64. Zurek, R. C.: Antibiotic-induced diseases. In Diseases of Medical Progress: A Study of Iatrogenic Disease, Ed. 3, p. 3, edited by R. H. Moser. Charles C Thomas Co., Springfield, Ill., 1969.

65. Morgan, L. K.: Nitrofurantoin pulmonary hypersensitivity. Med. J. Aust., 3: 136, 1970.

66. Horan, J. D., and Lederman, J. J.: Possible asthmogenic effect of oral contraceptives. Can. Med. Assoc. J., 99: 130, 1968.

67. Barnes, J.: Allergy to oral contraceptives. Practitioner, 198: 873, 1967.

68. Manten, A.: Antibiotic drugs. In Side Effects of Drugs, Vol. 7, p. 335, edited by L. Meyler and A. Herxheimer. Excerpta Medica, Amsterdam, 1972.

69. Weinstein, L.: The penicillins. In The Pharmacological Basis of Therapeutics, Ed. 4, p. 1204, edited by L. S. Goodman and A. Gilman. Macmillan Co., New York, 1970.

70. Stafford, A.: Drugs acting on the heart. In Side Effects of Drugs, Vol. 7, p. 269, edited by L. Meyler, and A. Herxheimer. Excerpta Medica, Amsterdam, 1972.

71. Moe, G. K., and Abildskov, J. A.: Antiarrhythmic drugs. In The Pharmacological Basis of Therapeutics, Ed. 4, p. 709, edited by L. S. Goodman and A. Gilman. Macmillan Co., New York, 1970.

72. Rosenoer, V. M.: Radiological contrast media. In Side Effects of Drugs, Vol. 7, p. 653, edited by L. Meyler and A. Herxheimer. Excerpta Medica, Amsterdam, 1972.

73. Wise, J. R.: Inquiry: bronchospasm after reserpine? N. Engl. J. Med., 281: 563, 1969.

74. Atuk, N. O., and Owen, J. A.: Bronchospasm after reserpine. N. Engl. J. Med., 281: 908, 1969.

75. Segal, M. S.: Bronchospasm after reserpine. N. Engl. J. Med., 281: 1426, 1969.

76. Koelle, G. B.: Neuromuscular blocking agents. In The Pharmacological Basis of Therapeutics, Ed. 4, p. 601, edited by L. S. Goodman and A. Gilman. Macmillan Co., New York, 1970.

77. Fellner, M. J., and Baer, R.: Anaphylactic reaction to tetracycline in penicillin-allergic patient. J.A.M.A., 192: 997, 1965.

78. Takki, S., and Tammisto, T.: Severe bronchospasm and circulatory collapse following the administration of d-tubocurarine. Ann. Clin. Res., 3: 112, 1971.

chapter 17

CHRONIC OBSTRUCTIVE PULMONARY DISEASE

Peter M. Penna, Pharm.D.

Chronic obstructive pulmonary disease (COPD) encompasses a number of pathologically distinct disease entities. In this discussion, the major emphasis will be given to emphysema, chronic bronchitis and bronchiectasis. Asthma was discussed in Chapter 16. In all of the diseases included under the heading of COPD, there is the common finding of resistance to the outflow of air from the lungs due to intrapulmonary lesions. The usual cause of the resistance is either chronic bronchitis, bronchiectasis, emphysema or chronic asthma. These diseases cause either a narrowing of the bronchi and bronchioles or destruction of the smaller units (alveoli, alveolar sacs, respiratory bronchioles, etc.) of the lung causing enlargement of the terminal air spaces. In many individuals, the two processes exist together. There has been a good deal of confusion concerning the definition of these disease states. For our purposes we will use the following definitions.

1. Emphysema, according to the World Health Organization, is defined as "a condition of the lung characterized by increase beyond the normal in the size of air spaces distal to the terminal bronchiole, with destructive changes in their walls."[1] The important points here are that there is destruction of lung tissue (especially alveolar walls) and enlargement of the air spaces (distal to the nonrespiratory bronchiole). Therefore, the process is irreversible, but not necessarily progressive.

2. Chronic bronchitis is defined as the continuous excessive production of mucus in the bronchi due to chronic inflammation resulting in a productive cough. Also, by definition, this process must occur for at least 3 months out of the year for 2 or more successive years. The obstruction which occurs may be reversible at first.[1,2]

3. Bronchial asthma is defined as a hypersensitivity reaction of the bronchial tree producing bronchoconstriction, mucosal edema and excess mucus in predisposed people. Family history is more important here than with either of the other diseases. This disorder may be reversible, either spontaneously, or with treatment, or it may develop into a chronic state which is irreversible.[1,2]

4. Bronchiectasis refers to a state in which there is chronic dilation of the bronchi accompanied by infection and hypersecretion of mucus.[1,3]

The above definitions delineate very specific disease states, but in actual clinical practice the lines of demarcation are not that clear, and patients classified as having chronic bronchitis in one country may be diagnosed as having emphysema in another. For example, patients with COPD in Britain are generally said to have chronic bronchitis. In the U.S., the same patients are just as likely to be diagnosed as having emphysema. While there are distinct differences in classical cases of these diseases, they are more academic than practical, particularly as far as pharmacists are concerned. In addition, there is probably a good deal of overlap between these diseases, so that a given individual can actually have chronic bronchitis and emphysema, emphysema and chronic asthma etc.

There are several important generalities that can be made about these conditions:

1. The disease processes usually begin years before the onset of signs and symptoms.

2. All are usually slowly progressive, with acute exacerbations which can cause respiratory failure.

3. Exacerbations may be caused by such things as increased air pollution, infections, alcoholism, diabetes, anemia or any debilitating disease.

4. Finally, the treatment regimens for any of these conditions have a great deal in common.

ANATOMY

In order to have an understanding of these diseases, it is necessary to review briefly some of the anatomy of the respiratory tract. Starting from the trachea, there is a continuous branching of the bronchial tree through about

50 generations until it reaches the alveolar sacs and alveoli (Fig. 17.1). The important structures are the following.

1. The bronchi, which are lined by ciliated cells and contain a large number of mucus glands. The bronchi are also lined by a diagonal layer of smooth muscle.

2. The bronchioles, which are simply bronchi less than 1 mm in diameter and which contain no mucus glands.

3. The terminal bronchioles, which contain no ciliated cells but still retain the smooth muscle layer.

4. The respiratory bronchiole, which has an incomplete layer of smooth muscle, such that the walls may bulge out to form alveoli.

5. The alveolar ducts, which are simply ducts completely lined with alveoli.

6. The alveolar sac, which contains many alveoli and which forms the tip of the pulmonary tree.

7. The alveolus, which is the functional unit of the lung where gas exchange takes place.

ETIOLOGY

A number of things have been implicated as possible causative agents for these diseases. The three major factors are smoking, pollution and infection. There is little doubt that smoking and atmospheric pollution have contributed to the disease processes. Cigarette smoking is probably the most important cause of chronic bronchitis in this country. In a similar manner, the increases in environmental and occupational pollutants (e.g., dust in mills and factories) have played a major role in the increased incidence of these diseases. For example, in England the incidence of chronic bronchitis is much greater in the polluted industrial areas than in the nonpolluted rural areas. Many people feel that climate plays a very important role because there is some evidence that these diseases are more prevalent in cold damp climates. However, it is more likely that some of the early observers mistook the effects of pollution for climatic effects.[4-10]

Pulmonary infection has been shown to have a part in the development of COPD, particularly bronchiectasis. It is generally felt that infections are rarely the initiating cause but that they deal significantly in the process once

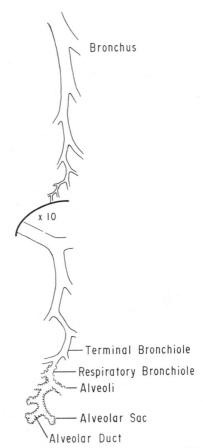

FIG. 17.1. The basic anatomy of the bronchial tree.

it has been initiated by some other mechanism, usually smoking or pollution. Once infection takes place, however, a great amount of lung tissue can be destroyed. It is readily recognized that these latter two conditions, either singly or in combination, are irritating to pulmonary tissue and thereby cause an increase in mucus production often accompanied by a persistent cough. In this situation, it is likely that infections can take hold more readily in the upper respiratory tract where they very easily spread to the lower respiratory tract. The symptoms produced at this time—severe cough, wheezing and purulent sputum—very often bring the person to a physician, who then discovers the underlying COPD. In bronchiectasis, infection of the bronchi may produce weakening of the wall which allows it to bulge in and out during expiratory movements. In addition, the infection will cause large amounts of mucus to be produced which will cause obstruction. It is also a well known fact that infections are often responsible for exacerbation of a patient's symptoms of COPD. It is for this reason, as we shall see later, that part of the therapy used in an attempt to control these diseases is aimed at protection against pulmonary infection.[1,3,5,11,12]

Recently, there has been some very good evidence that a certain type of emphysema is associated with an inherited deficiency (carried by an autosomal recessive gene) of the enzyme a_1-antitrypsin. This low molecular weight glycoprotein is normally found in human serum, and it has the property of inhibiting proteolytic enzymes. This type of emphysema occurs mainly in the lower lobes of the lung, causing diffuse panacinar destruction in these areas. In addition, the onset of the symptoms of this type of emphysema is usually earlier than with the other types, and it affects women much more commonly than the others. Finally, there is a very distinct familial history of the disease because deficiency of the enzyme is genetically determined. It should be noted, however, that some familial distribution of emphysema has been found where no deficiency of this enzyme could be demonstrated.

It is theorized that proteases (e.g., from bacteria, macrophages, etc.) may be responsible for damage to the lungs. Since a_1-antitrypsin inhibits proteases, a deficiency of the enzyme will allow the proteases to do more damage to the lung. However, much more work needs to be done in this area before the exact mechanisms are defined.[13-17]

INCIDENCE

The incidence of chronic bronchitis and emphysema has been increasing in the U.S., while bronchiectasis has been declining. The increase seen in emphysema and chronic bronchitis can be attributed to two factors. The first is that the amounts of air pollution and cigarette smoking (particularly after World War II) have increased. The second is that diagnostic procedures have improved to the point where more people can be diagnosed who have minimal amounts of the disease. The death rate for men due to emphysema in the U.S. increased from 1.3 per 100,000 population in 1950, to 12.6 per 100,000 in 1964. During the same period, the death rate attributed to chronic bronchitis doubled. In England there has not been much of a change in the mortality rate due to either of these diseases, but it has been uniformly high for many years, averaging about 85 per 100,000 since 1945. In the U.S. at the present time, COPD is second only to heart disease as a cause of disability.[5,6]

In one study of 6,000 persons in the eastern U.S., evidence of chronic bronchitis was found in 8%, emphysema in 3% and a combination of the two in 5%.[6] In another study in Britain on people 40 to 54 years old, 17% of the men and 9% of the women had signs and symptoms of chronic bronchitis.[18] Some authorities anticipate that the mortality rate due to emphysema will double every 5 years.[19]

The incidence of bronchiectasis has been declining mainly due to the development of effective antibiotics. It still occurs following pulmonary infections and sometimes after aspiration of foreign objects. The incidence in England during the period from 1946 to 1955 has been estimated at 10.6 per 100,000 children.[1,3]

PATHOLOGY

As mentioned previously, the basic problem in COPD is resistance to air flow, especially flow of air out of the lungs.

In bronchitis, the bronchial tree responds to irritation from smoke, infection, etc., with an increase in the amount of mucus production accompanied by edema of the mucosal lining of the bronchi. If the irritation is removed, the process is entirely reversible. However, if the source of irritation remains, the mucus glands in the large airways hypertrophy, and the goblet cells in the smaller airways increase in number. The increased amount of sputum, which usually must be removed by coughing and ciliary action, makes a very fertile medium for bacterial growth. Undoubtedly, infections of the smaller air passages extending into the alveolar sacs are responsible for breakdown of lung tissue and scarring in some individuals. A more significant finding, however, is that the mucus is often thick and difficult to remove, and, therefore it may act to cut down the effective diameter of the bronchi and cause turbulence in air flow. Also, the bronchi normally expand on inspiration and contract (or relax) on expiration. Therefore, a glob of mucus lining the bronchi will not have much effect on inspiration, but it may significantly affect expiration. In this situation, expiratory effort will be increased. In addition, excess mucus lining the wall may act as an irritant and cause bronchospasm thereby reducing the diameter even further (Fig. 17.2).

As more mucus is produced, it may coalesce and consolidate to produce a mucus plug, especially in the smaller bronchi and bronchioles. These plugs very effectively trap air in the distal areas of the lung (alveoli, alveolar sacs, terminal bronchioles and respiratory bronchioles). As pressure is built up in the thoracic cavity in the process of expiration, this trapped air exerts pressure on the walls of the alveoli, etc. and may cause a breakdown in tissue in these areas. In many instances, all of the alveoli in an alveolar sac may be broken down so that there is only one large air space left. There is much less functional surface area left for gas exchange in this large air space than in the normal structure. Another complication of the obstructive and destructive processes that take place here is that elastic fibers in the alveolus are lost. They are necessary in aiding the expulsion of air from the alveolus.

Essentially what is happening, then, with chronic bronchitis in many patients, is that the obstruction caused by the mucus eventually leads to emphysematous changes in the lung (destruction of tissue and expansion of air spaces). At autopsy it is not at all uncommon to find bronchitic and emphysematous changes in the same patient.[11,20,21]

In emphysema the basic problem is destruction of tissue and expansion of air spaces. There are several pathologically distinct forms of pulmonary emphysema. Very briefly they are as follows:

1. Centrilobular emphysema refers to the condition resulting from destruction of tissue in the respiratory bronchioles. This weakened tissue collapses very easily during expiration (Fig. 17.3).

2. Panacinar or panlobular emphysema is diffuse destruction of the smaller structures in the lung—the respiratory bronchiole, alveolar ducts, alveolar sacs and alveoli. Panacinar and centrilobular emphysema may be found in the same patient.

3. Aging lung or senile emphysema, used interchangeably, really refer to definite disease entities. Specifically, aging lung emphysema refers to supposed emphysematous changes that occur simply as a result of aging. The term "senile emphysema" refers to the condition where kyphotic changes in the thoracic spine cause the ribs to bow outward, thereby producing the so-called classic barrel chest of emphysema. Usually, there will be some enlargement of air spaces, but there is not much impairment of pulmonary function in these patients. This is not to say that people with panacinar or centrilobular emphysema don't often have "barrel chests," because many of them do. The major point is that a barrel chest is not always diagnostic of emphysema.

4. Focal or localized emphysema results when changes are localized in a specific area of the lung due to such things as tumors causing obstruction of a bronchus. There are several other types of emphysema which may attack the lung, but the ones of most interest to us are the first two in the above classification. It is also important to realize that various authors

  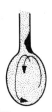

Normal   Obstruction

FIG. 17.2. Inspiration into and expiration from normal and diseased units of the lung. The "glob" of mucus will not affect inspiration, but may decrease expiration.

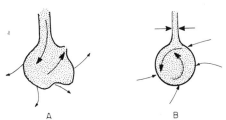

A   B

FIG. 17.3. Inspiration creates no problems into an area of the lung in which disease has weakened the bronchiolar walls. On expiration, however, the weakened walls may collapse, trapping air. Note that on inspiration air may leak through damaged walls into adjacent alveoli or alveolar sacs.

classify pulmonary emphysema differently. The classification given here is an oversimplified compromise of a much more complex subject.[9,21-24]

Besides the theory that chronic bronchitis can lead to emphysematous changes by causing simple obstruction to outflow of air in the lungs, there is another interrelated theory concerning the changes that take place in emphysema. This is the idea that the elastic recoil of the lung is diminished in emphysema due to infection, dust particles causing inflammation, or breakdown due to mucus plug obstruction. The elastic recoil of the lung is the major force behind expiration. It raises the intrabronchial pressure above that in the thoracic cavity. When the pressure inside a bronchiole or bronchus is lower than the pressure inside the chest cavity, the bronchiole or bronchus may collapse or narrow because of the external pressure exerted on it. As illustrated in Figure 17.3, there is no problem on inspiration, but on expiration the walls of the bronchiole may collapse, especially if the elastic fibers in the distal alveoli have been destroyed.[1,21,25] Figure 17.4 gives an overview of how a normal group of alveolar sacs and their cross-section compares to diseased structures.

Bronchiectasis often begins in childhood. It usually affects the bronchi in just one area of the lung. The walls of these bronchi may exhibit destruction, which allows the wall to bulge in or out during respiratory movements. The bronchi distal to the primary affected area may become completely occluded with mucus or may even be obliterated by inflammatory processes. This area then is particularly susceptible to infection, and abscesses may develop along with collapse of the affected areas and emphysematous changes.[3,7,26]

DIAGNOSIS AND CLINICAL FEATURES

The diagnosis of emphysema during life is extremely difficult. Emphysema is defined by its pathology and by the changes that occur in the lung. While these changes will in time produce signs and symptoms of COPD, it is very difficult to say that the clinical state of the patient is due, for example, to panacinar emphysema. With our present knowledge, it does not make too much difference to us, as pharmacists, whether a patient has emphysema or chronic bronchitis, because the treatment regimens are very similar. Nevertheless, patients with COPD have been categorized into two different types, depending on their presenting signs and symptoms. These are the emphysematous types (type A or the "pink-puffers") and the bronchitic types (type B or the "blue-bloaters").

Generally speaking, the "pink-puffers" are thin, anxious and dyspneic on exertion. There is usually no cyanosis (hence, the term "pink"), and they appear well aerated during minimal activity. However, they may become breathless very easily when called upon to perform even the lightest tasks.

The "blue-bloater," on the other hand, is typically obese, quiet, cyanotic at rest and has a cough producing a great deal of mucus. While there is some correlation between clinical presentation and primary disease, many, if not most, patients combine attributes of each (Table 17.1).

The usual patient with COPD is a 50- or 60-year-old cigarette-smoking male. He usually complains of a chronic, often productive cough, particularly in the winter. He becomes breathless very easily and may suffer from dyspnea, orthopnea and wheezing.[1,27]

Very often these patients will present with shortness of breath (SOB) due in part to a pulmonary infection. Upon questioning, it becomes evident that many of them have a long history of cigarette cough and excess sputum production, particularly in the winter months. Gradually, the cigarette cough worsens, and the

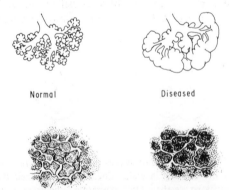

Normal   Diseased

FIG. 17.4. An overview of normal bronchioles and alveolar sacs, with a cross section of this tissue. This is contrasted with the appearance of the same structures in an emphysema patient.

TABLE 17.1[a]

Clinical Patterns and Laboratory Finding in Patients with Emphysema and Chronic Bronchitis

	Bronchitis	Emphysema
Synonyms	Blue-bloater	Pink-puffer
	Type B	Type A
Age at onset	Younger (45-65)	Older (55-75)
Major onset symptom	Tussive	Dyspneic
Body type	Obese	Lean, or history of wt. loss
Heart	Enlarged	Normal
Sputum	Copious, mucopurulent	Scanty
Hematocrit	Polycythemic	Normal
$PaCO_2$	High	Normal
PaO_2	Low	Near normal
Vital capacity	Decreased	Low normal
Residual volume	Increased	Increased
Total lung capacity	Low normal	Increased

[a]Reprinted with permission from Ref. 28.

patient may suffer from it continuously. Mild upper respiratory tract infections become more severe, and the mucus may appear purulent. Wheezing will often be noticed at this time.

In other cases, however, the patient is experiencing dyspnea but accepts it as a result of the aging process and, therefore, does not seek medical attention. Eventually he gets to a point where even the slightest physical exertion leaves him breathless, at which time he will seek aid. In either of these cases, a great deal of damage already may have occurred in the pulmonary system.

In the diagnosis of bronchiectasis, many of the signs and symptoms are the same as for emphysema and chronic bronchitis. The major findings are those of chronic productive cough, especially with changes in posture. The sputum which is produced (up to 500 ml per day) may have a foul odor and may be streaked with blood. In untreated cases, the sputum production does not vary with the seasons of the year. If there is significant obstruction, wheezing, dyspnea and cyanosis may be noted.[1,3]

TREATMENT

Unfortunately, there is no one specific treatment or cure for COPD at the present time. With multiple causes for this condition, it is doubtful that there will ever be one specific cure to cover the various types of these diseases.

The treatment of COPD is such that a number of different measures are employed in order to stop or slow down the disease process and to make life more comfortable for these patients. There are six different objectives involved in this. They are: to prevent or eradicate or reduce bronchial and alveolar inflammation; to alleviate bronchial obstruction; to train the patient to breathe properly; to rehabilitate the patient physically; to manage complications (*e.g.*, respiratory failure brought on by an infection); and, finally, to educate the patient concerning his disease, how he can live with it and treat it.

As shall be demonstrated, these objectives and the means by which they are achieved have a great deal of overlap.

1. In order to eliminate or decrease inflammation and irritation in the pulmonary tree, several things can be done. First of all, these patients should stop smoking. Often, this is enough to cause significant improvement in early chronic bronchitis. Obviously, there may be some psychological problems when a patient who has been smoking for 20 to 40 years is forced to stop. With some disease states, a fairly good argument can be made that the psychological stress involved with trying to stop smoking is more severe than the damage that would be done if that person were to continue to smoke. This is not the case with COPD. It has been shown that continuation of smoking causes a more rapid development of the disease. In addition, those patients who are able to quit

usually fare much better than those who continue.

Another thing that can be done is to avoid air pollution if at all possible. Many patients with COPD have benefited greatly by moving into areas where there is less atmospheric pollution.

Finally, many people are able to relieve pulmonary inflammatory problems by adjusting the atmospheric environments in their homes. It is desirable to keep the rooms well humidified and to have the temperature stabilized. Proper humidification helps in liquefying and removing the tenacious mucus secretions which often lead to the destructive changes.[3,28,29]

2. The relief of bronchial obstruction is often referred to as "bronchial hygiene." The bronchodilators are used with some success, and they work very well in patients with COPD who do have bronchospasm playing a part in their disease, but generally they are not as effective as they are in patients with asthma. Bronchodilators usually are given orally or by inhalation with pressurized aerosols, hand-held nebulizers, pump-driven nebulizers and intermittent positive pressure breathing (IPPB). The drugs used in this country include isoproterenol, epinephrine, ephedrine, phenylephrine, and a few others. Phenylephrine has very little bronchodilating activity and is rarely used alone. It does cause constriction of the bronchial vessels, however, and therefore helps relieve any edema which may be present. Ephedrine is the drug of choice for oral administration and appears to work very well for controlling the mild symptoms of bronchospasm. The normal dose is 25 mg 3 or 4 times daily. It is ineffective for the more serious conditions. The problem of abuse of the small pressurized aerosols of these drugs, particularly isoproterenol, has been mentioned in Chapter 16. It should be stressed that these same problems can occur just as easily in patients with chronic bronchitis and emphysema.

There is a new drug called salbutamol, not yet released in the U.S., which selectively stimulates the beta-2 receptors of the lungs to cause bronchodilation. The beta-adrenergic system has been subdivided into two categories: the beta-1 system, which controls the heart and several other structures, and the beta-2 system, which controls the smooth muscle of the lungs. Since salbutamol does not affect the beta-1

receptors, it should have little effect on the heart compared to isoproterenol. The studies done thus far indicate that it is both safe and effective, and it has less cardiovascular effects and a longer duration of action than isoproterenol. It will be interesting to see if any new adverse effects occur when it is released for general use.[30-32] The concept of the existence of more than one type of beta-receptor is the newest refinement of Ahlquist's theory of adrenergic neuronal function. If the separation of beta-1 and beta-2 receptors can indeed be achieved clinically, it will be a significant therapeutic advantage.

When isoproterenol or the other drugs are given by nebulizer or IPPB, they are diluted usually in half with water or saline and given 2 or more times daily as needed. The actual dilutions used and the techniques are individualized for each patient.

Aminophylline or other methylxanthines may be used when a long acting bronchodilator is needed. The doses required are from 200 to 600 mg of aminophylline up to 6 times a day orally, or 250 to 500 mg rectally. Tablets and suppositories may not give good absorption. When prompt onset of action is desired, theophylline elixir will give very good results. The most effective method of administration, however, is I.V., preferably by slow I.V. drip after a loading dose (must be given over 10 to 15 min to prevent vascular collapse). The major problem with aminophylline is that it is irritating to the gastrointestinal (GI) tract due to local and systemic effects. This is particularly important because many patients with emphysema have peptic ulcers and, therefore, should not receive methylxanthines except in emergency situations.

The corticosteroids may be lifesaving in the critically ill patient in whom the standard bronchodilators have not worked. They may be very effective in relieving bronchospasm, but they should not be used casually or chronically in patients who benefit from other modes of therapy. In the acutely ill patient, large doses may be required (e.g., 300 mg of hydrocortisone daily or equivalent doses of the other corticosteroids). These drugs may be continued at high doses for 3 to 5 days, then tapered over 7 to 10 days.[5,28,33] If it is deemed necessary to place the patient on chronic steroid therapy, the lowest possible dose should be used, and alternate day therapy should be tried (*e.g.,* 20 mg prednisone every other day). As with aminophylline, the effects of the corticosteroids on the GI tract must also be considered.

Humidification of the atmosphere is extremely useful in helping to remove mucus secretions. Besides adjusting the humidity of the rooms of the home, many patients will inhale highly moisturized air (*e.g.,* from a vaporizer, ultrasonic nebulizer etc.) for about 10 min after each use of a bronchodilator. They may follow this with careful coughing or postural drainage to aid in the removal of the mucus.[1,29,33]

The mucolytic agent, *N*-acetylcysteine, has been used with some success in these people. There is no doubt that the drug will help to liquefy mucus *in vitro,* but there is some question concerning its effectiveness *in vivo* when compared to nebulized water or saline. Most authorities seem to feel that it is effective, and many patients experience great relief in their symptoms after treatment with the drug. There are three major problems associated with its use. The first is that it has a very foul odor and frequently causes nausea. Secondly, a number of patients, particularly asthmatics, are hypersensitive to it and respond with bronchospasm. If the drug is to be used at all in these patients, they should be pretreated with a bronchodilator. The third problem is that some patients may experience a massive liquefaction of mucus after *N*-acetylcysteine, and they may have trouble removing it by ciliary motion and coughing. Suction may have to be used. The usual dose is 3 to 5 ml of a 20% solution or 6 to 10 ml of a 10% solution, given 3 to 4 times daily by mouthpiece, face mask or tracheostomy. It may also be instilled directly into various segments of the bronchial tree with a catheter, which will also aid in the removal of the liquefied secretions. Two to 5 ml of a 20% solution are used for this purpose. Postural drainage after use of the drug will help in removing the mucus. The pH of the solution should be kept between 7.0 and 9.0 for maximal effectiveness.[34-36]

Bromhexine HC1 is a relatively new drug which has not yet been approved for general use in this country. It is an orally active alkaloid which aids in the liquefaction of mucus by fragmenting the mucopolysaccharide fibers present. While there is conflicting evidence at this point concerning its effectiveness, the majority of opinion seems to be that it does produce significant improvement in patients who use it. The side effects which have been noted are rare, consisting of nausea, mild elevations of serum glutamic-oxaloacetic transaminase and a worsening of ulcer symptoms. The drug has promise of being a very useful additon to the treatment regimens now used for patients with COPD, particularly since it is effective after oral administration. It will require more experimentation to define its true place, adverse effects, etc.[37,38]

There are several other agents which have been used to help remove mucus in these patients. Propylene glycol, given as a mist, may be slightly effective. The expectorants, saturated solution of potassium iodide (SSKI), hydriodic acid (HI) and glyceryl guaiacolate likewise may be of some benefit, but generally their effectiveness has been disappointing. Finally, the detergent aerosols, such as Alevaire, have been shown to be no more effective than saline or water mists. Some commercial products for COPD contain antihistamines. Because of their ability to dry mucus secretions, they are contraindicated.

In general, the most effective way to help remove these secretions is to make sure that the patient is well hydrated from an adequate fluid intake. This, along with the inhalation of water or saline mist, and with the use of *N*-acetylcysteine in severe cases should take care of the majority of patients.

3. Training these patients to breathe properly can add greatly to their enjoyment of life. They must be taught to breathe in a slow and relaxed manner. Dyspnea can be terrifying, and many patients, when they become dyspneic, try to increase their inspiratory and expiratory efforts. Because of the nature of the disease, they have no trouble with inspiration, but they are unable to expire properly. Therefore, they are taught to breathe slowly, preferably inspiring through the nose and expiring through pursed lips. Breathing control is essential to prevent overdistention and dyspnea.

When lying down, they can place a heavy weight on their abdomens to displace the viscera and, therefore, the diaphram upward. This aids in causing a more complete expiration of air. Some patients benefit from an "emphysema belt," which is a large wide belt fixed tightly around the abdomen to displace the viscera and diaphram upward.

They are taught to let the natural rhythm of their breathing determine the amount of activity they can undertake. In normal individuals, the opposite occurs. Finally, they are taught to cough properly. Coughing is one of the main mechanisms whereby sputum is removed, and it is rarely, if ever, justified to suppress the cough in these patients. On the other hand, it is important that they be taught to cough moderately and not too forcefully, since vigorous coughing can cause further breakdown of alveolar walls.[39-41]

4. Physical rehabilitation, like breathing training, can greatly extend the amount of work that these patients can attempt. In the usual patient, shortness of breath upon exertion removes the desire to attempt that type of exertion again. This leads to atrophy of the skeletal muscles which causes an even greater decrease in tolerance to exertion or exercise. This sets up a vicious circle which eventually results in a state of invalidism which is not really warranted, if the actual disease state is considered. Therefore, these patients are subjected to graded exercises in order to increase their stamina. Many people have benefited greatly from oxygen support while they are initiating these exercises. Some people even carry portable oxygen supplies with them to be used when needed. In general, physical rehabilitation has worked very well in allowing these patients to continue useful productive lives.[39-41]

Oxygen therapy is very important in the treatment of COPD. Hypoxia can be severe and sudden in onset, or it can develop slowly over a long period of time. Many patients will have a pO_2 as low as 40 mm Hg (normal is above 80 mm Hg) with significant retention of carbon dioxide. When oxygen is administered, there are several problems which may occur. First of all, if the gas mixture is improperly humidified, it may be drying to the mucous membranes. Secondly, if the concentration of administered oxygen is too high, it may depress the respiration by suddenly removing CO_2 and saturating the blood with oxygen. It is important, therefore, to monitor blood gases carefully during oxygen therapy.[42,43]

Many patients will react to hypoxia by becoming agitated, restless, etc. When a patient with COPD exhibits these symptoms, it is vitally important to make sure that he is not hypoxic before initiating therapy with a "tranquilizer." Obviously, if hypoxia is the cause of the agitation, oxygen therapy is indicated. Hypoxic patients are extremely sensitive to even low doses of the commonly used "tranquilizers." These include phenothizines, barbiturates and benzodiazepines. In hypoxia, these drugs (and probably any CNS depressant) can depress the respiratory center enough to completely obliterate respiratory drive resulting in death. In the absence of hypoxia, these same drugs may be safe in normal doses in COPD patients. However, it would be wise to use depressants very cautiously, if at all.[44,45]

5. Managing complications as they occur is one of the most important aspects of controlling these diseases. The major thing here is pulmonary infection. Obviously, many of the other things that have been mentioned, e.g., bronchial hygiene, will aid in preventing infections. There are a few specifics, however, which should be mentioned. First of all, these patients should try to avoid crowds when respiratory infections are prevalent. Secondly, they should receive polyvalent flu vaccine yearly. Thirdly, they should be very careful to practice proper oral hygiene since this may be a portal of respiratory infection.

When bacterial infections do occur, they should be treated vigorously, preferably with a bacteriocidal agent. Also, the treatment may need to be prolonged when compared with treatment in a "normal" individual. Material for culture and sensitivity should be collected before treatment is started. However, treatment must be started before the results are back. In many situations, past experience with a given patient or experience with many patients in the area may give a clue to the most likely offending organism. Also, a Gram stain of the mucus may provide some information. Recurrent infections are often due to viruses, or *Diplococcus pneumoniae*. In diplococcal infections, penicillin or ampicillin is the drug of choice, followed by erythromycin. In patients who do not practice good bronchial hygiene or who have been on prophylactic antibiotic therapy, it is not uncommon to see infections caused by *Klebsiella, Escherichia coli*, anerobic streptococci etc.

There is some controversy concerning the use of prophylactic antibiotics in these patients.

The proponents of prophylaxis claim that this will stop many infections from occurring; the opponents claim that prophylactic therapy will only prevent infection by sensitive organisms and that infection with some other organisms will result. Certainly, prophylactic treatment with low doses of penicillin or tetracycline may prevent a few infections by sensitive organisms. If it has been the experience of a physician with an individual patient that he does develop diplococcal pneumonia several times every winter, perhaps it may be worthwhile to try prophylaxis. In the majority of patients, however, prophylaxis should be discouraged because it simply encourages growth of resistant strains, colonization by resistant bacteria, or sensitivity to the antibiotics being used.[5,12,20,42,46]

There are several other complications which can occur. Congestive heart failure, especially right-sided heart failure (cor pulmonale), is a fairly common finding and may require treatment with digitalis, diuretics, etc. Polycythemia occurs frequently and may cause problems if the hematocrit gets too high. In these cases, venesection may be required to keep it at 55% or less. Acute respiratory failure and respiratory acidosis may occur, often as a result of pulmonary infections. The aim of treatment is to reduce bronchospasm, remove mucus secretions, treat infection (if present), correct hypoxemia, hypercapnia and heart failure. This involves the vigorous use of some of the things already mentioned, including oxygen, humidification, bronchodilators, mucolytics, corticosteroids, antibiotics, etc.[5,28]

6. It is vitally important that the patient be educated concerning his disease. He should have an understanding of what is happening to him and how the disease process can be slowed or halted. The treatment of COPD involves many processes, procedures and drugs. If the patient is to comply with all of this, he must understand why it is important that he do so. Also, the patient must learn to recognize problems or potential problems which might arise. For example, it is extremely important that infections be treated promptly and vigorously. For this reason, the patient has to be aware of not only the first signs and symptoms of the infection, but also what might happen if he delays seeking proper treatment.

The treatment of bronchiectasis will involve many of the same principles and procedures mentioned above. Postural drainage will usually afford significant improvement in the symptoms. Antibiotics are used to treat acute exacerbations. The problems associated with prophylactic treatment in patients with emphysema or acute bronchitis apply equally well here. Surgery may be used in an effort to resect the diseased areas. Significant improvement has been demonstrated in some patients in whom the disease was localized, thereby allowing easy resection of the lesions.[1,3]

PROGNOSIS

The prognosis of COPD is extremely variable. Death due to the disease may occur within several years after the onset of symptoms; likewise, some patients will live for many decades and will eventually die from some unrelated cause. The usual case is slowly progressive with acute exacerbations which may cause death. The average 5-year mortality rate is 50%.

There are several processes which relate particularly to a poor prognosis. These are: a sudden loss of weight, severe dyspnea, and one or more episodes of right-sided heart failure. In addition to these the following may affect or give a clue to the prognosis:

1. The height above sea level at which the patient lives is important. Generally speaking, the higher the elevation, the shorter the lifespan. This is thought to be due to an increased hematocrit which will occur at higher elevations and which may precipitate heart failure.

2. Women seem to fare better than men.

3. Patients in whom the disease develops later in life do better than patients in whom the signs and symptoms occur earlier in life.

4. Patients who must work at physically taxing jobs do not fare as well as those who have less demanding work.

5. Patients who continue to smoke do not do as well as those who quit.

6. Finally, the type of onset of this disease can be important. Those in whom the first symptoms were related to dyspnea had the poorest prognosis; those in whom overproduction of mucus was the first sign did moderately well; and those in whom the first signs were asthmatic did the best.[47-49]

The prognosis of bronchiectasis is much

better than that of emphysema or chronic bronchitis. If infection is adequately treated, or if the disease is amenable to surgical intervention, the prognosis for a normal life is very good. If the infectious processes can not be controlled or if the disease is widespread, the mortality rate is 30% in 10 years.[1,3]

CONCLUSION

COPD involves a number of interrelated disease processes. The basic abnormality is resistance to flow of air in the lungs, particularly on expiration. Recognition of the etiological factors is important because it allows us to institute programs to reduce the very high incidence of these diseases. The treatment program involves a number of related processes which may aid in slowing or stopping the progression of the disease. The usual case, however, is slowly progressive, and death may result within 5 to 10 years after onset of symptoms.

REFERENCES

1. Howell, J. B. L.: Airway obstruction. In Cecil-Loeb Textbook of Medicine, Ed. 13, p. 881, edited by P. B. Beeson and W. McDermott. W. B. Saunders Co., Philadelphia, 1971.
2. American Thoracic Society: Chronic bronchitis, asthma, and pulmonary emphysema. Am. Rev. Respir. Dis., 85: 762, 1962.
3. Crofton, J., and Douglas, A.: Respiratory Diseases, p. 347. Blackwell Scientific Publications, Oxford, England, 1969.
4. Fletcher, C. M., Jones, N. L., Burrows, B., and Niden, A. H.: American emphysema and British bronchitis. Am. Rev. Respir. Dis., 90: 1, 1964.
5. Crofton, J., and Douglas, A.: Respiratory Diseases, p. 300. Blackwell Scientific Publications, Oxford, England, 1969.
6. Belinkoff, S.: Emphysema and Chronic Bronchitis, p. 1. Little, Brown and Co., Boston, 1971.
7. Spencer, H.: Pathology of the Lung, Ed. 2, p. 116. Pergamon Press, Oxford, England, 1968.
8. Auerbach, O., Hammond, E. C., Garfinkel, L., and Benante, C.: Relation of smoking and age to emphysema. N. Engl. J. Med., 286: 853, 1972.
9. Knowles, J. H.: Chronic obstructive pulmonary disease. Bronchitis and emphysema. In Harrison's Principles of Internal Medicine, Ed. 6, p. 1290, edited by M. W. Wintrobe, G. W. Thorn, R. D. Adams, I. L. Bennett, Jr., E. Braunwald, J. J. Iselbacher, and R. G. Peters-

dorf. McGraw-Hill Book Co., New York, 1970.
10. FitzGerald, M. X., Carrington, C. B., and Gaensler, E. A.: Environmental lung disease. Med. Clin. North Am., 57: 593, 1973.
11. Reid, L.: The Pathology of Emphysema, p. 158. Lloyd-Luke, Ltd., London, 1967.
12. Hallett, W. Y.: Infection: the real culprit in chronic bronchitis and emphysema? Med. Clin. North Am., 57: 735, 1973.
13. Anon.: Enzyme deficiency and emphysema. Br. Med. J., 3: 655, 1971.
14. Larson, R. K., Barman, M. L., Kueppers, F., and Fudenberg, H. H.: Genetic and environmental determinants of chronic obstructive pulmonary disease. Ann. Intern. Med., 72: 627, 1970.
15. Boggs, P. B., Stephens, A. L., and Jenkins, D. E.: Emphysema associated with a deficiency in alpha-1-antitrypsin globulin. South. Med. J., 64: 426, 1971.
16. Makino, S., Chosy, L., Valdinia, E., and Reed, C. E.: Emphysema with hereditary alpha-1-antitrypsin deficiency masquerading as asthma. J. Allergy Clin. Immunol., 46: 40, 1970.
17. Black, L. F., Hyatt, R. E., and Stubbs, S. E.: Mechanism of expiratory airflow limitation in chronic obstructive pulmonary disease associated with alpha-1-antitrypsin deficiency. Am. Rev. Respir. Dis., 105: 891, 1972.
18. College of General Practitioners: Chronic bronchitis in Great Britain. Br. Med. J., 2: 973, 1961.
19. Rosenblatt, M. B.: Emphysema. J. Am. Geriatr. Soc., 18: 517, 1970.
20. Belinkoff, S.: Emphysema and Chronic Bronchitis, p. 27. Little, Brown and Co., Boston, 1971.
21. Macklem, P. T.: The pathophysiology of chronic bronchitis and emphysema. Med. Clin. North Am., 57: 669, 1973.
22. Mitchell, R. S., Silvers, G. W., Goodman, N., Dart, G., and Maisel, J. C.: Are centrilobular emphysema and panlobular emphysema two different diseases? Hum. Pathol., 1: 433, 1970.
23. Spencer, H.: Pathology of the Lung, Ed. 2, p. 517. Pergamon Press, Oxford, England, 1968.
24. Thurlbeck, W. M.: Chronic bronchitis and emphysema. Med. Clin. North Am., 57: 651, 1973.
25. Duffell, G. M., Marcus, J. H., and Ingram, R. H.: Limitation of expiratory flow in chronic obstructive pulmonary disease. Ann. Intern. Med., 72: 365, 1970.
26. Knowles, J. H.: Bronchiectasis, bronchial obstruction, and lung abscess. In Harrison's Principles of Internal Medicine, Ed. 6, p. 1332, edited by M. W. Wintrobe, G. W. Thorn, R. D. Adams, I. L. Bennett, Jr., E. Braunwald, J. J. Isselbacher, and R. G. Petersdorf. McGraw-Hill Book Co., New York, 1970.
27. Filley, G. F.: Emphysema and chronic bronchitis: clinical manifestations and their physiologic

significance. Med. Clin. North Am., 51: 283, 1967.

28. Bocles, J. S., and Llamas, R.: Airway obstruction. Med. Clin. North Am., 55: 445, 1971.

29. Petty, T. L.: Ambulatory care for emphysema and chronic bronchitis. Chest, 58: 441, 1970.

30. Spitzer, S. A., Goldschmidt, Z., and Dubrowsky, C.: The bronchodilator effect of salbutamol administered by IPPB to patients with asthma. Chest, 62: 273, 1972.

31. Vale, J. R.: Oral salbutamol as a supplement to inhaled aerosol in obstructive respiratory disease. Scand. J. Respir. Dis., 52: 58, 1971.

32. Chervinsky, P.: Evaluation of a new selective beta-adrenergic receptor stimulant. Ann. Allergy, 29: 627, 1971.

33. Petty, T. L., Hudson, L. D., and Neff, T. A.: Methods of ambulatory care. Med. Clin. North Am., 57: 751, 1973.

34. Lieberman, J.: The appropriate use of mucolytic agents. Am. J. Med., 49: 1, 1970.

35. Swinyard, E. A.: Demulcents, emollients, protectives and absorbents, antiperspirants and deodorants, absorbable hemostatics, astringents, irritants, sclerosing agents, caustics, keratolytics, antiseborrheics, melanizing and demelanizing agents, mucolytics, and certain enzymes. In The Pharmacological Basis of Therapeutics, Ed. 4, p. 987, edited by L. S. Goodman and A. Gilman. The MacMillan Co., New York, 1970.

36. Hurst, G. A., Shaw, P. D., and LeMaistre, C. A.: Laboratory and clinical evaluation of the mucolytic properties of acetylcyteine. Am. Rev. Respir. Dis., 96: 962, 1967.

37. Cobbin, D. M., Elliott, F. M., and Reback, A. S.: The mycolytic agent bromhexine (Bisolvon) in chronic lung disease. Aust. N. Z. J. Med.,

2: 137, 1971.

38. Thompson, K. J., and Reeve, J.: A clinical trial of bromhexine. N. Z. J. Med., 76: 73, 1972.

39. Kass, I., and Rubin, H.: Chest physiotherapy for chronic obstructive pulmonary disease. Postgrad. Med., 48: 145, 1970.

40. Miller, W. F.: Treatment of chronic pulmonary emphysema. Postgrad. Med., 39: 230, 1966.

41. Webster, Jr., and Addington, W. W.: Chronic bronchitis and emphysema. Postgrad. Med., 50: 113, 1971.

42. Bruce, R. M., and Hirst, R. N.: Pulmonary disease. In Manual of Medical Therapeutics, Ed. 20, p. 191, edited by M. G. Rosenfeld. Little, Brown and Co., Boston, 1971.

43. Petty, T. L.: Misunderstanding concerning the proper clinical use of oxygen. Ann. Intern. Med., 70: 645, 1969.

44. Clark, T. J. H., Collins, J. V., and Tong, D.: Respiratory depression caused by nitrazepam in patients with respiratory failure. Lancet, 2: 737, 1971.

45. Hilton, A. M.: Sedative drugs in respiratory failure. Lancet, 2: 922, 1971.

46. Burrows, B., and Nevin, W.: Antibiotic management in patients with chronic bronchitis and emphysema (editorial). Ann. Intern. Med., 77: 993, 1972.

47. Mitchell, R. S., Webb, N. C. and Filley, G. F.: Chronic obstructive broncho-pulmonary disease. Am. Rev. Respir. Dis., 89: 878, 1964.

48. Emirgil, C., and Sobol, B. J.: Long-term course of chronic obstructive pulmonary disease. Am. J. Med., 51: 504, 1971.

49. Burrows, B., and Earle, R. H.: Course and prognosis of chronic obstructive lung disease. N. Engl. J. Med., 280: 397, 1969.

Endocrine diseases

chapter **18**

HYPERTHYROIDISM

Barbara Sauer, Pharm.D.

Hyperthyroidism is a condition due to increased activity of the thyroid gland which results in excess secretion of the thyroid hormones. It may range in severity from a very mild, hypermetabolic state to a serious, life-threatening crisis, although most patients with the disease have symptoms somewhere in between. The symptoms are generalized, affecting nearly every organ system in the body, especially the cardiovascular, neuromuscular and gastrointestinal systems. The presenting symptoms are often vague and suggestive of other diseases, eluding proper diagnosis.

A basic understanding of the etiology of the disease, methods of detection and optimal treatment enables the pharmacist to participate in achieving the goal of therapy for the patient. The patient who is managed medically requires education about the drugs employed, dosing schedules and possible side effects which may occur. Because many of the symptoms of the disease are overt, yet nonspecific, the alert pharmacist may be involved in the detection of previously undiagnosed cases. He or she may also be called upon to recommend proprietary products for colds, hay fever or sinus congestions, many of which contain sympathomimetics and are cautioned against in thyroid disease.

PHYSIOLOGY

The thyroid gland secretes two metabolically active hormones: triiodothyronine (T_3) and thyroxine (T_4). Synthesis of the hormones is dependent upon an anterior pituitary hormone, thyrotrophin (thyroid-stimulating hormone, TSH), which is a glycoprotein of molecular weight 25,000.[1] TSH secretion is regulated by thyrotrophin-releasing factor (TRF), which is a tripeptide formed in the hypothalamus and transported to the pituitary via portal vessels[1] (Fig. 18.1). The secretion of TSH is regulated by a negative feedback mechanism: high circulating levels of thyroid hormones suppress TSH release and render the pituitary unresponsive to TRF. As the hormone levels drop, the pituitary becomes responsive to TRF once again and TSH is secreted.

Three major steps are involved in the production of the hormones, all of which are stimulated by TSH (or perhaps long acting thyroid stimulator [LATS] in Graves' disease): iodine trapping, hormone biosynthesis and storage, and hormone release.[2] Iodine is absorbed from the gastrointestinal (GI) tract as iodide and dispersed throughout the total body iodide pool. The thyroid gland traps iodide via a peroxidase enzyme system, and tyrosine molecules in the gland are subsequently iodinated to form monoiodotyrosine (MIT) and diiodotyrosine (DIT). MIT and DIT undergo a coupling reaction to form T_3 and T_4, which is facilitated by a stereochemical relationship in the thyroglobulin molecule, rather than an enzymatic process.[1,2] Triiodothyronine and thyroxine are stored within the colloid cells in the gland until released by a proteolytic hydrolysis. Other iodotyrosines (MIT, DIT, etc.) also released are deiodinated enzymatically, contributing about 2/3 of the iodide available for new hormone synthesis, the remaining 1/3 coming from newly trapped iodide.[2]

The released hormones are bound extensively to plasma proteins, to be slowly released as the active or "free" hormones. Thyroxine binds primarily to thyroid-binding globulin — TBG (60%), thyroid-binding prealbumin — TBPA (30%), and to a small extent, albumin (10%). Triiodothyronine is less extensively bound to TBG and albumin but does not bind to TBPA.[1] The serum half-life of T_4 is about 6 days, while that of T_3 is about 1 day.[3] Approx-

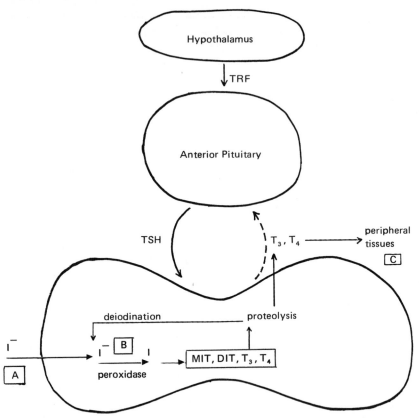

FIG. 18.1. Hormone synthesis in the thyroid gland, showing sites of action of antithyroid agents. A. Thiocynate; B, thioamides, thiocynate, perchlorate, iodide; C, beta adrenergic blocking agents; →, stimulatory pathway; - - - →, inhibitory pathway.

imately one-third of the circulating thyroxine is metabolized to triiodothyronine daily, accounting for as much as 40% of the daily production of T_3.[3,4]

In hyperthyroidism, excess production of thyroid hormones leads to increased serum concentrations of hormones, which is augmented by decreased levels of TBG and TBPA. The hepatic thyroxine pool is elevated, which may account for the stimulation of the hepatic microsomal enzyme system which degrades thyroxine and its binding proteins.[2] The net effect is an increase in "free" thyroxine at the cellular level.

Thyrotoxicosis is characterized by an increase in oxygen consumption as reflected by an elevated basal metabolic rate (BMR). Originally, this was thought to be due to uncoupling of oxidative phosphorylation, a process which utilizes energy from mitochondria for the formation of adenosine triphosphate (ATP). Recent studies have shown the increased oxy-

gen consumption to be more likely due to an increase in mitochondrial mass in skeletal muscle, rather than an increase in the rate of oxygen consumption.[5,6]

As with other hormones, thyroid stimulates the adenosine 3'5'-monophosphate (cyclic AMP) system via the enzyme adenyl cyclase, which converts ATP to cyclic AMP, thereby initiating a physiological response at the cellular level.[6,7] It is known that catecholamines stimulate adenyl cylase as well, probably by an independent mechanism since thyroid status has no effect on the norephinephrine stimulation of cyclic 3', 5'-AMP.[6] This could explain the clinical increased sensitivity to circulating catecholamines in thyrotoxicosis, although more studies in this area are needed.

Many of the clinical symptoms of thyrotoxicosis reflect an increase in the activity of the adrenergic nervous system, primarily cardiovascular and neuromuscular. Frequently encountered symptoms include palpitations, tachycardia, tremors, nervousness, irritability, fatigue, muscle weakness, weight loss despite increased appetite, rapid deep tendon reflexes, lid lag and stare, menstrual irregularities and increased frequency of bowel movements. Since many of these symptoms are seen in other diseases (GI diseases, pheochromocytoma, myasthenia gravis), proper diagnosis necessitates demonstration of hyperfunction of the thyroid gland.

LABORATORY TESTS

Laboratory tests to measure thyroid function are an integral component of the diagnosis of thyroid disease. Generally, they are designed to measure the levels of the circulating hormones or to assess the degree of activity of the gland. Formerly, assessment of the basal metabolic rate (BMR) was also included in the diagnosis of thyroid disease, but it is rarely used now because of its nonspecific nature. The BMR measures the ability of the thyroid gland to stimulate oxygen consumption,[8] and in addition to being elevated in hyperthyroidism it may be elevated with fever, hypertension, pheochromocytoma and malignancies.

Another test of metabolic status which may be useful in assessing a patient's clinical response to therapy is the ankle tendon reflex time as measured on a photomotograph or similar device. It is of limited usefulness in the diagnosis of hyperthyroidism because, although the reflexes are rapid, there is a significant degree of overlap within the normal range.[8]

Tests Measuring Circulating Hormones

Tests measuring the serum hormone concentrations are either direct or indirect with respect to measuring the metabolically active hormone. Most frequently, indirect tests (PBI, BEI, T_4I by column or Murphy-Pattee and resin T_3 uptake) measuring circulating hormone bound to plasma proteins or degree of saturation of hormone on the protein, are utilized and are elevated in hyperthyroidism. Recently, techniques have been developed to measure the free hormones directly, which are much more accurate. The following is a brief description of the more commonly used tests and possible mechanisms of interference (Table 18.1).

Protein-bound Iodine. The PBI measures the iodine content of precipitated plasma proteins. Since the circulating thyroid hormones are highly protein-bound, an approximation of the level of thyroxine in the body may be made from the amount of iodine extracted from plasma proteins.[9] Unfortunately, inorganic and organic iodine contaminants are also measured and may be a cause of a falsely elevated PBI.[9] Misleading values are also obtained in the presence of abnormal thyroid-binding protein levels, which are increased in pregnancy and depressed in nephrosis and certain idiopathic conditions,[8,9] although the metabolic status remains unchanged.

Many drugs interfere with the determination of thyroxine-iodine by the PBI method. Iodide or iodine-containing medicinals, including expectorants, amoebacides and radiocontrast material, elevate the PBI.[9,10] Estrogens and oral contraceptives increase thyroid-binding proteins, resulting in elevation of T_4I, while androgens and anabolic steroids depress thyroid-binding protein levels and T_4I. Other drugs which lower the PBI include diphenylhydantoin and large doses of salicylates, which displace thyroxine from its binding proteins.[9,10]

Butanol-extractable Iodine. The BEI parallels the PBI, although inorganic iodide contaminants will not interfere with the test due to the extraction procedure. Other organic iodides (radiocontrast agents) and drugs interfering with the PBI will also influence the BIE.[9]

Thyroxine-Iodine by Column. A more specific measurement of the thyroxine-iodine is achieved with the use of an anion-exchange resin and column chromatography. The major advantage of this technique is the exclusion of the contamination due to iodoproteins and iodine-containing medicinals, with the exception of some radiocontrast agents.[9] Any abnormalities in the level of circulating thyroid-binding proteins, or alterations in the nature of protein binding will influence the T_4I by column in the same manner as with the PBI.

Thyroxine by Murphy-Pattee – True T_4. The most specific indirect measurement of thyroxine is the Murphy-Pattee technique, which is not influenced by any organic or inorganic iodines.[11] Thyroxine is extracted from a sample of the patient's serum and added to TBG labeled with radioactive T_4. The amount of labeled T_4 displaced is measured and compared to a standard curve to determine the amount of T_4 in the patient's serum,[11,12]

TABLE 18.1

Effects of Various Conditions and Drugs On Laboratory Tests

Test	Normal Values	Inorganic Iodide	Organic Iodide	Pregnancy, Estrogens	Androgens, Anabolic Steroids, Nephrosis	Dilantin Salicylates (large doses)
PBI	4-8 µg/100 ml	↑	↑	↑	↓	↓
BEI	2.9-6.5 µg/100 ml	—	↑	↑	↓	↓
T_4-I (column)	2.9-6.5 µg/100 ml	—	↑	↑	↓	↓
TT_4 (Murphy-Pattee)	5-14.5 µg/100 ml	—	—	↑	↓	↓
Free T_4	2.75±0.5 µg/100 ml	—	—	—	—	—
RT_3U	25-35%	—	—	↓	↑	↑
RAIU	15-40% at 24 hr	↓	↓	—	—	—

which is reported as the true T_4 (TT_4), or T_4I which is 65% of the TT_4 by molecular weight. As with other indirect tests of thyroxine, this test is also influenced by abnormal levels of thyroid-binding proteins or alterations in the nature of protein binding.

Resin T_3 Uptake. The T_3 uptake utilizes the differences in the binding characteristics of T_3 and T_4 to estimate the degree of saturation of T_4 on TBG. A resin containing radioactive T_3 is added to a sample of the patient's serum and allowed to equilibrate. Since T_3 is less tightly bound to TBG than T_4, it will not displace endogenous T_4 and must occupy the unbound protein sites.[13] The radioactivity remaining on the resin after equilibration is measured and is indirectly proportional to the number of unbound sites available to T_3. In hyperthyroidism, the degree of saturation of thyroxine on protein is increased, with fewer binding sites available to T_3, resulting in increased levels of labeled T_3 on the resin.[9,12,13] If TBG levels are elevated (pregnancy, estrogens, oral contraceptives), there is a corresponding increase in available binding sites, and the T_3 uptake on the resin is decreased. The reverse is true with depressed TBG levels (nephrosis, androgens, anabolic steroids).[9,12,13] Occupation of available binding sites on TBG with diphenylhydantoin, or shift of T_4 from TBPA to TBG due to displacement by salicylates also results in increased T_3 resin uptake values.[9,13]

Free Thyroxine. Unbound thyroxine may be measured directly utilizing a dialysis technique after labeling the patient's serum *in vitro.*[11] Although technically difficult, direct measurement of the unbound or metabolically active hormone has the advantage of reflecting true physiological status and is not influenced by any thyroid-binding protein abnormalities. Only hyperthyroidism produces an elevation of the free thyroxine.

Serum Triiodothyronine. The measurement of serum triiodothyronine has been developed in recent years and involves the displacement of T_3 from TBG by a technique similar to the Murphy-Pattee method for T_4.[11] Although the procedure is difficult, the results of this method are very useful in the diagnosis of hyperthyroidism due to preferential T_3 toxicity, when other laboratory results are often not elevated.[14]

Tests of Glandular Activity

Radioactive Iodine Uptake. An approximation of the function of the gland may be made by its ability to incorporate iodine. The percentage glandular uptake of a trace oral dose of radioactive iodine is measured at intervals of about 1, 5 and 24 hr after ingestion of the tracer.[13] In hyperthyroidism, where the gland is rapidly incorporating iodine and synthesizing hormone, these values are elevated. A scintillation scan may be taken simultaneously at 24 hr and any nodules present may be visualized.

Many drugs and foods are known to interfere with the RAIU owing to alterations in the total body iodine pool. Ingestion of substances high in iodine or iodide result in expansion of the iodide pool, delivering a smaller percentage of the pool to the thyroid gland and decreasing the RAIU.[9,13] Contraction of the pool, as seen in chronic iodine deficiency or with vigorous diuretic therapy, results in a greater daily percentage uptake or increased RAIU.[9,13]

Triiodothyronine Suppression Test. The T_3 suppression test is useful in the diagnosis of an autonomously functioning gland. Suppressive doses of triiodothyronine (50 to 100 μg per day in divided doses) are administered for 5 to 7 days to suppress TSH. Normally, a 24-hr RAIU will drop to below 50%[11] of the baseline value; failure to do so indicates autonomous function or nonsuppressibility by endogenous TSH.[8,11] It is primarily used to determine the suppressibility of the gland and to evaluate the success of antithyroid drug therapy, since remission is more frequently associated with a return of suppressibility.[8]

ETIOLOGY

Hyperthyroidism may be classified according to the physical characteristics of the gland into one of three types: Graves' disease, which is characterized by a diffusely enlarged, soft-to-rubbery gland; Plummer's disease, typified by a single, hyperactive nodule; and multinodular goiter, which may be characterized by activity in the nodules or in the diffuse intranodular tissue.[15] It may also be transiently associated with subacute thyroditis due to release of stored hormones in the damaged cells, or with thyrotoxicosis factitia, which is the result of an overdose of exogenous thyroid. Other causes include stimulation of the gland by thyrotrophin-like substances released by some tumors, such as some choriocarcinomas and hydatiform moles.[15]

Graves' Disease

The syndrome of diffuse thyroid enlargement, exophthalmos and thyrotoxicosis was reported by Parry in 1825, Graves in 1835 and Basedow in 1940 and has subsequently acquired the name of Graves' disease. It is the most frequent cause of hyperthyroidism and occurs primarily in women with the peak onset between the ages of 30 and 40.[15]

In addition to the hypermetabolic symptoms of thyrotoxicosis described previously, Graves' disease is unique in that it may also be associated with infiltrative ophthalmopathy, dermopathy and the presence of long acting thyroid stimulator.(LATS.)[5,15]

Exophthalmos is characterized by periorbital edema, conjunctivitis and mucopolysaccharide and lymphocytic deposition in retro-orbital tissue and muscle, which may lead to proptosis and ophthalmoplegia. It may be severe despite treatment of underlying thyroid disease and result in loss of eyesight.[15] Dermopathy, which is less frequently encountered and generally less severe, is characterized by skin thickening and intradermal deposition of a mucin-like substance, usually in the pretibial area, which is often called pretibial myxedema.[5,15] It rarely occurs in the absence of ophthalmopathy, which occurs in about 70% of the patients with Graves' disease.[15]

The exact etiology of Graves' disease is unknown, although an immune mechanism is strongly suspected. LATS was discovered by Adams and Purves in 1956 and has been shown to be immunoglobin of the IgG type[5,16,17] (Table 18.2). It has been found in the blood of 50[5] to 80[16] percent of the patients with Graves' disease and in 90% of patients with the additional presence of dermopathy.[5] The fact that it is not present in all patients with Graves' disease is evidence that there is probably a more complex etiology. Recently, there has been evidence for a thyroid-stimulating substance in LATS-negative Graves' patients, which may be the result of a more sensitive assay,[17] although it is generally agreed that additional etiological factors are present as well.

Plummer's Disease

A single hyperfunctioning nodule causing thyrotoxicosis was first described by Plummer in 1928. Unlike Graves' disease, there seems to be no difference in occurrence in either sex, and it may occur at any age.[18] The nodule is usually 3 to 5 cm in diameter, releasing supraphysiological doses of the thyroid hormones and resulting in TSH suppression and hypofunctioning of the remainder of the gland.[19] This accounts for the lack of goiter seen with this type of hyperthyroidism, which is the least common of the three major types.

TABLE 18.2
Comparison of TSH and LATS

Characteristic	TSH	LATS
Origin	Anterior pituitary	Uncertain
Composition	Glycoprotein	IgG immunoglobulin
Sedimentation constant	45	75
Molecular weight	25,000	160,000
Biological half-life	30 min	1-2 weeks
Administration of thyroxine	Depressed serum level	No effect on serum level
Placental transport	No	Yes

Toxic Multinodular Goiter

A multinodular gland is frequently asymptomatic for many years and only progresses to hyperthyroidism in about 13% of the patients.[15,18] Usually by the time these patients become symptomatic, they are in their 40's or 50's and more prone to cardiac manifestations. As with Graves' disease, there seems to be a higher incidence of the disease in females.[15,18]

Triiodothyronine Toxicosis

Rarely, a variant form of hyperthyroidism is seen which is identical clinically to thyrotoxicosis although unsubstantiated by routine laboratory tests. It has been suggested that these patients suffer from a preferential secretion of T_3, producing T_3 toxicosis.[14] It may occur in any of the three types of hyperthyroidism described above and is confirmed with a T_3 suppression test and measurement of the level of circulating T_3 Shenkman *et al.*[20] have reported a group of patients with recurrent hyperthyroidism presenting the second time as T_3 toxicosis, suggesting that perhaps preferential T_3 secretion occurs prior to the development of T_4 toxicosis.

Apathetic Hyperthyroidism

Another unusual type of hyperthyroidism frequently misdiagnosed is apathetic hyperthyroidism.[21,22] It usually occurs in the elderly, especially in women and frequently in patients who have had a multinodular goiter for many years. The presenting symptoms obscure the diagnosis and include lethargy, senility, slowed speech and mentation, muscle wasting, weight loss and other general symptoms of cardiovascular, neuromuscular or gastrointestinal disease. Hypermetabolic symptoms of the classical disease are clinically absent or obscure. Unless diagnosed properly and treated, these patients become comatose and expire, without the agitation associated with thyroid crisis.

Thyroid Storm

Acute thyroid crisis or storm is a life-threatening episode characterized by fever, tachycardia, gastrointestinal and cardiac manifestations, agitation, psychoses and coma. It may be precipitated by stress or infection or other underlying diseases characterized by excessive metabolic demands. Unless treated, the mortality is high, approaching 60%.[23]

Therapy is aimed at supporting vital functions, blocking synthesis and release of thyroid hormones and correcting the underlying disease. Sodium iodide, 1.0 to 2.0 g daily, in divided doses, is administered intravenously to block the release of preformed hormones. Propylthiouracil, 1.0 g daily in divided doses every 2 to 3 hr, may be given orally or by nasogastric tube to disrupt subsequent hormone synthesis.[23] Although there are no parenteral products available, methimazole can be dissolved in saline and heat sterilized[24] should the necessity arise, equivalent doses being 1/10 that of propylthiouracil. Sympatholytic agents may also be employed for symptomatic control of the disease. Propranolol, a beta-blocking agent, seems to be quite efficacious for this purpose[25] and may be slowly administered intravenously in divided doses of 40 to 160 mg daily. Reserpine and guanethidine have also been employed for this purpose but offer no advantages over propranolol and seem to be associated with more side effects and a mortality rate of 30 to 50% despite therapy.[24,25]

PEDIATRIC ASPECTS

Hyperthyroidism is occasionally seen in children, accounting for 1 to 5%[15,26] of the cases presented, excluding neonatal thyrotoxicosis. The peak incidence in children occurs in prepubertal age groups between the ages of 10 and 12,[26-28] and the onset is frequently associated with stress due to acute infections, trauma and fractures.[26] Like adult forms of the disease, there is a greater incidence in females.[27,28]

The presenting symptoms of juvenile hyperthyroidism are similar to those of adult forms (nervousness, weight loss, tremors, eye signs) with the notable exception of cardiovascular manifestations. Additionally, children frequently complain of excessive thirst and often suffer from restlessness and inability to concentrate, as reflected by poor grades in school.[26]

Management of the disease in children is similar to that for adults except that radioactive iodine is not used because of its high rate of production of secondary hypothyroidism. There is also a reluctance to employ the isotope because of uncertain effects on germinal tissue and progeny and the remote possibility of subsequent malignancy, especially leukemia. It is known that external radiation to the head and neck areas of children is associated with a high risk of subsequent thyroid carcinoma[28,29] although this has not been shown with internal radiation. A strong association between hyperthyroidism and leukemia has been demonstrated, but it has not been shown to be statistically higher after radioactive iodine therapy.[28,30]

Another consideration important in this age group is compliance. Active school-aged children who are managed medically may have trouble adhering to rigid dosing schedules, requiring an alternate mode of therapy.[28,29]

NEONATAL THYROTOXICOSIS

Neonatal thyrotoxicosis, unlike spontaneous juvenile hyperthyroidism, is an acute disease characterized by severe cardiovascular and respiratory symptoms. It accounts for most cases of the disease under the age of 2, although there have been occasional reports of idiopathic disease in infancy.[31,32] It is an hereditary disease occurring in infants of mothers with Graves' disease, and it may occur in either sex. Although frequently severe, the disease is self-limiting.[32]

High LATS titers are usually found in the serum of both the mother and infant, suggesting the etiology of the disease. A fall in the LATS titer is associated with spontaneous remission and generally occurs in 1 to 2 months. This is consistent with the half-life of LATS, which has been reported to be from 6 days to 1 to 2 weeks.[16]

Therapy is generally limited to symptomatic control with iodides to prevent subsequent hormone release and propranolol to control peripheral manifestations. Thioamides are seldom used because of the self-limiting nature of the disease.

PREGNANCY

Occasionally a woman with hyperthyroidism becomes pregnant or a pregnat woman develops hyperthyroidism—a rare event regardless of sequence.[33] Hyperthyroidism in the pregnant woman creates special problems with respect to management of the disease because most of the agents used to treat thyrotoxicosis cross the placenta. Thioamides readily cross the placenta and have been associated with spontaneous abortion[34,35] or significant morbidity to the fetus, including goiter which may cause asphyxiation. Iodides also cross the placenta, affecting the fetal gland when it begins to incorporate iodide at 12 weeks.[33] However, if the maternal disease is left untreated, the fetal mortality rate may reach 10%.[36]

Maternal thyroid-binding proteins are elevated in the pregnant woman and may be twice the concentration of those in the fetus at term.[33,34] If the mother is receiving antithyroid medication, the fetus may become hypothyroid owing to delayed placental transport of

T_3 and T_4 and the decreased binding of the proteins for the hormones.[33-35] Coadministration of physiological doses of thyroxine or triiodothyronine has been proposed to protect the mother against hypothyroidism; however, this is not sufficient to prevent hypothyroidism in the fetus.[33-35] Additionally, this practice obscures the clinical status of the mother, which otherwise allows titration of the drugs to the lowest dose effective for the control of symptoms.[35]

Surgery in the 1st or last trimester may induce premature labor,[36] although it is generally safe in the 2nd trimester of pregnancy. It is usually recommended that the goal of therapy be surgery in the late 2nd or early 3rd trimester[33,34] after rendering the patient euthyroid with thioamides. If unable to prepare the patient properly for surgery, thioamides may be continued throughout the pregnancy. Initial doses of propylthiouracil (PTU) should be as low as possible (300 mg daily) with gradual tapering to 100 to 150 mg daily or less. Single daily doses may be attempted since some recovery from the antithyroid effects may suppress goiter formation in both mother and fetus.

Both PTU and iodides are also excreted in breast milk[36]; hence the pharmacist should caution the mother against nursing.

TREATMENT OF HYPERTHYROIDISM

Management of the disease may be achieved with one of three methods: antithyroid drugs, radioactive iodine, or surgery. Each has its advantages and limitations (Table 18.3), and so the specific mode of therapy must be selected for each patient individually. The decision is usually based upon the type and severity of hyperthyroidism present, the patient's age, cosmetic considerations, presence of underlying disease and response to previous therapy. Patients with Graves' disease may have cyclical disease that is able to be controlled medically until remission occurs, whereas Plummer's disease is progressive and requires definitive therapy with radioactive iodine or surgery.[37] Severe ophthalmological, cardiac or psychotic complications also require ablation of the gland, preferably with radioactive iodine since these patients are frequently also poor surgical risk patients.

ANTITHYROID DRUGS

Antithyroid drugs fall into three categories: thioamides, monovalent anions (perchlorate, thiocynate) and iodine. The thioamides are used routinely in the control of thyrotoxicosis; however, perchlorate and iodides are of limited usefulness, as described in Table 18.4.

Thioamides

The thioamides are thiourea derivatives which interfere with the organification (oxidation) of iodine, probably owing to antagonism of the peroxidase enzyme system. To a lesser extent, they block the coupling of MIT and

TABLE 18.3
Comparison of Treatment of Hyperthyroidism

Treatment	Indications	Contraindications
Thioamides	Children, young adults, pregnancy	Hypersensitivity
Surgery	Pregnancy, children, Plummer's disease, multinodular goiter	Debilitating disease, patient unable to be prepared, previous thyroid surgery
Radioactive iodine	Adult Graves', Plummer's disease; young adults with serious cardiac complications	Children, pregnancy

TABLE 18.4
Antithyroid Drugs

Drug	Mechanism of Action	Dose	Available Preparations	Toxicity
Propylthiouracil	Blocks organification of iodides, coupling of iodotyrosines	300-600mg/day initially, divided doses	50 mg tablets	Skin rash, leukopenia, thrombocytopenia, agranulocytosis (0.12%)
Methimazole	Blocks organification of iodides, coupling of iodotyrosines	15-60mg/day initially, divided doses	5, 10 mg tablets	Skin rash, leukopenia, thrombocytopenia, agranulocytosis (0.44%)
Iodide	Blocks organification of iodides, prevents release of stored hormones	6.0mg of iodide daily, Lugols or SSKI, qtts iii po tid; sodium iodide 1-2g I.V.	Lugol's Sol'n., SSKI, sodium iodide for injection	Hypersensitivity; skin rash, serum sickness, iodism
Perchlorate	Competes with iodide, interfering with iodide trapping, promoting discharge of unorganified iodide	Up to 250 mg qid	Sodium or potassium perchlorate	Nausea, vomiting, skin rash, lymphadenopathy, leukopenia, agranulocytosis, aplastic anemia
Propranolol	Beta-adrenergic blocking agent, no effect on underlying thyroid disease	40 mg qid	10, 40 mg tablets	Heart failure, increased airway resistance, hypoglycemia, nausea, vomiting, diarrhea, constipation, lightheadedness, rash

DIT but have no effect on the ability of the gland to trap iodine.

Propylthiouracil and methimazole are currently used in this country, while another derivative, carbimazole, is available in Great Britain. The drugs are rapidly absorbed from the gastrointestinal tract, with peak effect of PTU around 2 hr and decline of activity after 6 to 8 hours.[24]

The usual dose of PTU is 300 to 600 mg initially in divided doses. The dose of methimazole is about 1/10 that of PTU. Although a divided dosing schedule is usually recommended initially, there have been reports of success with the total daily dose in one single dose,[38,39] although not all patients in the groups reported could be managed in such a manner.

Recently, the perchlorate discharge test, originally described by Astwood in 1948, has been re-evaluated[40] as an aid in predicting the patient's response to thioamides. Perchlorate blocks the trapping of iodide into the gland and causes discharge of nonorganified iodide. Normally, an elevation of the RAIU is seen 1 hr after ingestion of the isotope, which increases during the 2nd hr. After administration of 1.0 g of potassium perchlorate, the 1-hr RAIU plateaus since no discharge occurs. However, if the patient is successfully blocked with thioamides, a 95% discharge of RAI occurs by the 2nd hr, indicating that the tracer was trapped, but not organified. By administration of this test at 12 hr after the last dose of thioamide, Barnes and Bledsoe were able to predict the optimal dosing schedule for their patients with 91% accuracy.[40] Although further study is necessary in this area, the perchlorate-discharge test may prove to be very useful in determining which patients require divided doses and which may be controlled with one or two daily doses.

The toxicities of PTU and methimazole occur in about 3 and 5% of the patients, respectively, with agranulocytosis occuring in 0.1 to 0.4%.[5,37] Skin rashes are most frequently encountered and often disappear with continued therapy, although another agent may be substituted, since there is little cross reaction between thioamides. Serious side effects include agranulocytosis, leukopenia and thrombocytopenia, which may occur so rapidly as to elude detection in routine white blood count.[37] For this reason, it is necessary that the pharmacist educate the patient about the importance of reporting sudden fever and sore throat to the physician.

Therapy is usually continued for 12 to 18 months and clinical response may be monitored with routine lab tests such as PBI, T_4I and T_3, uptake. Since the rate of relapse is high (about 50 to 70% relapse within the 1st year[5,37]), attempts have been made to predict the degree of success. Return of suppressibility of the gland, as measured by a 20-min radioactive uptake test (unaffected by thioamides) with a drop in the uptake of at least 50%, carries a much more favorable prognosis.[37] Remissions on drug therapy are also more likely to occur with mild disease of short duration and when a reduction in goiter occurs during treatment.[5,41] An increase in the goiter during therapy may be a sign of overtreatment and is treated by either reducing the dose or administering physiological doses of thyroid hormone.

Ionic Inhibitors

Anions which resemble iodine in size and valence interfere with iodine trapping by the thyroid gland, effectively blocking hormone synthesis. Thiocynate and perchlorate have been used for this purpose in this country, although they are rarely used therapeutically today.

Thiocynate is not concentrated by the gland but is metabolized in the gland and found to inhibit the uptake and organification of iodide.[24] Addition of iodide will reverse its action. Perchlorate, on the other hand, is concentrated by the gland and is a competitive inhibitor of iodide, interfering with its binding and promoting the discarge of iodide taken up by the gland.[24] Sodium or potassium perchlorate in doses of 1.0 g per day are efficacious for controlling hyperthyroidism and are tolerated well by most patients. Usual side effects include nausea, gastrointestinal disturbances, rashes and lymphadenopathy. Serious toxicities include leukopenia, agranulocytosis and aplastic anemia (potentially fatal), although they are rarely seen at doses below 1.0 g daily.[24] For this reason, perchlorate is not used routinely, although it may be used for the perchlorate-discharge test described above.

Iodide

Iodide ion has a paradoxical effect on the thyroid gland; it is necessary for hormone production, yet, in excess it may suppress hormone release in susceptible persons. The normal gland requires 50 to 500 μg[42] of iodide daily for hormone synthesis and is insensitive to the antithyroid effect of larger doses because high intracellular concentrations of iodide are not maintained. In the abnormal thyrotoxic gland, high intracellular concentrations are maintained with excessive doses of iodides, causing a block in the organification of iodide and prevention of the release of synthesized hormone.[042]

The maximal effect is seen in 10 to 14 days, after which time there may be an escape from the effects. For this reason, iodides are primarily used as adjuvants to surgery to decrease the vascularity and increase the firmness of the gland. The major toxicity of iodides is due to hypersensitivity, ranging from skin rash to angioedema. Various preparations containing iodide are available, all being equally efficacious in therapeutic doses of at least 6.0 mg daily.[24] Usually Lugol's solution or saturated solution potassium iodide (SSKI) are administered, in doses of 0.3 ml 3 times a day for 10 to 14 days prior to surgery. In acute situations, sodium iodide may be administered intravenously in doses of 1.0 to 2.0 g daily.

Sympatholytic Agents

The association of hyperthyroidism and hyperfunction of the adrenergic nervous system has long been recognized, which has led to the proposal of adrenergic blocking agents for the treatment of thyrotoxicosis. Although they may effectively control symptoms associated with hyperthyroidism, adrenergic blockers have no effect on underlying thyroid disease or its progression. Reserpine and quanethidine, which interfere with the uptake and release of catecholamines in the adrenergic neuron, have been used in the past for this purpose. They have not proven satisfactory because of their slow onset (up to several weeks) and frequent side effects (mental depression, diarrhea, postural hypotension). They have been largely replaced by propranolol, a specific beta-blocking agent.

Although there have been isolated reports of success with propranolol alone[43], its use is limited to combination with more conventional agents to treat the underlying disease. It may be useful for symptomatic control of the disease until the effect of RAI takes place.

Effective beta-adrenergic blockade may improve tachycardia, tremor, hyper-reflexia, excessive perspiration, palpitations and heat intolerance, as displayed with both propranolol[44] and sotolol[45] but it has no effect on infiltrative ophthalmopathy or dermopathy, weight loss or serum cholesterol.[45] The doses of propranolol usually recommended are 40 mg 4 times daily. Propranolol should be used very cautiously in patients with asthma, congestive heart failure or recent history of myocardial infarction, as it may increase airway resistance and have direct cardiac depressant effects.

Radioactive Iodine

Since its initial application in the 1950's, radioactive iodine has remained an effective alternative for the treatment of hyperthyroidism. The isotope most frequently used is ^{131}I, which has a half-life of 8 days and delivers beta-radiation about 2 mm.[46]

The effects of internal radiation are 2-fold: initially the radiation is delivered at a diminishing rate over a period of 4 weeks causing cellular destruction and disruption of hormone synthesis; later, chromosomal damage interrupts cell division, which contributes to the development of secondary hypothyroidism.[5,46] Secondary hypothyroidism is a frequent occurrence, usually appearing in about 10% of the patients within the 1st year and an additional 2 to 4% each year thereafter,[5,46] accounting for 20-year incidences of 30 to 70%.[46]

Radioactive iodine is contraindicated in young children and pregnant women as described previously. It is primarily indicated in patients over 40 years of age with Graves' disease, with Plummer's disease and in the presence of increased surgical risks—as in cardiovascular disease and for recurrent hyperthyroidism previously treated with surgery.[5,36]

Surgery

Another effective alternative for controlling hyperthyroidism is subtotal thyroidectomy where a portion of the gland is removed. The procedure is associated with a low mortality and morbidity rate (vocal cord paralysis, hypoparathyroidism), although secondary hypothyroidism seems to be cumulative, as with radioactive iodine therapy, approaching 30%.[36]

Surgery is indicated in children and pregnant women and in adults with Plummer's disease or with Graves' disease who are unlikely candidates for pharmacological cure because of large goiters. Whenever malignancy is suspected, surgery is necessary for confirmation of the diagnosis. It is not recommended for elderly patients, patients unable to be brought under control in preparation for surgery and in recurrent disease previously managed surgically.[34]

CONCLUSION

As apparent from this discussion, hyperthyroidism is not one disease with one ideal mode of treatment. The etiology of the disease is varied, as is the patient's response to treatment. Many considerations influence the choice of treatment for an individual patient.

The pharmacist is in a unique position to monitor the medically managed patient since treatment often continues for several years. Both hypothyroidism and recurrence of the hyperthyroidism may occur, necessitating evaluation by the physician and often a change in the dose of medication. Additionally, the pharmacist may reiterate the necessity of adhering to dosing schedules and the importance of contacting the physician if serious symptoms of toxicity occur. He or she may also be alert for the symptoms of hypothyroidism in a patient he knows has received radioactive iodine or thyroidectomy in the past.

REFERENCES

1. Catt, K. J.: ABC of endocrinology: the thyroid gland. Lancet, 2: 1383, 1970.
2. Fisher, D.: Abnormalities in thyroid hormone production and metabolism in hyperthyroidism. In Symposium on Hyperthyroidism, W. Odell (moderator). Calif. Med., 113: 35, 1970.
3. Pittman, C., Chambers, J., and Mead, V.: The extrathyroidal conversion rate of thyroxine to triiodothyronine in normal man. J. Clin. Invest., 50: 1187, 1971.
4. Sterling, K., Brenner, M., and Newman, E.: Conversion of thyroxine to triiodothyronine in normal subjects. Science, 169: 1099, 1970.
5. Solomon, D. (moderator), Bennett, R., Brown, J., Peter, J. B., Pollock, W., and Richards, J.: Hyperthyroidism (U.C.L.A. Interdepartmental Conference). Ann. Intern. Med., 69: 1015, 1968.
6. Korenman, S.: The actions of thyroxine and triiodothyronine. In Symposium on Hyperthyroidism, W. Odel (moderator). Calif. Med., 113: 35, 1970.
7. Lefkowitz, R.: Isolated hormone receptors — physiologic and clinical implications. N. Engl. J. Med., 288: 1061, 1973.
8. Schussler, G.: Diagnostic tests and physiologic relationships in thyroid disease. Mod. Treat., 6: 443, 1969.
9. Sisson, J.: Principles of, and pitfalls in, thyroid function tests. J. Nucl. Med., 6: 853, 1965.
10. Anon.: Thyroid function tests. Med. Lett. Drugs Ther., 12: 59, 1970.
11. Greenspan, F.: Thyroid physiology in relation to tests of thyroid function. In Laboratory Tests in Diagnosis and Investigation of Endocrine Function, Ed. 2, Chap. 6, p. 63, edited by R. Escamilla. F. A. Davis Co., Philadelphia, 1971.
12. Gorman, C., and McConahey, W.: Diagnosis of hyperthyroidism and hypothyroidism by laboratory methods. Med. Clin. North Am., 54: 1037, 1970.
13. Thoma, G., and Leightner, W.: Dynamic clinical laboratory tests of thyroid function. Med. Clin. North Am., 52: 463, 1968.
14. Sterling, K., Refetoff, S., and Selenkow, H.: T_3 thyrotoxicosis — thyrotoxicosis due to elevated serum triiodothyronine levels. J.A.M.A., 213: 571, 1970.
15. Odell, W.: Symptoms, physical findings and etiology of hyperthyroidism. In Symposium on Hyperthyroidism, W. Odell (moderator), Calif. Med., 113: 40, 1970.
16. Kreiss, J.: The long acting thyroid stimulator. Calif. Med., 109: 203, 1968.
17. Volpe, R.: The immunological basis of Graves' disease. N. Engl. J. Med., 287: 463, 1972.
18. Werner, S.: Hyperthyroidism — introduction. In The Thyroid, Ed. 3, Chap. 32, p. 491, edited by S. Werner and S. Ingbar. Harper and Row, New York, 1971.
19. Solomon, D. (moderator), Bennett, R., Brown, J., Peter, J. B., Pollock, W., and Richards, J.: Hyperthyroidism (U.C.L.A. Interdepartmental Conference). Ann. Intern. Med., 69: 1023, 1968.
20. Shenkman, L., Mitsuma, T., Blum, M., and Hollander, C.: Recurrent hyperthyroidism presenting as triiodothyronine toxicosis. Ann. Intern. Med., 77: 410, 1972.
21. Thomas, F., Mazzaferri, E., and Skillman, T.: Apathetic thyrotoxicosis: a distinctive clinical and laboratory entity. Ann. Intern. Med., 72: 679, 1970.
22. Anon.: Apathetic thyrotoxicosis (editorial). Lancet, 2: 809, 1970.
23. Roizan, M., and Becker, C.: Thyroid storm. Calif. Med., 115: 4, 1971.
24. Astwood, E. B.: Thyroid and antithyroid drugs. In The Pharmacological Basis of Therapeutics, Ed. 4, Chap. 66, p. 1466, edited by L.

Goodman and A. Gilman. The MacMillan Co., New York, 1970.

25. Das, G., and Kreiger, M.: Treatment of thyrotoxic storm with intravenous administration of propranolol. Ann. Intern. Med., 70: 985, 1969.

26. Maenpää, J., Hiekkala, H., and Lamberg, B.-A.: Childhood hyperthyroidism. Acta Endocrinol., 51: 321, 1966.

27. Hayles, A., Chaves-Carballo, E., and McConahey, W.: The treatment of hyperthyroidism in children. Mayo Clin. Proc., 42: 218, 1967.

28. Kogut, M., Kaplan, S., Collipp, P., Tiamsic, T., and Boyle, D.: Treatment of hyperthyroidism in children. N. Engl. J. Med., 272: 217, 1965.

29. Green, W., Wessler, S., and Avioli, L.: Management of juvenile hyperthyroidism. J.A.M.A., 213: 1652, 1970.

30. Saenger, E., Thoma, G., and Tomkins, E.: Incidence of leukemia following treatment of hyperthyroidism. J.A.M.A., 205: 855, 1968.

31. Park, R., and Frasier, D.: Hyperthyroidism under 2 years of age. Am. J. Dis. Child., 120: 157, 1970.

32. Leszynsky, H., Gross-Kielselstein, E., and Abrahamov, A.: Hyperthyroidism in a 3 month old baby. Pediatrics, 47: 1069, 1971.

33. Smith, L. (Ed.), and Greenspan, F.: Thyrotoxicosis and pregnancy. Calif. Med., 112: 41, 1970.

34. Talbert, L. M., Thomas, C. G., Holt, W. A., and Rankin, P.: Hyperthyroidism during pregnancy. Obstet. Gyn., 36: 779, 1970.

35. Hamburger, J.: Management of the pregnant hyperthyroid. Obstet. Gynecol., 40: 114, 1972.

36. Reinfrank, R.: Hyperthyroidism in pregnancy. South. Med. J., 64: 299, 1971.

37. Swerdloff, R.: Treatment of thyrotoxicosis. In Symposium on Hyperthyroidism, W. Odell (moderator). Calif. Med., 113: 55, 1970.

38. Greer, M., Meijoff, W., and Studer, H.: Treatment of hyperthyroidism with a single daily dose of propylthiouracil. N. Engl. J. Med., 272: 888, 1965.

39. Kammer, J., and Srinivasan, K.: The use of antithyroid drugs in a single daily dose. J.A.M.A., 209: 1325, 1969.

40. Barnes, H. V., and Bledsoe, T.: A simple test for selecting the thioamide schedule in thyrotoxicosis. J. Clin. Endocrinol. Metab., 35: 250, 1972.

41. Wool, M.: The investigation and treatment of hyperthyroidism. Surg. Clin. N. Am., 50: 545, 1970.

42. Utiger, R.: The diverse effects of iodide on thyroid function. N. Engl. J. Med., 287: 562, 1972.

43. Pimstone, N., Marine, N., and Pimstone, B.: Beta adrenergic blockade in thyrotoxic myopathy. Lancet, 2: 1219, 1968.

44. Shanks, R. G., Hadden, D., Lowe, D., McDevitt, D., and Montgomery, D.: Controlled trial of propranolol in thyrotoxicosis. Lancet, 1: 993, 1969.

45. Grossman, W., Robin, N., Johnson, L., Brooks, M., Jelenkow, H., and Dexter, L.: Effects of beta blockade on the peripheral manifestations of thyrotoxicosis. Ann. Intern. Med., 74: 875, 1971.

46. Hagan, G.: Treatment of thyrotoxicosis with ^{131}I and post-therapy hypothyroidism. Med. Clin. North Am., 52: 417, 1968.

chapter 19

HYPOTHYROIDISM

Eric T. Herfindal, Pharm.D.

Joseph L. Hirschman, Pharm.D.

From the point of view of the pharmacist, it would appear that a great proportion of the American public is suffering from hypothyroidism. Sometimes it seems as if every other slightly overweight, middle-aged female who appears at our counter has a prescription for one of the thyroid preparations. The only proven therapeutic indications for thyroid hormones are for diagnosable thyroid deficiencies and as suppressants of thyrotropin (TSH) production by the anterior pituitary. Even so, these drugs continue to be prescribed for a number of conditions such as the "tired housewife syndrome," obesity, metabolic insufficiency and a number of gynecological conditions.[1] There is no convincing evidence that thyroid hormones have a clear indication in these cases. Because of the extensive use of these medications, it behooves the pharmacist to review this disease and become familiar with the proper use of thyroid hormones.

Thyroid deficiency may range in severity from a mild hypothyroid state that is difficult to diagnose to a severe emergency state called myxedema coma. The severity of the disease depends upon the ability of the thyroid gland to produce and secrete the thyroid hormone and the age of the patient. The treatment of hypothyroidism is generally very satisfactory, especially if started early enough.

PHYSIOLOGY

The thyroid gland is a highly vascular organ weighing 20 to 25 g in the average adult. It has one of the highest rates of blood flow of any organ in the body. The gland consists of two lobes connected by the thyroid isthmus and is made up of follicles containing a proteinaceous material called colloid. The two principle hormones secreted by the thyroid, thyroxine (T_4) and triiodothyronine (T_3), are synthesized in the colloid. For a detailed discussion of the biosynthesis and regulating factors of thyroid hormones, refer to Chapter *18*.

The thyroid hormones are not essential to life, but in their absence there is poor resistance to cold, mental and physical slowing and, in children, mental retardation and dwarfism. Thyroid hormones stimulate the oxygen consumption of most cells of the body, help regulate lipid and carbohydrate metabolism and are necessary for normal growth and maturation. Most of the effects of T_3 and T_4 are related to their calorigenic action; in other words, the ability to increase oxygen consumption. This is reflected in the metabolic rate. When the metabolic rate is increased, weight is lost if food intake is not increased. This weight loss is due to breakdown of fat and protein stores. The thyroid hormones also affect the following.[2,3]

1. Heat production. Thyroid secretion is increased in a cold environment. Large doses of thyroid can cause an increase in body temperature. Hypothyroid patients tend to have subnormal body temperatures.

2. Cardiac output. Pulse pressure and cardiac output are increased owing to the effects of thyroid and catecholamines on the heart.

3. Vitamin absorption and requirements. In the absence of thyroid, vitamin B_{12} absorption is reduced, which may lead to an anemia associated with decreased bone marrow metabolism. In thyrotoxicosis, vitamin requirements are increased owing to higher metabolic rate. Thyroid is required for the liver conversion of carotenes to vitamin A. Carotenmia with yellowing of the skin may be seen in hypothyroidism.

4. Milk secretion. Milk secretion is decreased in hypothyroidism.

5. Nervous system. Lack of thyroid hormone produces slowing of mentation. The

effect of thyroid may be due to the increased sensitivity of the brain to catecholamines. In infants, lack of thyroid seriously retards the development of the nervous system. The peripheral nervous system is also affected by thyroid hormone. Reaction time of reflexes is faster in hyperthyroid and slower in hypothyroid patients.

6. Carbohydrate metabolism. Thyroid increases carbohydrate absorption from the gastrointestinal tract, resulting in a transient hyperglycemia and glycosuria after meals.

7. Cholesterol metabolism. Thyroid stimulates cholesterol synthesis, but it also stimulates removal of cholesterol from the circulation by the liver. The rate of removal is greater than the increase in synthesis, so a net reduction in serum cholesterol is seen. The d-form of T_4 has little "thyroid" effect but still retains the ability to reduce cholesterol.[4,5]

8. Action of catecholamines. Thyroid potentiates the effect of norepinephrine and epinephrine by an unknown mechanism. Catecholamine secretion is usually normal in hyperthyroidism, but the increased cardiovascular effects, tremulousness and sweating, can be blocked by catecholamine depleters such as reserpine or quanethidine.

9. Growth and development. Thyroid hormone potentiates the effect of growth hormone. In the absence of thyroid, the secretion of growth hormone by the pituitary is decreased.

ETIOLOGY

A lack of the appropriate amounts of thyroid hormone may be due to a number of causes. The Committee on Nomenclature of the American Thyroid Association[6] lists the following diseases as being primarily characterized by hypothyroidism:

1. Idiopathic myxedema
2. Cretinism
   a. Endemic
   b. Congenital goitrous
3. TSH deficiency
   a. Isolated
   b. Panhypopituitary
4. Thyrotropin-releasing factor (TRF) deficiency due to hypothalamic injury or disease
5. Thyroid destruction

a. Postoperative
b. Postradioiodine
c. Post-x-ray
6. Congenital aplasia

No matter what the etiology of the deficiency, the manifestations of the disease are relatively constant depending on the age of the patient and degree of deficiency.

Thyroid deficiency in fetal or neonatal life is manifested in the condition of cretinism. The cause of the lack of hormone may be:

1. Endemic—lack of iodine in the diet
2. Congenital
   a. Failure of the gland to develop
   b. Defective hormone secretion
   c. Failure of gland to synthesize hormone
   d. Maternal ingestion of goitrogenic substances

In a majority of cases the cause of primary myxedema (not due to pituitary insufficiency) is not known. There is some reason to believe that in most cases the destruction of the thyroid is due to autoimmune mechanisms.[3] Antibodies to thyroid may be detected in most patients with spontaneous hypothyroidism. However, hypothyroidism may result as a complication of thyroidectomy, the use of radioactive iodine or the exposure of the patient to goitrogenic substances. The thiocarbamides (methimazole and propylthiouracil) block the oxidation of iodide to iodine and are used clinically in hyperthyroidism (Chapter *18*). Because they block thyroid activity, they are referred to as goitrogens (Table 19.1). A number of other substances also block thyroid activity by different mechanisms. Anions such as sodium and potassium perchlorate are potent

goitrogens but are too toxic to use therapeutically. Administration of agents such as *para*-aminobenzoic acid and sulfonamides have also been reported to produce decreased thyroid activity in rare cases. In addition to the antithyroid drugs, certain vegetables such as rutabagas, cabbage and turnips have antithyroid activity. Large amounts ingested daily over a long period of time are necessary to produce any significant degree of hypothyroidism.[10]

Secondary hypothyroidism is due to a disorder of the pituitary gland. Consequently, concomitant disorders of the adrenals and gonads are also seen.

SIGNS AND SYMPTOMS, CRETINISM

The failure to feed properly may be the first sign of cretinism. This may be observed as early as 4 weeks after birth. In addition, a swollen tongue, dry, yellow, cold skin, a "pot belly" with umbilical hernia, hyporeflexia and constipation may be seen. Later, delayed skeletal maturation, mental retardation, hoarseness, a round face and dark brittle hair may also be observed. If thyroid therapy is not initiated immediately upon diagnosis, irreversible mental retardation may result.[11]

SIGNS AND SYMPTOMS, MYXEDEMA

Early in the course of adult myxedema, signs and symptoms may be few or absent. If symptoms are present, they are likely to be lethargy, menstrual disturbances, weakness, fatigue, headache, cold intolerance, nervousness, thinning, coarse hair, brittle nails and delayed deep tendon reflexes. Later, slow speech, weight gain, constipation, anginal pain, absence of sweating and deafness may be seen. The pulse is slow and regular and elevated blood pressure may be seen in elderly patients. The circulation time is slow and anemia may be present.

Myxedema coma is an emergency condition that must be treated vigorously. This is a condition that is mostly seen in elderly patients, characterized by a sudden onset of coma associated with seizures. Normally these are patients with a long history of myxedema. The emergency can be precipitated by a number of factors such as infection, drug overdose, myo-

TABLE 19.1
Goitrogenic Substances

Thiocarbamides	Vegetables
Methimazole	Turnips
Propylthiouracil	Rutabagas
	Cabbage
Iodides	
	Miscellaneous agents
Radioiodine	Lithium carbonate
	para-Aminobenzoic acid
Anions	Sulfonamides
Thiocyanates (SCN–)	
Perchlorates (ClO$_4$–)	
Nitrates (NO$_3$–)	

cardial infarction, hypoglycemia and congestive heart failure (CHF).[11]

LABORATORY FINDINGS

There are a number of laboratory tests available with which to measure thyroid activity. These tests are based on the physiological and chemical characteristics of the thyroid hormone. Refer to Chapter *18* on hyperthyroidism for a discussion of common thyroid function tests. Nonspecific tests such as serum cholesterol, glucose tolerance, 17-ketosteroids and serum triglycerides are also useful in diagnosing hypothyroidism.

TREATMENT

The treatment of hypothyroidism (Table 19.2) is generally effectively carried out by the careful administration of thyroid hormone. All of the commercially available preparations of thyroid hormone are effective. However, there are a number of qualities of each drug that should be considered before a selection is made.

Thyroid USP. Desiccated thyroid is made from the dried and defatted thyroid glands of slaughtered cows and pigs. This preparation is standardized only with respect to iodine content. Since no requirements are made as to thyroxine and triiodothyronine, the ratio of hormones and the total amount of hormones may vary.[12] However, with very few exceptions, this preparation has been shown to be satisfactorily uniform in potency.[13] However, the preparation may deteriorate under poor storage conditions and produce unsatisfactory results.[12] Absorption of thyroid hormone is generally good, although variations in total amounts absorbed have been reported.[14,15] Enteric-coated preparations produce more variation in response than compressed tablets.[16] Since thyroid USP contains both T_4 and T_3, the plasma-bound iodine (PBI) can be monitored, and it produces euthyroid levels when the patient has achieved a normal metabolic rate. The other laboratory tests also produce predictable levels. Because of its low price, thyroid USP remains the most heavily prescribed thyroid preparation.

Thyroglobulin. This drug consists of the partly purified, denatured thyroglobulin derived from slaughtered pigs. In addition to being standardized by iodine content, thyroglobulin is also bioassayed.[12] Thyroglobulin has no apparent advantages over thyroid USP and is slightly more expensive.

Sodium Levothyroxine USP. Sodium levothyroxine is the sodium salt of synthetic L-thyroxine (T_4). As such, the amount of hormone present is certain.[12] Because it contains no T_3, this preparation has the tendency to produce higher than normal euthyroid PBI levels when normal metabolic activity is established. This is no real disadvantage if the physician is cognizant of this fact. The absorption of the drug is varied, and 40 to 50% has been recovered from the stool.[20] The preparation is also available for intravenous administration.

Sodium Liothyronine. Sodium liothyronine is the sodium salt of synthetic L-triiodothyronine (T_3). It is thus a pure form of T_3 that has been chromatographically assayed.[12] The major advantage and disadvantage of this drug are its relatively short half-life and rapid onset of activity. In emergency conditions (myxedema coma) where a rapid onset is mandatory, sodium liothyronine is the drug of choice.[8] It is not commercially available in intravenous form, but many physicians consider it the drug of choice in myxedema coma. There are few indications for the use of this drug on a chronic basis. Because of its short half-life it should be given 3 times a day. In rare cases in which relatively rapid abatement of action (severe angina, CHF) may be desired, this drug could be used for maintenance.[11] Because T_3 is poorly bound to serum protein, the PBI levels are barely raised from hypothyroid levels.

Liotrix. Liotrix is a 4 : 1 mixture of the sodium salts of T_4 and T_3. The two commercially available preparations vary slightly in composition, and they should not be considered generically equivalent (Table 19.3). After a patient has been stabilized on one preparation, it would be unwise to change to the other. The major advantage of liotrix is that the two hormones are present in a uniform ratio and of known strength.[18,21] As with thyroid USP and thyroglobulin, PBI levels are in the euthyroid range when a normal metabolic rate has been achieved. Because of its higher cost, this preparation should generally be reserved until the less expensive natural preparations have been shown to produce erratic results in a particular patient.

TABLE 19.2
Available Thyroid Preparations

Drug	Dose to Maintain Normal BMR[a] (euthyroid) mg	Route	Preparation	$t_{1/2}$ (biol.) days	Peak	Duration	Euthyroid PBI μg/100 ml	Standardized	Advantages	Disadvantages
Thyroid, USP	60-240 (av = 120)	P.O.	$T_3 + T_4$ (cow and pig)	6-7	1-3 weeks	3 weeks	4-8	Iodine content (0.17-0.23%)	Inexpensive / Can monitor T_4 / Has $T_3 + T_4$	Variations in lots / Poorly standardized / Unknown T_4/T_3 ratio / Deterioration on storage
Thyroglobulin	60-240 (av = 120)	P.O.	Purified thyroglobulin (pig)	6-7	1-3 weeks	3 weeks	4-8	Iodine content, bioassay, chromatographic assay	Relatively inexpensive / Can monitor T_4 / Has T_3 and T_4	Variable T_3/T_4 ratio
Sodium levothyroxine (T_4)	0.1-0.4 (av = 0.2)	P.O. I.V.	Synthetic T_4	6-7	1-3 weeks	3 weeks	7-10	Chromatographic assay	Long acting / Can monitor T_4 / Known potency	Slow excretion: disadvantage in toxicity / Expensive
Sodium liothyronine USP (T_3)	0.025-0.1 (av = 0.05)	P.O.	Synthetic T_3	2.5	24-72 hr	5-6 days	1-2	Chromatographic assay	Good absorption / Rapid onset / Known potency	Difficult to monitor by lab tests / Expensive / Short duration: divided dosage
Liotrix ($T_3 + T_4$)	"1" - "4" av = "2"	P.O.	Synthetic T_4 and T_3 ratio: 4:1	6-7	1-3 weeks	3 weeks	4-8	Chromatographic	Known potency / Known ratio of T_4 to T_3 / Can monitor T_4	Expensive

[a] BMR: basal metabolic rate.

TABLE 19.3
Available Liotrix Preparations

Tablet	T_4/T_3 μg	Tablet	T_4/T_3 μg
Thyrolar - 1/2	25/6.25	Euthroid - 1/2	30/7.5
Thyrolar - 1	50/12.5	Euthroid - 1	60/15
Thyrolar - 2	100/25	Euthroid - 2	120/30
Thyrolar - 3	150/37.7	Euthroid - 3	180/45

Toxicity. The toxicity of thyroid hormones mimics hyperthyroidism. One can expect to see hyperirritability, nervousness, insomnia, tachycardia, cardiac arrhythmias, angina pectoris, intolerance to heat, increased pulse and blood pressures, diarrhea, cramps, weight loss, vomiting and tremors.[22] In children, accelerated rate of bone maturation is an early manifestation of toxicity. At the earliest sign of toxicity, the drug should be discontinued for 2 to 6 days when thyroid, thyroglobulin and sodium levothyroxine are used and 2 to 3 days if sodium liothyronine is used. The drug should be restarted at a lower dose following abatement of toxicity.

THERAPY, CRETINISM

Immediately upon diagnosis of hypothyroidism, thyroid replacement therapy should be initiated. The drug of choice is either thyroid USP or equivalent doses of liotrix. Sodium levothyroxine and sodium liothyronine will give unpredictable values of thyroid function tests, making monitoring difficult. The more myxedematous infants are more sensitive to the action of thyroid hormone, necessitating the initiation of treatment with very small doses followed by gradual dose increases.

An initial dose of 30 mg per day is the starting dose, increased by 15 mg a day every 3 weeks. The maintenance dose should not be less than 60 mg a day of thyroid or equivalent (Table 19.4). A 1-year old usually will require 90 mg a day. Three-year-old children will require 90 to 120 mg per day; 5-year-old children, 120 to 150 mg, 10-year-old children 150 to 180 mg. Older patients require proportionally higher doses, up to 240 mg per day of thyroid or equivalent.[23] Treatment must be continued for life.

THERAPY, MYXEDEMA

The drug of choice in myxedema depends on a number of factors:
1. Patient's age
2. Severity and duration of disease
3. Presence of other disease such as congestive heart failure, angina or diabetes

Generally, older patients with severe myxedema and concomitant heart disease must be started with small doses of thyroid—8 to 15 mg for 1 week and increased by 15 mg every week up to 120 to 180 mg.[8,23] The dose is increased until the clinical signs of the disease have disappeared or signs of toxicity appear. The laboratory findings should reflect a euthyroid state. Younger patients can generally tolerate higher initial doses: 30 mg for 1 week, then increased by 30 mg every week until euthyroid levels are reached. In postradioiodine, post-thyroidectomy and post-x-ray hypothyroidism, maintenance levels can be reached sooner than in long standing myxedema. The more severe the deficiency, the more sensitive is the patient to the effect of thyroid hormone. Although some patients may require more than 300 mg of thyroid or equivalent per day, most patients become euthyroid below this level. Because of this, the diagnosis of hypothyroidism is questionable in patients receiving massive doses of thyroid.[24]

In patients with severe angina or congestive heart failure, the use of sodium liothyronine should be considered. If toxicity symptoms appear, the effect can be terminated relatively rapidly because of the drug's short half-life. Increments of 5 μg are generally employed.[8]

Myxedema coma is an emergency condition requiring the use of intravenous sodium levothyroxine 200 to 500 μg. This dose may be repeated in 24 hr. Some physicians prefer sodium liothyronine 10 to 20 μg intravenously every 8 hr (not available commercially).[8] Prolonged hypothyroidism leads to adrenocortical

TABLE 19.4
Equivalent Doses of Thyroid Preparations

Thyroid, USP	60 mg
Thyroglobulin	60 mg
Sodium levothyroxine, USP	0.1 mg
Sodium liothyronine, USP	25 μg
Liotrix	"1"

depression, and so hydrocortisone should be given in doses of 100 mg intravenously every 8 hr until the crisis is over. In addition, precipitating factors such as infection, drug overdosage, myocardial infarction, hyponatremia, hypoglycemia and congestive heart failure should be treated immediately.[25] Care must be taken to avoid overhydration, which can worsen the hyponatremia. The patient should be warmed, but too rapid correction of the hypothermia may lead to peripheral vasodilation and worsening of the shock.[26]

SPECIAL CONSIDERATIONS

Myxedematous patients metabolize drugs very slowly and are thus very sensitive to overdosages. Sedatives and opiates must be used with caution since normal doses may produce signs of overdosage. Signs of Cushing's syndrome have been produced in hypothyroid patients with relatively low doses of corticosteroids.[27] Patients requiring digitalis may require lower maintenance doses than euthyroid patients.[28] Thyroid hormones may potentiate the action of oral anticoagulants, and the dose may have to be adjusted when thyroid therapy is initiated.[29,30] The initiation of thyroid therapy in diabetic patients is usually accompanied by an increased requirement of insulin or oral hypoglycemics. This may be due to the enhanced carbohydrate absorption produced by thyroid hormones.[31] It has also been demonstrated that hypothyroid patients respond poorly to tricyclic antidepressants such as imipramine and that the addition of thyroid hormones increases the percentage of patients responding to these drugs.[32,33]

PROGNOSIS, CRETINISM

Even with early treatment, the chances of a congenital cretin reaching full mental development is poor. However, full skeletal and sexual maturation may be achieved with optimal thyroid therapy.

PROGNOSIS, MYXEDEMA

Hypothyroidism of later onset generally responds excellently to thyroid therapy. Improvement can be very striking with early treatment and can be maintained indefinitely with continued therapy. Relapses will occur if treatment is interrupted. Myxedema coma has a high mortality rate, but with prompt recognition of the cause and the immediate initiation of appropriate therapy, a significant number of patients survive.

CONCLUSION

Hypothyroidism is a relatively easy disease to diagnose. A large number of specific laboratory tests are available to substantiate clinical findings. However, these tests may be altered by a number of disease states and drugs. Subtle differences between the available thyroid preparations make the selection of the proper drug important. Myxedematous patients have altered metabolism of drugs such as digitalis, narcotics, hypnotics and corticosteroids. The initiation of thyroid therapy may alter the patient's requirements of oral hypoglycemics, insulin and anticoagulants. By being aware of all these factors and conveying his knowledge to the physician and the patient, the pharmacist can play an important role in the rational therapy of hypothyroidism.

REFERENCES

1. Meyers, F. H., Jawetz, E., and Goldfein, A.: Review of Medical Pharmacology, Ed. 3, p, 323, Lange Medical Publications, Los Altos, 1972.
2. Ganong, W. F.: The thyroid gland. In Review of Medical Physiology, Ed. 6, Chap. 18, p. 232. Lange Medical Publications, Los Altos, 1973.
3. Tepperman, J.: Metabolic and Endocrine Physiology, Ed. 2, p. 86. Year Book Medical Publishers, Chicago, 1968.
4. Cohen, B. M.: The clinical use of dextrothyroxine in hypercholesteremic states. An eight-year appraisal. J. Clin. Pharmacol., 9: 45, 1969.
5. Wadman, B., Werner, I., Dano, G., and Levander-Lindgren, M.: Treatment with sodium dextrothyroxine in hypercholesterolaemia; an attempt at critical evaluation. Nord. Med., 81: 691, 1969.
6. Werner, S. C.: Classification of thyroid disease (letter to the editor). J. Clin. Endocrinol. Metab., 29: 860, 1969
7. Luby, E. D., Schwartz, D., and Rosenbaum, H.: Lithium-carbonate-induced myxedema. J.A.M.A., 218: 1298, 1971.
8. Anon.: Current practice: today's drugs, thyroid hormones. Br. Med. J., 2: 561, 1969.

9. Fieve, R. R., and Platman, S. R.: Follow-up studies of lithium and thyroid function in manic-depressive illness. Am. J. Psychiatry, 125:' 1443, 1969.

10. Greer, M. A.: The natural occurence of goitrogenic agents. Recent Prog. Horm. Res., 18: 187, 1962.

11. Wintrobe, M. M., Thorn, G. W., Adams, R. D., Bennett, I. L., Braunwald, E., Isselbacher, K. J., and Petersforf, R. G.: Harrison's Principles of Internal Medicine, Ed. 6, p. 454. McGraw-Hill Book Co., New York, 1970.

12. Anon.: Thyroid and antithyroid, Sect. 68: 36. In American Hospital Formulary Service, edited by M. J. Reilly. American Society of Hospital Pharmacists, Washington, D.C., 1970.

13. Astwood, E. B.: Hormones and hormone antagonists. In The Pharmacologic Basis of Therapeutics, Ed. 4, p. 1464, edited by L. S. Goodman and A. Gilman. The MacMillan Co., New York, 1970.

14. Anon.: Thyroid, thyroxine and triiodothyronine. Med. Lett. Drugs Ther., 5: 69, 1963.

15. Anon.: Armour's "Letter" for hypothyroidism. Med. Lett. Drugs Ther., 8: 41, 1966.

16. Anon.: A.M.A. Drug Evaluations, 1971, Ed. 1, p. 325. American Medical Association, Chicago, 1971.

17. Johnson, P. C.: The effect of thyroid replacement therapy on the protein bound iodine levels. Med. Times, 95: 1312, 1967.

18. Alley, R. A., Danowski, T. S., Robbins, T. J. L., Weit, T. T., Sabeh, G., and Moses, C. L.: Indices during administration of T_4 and T_3 to euthyroid adults. Metabolism, 17: 97, 1968.

19. Farmer, T. A., Jr., Smitherman, T. C., Beschi, R. J., and Pittman, J. A.: Effect of triiodothyronine administration on serum PBI in hypothyroid patients maintained on constant doses of thyroxine. J. Clin. Endocrinol. Metab., 29: 781, 1969.

20. Hays, M. T.: Absorption of oral thyroxine. Amer. Fed. for Clin. Res., Ann. Meeting, Atlantic City, N. J., May 1966, Abst., Clin. Res., 14: 281, 1966.

21. Bakke, J. L., and Klotz, L. J.: Treatment of hypothyroidism with synthetic thyroid hormones. Northwest Med., 68: 651, 1969.

22. Schottstaedt, E. S., and Smoller, M.: "Thyroid storm" produced by acute thyroid hormone poisoning. Ann. Intern. Med., 64: 847, 1966.

23. Beeson, P. B., and McDermott, W. (editors): Cecil-Loeb Textbook of Medicine, Ed. 12, p. 1299. W. B. Saunders Co., Philadelphia, 1967.

24. Kolb, F. O.: Endocrine disorders. In Current Diagnosis and Treatment 1973, p. 608, edited by M. A. Krupp and M. J. Chatton. Lange Medical Publications, Los Altos, 1973.

25. Robin, N. I.: Hypothyroidism. In Current Therapy 1973, Vol. 25, p. 467, edited by H. F. Conn. W. B. Saunders Co., Philadelphia, 1973.

26. Williams, H. E., and Becker, C. E.: Endocrine disorders. In Clinical Pharmacology, Ed. 1, p. 290, edited by K. L. Melmon and H. F. Morrelli. The MacMillan Co., New York, 1972.

27. Parfitt, J. C.: Cushing's syndrome with normal replacement dose of cortisone in pituitary hypothyroidism. J. Clin. Endocrinol. Metab., 24: 560, 1964.

28. Doherty, J. E., and Perkins, W. H.: Digoxin metabolism in hypo- and hyper-thyroidism. Ann. Intern. Med., 64: 489, 1966.

29. Solomon, H. M., and Schrogie, J. J.: Change in receptor site affinity: a proposed explanation for the potentiating effect of D-thyroxine on the anticoagulant response of warfarin. Clin. Pharmacol. Ther., 8: 797, 1967.

30. Azarnoff, D. L., Hurwitz, A.: Drug interactions. Pharmacol. Physicians, 4: 1, 1970.

31. Zinn, J., and Schleissner, L. A.: The effects of dextrothyroxine in diabetes. Calif. Med., 101: 240, 1964.

32. Earle, B. V.: Thyroid hormone and tricyclic antidepressants in resistant depression. Am. J. Psychiatry, 126: 1667, 1970.

33. Prange, A. J., Wilson, I. C., Rabon, A. M., and Lipton, M. A.: Enhancement of imipramine antidepressant activity by thyroid hormone. Am. J. Psychiatry, 126: 457, 1969.

chapter 20

ADDISON'S DISEASE

Fredric E. Jones

It has long been a practice in science to name discoveries or scientific phenomena in honor of the person or persons responsible for the work. Thomas Addison, the 19th Century English physician, earned his place in history by first elucidating the clinical manifestations of chronic adrenocortical insufficiency. Addison's disease is a gradual and usually progressive disease due to adrenocortical hypofunction, characterized by increasing weakness, abnormal pigmentation of the skin and mucous membrane, weight loss, hypotension, dehydration, gastrointestinal upsets and occasional hypoglycemia.

ETIOLOGY AND INCIDENCE

Addison's disease is a condition which is seen in less than 1 per 200,000 population. The Massachusetts General Hospital saw 12 cases in 1968. There are two major groups[1] in which to classify these cases etiologically. The first group is of unknown etiology and accounts for slightly over 70% of the cases. The remainder of the cases are the result of the partial destruction of the adrenal gland by various mechanisms such as tuberculosis, neoplasm, amyloidoses or inflammatory necrosis. The condition may also manifest itself after bilateral adrenalectomy. Inadequate hormone-replacement therapy is usually the cause. Also, in unilateral adrenalectomy, the remaining adrenal gland may be suppressed.

The adrenocortical reserve represents one of the greatest organ reserves of the human body. At least 90 to 95% of the adrenocortical tissue must be destroyed in order for adrenal insufficiency to become manifest.[2]

PATHOGENESIS

As might be expected in adrenal destruction, hydrocortisone and aldosterone production, function and metabolism are altered. The reduction or loss of aldosterone results in the exchange of extracellular sodium and intracellular potassium. These major changes in the electrolyte balance produce increased water excretion, causing severe dehydration, a concentration of the blood plasma, a decrease in circulatory volume and, if left untreated, hypotension and circulatory collapse.

The problems caused by the decrease or loss in hydrocortisone levels are equally as devastating. Disturbances in protein and intermediate carbohydrate and fat metabolism occur. A severe sensitivity to insulin also develops. In the absence of hydrocortisone, too little fat and too much carbohydrate are broken down. The carbohydrate breakdown is due mainly to a reduced carbohydrate production from protein. These altered metabolic effects give rise to hypoglycemia and diminished liver glycogen production. The combined total of these metabolic and electrolytic disturbances create a condition of general weakness due in part to reduced neuromuscular function, decreased resistance to infection and an increased probability of circulatory collapse. The pituitary gland reacts to the fall in hydrocortisone levels by increasing the output of corticotrophin (ACTH).[3] This increase in ACTH causes hyperpigmentation to occur owing to increased plasma levels of melanocyte-stimulating hormone (MSH).

SIGNS AND SYMPTOMS

Weakness and fatigability are two of the primary symptoms that may be seen in patients with adrenocortical insufficiency. Increased pigmentation is also seen in almost every case. The exception to this is adrenal insufficiency secondary to pituitary failure. This increased pigmentation is characterized by diffuse tanning, primarily in the area of bony prominences, skin folds, scars and extensor surfaces. The mucous membranes of the lips, mouth, rectum and vagina commonly display bluish black discolorations. Other characteristic symptoms which may indicate adrenal cortical insufficiency include weight loss, dehydration, hypotension, decreased tolerance to cold and small heart size. These symptoms and signs are present in the benign development of stages of Addison's disease and are intensified in an adrenal crisis. An adrenal crisis may be brought about by acute infection; stress; accidental or surgical trauma; or electrolyte loss through excess sweating, emesis or diarrhea.[1] The symptoms associated with Addisonian crisis are marked asthenia, severe abdominal pain, low back and leg pains, possible peripheral vascular collapse and, if untreated, renal shutdown with azotemia. The body temperature during the crisis is generally subnormal.[4]

DIAGNOSIS

The most definite diagnostic procedure is the demonstration of a lack of adrenal cortical response to the administration of ACTH. This can be accomplished as an office or outpatient procedure with the ACTH moiety cosyntropin.[5] This agent is intended for use as a diagnostic agent in screening patients presumed to have adrenocortical insufficiency. An effective diagnostic method for demonstrating the lack of adrenocortical response in patients is the 8-hr intravenous corticotropin test.[6] This test requires that 25 to 50 units of ACTH be infused intravenously with 500 ml of normal saline over an 8-hr period for each of 3 successive days. Urinary output determinations for 17-ketosteroids and 17-hydroxycorticosteroids for 4 24-hr collection periods, 1 control period and 3 ACTH administration periods, are then made (Fig. 20.1). Under these clinical circumstances, a patient with normal adrenal cortical function will have an 8 to 16 mg per day increase in the excretion of 17-hydroxycorticosteroids and a 4 to 8 mg per day increase in 17-ketosteroids excretion. The Addisonian patient will show virtually no response.[7] Blood is also taken at the beginning and end of each ACTH infusion for an eosinophil count. Normal patients will respond with an eosinopenia of 80 to 90%, whereas patients with adrenocortical

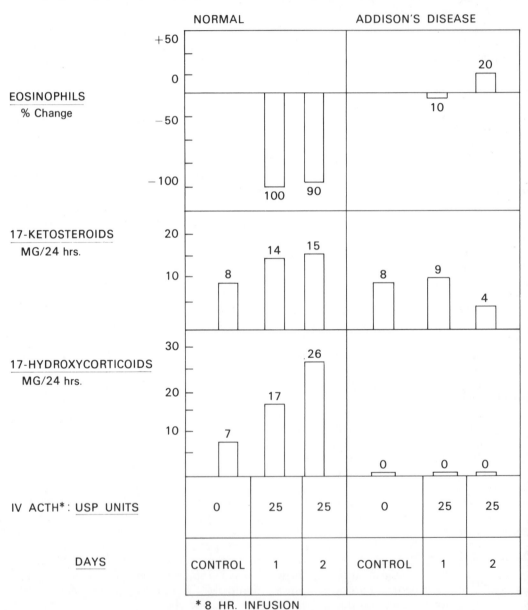

FIG. 20.1. Adrenal responses to intravenous corticotropin.

insufficiency will exhibit little or no change. The lack of glucocorticoid production in this disorder leads to lymphocytosis and eosinophilia (Table 20.1), a decrease in gluconeogenesis and reduced intestinal absorption of glucose. An elevated serum magnesium is also seen in these patients. When the diagnosis of adrenal insufficiency is probable and the corticotropin test is performed for verification, certain precautions should be exercised.[1] A preinfusion dose of 1.0 mg fluorohydrocortisone or dexamethasone should be administered to the patient to protect against a reaction to the infusion. A 1.0-mg fluorocortisone dose is just enough to prevent serious sodium excretion. Normal saline is the intravenous fluid of choice. Dextrose 5% in water should be excluded because of occasional reports of pyrogenic effects caused in patients with adrenal insufficiency. Various chronic infections or other conditions often resemble Addison's disease. Weakness, common to both adrenocortical insufficiency and myasthenia gravis, can be differentiated by therapeutic tests with neostigmine methylsulfate.[8] This test is specific for myasthenia gravis. Iron-deficiency anemia associated with increased pigmentation can be differentiated by good responses to iron therapy. The eosinophils in Addison's disease also usually present with a normocytic, normochromic morphology, while eosinophils characteristic of iron-deficiency anemia present a microcytic hypochromic morphology.[9]

TABLE 20.1[a]
Laboratory Findings Suggestive of Addison's Disease

Blood chemical	Low serum Na (<130mEq/liter); high serum K (>5 mEq/liter); ratio of serum Na:K (<30:1); Low fasting blood sugar (<50mg/100 ml); decrease in CO_2 combining power (28mEq/liter); Elevated BUN (>20mg/100ml)
Hematological	Elevated hematocrit; low W.B.C.; relative lymphocytosis
Basal metabolic	BMR of −15 to −20
X-ray	Evidence of: calcifications in the adrenal areas; renal tuberculosis; pulmonary tuberculosis; small heart

[a]Reprinted with permission from the Merck Manual, Ed. 11.

TREATMENT

Once the diagnosis of adrenal cortical insufficiency has been established, a search should be made for tuberculosis or a fungal disease. The determination of etiology is important for treatment. Appropriate therapy should be instituted if an active infection is discovered. To correct the glucocorticoid deficiency, the oral[10] administration of 25 to 37.5 mg of cortisone, or 20 to 30 mg of hydrocortisone may be given orally. In an attempt to mimic the normal circadian rhythm of glucocorticoid secretion, 2/3 of the total dose should be given in the morning and 1/3 of the total dose in the late afternoon. During the first few days of treatment some patients may develop insomnia, mental excitation, irritability and even frank psychosis. In these circumstances, steroid doses should be reduced temporarily. Later in the course of treatment, complications of glucocorticoid administration in the doses used are rare. Excessive appetite and weight gain may occur occasionally and require the reduction of the dose. Aside from these early complications or side reactions, administration and implementation of hormone replacement leads to restoration of appetite, muscle strength and body weight and a general feeling of well being. The anemia is soon corrected, the electrocardiogram returns to normal, the tendency towards hypoglycemia is reduced, pigmentation is lightened and the capacity to withstand the stress of intercurrent infections and trauma is greatly enhanced. It is interesting to note that the above mentioned doses of cortisone and hydrocortisone, when given daily to Addisonian patients with active tuberculosis, do not appear to promote the spread of the infectious tuberculosis. During periods of intercurrent illness, it is essential that the dose of cortisone or its congener be increased to a level comparable to a cortisone dosage of at least 75 to 100 mg per day. If oral administration is not possible, parenteral administration with equivalent drugs may be used.

The amounts of cortisone or hydrocortisone required to restore to normal the metabolism of carbohydrate, protein and fat are unfortunately too small to assure normal electrolyte and water balance. Adequate hydration and blood pressure stabilization are thus required either with the use of 10 to 15 g of supplementary sodium chloride per day, or, in the vast majority of cases, the use of small amounts of mineralocorticoid. The use of small amounts of fluorocortisone[10] in dosages in 0.1 to 0.2 mg orally or injections of 2.5 to 5 mg of deoxycorticosterone will usually prevent excess sodium loss. This may be done on a daily or every other day schedule, depending upon the patient. Most patients naturally prefer the simple oral route to obtain the mineralocorticoid-replacement therapy. Body weight, blood pressure, heart size and serum potassium are followed closely and the doses of the hormone-replacement therapy are titered to bring these measurements within normal limits. In elderly patients or in the presence of hypertension, edema or cardiac enlargement, all salt-retaining steroid hormone therapy should be discontinued, and the patient's mineral requirement should be regulated by diet alone. Because of the relatively small doses of cortisone employed in maintenance therapy, undesirable effects are rarely seen. Gastric irritation may occasionally occur in patients taking cortisone acetate by mouth. This is overcome in most instances by giving the hormone during meals. Increased excitability and sleeplessness are only rarely encountered, and, if the last dose of cortisone is given no later than 4:00 p.m., this usually does not happen.

THERAPY FOR STRESS CONDITIONS

In the anticipation of surgery, or with the onset of an acute illness, adrenal crisis is prevented by increasing glucocorticoid dosage.[11] The Addisonian patient who undergoes surgery should be adequately prepared with hormone therapy. It is recommended that for major surgery a therapeutic program similar to that used in patients with Cushing's syndrome be instituted (Table 20.2). With mild illness, such as an upper respiratory infection, the patient can double the daily dose of his hormone therapy. With an illness complicated by severe vomiting or diarrhea of more than 12-hr duration, the patient is urged to contact his doctor. These circumstances require the injection of 50 to 100 mg daily of hydrocortisone. It may occasionally become necessary for the patient himself to administer this injection. This has not proved to be a problem for patients with Addison's disease since this circumstance is similar to the many diabetic patients who ad-

TABLE 20.2
Hormone Therapy Following Complete Adrenalectomy

Preoperatively	Postoperatively
Cortisone acetate 100 mg I.M. 12 hr and 2 hr preoperatively	Day 1—cortisone acetate 50 mg I.M. q 6 hr
During operation Hydrocortisone 100 mg I.V. Repeated 6 and 12 hr postoperatively	Days 2, 3—50 mg I.M. q 8 hr
	Days 4, 5, 6, 7a—50mg P.O. q 12 hr
Cortisone acetate 50 mg I.M. q 6 hr	Days 8, 9, 10—25mg P.O. q 8 hr
	Thereafter taper cortisone acetate P.O. slowly to maintenance needsb

[a] Salt-retaining hormone (desoxycorticosterone or fluorocortisone) may be required after 7th day.

[b] In patients with severe Cushing's disease and excreting large quantities of 17-hydroxycorticoids into urine, it is essential to reduce the cortisone dosage somewhat more slowly than is shown in the table.

minister their own insulin. Ordinarily it is not necessary to alter steroid doses during pregnancy in an Addisonian patient; however, if edema should occur in the 3rd trimester, the mineralocorticoid dosage should be reduced. Once labor begins, administration of 100 mg of hydrocortisone every 8 hr should be given until delivery. With minor surgical procedures such as dilation and curettage, it is necessary merely to give 100 mg of hydrocortisone 1 hr before anesthesia induction. Following the operation, the patient is returned to his normal dosage regimen. With a major operation, 100 mg of hydrocortisone is administered I.M. 1 hr before the procedure, and 100 mg in 500 ml of normal saline is given intravenously every 8 hr beginning with the administration of anesthesia and continuing throughout the operative day. Over the next 4 to 5 days, the hydrocortisone dose is regularly tapered to oral maintenance levels, at which time mineralocorticoid treatment is resumed. The hydrocortisone infusion should not be interrupted; if blood is required, it should be given through another vein. The only stressful occasion during which it is desirable to increase mineralocorticoid dosage is a period of excessive perspiration or in extremely hot weather. When severe salt depletion gets to be a problem, either from surgical stress or from extremely hot weather, the hospitalized patient may require as much as 4 liters of isotonic saline solution on the 1st day of therapy. It is to be emphasized, however, that in the absence of appreciable salt deficiency, excessive saline infusion may induce cardiac failure in the Addisonian patient. If shock is present, or if the patient goes into shock, pressor agents such as metaraminal or angiotensin should be given along with the intravenous hydrocortisone. It should be emphasized that, because of slower absorption from the site of injection, I.M. therapy should never be used in the treatment of acute adrenal insufficiency. In patients who have undergone partial and, in many instances total, adrenalectomy, the required adrenocortical hormone-replacement therapy is similar to that prescribed for Addison's disease.

PROGNOSIS

In the absence of active tuberculosis, the future for Addisonian patients is good. They may continue to lead normal, healthy, active lives much as diabetics do. Current hormone-replacement therapy is quite sufficient for the control and maintenance of these patients. The only time that dosage regimens need be altered or modified is in emergency situations or hospitalization. The experience with female patients with Addison's disease is such that they generally do not experience any difficulty with pregnancy, provided their corticoid dosage has been increased.[1]

INTERACTIONS

The potential interactions during corticosteroid therapy are quite numerous. The following examples[12] represent some of the different interactions.

Antihistamine preparations increase the rate of metabolism of hydrocortisone. This is especially important to remember for nonhospitalized Addisonian patients. The abundance of over-the-counter items available that contain antihistamines afford the Addisonian patient an easy chance to get into trouble.

It has been shown that barbiturate sedative action is potentiated by the glucocorticoids. This is thought to occur owing to plasma protein-binding site competition. Conversely, the sedative chlorol hydrate, through the action of enzyme induction, causes a decrease in hydrocortisone activity.

Indomethacin represents another example of hydrocortisone potentiation due to plasma protein-binding site competition.

Thyroid preparations create an increased tissue demand for adrenocortical hormones. The concomitant administration of thyroid preparations with hydrocortisone may precipitate an acute adrenal crisis.

The hypoglycemic effect of insulin[3] is antagonized by corticosteroid administration. This, in addition to increased gluconeogenesis caused by hydrocortisone administration, again presents an area in which Addisonian patients may inadvertently get into trouble.

These few examples represent only some of the interaction areas of which pharmacists should be aware. These specific drugs and drug classes were selected because they represent some of the more frequently prescribed therapeutic agents.

Narcotic analgesics are contraindicated in Addisonian patients. Even small amounts of these preparations may cause stupor or precipitate coma and respiratory collapse.[13]

CONCLUSION

Chronic adrenocortical insufficiency (Addison's disease) is a rarely encountered medical entity. The majority of these cases are satisfactorily controlled and maintained with substitution therapy of a glucocorticoid (hydrocortisone) and a mineralocorticoid (fluorocortisone). It is important that the Addisonian patient adhere to his daily therapy. This patient should always carry a medical identification card bearing the doctor's name, address and phone number; the next of kin's name, address and phone number; and the following instructions: "In the event of illness, administer 25 mg of cortisone acetate every six hours by mouth unless the patient is unconscious, then 100 mg of the hormone should be given by intramuscular injection."

REFERENCES

1. Beeson, P. B., and McDermott, W.: Cecil Loeb Textbook of Medicine, Ed. 7. W. B. Saunders Co., Philadelphia, 1971.
2. Sparagana, M.: Addison's disease due to reticulum-cell sarcoma apparently confined to the adrenals. J. Am. Geriatr. Soc., 18: 553, 1970.

3. Lyght, C. E., Keefer, C. S., Lukens, F. D. W.,
   Richards, D. W., Sebrell, W. H., and Trapnell,
   J. M.: The Merck Manual of Diagnosis and
   Therapy, p. 467. Merck Sharpe and Dohme
   Research Laboratories, Rahway, N.J., 1966.
4. Conn, H. F., and Conn, R. B.: Current Diagnosis,
   Ed. 3, p. 736. W. B. Saunders Co., Philadelphia, 1971.
5. Cosyntropin package insert, Organon, Inc., West
   Orange, N.J., 1969.
6. Riley, M. J.: American Hospital Formulary Service. American Society of Hospital Pharmacists, Washington, D.C., 36: 4, 1972.
7. Davidsohn, I., and Henry, J. B.: Clinical Diagnosis
   by Laboratory Methods, Ed. 14, p. 279. W.
   B. Saunders Co., Philadelphia, 1967.
8. Riley, M. J.: American Hospital Formulary Service. American Society of Hospital Pharmacists, Washington, D.C., 36: 56, 1972.
9. Collins, R. D.: Illustrated Manual of Laboratory
   Diagnosis, Ed. 1, p. 225. J. B. Lippincott Co.,
   Philadelphia, 1968.
10. Riley, M. J.: American Hospital Formulary Ser-
    vice. American Society of Hospital Pharma-
    cists, Washington, D.C., 68: 4, 1972.
11. Conn, H. F.: Current Therapy, Ed. 24, p. 440. W.
    B. Saunders Co., Philadelphia, 1972.
12. Martin, E. W.: Hazards of Medication, Ed. 1, p.
    491. J. B. Lippincott Co., Philadelphia, 1971.
13. Anon.: AMA Drug Evaluations, Ed. 1, p. 171.
    American Medical Association, Chicago,
    1971.

chapter 21

CUSHING'S SYNDROME

Donald T. Kishi, Pharm. D.

In 1932, Cushing described the characteristic clinical manifestations found in a series of 12 patients with either documented or presumptive basophilic adenomas of the pituitary gland. The syndrome which he described and which was eventually to bear his name was most consistently characterized by the following features: adiposity of the face, neck and trunk; hypertrichosis of the face and trunk in females and preadolescent males; amenorrhea; cutaneous striae; hypertension; polycythemia; kyphosis and backaches; and fatigabilty and weakness.[1] Cushing's work delineated one possible pathological abnormality which could account for the development of the syndrome.

Cushing, however, could not elucidate the fundamental hormonal basis for the development of the syndrome. Subsequent work by endocrinologists revealed not only the basic hormonal disturbance, hypercortisolism, but also other pathological abnormalities which could lead to this hormonal disturbance and to the development of Cushing's syndrome. Consequently, this syndrome can now be defined as the group of clinical and metabolic abnormalities resulting from a chronic overproduction of cortisol (hydrocortisone).[2]

Approximately 25 years ago, exogenous glucocorticoids were introduced into the physician's armamentarium of medical therapy. Consequently, an iatrogenic cause of Cushing's syndrome also exists. Aside from this iatrogenic hyperglucocorticoidism, Cushing's syndrome occurs in the general population at a rate of 1 per 1,000. Females are afflicated 3 to 5 times more often than males. There is also a predominance in the age of onset; that is, over 50% of cases occur between 20 and 40 years of age.[3]

PHYSIOLOGY

Cortisol is the major endogenous glucocorticoid produced in the body. In the normal individual, cortisol production and secretion are governed by the hypothalamic-anterior pituitary-adrenocortical (HPA) axis. It is the primary function of this axis to maintain and control the level of circulating cortisol (Fig. 21.1).

The adrenal cortex consists of three zones: the zona glomerulosa, reticularis and fasiculata. The zona reticularis and fasiculata comprise the inner zones responsible for cortisol production and secretion. The adrenal androgens are also produced and secreted from these inner zones. The zona glomerulosa is responsible for the production and secretion of aldosterone.[4]

The production of cortisol is, in the normal individual, controlled by adrenocorticotrophic hormone(ACTH) which is secreted from the anterior pituitary gland in response to low plasma cortisol levels. Conversely, high plasma cortisol levels result in an inhibition of pituitary ACTH secretion. This relationship between ACTH and corisol manifests as a diurnal variation in their plasma levels.[5]

The synthesis of cortisol is initiated by an ACTH stimulus to the conversion of cholesterol and its esters to form pregnenolone. Pregneno-

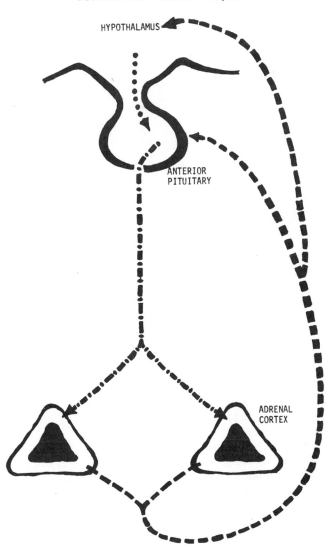

FIG. 21.1. Normal hypothalamic-anterior pituitary-adrenal cortex axis. Note: cortisol negative feed-back on hypothalamus and anterior pituitary. ...., CRF;.-.-.-.-., ACTH; - - - -, cortisol.

lone is converted by a series of enzymatic steps to form cortisol and some intermediary products such as the adrenal androgens. The final enzymatic step involves 11-hydroxylase, which will be discussed later in this chapter.

As mentioned previously, the secretion of ACTH follows a diurnal pattern; that is, there is a peak and valley effect of plasma ACTH each 24 hr. Consequently, it follows that cortisol production and secretion follow a diurnal pattern. Maximal ACTH levels occur between 2 a.m. and 6 a.m. During this time period, the stimulus to cortisol production is also at its maximum. After 8 a.m., ACTH and cortisol secretion gradually decline until the low point is reached—approximately 12 midnight. The low plasma cortisol level stimulates ACTH production and the diurnal pattern begins to repeat itself (Fig. 21.2).

The diurnal pattern of ACTH and cortisol secretion is a function of the sleep-wake or in-activity-activity pattern of an individual and not necessarily a function of daylight and night. For example, a person who works during the night and sleeps during the day will have an inverted diurnal pattern.[6] Upon initiating this altered wake-sleep pattern, 1 to 3 weeks is required to completely invert the diurnal

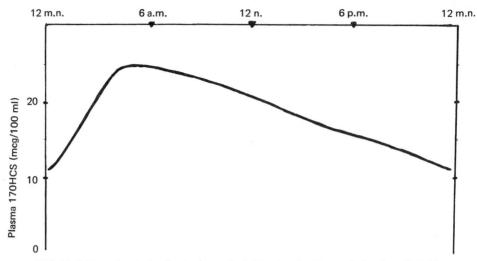

FIG. 21.2. Diurnal variation in plasma cortisol. (Reprinted with permission from Ref. 8.)

rhythm of ACTH and cortisol secretion.[7] Individuals who have been comatose for any length of time lose the rhythmicity of ACTH and cortisol secretion.[8]

The negative feedback relationship between the adrenal cortex and the anterior pituitary can be interrupted by the activation of the hypothalamic corticotrophin-releasing center. This activation is mediated by stressful stimuli which may be emotional, physical or chemical.

Stress activates the center and causes the corticotrophin-releasing factor (CRF) to enter the portal system of the pituitary. ACTH is then released from the anterior pituitary and, consequently, cortisol from the adrenal cortex. Sufficient cortisol, up to 300 mg in 24 hr is secreted to deal with the stress. Normal cortisol production ranges from 5.0 to 27.9 mg/24 hr.[9]

Once cortisol enters the circulation, it is bound primarily to an alpha-2 globulin known as corticosteroid-binding globulin (CBG) or transcortin and secondarily to albumin. In the normal individual, approximately 90% of the circulating cortisol is bound. The remaining unbound 10% is physiologically active and available for metabolism and excretion. It should be noted that pregnancy or estrogen therapy increases the amount of CBG available for cortisol binding. Conversely, CBG is decreased in conditions associated with decreased protein production or increased protein loss, e.g., cirrhosis and nephrosis.[10]

Free cortisol is metabolized by the liver by conjugation with glucuronide. This glucuroni-dated form is physiologically inactive. The metabolism of cortisol can be enhanced by concurrent hyperthyroidism and by enzyme induction by diphenylhydantoin, phenobarbital and phenylbutazone.[10, 11] Hypothyroidism and severe liver impairment inhibit the metabolism of cortisol.[10] Free cortisol to the extent of approximately 1% is excreted unchanged in the urine.[12]

PATHOPHYSIOLOGY

The fundamental hormonal defect in Cushing's syndrome is the overproduction and secretion of cortisol.[2] The overproduction of cortisol is the net result of pathological processes which relate primarily or secondarily to the adrenal cortex. Primary hypercortisolism relates to the overproduction of cortisol from an intrinsic disorder of the adrenal cortex. Secondary hypercortisolism relates to the excessive stimulation of normal adrenal cortices by an overproduction of ACTH.[13]

Primary hypercortisolism is indicative of an adrenocortical tumor, usually an adenoma or carcinoma. The adenomas and carcinomas are usually unilateral and represent 15% and 10% of the cases of Cushing's syndrome, respectively.[14, 13] The adrenocortical tumors are usually autonomous; that is, the production and secretion of cortisol by the adrenal cortex is independent of ACTH stimulation. In fact, the elevation of the cortisol levels results in a negative feedback on the normal pituitary.

Plasma levels of ACTH in the presence of these autonomously functioning tumors are subnormal and may be undetectable.[15, 16] The subnormal ACTH levels result in the atrophy of the contralateral adrenal cortex[14] (Fig. 21.3). However, even in patients with negligible ACTH, the conversion of cholesterol to pregnenolone and, eventually, to cortisol occurs but at a very slow rate. The net result is the production of 0.5 mg per day of cortisol in these individuals.[17]

Adrenocortical carcinomas occur in all age groups: however, the majority of cases occur in the 4th decade of life. There also appears to be a higher incidence in females—approximately 68% of the cases of adrenocortical carcinomas.[18]

The adrenocortical carcinomas can metastasize to other tissues. The two most common sites of distant metastases are the lung and liver. Metastatic lesions have also been reported in bone, brain, skin, spleen, myocardium, ovary, bone marrow, thoracic duct and pelvis. The metastatic lesions usually manifest the same hormonal pattern as the primary tumor.[18] Tissues adjacent to the primary tumor may also be involved.

Secondary hypercortisolism is related to the overproduction of ACTH. The excess ACTH can be from a pituitary origin or from an ectopic tumor. Although the adrenal cortex is fundamentally normal, the excess ACTH stimulation results in a hyperplasia of both adrenal cortices. Secondary hypercortisolism

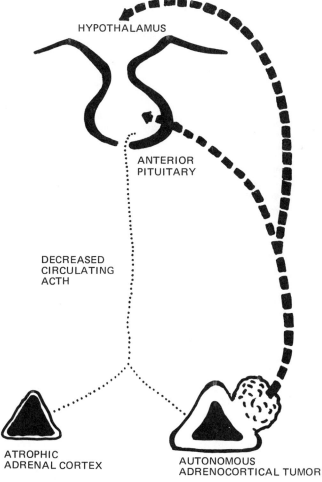

HYPOTHALAMUS

ANTERIOR PITUITARY

DECREASED CIRCULATING ACTH

ATROPHIC ADRENAL CORTEX

AUTONOMOUS ADRENOCORTICAL TUMOR

FIG. 21.3. Autonomous adrenocortical tumor. Note: negative feedback inhibition of ACTH and consequent atrophic contralateral adrenal cortex.

accounts for approximately 75% of the cases of Cushing's syndrome.[14]

The pituitary origins of Cushing's syndrome are often referred to as Cushing's disease.[13] The basophilic adenoma, carcinoma and the chromophobe adenoma represent primary anterior pituitary lesions which result in excess ACTH secretion.[14] Secondary or nontumorous pituitary ACTH overproduction is the result of an overactive hypothalamus.[19] The basophilic adenoma of the anterior pituitary and hypothalamic overactivity result in moderately elevated ACTH production. The chromophobe adenoma, in contrast, is associated with marked elevation of ACTH secretion. In the latter case, the minor melanocyte-stimulating properties of ACTH become significant. Consequently, the skin of patients with chromophobe adenomas is pigmented. Another contrasting feature which distinguishes the chromophobe adenoma from basophilic adenoma and hypothalamic overactivity is the size of the sella turcica. The chromophobe adenoma is associated with radiological evidence of sella turcica enlargement, whereas the hypothalamic overactivity and basophilic adenoma generally are not[14] (Fig. 21.4)

The ectopic nonendocrine tumors, which secrete an ACTH-like substance, result in mean cortisol secretion rates 3 times higher than that found in other forms of Cushing's syndrome.[20] This is perhaps the most insidious cause of Cushing's syndrome since the clinical picture may not always suggest adrenocortical overactivity. The most common findings are progressive weakness, muscle wasting, edema and severe hypokalemic alkalosis. The severity of hypokalemic alkalosis appears to be a function of the degree of hypercortisolism and cortisol renal effect and may not relate to hyperaldosteronism. Death has been reported within days of the onset of these nonclassical findings.[20]

The two most common ectopic ACTH-producing tumors are the oat cell carcinoma of the lung and pancreatic carcinomas. The former represents greater than 50%, and the latter 20%, of reported cases of ectopic ACTH-producing tumors. Other common sites of these ectopic tumors include the gall bladder, thymus and fibrosarcomas located retroperitoneally. Rarely reported sites include the breast, colon, ovaries, testes, prostate, kidney, thyroid, parotids, trachea and parathyroids. The metastatic lesions from these primary ectopic ACTH-producing tumors manifest the same hormonal patterns as the primary tumors.[20]

The ectopic ACTH-producing tumors are usually autonomous. The tumors of the anterior pituitary and the hyperfunctioning hypothalamus lack this autonomous behavior and are responsive to high glucocorticoid plasma levels. It appears that the HPA negative feedback threshold for plasma glucocorticoid is abnormally elevated.[20]

It should be noted that the etiologies of Cushing's syndrome are not as clear-cut as defined in this section. There appears to be a definite intermediate form of adrenocortical hyperplasia and adenoma.[21, 22] This rare intermediate form is termed "primary adrenocortical nodular dysplasia."[22] Gross pathological examination reveals adrenocortical hyperplasia with multiple small adenomas. Characteristically, this intermediate form is resistant to dexamethasone suppression, may show either a hyperactive or no response to exogenous ACTH stimulation and is associated with low plasma ACTH levels[22] (Fig. 21.5).

The manifestations of Cushing's syndrome can result from the therapeutic use of exogenous ACTH and/or glucocorticoids in the patient with an intact, normally functioning HPA axis or from the use of supraphysiological glucocorticoid replacement. The predictability or assignment of a minimal total daily dose of glucocorticoid or ACTH necessary to induce a given symptom, finding or the entire syndrome complex is not feasible. This lack of predictability is based on the individual variability of cortisol synthesis and secretion. Although the total daily dose is a major factor in the development of some of the signs and symptoms of Cushing's syndrome, other factors also play a major role. Factors such as the dosage regimen, total dose and duration of therapy are also major factors in the rate of the development of specific findings or manifestations of Cushing's syndrome. The picture of iatrogenic Cushing's syndrome is further complicated by the fact that a patient may have a predisposition for a given finding or manifestation.

ELECTROLYTES

Cortisol and other glucocorticoids have varying degrees of mineralocorticoid properties. However, the serum sodium in Cushing's syn-

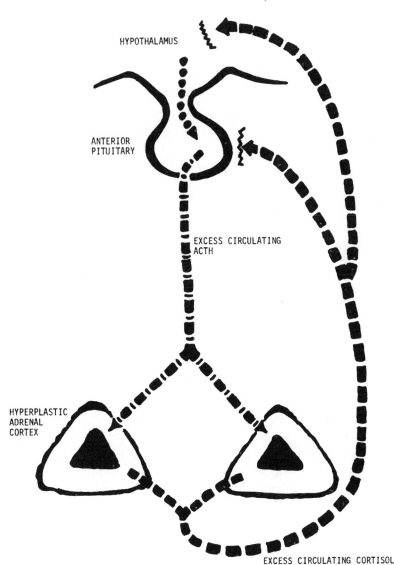

HYPOTHALAMUS

ANTERIOR
PITUITARY

EXCESS CIRCULATING
ACTH

HYPERPLASTIC
ADRENAL
CORTEX

EXCESS CIRCULATING CORTISOL

FIG. 21.4. Bilateral adrenocortical hyperplasia due to excess anterior pituitary ACTH production. Note: relative loss of negative feedback effect of excess cortisol.

drome is usually normal.[14],[23],[24]. Exogenous glucocorticoid therapy is associated with a positive sodium balance. With continued therapy, however, an escape from the abnormal sodium retention occurs.[25] The latter mechanism might also explain the normal serum sodium in Cushing's syndrome.

Hypokalemic alkalosis is associated primarily with Cushing's syndrome due to an ectopic ACTH-producing tumor and high dose glucocorticoid therapy.[23],[24]

Calcium balance is negative owing to an inhibition of vitamin D and decreased calcium renal tubular reabsorption which result in increased fecal calcium and hypercalciuria. In spite of the negative calcium balance, serum calcium levels are normal. However, serum phosphate is reduced in 50% of Cushing's syndrome patients and is based on increased fecal and urinary phosphate clearance.[23],[26],[27]

It is now recognized that a continued elevation of plasma glucocorticoid—loss of diurnal variation—is a basic characteristic of Cushing's syndrome. Consequently, iatrogenic Cushing's syndrome would occur more rapidly in the patient with a divided daily dose regimen than

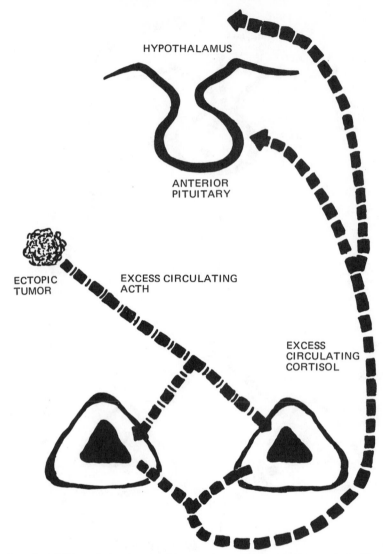

FIG. 21.5. Ectopic ACTH-producing tumor with secondary adrenocortical hyperplasia. Note: negative feedback inhibition of anterior pituitary ACTH secretion.

in the patient on a single morning dose, alternate day or intermittent dosing regimen. At the same time, the particular glucocorticoid preparation used is important since there is a difference in duration of tissue effects as exemplified by their variation in HPA axis suppression. With respect to this latter example, dexamethasone and betamethasone suppress the HPA for greater than 2.5 days, triamcinolone and paramethasone for 2.0 to 2.5 days and cortisol prednisolone for less than 1.5 days.[28]

Systemic effects have also been reported during topical,[29] ophthalmic,[30] aerosol,[31] and rectal[32] administration of glucocorticoids. Thus, the potential for development of iatrogenic Cushing's syndrome should not be thought of as being limited to systemic therapy. Rather, the possibility of iatrogenic Cushing's syndrome should be considered whenever a chronic course of glucocorticoid therapy by any route of administration is being considered.

DIAGNOSIS

Patients with the manifestations of classic Cushing's syndrome can be easily recognized.

Unfortunately, it is only the patient with long standing hypercortisolism who presents with these classic manifestations. Patients with a shorter history of hypercortisolism have variable signs and symptoms. This variability of presenting manifestations makes diagnosis of early Cushing's syndrome difficult. It is, therefore, recommended that patients even remotely suspected of hypercortisolism be tested.[23]

The diagnosis of Cushing's syndrome involves two phases: documentation that hypercortisolism exists and the elucidation of the etiology of the hypercortisolism.[33] In the normal adult, cortisol secretion rate varies from 5.0 to 27.9 mg/24 hr.[9] In normal, unstressed males the mean secretion rate is 20.4 mg/24 hr. In normal, unstressed females a mean secretion rate of 17.4 mg/24 hr has been reported.[34] In infants less than 5 days old, the cortisol secretion rate is 18 mg per meter^2 per day. By age 11, the secretion rate is 11 mg per meter^2 per day, essentially the same as an adult.[35] The diagnosis of Cushing's syndrome is based on direct or indirect evidence of hypercortisolism.

SCREENING TESTS

It would seem logical that the demonstration of a single, elevated plasma cortisol level 17-hydroxycorticosteroid (measured as [17-OHCS]) would be sufficient to document hypercortisolism. However, since cortisol secretion and production may be temporarily elevated by stress, a single plasma level may solely reflect such a temporary elevation and not sustained overproduction. It also should be noted that plasma levels of cortisol may be elevated by factors which elevate CBG, e.g., estrogens and pregnancy.[36] If, on the other hand, two plasma cortisol levels are drawn, one in the early morning and the second in the late evening, loss of diurnal rhythm in plasma cortisol level due to sustained overproduction of cortisol can be demonstrated. The presence of a diurnal rhythm in plasma cortisol levels, however, does not totally exclude the possibility that Cushing's syndrome exists.[37] In general, it can be stated that, while the early morning plasma cortisol levels may be elevated or normal, the evening plasma cortisol level is abnormally elevated in Cushing's syndrome. Indirect evidence of the overproduction of cortisol can be obtained by measurement of urinary 17-OHCS excretion. In the normal adult, 3 to 12 mg of 17-OHCS are excreted in the urine in 24 hr. In patients with a 17-OHCS urinary excretion which exceeds 12 mg/24 hr, Cushing's syndrome must be suspected.[38,39] Since obesity influences the rate of 17-OHCS excretion, a correction factor for body weight is made. This correction factor is based on urinary 17-OHCS excretion per g of urinary creatinine. In the normal adult, 3 to 7 mg of 17-OHCS is excreted per g of urinary creatinine. On the other hand, patients with Cushing's syndrome excrete greater than 10 mg of 17–OHCS per g of urinary creatinine.[38,39] Cortisol secretion rate can be measured by the radioisotope-dilution method. Unfortunately, although considered by some to be the definitive test for overproduction of cortisol, the limited availability of this test makes it an impractical method of testing.

Dexamethasone can be used as a diagnostic tool in the establishment of cortisol overproduction. The low dose dexamethasone-suppression test and the more simple dexamethasone-screening test are based on the negative feedback system of the HPA axis. Dexamethasone is used since it does not contribute significantly to the 17-OHCS levels, yet it has significant glucocorticoid activity. The dexamethasone-suppression test is performed by administering 1 mg of the drug orally between 11 p.m. and 12 midnight with subsequent measurement of plasma 17-OHCS at 8 a.m. the following morning. In normal individuals, the level of plasma 17-OHCS is suppressed to less than 5 μg% when measured by the Porter-Silber method.[40] If 17-OHCS is measured by the Eik-Nes method,[41] normal individuals have a level of less than 11 μg%; plasma levels between 11 and 19 μg% are indeterminate and a level of 20 μg% or greater is considered evidence of the existence of Cushing's syndrome. Regardless of the method of measurement, it is recommended that sedation with a barbiturate be given during the evening to eliminate the possibility of stress-induced activation of the HPA axis and resultant temporary increase in cortisol production.[40]

The low lose dexamethasone-suppression test[42] consists of collecting two baseline 24-hr urine samples for 17-OHCS. Dexamethasone 0.5 mg is administered orally every 6 hr for eight doses. During the administration of the dexamethasone, 24 hr urine samples for 17-OHCS are collected. The normal patient will have 17-OHCS levels less than 2.5 μg and/or lower levels than the controls. Patients with Cushing's syndrome will show no suppression of 17-OHCS when compared to the baseline collections. However, diagnosis of Cushing's syndrome is not based on one single finding or test. Rather, loss of diurnal variation in plasma cortisol levels, elevated urinary 17-OHCS levels, clinical manifestations and suppression of HPA by the dexamethasone screening or low dose suppression test all contribute to the diagnosis of Cushing's syndrome.

DIFFERENTIAL DIAGNOSIS

Once the diagnosis of Cushing's syndrome has been established, the underlying pathology producing the chronic overproduction of cortisol, i.e., hypothalamic-pituitary malfunction, adrenocortical tumor or ectopic ACTH-secreting tumor must be elucidated. There are a variety of diagnostic tests which can be used for the differential diagnosis. Currently, the high dose dexamethasone-suppression test is the most widely accepted.

The high dose dexamethasone-suppression test[42] is an extension of the low dose test. If the low dose test indicates the presence of Cushing's syndrome, the high dose suppression test is initiated. In the high dose suppression test, 2 mg of dexamethasone are administered orally every 6 hr for eight doses. During this time period, two consecutive 24 hr urine samples for 17-OHCS are collected. If suppression of the production of cortisol occurs, as reflected by a comparison of the base-like 24-hr urinary 17-OHCS and the final 24-hr urinary 17-OHCS, the etiology of the hypercortisolism is hypothalamic-pituitary malfunction with secondary bilateral adrenal hyperplasia. If no suppression occurs, the diagnosis may be either adrenocortical tumor or ectopic ACTH-producing tumor.

Metyrapone has also been used in the differential diagnosis of adrenocortical hyperplasia and adrenocortical tumors. The basis of the metyrapone test is the responsiveness of hyperplastic adrenals and the autonomous behavior of tumors to ACTH stimulation. Metyrapone is administered orally in a dose of 750 mg every 4 hr until a maximum of 4.5 to 5.0 g is reached

or intravenous infusion of 30 mg per kg body weight of metyrapone in normal saline or 5% dextrose in water over a 2-to 4-or 16-hr period.[43,44] At this dosage, metyrapone inhibits the 11-hydroxylation step of cortisol production. Consequently, plasma cortisol levels fall and initiate the stimulus for cortisol production via the HPA axis. In patients with normal or hyperplastic adrenal cortices, the response to the resultant increased ACTH production is a buildup of cortisol precursors which are measured as urinary 17-OHCS. Autonomously functioning adenomas and carcinomas of the adrenal cortex are not ACTH-dependent and do not respond to the ACTH stimulus. The metyrapone test is subject to interference by a number of drugs including diphenylhydantoin, meprobamate and chlorpromazine.[45]

The differential diagnosis of adrenocortical tumor versus ectopic ACTH-producing tumor is based on the plasma ACTH levels. Ectopic ACTH-producing tumors result in elevated ACTH levels. Adrenocortical tumors are autonomous and, consequently, are independent of ACTH stimulation for cortisol production. Autonomous adrenocortical tumors producing excess cortisol result in the inhibition of pituitary ACTH release.

The differential diagnosis of adrenocortical adenoma versus adrenocortical carcinoma is not as clear. In general, it can be said that carcinomas are associated with an elevated urinary 17-ketosteroid (17-KS) and an elevated or normal 17-OHCS excretion, whereas adenomas may be associated with slightly elevated, normal or even low 17-KS urinary excretion levels.[14,18] Normal 17-KS urinary excretion approximates 10 ± 5 mg/24 hr in females, and 15 ± 5 mg/24 hr in males. Adrenocortical carcinomas have been associated with urinary 17-KS ranging from 40 to 100 mg/24 hr. Another potential distinguishing characteristic of the adrenocortical carcinoma is its lack of response to ACTH stimulation.[14] Adrenocortical adenomas, on the other hand, may (rarely) respond to ACTH by increasing 24 hr urinary 17-OHCS excretion as compared to a control collection.[46,47]

The establishment of the diagnosis and the further delineation of the etiology of Cushing's syndrome are based primarily on the direct or indirect laboratory demonstration of hypercortisolism. The laboratory methods used in the determination of elevated cortisol levels are subject to interference by medications and chemicals. As a consequence, there must be an awareness by the diagnostician and his fellow clinicians of the possible interfering factors peculiar to his institution because variations in laboratory methods and facilities do exist. There are comprehensive tabulations available to assist in identifying potentially interfering substances[36] and physiological conditions.

Factors which alter the physiology and metabolism of cortisol should be sought out and corrected before evaluation begins. Drugs such as diphenylhydantoin and phenobarbital, which have been known to speed up the metabolism of cortisol, should be considered.[36] Alteration of the protein binding of cortisol, such as pregnancy or estrogen-induced elevation of CBG, and consequently circulating plasma cortisol, should be noted.[36] Patients who are acutely ill and/or under stress will also have an elevated plasma cortisol level.

CLINICAL MANIFESTATIONS

The clinical manifestations and pathologies of Cushing's syndrome are primarily the result of the actions of a chronic excess of cortisol, regardless of etiology. However, since adrenal androgens are intermediary by-products of cortisol biosynthesis, manifestations of excess androgens can contribute to the clinical presentation of patients with Cushing's syndrome. Since secondary hypercortisolism is attributable to chronic excess ACTH production, extra-adrenal manifestations as well as adrenal manifestations of ACTH can occur—transient aldosterone stimulation and melanocyte stimulation.[5] Although ACTH is only 1/100 as potent as melanocyte-stimulating hormone (MSH), ACTH in excess can cause pigmentation.

The patient with clinical manifestations of classic Cushing's syndrome is easily recognizable. However, since adrenocortical activity can be present in patients with few signs and symptoms suggestive of classical Cushing's syndrome, recognition of the existence of the syndrome may be difficult.

This difficulty may be attributable to the fact that cortisol possesses multiple actions which affect the metabolic processes of most tissues. These actions of cortisol on a given tissue can be augmented or counterbalanced by the actions of other hormones and other homeostatic mechanisms. Thus, the clinical manifestations and pathological findings due to excess cortisol are the net result of the interaction of cortisol and the counterbalancing hormone or other homeostatic mechanisms for the tissue and the metabolic process involved.[48] However, the severity of a given cortisol-induced problem is not related to the plasma cortisol level,[37] but certain signs, symptoms, effects or laboratory values may occur more frequently in relation to a higher cortisol level.[14] Thus, there is considerable variability in the clinical manifestation in patients with Cushing's syndrome.

As the term "glucocorticoid" implies, cortisol and other compounds in this group have an effect on glucose. This involvement is primarily manifest in the intermediary metabolism of carbohydrates. In general, cortisol causes a glucose-sparing effect and increased glucose production through its influences on protein, lipid and carbohydrate metabolism. The net result is a tendency toward hyperglycemia.

The effect of cortisol on the metabolism of proteins, lipids and carbohydrates can be either catabolic or anabolic. The action of cortisol on muscle, lymphoid, connective, and adipose tissue is catabolic and results in the release of fatty acids, glycerol and glucose. In addition, cortisol may exert an antianabolic action on these tissues by inhibiting the passage of amino acids and glucose into these tissues.[49,50] Cortisol exerts an anabolic action on the liver which through the utilization of amino acids, fatty acids, and glycerol results in the increased production of protein, ribonucleic acid (RNA) and glucose.[51] The clinical manifestations and frequency of appearance of these metabolic derangements in these and other tissues are noted in Table 21.1

Hyperglycemia

These metabolic breakdown products— amino acids, glycerol and fatty acids—provide raw materials for hepatic gluconeogenesis. Cortisol also has a direct anti-insulin effect.[52,53] Consequently, hyperglycemia, decreased glucose tolerance, a relative resistance to insulin and glycosuria may occur.[54] This hyperglycemic effect is dependent on the presence of excess cortisol for its persistence.[55] Patients with latent diabetes will exhibit diabetes in the

TABLE 21.1
*The Presenting Signs and/or Symptoms
in Cushing's Syndrome*

Sign or Sympton	$(N = 601)^a$ %	$(N = 50)^b$ %
Obesity	88	94
Generalized		60
Trunkal		40
Moonface	75	84
Menstrual irregularities	60	76[c]
Muscular Weakness	61	58
Bruising	42	36
Psychological difficulties	42	
Acne	45	
Hirsuitism	65	82
Backache	40	
Striae		52
Osteoporosis on x-ray		46
Hypertension		
BP 140/90		72
BP 100 diastolic		54
Renal calculi		16
Cholelithiasis		10

[a]Review of 601 patients.[2 3]

[b]Report on 50 patients.[2 1]

[c]Twenty-nine female patients.[2 3]

presence of hypercortisolism. Patients with diabetes who develop Cushing's syndrome will experience exacerbation of the diabetes. In general, the diabetes of hypercortisolism is mild, reversible and not associated with ketosis.

Obesity, Moon Face, Buffalo Hump

Cortisol causes a redistribution of fat without a major alteration in total body fat.[50] The manifestation of this redistribution of fat is the moon face, protuberant abdomen and buffalo hump of the classic Cushing's syndrome patient. The redistribution of fat results from the facilitation of lipolysis by cortisol and the lipogenic effect of insulin. The net result is deposition of fat in areas of the body where the lipogenic effect of insulin predominates—face, back, abdomen—and the loss of fat in tissues where the action of cortisol predominates.[50]

Myopathy

The myopathy which results from excess cortisol is characteristically found in the proxi-

mal musculature of the extremities as seen on electromyography and tissue biopsy. The negative nitrogen balance—protein wasting—which results from cortisol is the result of catabolism, as evidenced by an elevation of amino acids leaving the tissue, and an antianabolic effect, demonstrated as a decrease in amino acids entering the tissue.[51] Additionally, inhibition of glucose uptake into muscle tissue may be a contributing factor.[49]

The myopathy of Cushing's syndrome is usually moderate in severity, may not be progressive and clears upon correction of the endocrine defect. However, there are reports of persistent cases following the correction of hypercortisolism.[56]

Osteoporosis, Compression Fractures of the Vertebra, Low Back Pain, Nephrocalcinosis, Renal Stones

Cortisol-induced osteoporosis is generally accepted as being associated with prolonged elevations of cortisol. It can occur in all bones, but is primarily associated with vertebrae (2%), dorsal and lumbar vertebrae (54%), femoral neck (18%), ribs (12%), and other long bones (14%).[57]

The mechanisms responsible for cortisol-induced osteoporosis are several: inhibition of vitamin D and consequent reduction of intestinal calcium absorption,[58] increased glomerular filtration and direct tubular action which increase urinary calcium clearance,[26] and catabolism of the proteinaceous bone matrix with consequent decrease in surface area for calcium deposition.[27]

Psychological Changes

There is no specific psychological picture associated with elevated cortisol levels. Rather, hypercortisolism amplifies pre-existent psychological defects,[59] which run the gamut from simple nervousness through hallucinations and paranoid ideation.[60] Regestein et al.[59] reported such cases of Cushing's syndrome with associated mental aberrations. They noted the following correlations: organic brain syndrome occurs more commonly in individuals 65 years of age or older; the same type psychological aberrations caused by excess cortisol may have been precipitated in the same individual previously by stress; and only nervousness was exhibited by an individual with no previous psychological problems and a secure background.

Hypertension, Edema

Cortisol exerts a permissive action on catecholamine effects.[60] In the cardiovascular system, this permissive effect results in an increased heart rate, improvement in left ventricular efficiency and an increase in arterial pressure. Cortisol also enhances the hepatic production of angiotensinogen;[60] this may result in an increase in angiotensin and consequent stimulus for vascular contraction and aldosterone production. The mineralocorticoid properties of cortisol and the ACTH stimulus to aldosterone production also provide other mechanisms for hypertension and edema in Cushing's syndrome.

Acne, Hirsuitism, Amenorrhea

Adrenal androgens are produced in the zona fasciculata and reticularis of the adrenal cortex. The production of these androgens is initiated by ACTH. Thus the manifestations of excess androgen in Cushing's syndrome due to excess ACTH production are not unexpected. Adrenocortical tumors can secrete cortisol and androgens alone or in combination.[18] Therefore, manifestations of excess androgens can also occur simultaneously with Cushing's syndrome secondary to adrenocortical tumors. Hirsuitism, acne and amenorrhea are most commonly associated with increased androgens in Cushing's syndrome.

Short Stature

Short stature is found in all children with hypercortisolism.[61] The mechanism of cortisol-induced growth suppression has not been fully defined; however, it is known that growth hormone secretion is not suppressed by elevated cortisol levels.[62] This implies that there may be a block in the peripheral actions of growth hormone.

Ulcer

The incidence of peptic ulceration in Cushing's syndrome is no greater than that found in the general population—less than 10%.[63,64] This low incidence is contrary to the widely accepted belief that glucocorticoid therapy caused ulceration.[28] The literature also does not support this belief. Nonarthritic patients receiving glucocorticoids for ulcerative colitis,[65] asthma,[66] other pulmonary diseases[67] and pemphigus[68] do not experience ulceration at a greater incidence rate than that found in the general population. A review of early reports of glucocorticoid-induced ulceration reveals that the patients under consideration were rheumatoid arthritics. No consideration was given to the concomitant gastric irritants—salicylates, phenylbutazone or indomethacin—which these patients commonly use. Thus, it appears that the significance of glucocorticoid-induced ulceration is questionable with the exception of patients known to have a predisposition to gastric ulceration. Therefore, it is not surprising that the incidence of peptic ulceration in patients with Cushing's syndrome approximates that in the general population.

LABORATORY MANIFESTATIONS

Erythrocytes

In his original report, Cushing noted a tendency toward erythemia in five of nine patients studied. cushing defined erythemia as a red blood cell count of greater than 5,000,000 per cubic mm. However, based on their study and other reported cases, Ross et al.[23] concluded that polycythemia, if defined as a red cell count greater than 6,000,000, a hemoglobin concentration of 18 g/100 ml or a hemotocrit of greater than 55%, is a rare occurrence in Cushing's syndrome.

White Blood Cells

Polymorphonuclear leukocytosis is often noted in Cushing's syndrome. In contrast, the lymphocytopenia and an eosinopenia are also noted in this syndrome. A lymphocytopenia of less than 25% was noted by Ross et al.[23] in 50% of their patients. Similarly, an eosinopenia of less than 100 eosinophils per cubic mm was noted in 37 of 42 patients studied. Of these 37 patients, the absolute eosinophil count was less than 10 eosinophils per cubic mm. The authors concluded that an eosinophil count of less than

10 per cubic mm favors the diagnosis of Cushing's syndrome, and that an eosinophil count in excess of 100 per cubic mm precludes the diagnosis of Cushing's syndrome.

THERAPY

Adrenocortical Adenoma and Adrenocortical Carcinoma

In Cushing's syndrome due to an adenoma or a nonmetastatic carcinoma of the adrenal cortex, the recommended mode of therapy is total unilateral adrenalectomy of the involved gland. This procedure is preferred over partial resection of the involved gland since the latter frequently is associated with recurrence of the tumor in the adrenal remnant.[14]

In considerating surgical intervention, it must be recalled that adrenocortical adenomas and carcinomas function autonomously. Consequently, the contralateral adrenal cortex is atrophic owing to the lack of ACTH stimulation. Since surgical excision of the adenomatous or carcinomatous gland results in removal of the only source of corisol production in the body, supplemental exogenous glucocorticoid must be supplied to the patient until the atrophic contralateral adrenal cortex recovers. If supplemental therapy with exogenous glucocorticoids is not provided during and after surgery, collapse due to acute adrenal insufficiency—Addisonian crisis—can occur. A suggested regimen for providing exogenous glucocorticoids is noted in Table 21.2.[14]

Subsequent tapering of glucocorticoid replacement should be performed by eliminating the 4 p.m. dose. The morning dose should be tapered until there is no longer a need for exogenous glucocorticoid replacement owing to the recovery of the contralateral adrenal cortex. If tapering beyond that shown in Table 21.2 is not possible owing to development of symptoms and signs of adrenal insufficiency, permanent glucocorticoid replacement therapy and concomitant ACTH stimulation therapy may be indicated. If at any time during the tapering procedure the patient is subjected to stress, the dose of replacement glucocorticoid may have to be temporarily increased to avoid acute adrenal insufficiency.

Inoperative Adrenocortical Carcinoma

Patients who are debilitated or who have metastatic lesions are considered to be inoperable. In these patients, chemotherapy is indicated to alleviate the overproduction of cortisol. Currently, two agents which can be used for the chemotherapy of Cushing's syndrome are mitotane (o, p'-DDD) and aminoglutethimide.

Mitotane is a derivative of the insecticide, DDD. The latter chemical was noted to cause adrenocortical necrosis in the canine. However, it was also found to be too toxic. Consequently, mitotane was developed. This compound is 20 times more potent and less toxic than its parent compound, DDD.

The mechanism of mitotane adrenolysis remains to be elucidated. The theoretical possibilities of this agent's suppression or inhibition of cortisol synthesis and/or the stimulation of conversion of cortisol to a more polar compound remain to be established.[69] However, it has been demonstrated that the zona reticularis and the zona fasciculata of the canine adrenal cortex atrophy in response to mitotane. This atrophy, however, is not attributable to an inhibition of pituitary ACTH secretion.[70] Consequently, the action of this drug is primarily directed toward the adrenal cortex.

The primary use of mitotane is in the treatment of adrenocortical carcinomas. When it is being considered for use, the following guidelines are applicable[71]:

1. The use of mitotane in adrenocortical carcinomas should be reserved for those patients who are considered inoperable.
2. Metastatic lesions or local recurrences should be treated as early as possible to obtain remission.
3. Therapy should be pursued for 4 to 5 weeks following initiation of therapy, since 86% of patients require a minimum of 4 weeks to respond. If there is no response following a trial of 4 to 5 weeks of therapy, the prospect of obtaining response with continued therapy is poor.[69]
4. If a response is obtained, therapy should be continued at a maximal tolerable dose for as long as possible.
5. The daily dose should approximate 10 g per day.

TABLE 21.2

Pre, Intra, Postoperative Management of Glucocorticoid Replacement for Cushing's Syndrome[a]

Relative Time	Medication	Dose (mg)	Route	Regimen
Evening prior to surgery	Cortisone acetate	100	I.M.	Single dose
Day of surgery	Cortisone acetate	100	I.M.	Single dose, preoperatively
	Hydrocortisone phosphate or sodium succinate	300	I.V. Infusion	Intraoperatively, postoperatively, over the remainder of the operative day
Postoperative day 1	Cortisone acetate	50	I.M.	Single dose, evening of the operative day
	Cortisone acetate	50	I.M.	Morning and evening
	Hydrocortisone phosphate or sodium succinate	200	I.V.	Infusion, over the next 24 hr
Postoperative day 2	Cortisone acetate	50	I.M.	Morning and evening
	Hydrocortisone phosphate or sodium succinate	150	I.V.	Infusion, over the next 24 hr
Postoperative day 3	Cortisone acetate	50	I.M.	Morning and evening
	Hydrocortisone phosphate or sodium succinate	10	I.V.	Infusion, over the next 24 hr
Postoperative day 4	Cortisone acetate	50/25	I.M.	Morning and evening
	Cortisone acetate	25	P.O.	Q.I.D.
Postoperative day 5	Cortisone acetate	50	I.M.	Morning
	Cortisone acetate	25	P.O.	Q.I.D.
Postoperative day 6	Cortisone acetate	50-25-25-25	P.O.	Q.I.D.
Postoperative day 7	Cortisone acetate	25	P.O.	Q.I.D.
Postoperative day 8	Cortisone acetate	25-12.5-25-12.5	P.O.	Q.I.D.
Postoperative day 9 through 14	Cortisone acetate	25-12.5-2.5	P.O.	T.I.D. (last daily dose 4 p.m.)
Postoperative day 15 through 21	Cortisone acetate	25-12.5-12.5	P.O.	T.I.D. (last daily dose 4 p.m.)
Postoperative day 22	Cortisone acetate	25		Morning
	Cortisone acetate	12.5		4 p.m.

[a]Adapted with permission from Ref. 14.

Tumor regression is the most reliable method of evaluating response to mitotane. Urinary 17-OHCS can not be relied upon since the drug alters the ratio of cortisol metabolites.[72] In the normal individual, tetrahydrocortisone and tetrahydrocortisol metabolites predominate over the more polar 6- p-hydroxy metabolite.

In pateints receiving mitotane therapy, the 6-p-hydroxy metabolite predominates. Since this latter metabolite is not extracted by the conventional methods for quantification of 17-hydroxycorticoids, values obtained are spuriously low and thus do not accurately reflect plasma cortisol levels.

Using objective evidence of tumor regression as criteria for response, Hutter and Kayhoe[69] noted a 34% response rate in a series of 138 patients treated with mitotane. A 35% response rate was noted when subjective symptomatic criteria were evaluated. The average dose required to obtain objective evidence of tumor regression was 8.1 g per day. Although the authors noted no correlation between age, sites or location of metastases and effectiveness of therapy, they did note that females responded to mitotane better than their male counterparts.

The adversities of mitotane therapy are most frequently associated with the gastrointestinal and neuromuscular systems. In the study by Hutter and Kayhoe[69] approximately 80% of 138 patients that were treated manifested anorexia, nausea, vomiting or diarrhea. Diarrhea occurred in 20% of the patients. Neuromuscular side effects appeared in 41% of the 138 patients. Lethargy and somnolence appeared in 26% and dizziness and vertigo in 14%. Muscle tremors, headache, confusion and weakness were also noted. The gastrointestinal and neuromuscular side effects are dose-related and are alleviated by discontinuance or reduction in the dose of the drug.

Dermatological reactions—skin rash—appeared in 14% of the patients. This reaction was not dose-related and can resolve itself spontaneously with continued therapy.

Other adverse reactions which were noted by Hutter and Kayhoe were: visual blurring, diplopia, reversible lens opacities, toxic actinopathy with papilledema and retinal hemorrhages, alopecia, erythema multiforme, hematuria, hemorrhagic cystitis, albuminuria, hypertension, orthostasis, aching pain and a decrease in protein-bound iodine (PBI).[69]

Aminoglutethimide was originally introduced as an anticonvulsant in the early 1950's. It was subsequently withdrawn from the market owing to the adverse reactions associated with the drug. The toxicities of aminoglutethimide include hypothyroidism and hypocortisolism which paradoxically may prove to be beneficial in Cushing's syndrome due to adrenocortical carcinoma.

Aminoglutethimide is a general adrenocortical poison as evidenced by vacuolization of the adrenal cortex in patients treated with the agent. There is also evidence for an inhibitory effect on cortisol sythesis which has been attributed to aminoglutethimide inhibition of the adrenocortical enzyme 20-hydroxylase.[73] Thus, cholesterol is not converted to pregnenolone, the first step in adrenocortical cortisol synthesis.[74]

Aminoglutethimide is used in doses of 1 g per day in divided doses. Higher doses may be required to obtain control or recapture control if escape has occurred. Used in the appropriate doses, aminoglutethimide, in contrast to mitotane, is rapid acting. The onset of action occurs within days rather than weeks as is the case with the latter drug. Similarly to mitotane, tumor regression and not urinary 17-OHCS levels should be used to monitor the effectiveness of the compound. Unlike mitotane, aminoglutethimide only transiently affects the zona glomerulosa and, consequently, aldosterone production and secretion.[75]

Ectopic ACTH-producing Tumors

The primary therapy for ectopic ACTH-producing tumors is surgical excision or radiotherapy. The majority of these tumors are malignant and nonresectable. Alternative therapy includes the adrenolytic agents, mitotane and aminoglutethimide, or in the early stages of the disease, bilateral total adrenalectomy. The alternative modes of therapy involve therapeutic maneuvers to correct the hypercortisolism and not the primary problem—the ectopic ACTH-producing tumor. The effectiveness of the adrenolytic agents in this type of Cushing's syndrome remains questionable.[13,20]

CUSHING'S DISEASE

The primary therapy for Cushing's disease is pituitary irradiation in doses of 4,000 to 5,000 rads over a 1-month period. Pituitary irradiation is effective in approximately 48% of the cases treated. Bilateral total adrenalectomy is the alternative approach and should be used in radiotherapy failures.[13]

If bilateral total adrenalectomy is to be performed, it should be emphasized that these patients will require permanent glucocorticoid and mineralocorticoid-substitution therapy. The patient should be prepared preoperatively and intraoperatively as described in Table 21.1. Postoperative management is the same with the following exceptions: On the 4th postoperative day, fludrocortisone 0.1 mg daily is initiated. Dosage of fludrocortisone must be titrated subsequently to provide adequate mineralocorticoid-replacement therapy permanently.[14] It must be emphasized that the patient who is on permanent substitution therapy must be given an increased dose of cortisone acetate or other glucocorticoid during stress situations as they occur during the remainder of his life.

In patients who are not surgical candidates, mitotane therapy may be attempted. Mitotane therapy has only a minor effect on the zona glomerulosa of the adrenal cortex. Consequently, in contrast to surgical intervention, no mineralocorticoid replacement is required. The dose of mitotane required usually ranges from 3 to 6 g daily in divided doses. Therapy is usually continued for 4 to 6 months. If necessary, smaller maintenance doses may be continued for a longer period. In the 3 to 6 g per day dosage range, the primary side effects noted are nausea and ataxia.[13]

Hypophysectomy is another therapeutic alternative in the treatment of Cushing's disease. However, it is viewed unfavorably owing to a high operative complication rate and the necessity of substitution therapy for varying degrees of hypopituitarism which result.[13]

PROGNOSIS

Prior to the introduction of glucocorticoids as pharmacological agents, the prognosis for patients with Cushing's syndrome was poor. Indeed, the 5-year survival was reported to be less than 50%. Currently, the survival of patients with Cushing's syndrome due to adrenal adenoma and Cushing's disease has improved markedly owing to the introduction of glucocorticoid replacement therapy. In a recent report,[13] a 100% cure was reported in 17 patients with adrenal adenoma following adrenalectomy. Patients with Cushing's disease were treated with pituitary irradiation (51 patients), adrenalectomy (28), mitotane (8), and hypophysectomy (3). The following results were obtained: pituitary irradiation—10 patients cured, 13 patients improved, 21 patients unimproved and 7 patients were followed less than one year; adrenalectomy—21 patients cured, 1 patient improved and the remaining patient did not improve; mitotane—8 patients cured; and hypophysectomy—1 patient cured and 2 patients did not improve. The basic factor for improved survival may be the development of an exogenous glucocorticoid source and, consequently, temporary or permanent replacement therapy.

Patients with Cushing's syndrome due to adrenocortical carcinoma or the ectopic ACTH syndrome continue to have a poor prognosis. In the study previously noted in this section, 17 patients with the ectopic ACTH syndrome all died within 18 months of diagnosis in spite of surgery, radiation or chemotherapy. Of 12 patients with adrenocortical carcinoma, 9 were treated with adrenalectomy and 3 were treated with mitotane. The following results were obtained: adrenalectomy—3 patients cured, 2 patients improved but with recurrent tumors and 4 died; mitotane—all 3 patients improved; however, 1 died after 10 months of therapy.[13]

SUMMARY

The basic hormonal defect in Cushing's syndrome is the overproduction of cortisol. The etiology of this hypercortisolism may be associated either primarily or secondarily with the adrenal cortex. Adrenocortical tumors comprise the primary lesions. Adrenocortical hyperplasias due to a defect in ACTH production of the anterior pituitary gland or from an ectopic nonendocrine tumor comprise the secondary lesions involved in the excess production of cortisol.

The clinical manifestations are primarily those of excess cortisol. The most frequently encountered manifestations include: hyperglycemia, osteoporosis, adiposity, stunted growth in children, menstrual irregularity, weakness, hirsuitism, psychological difficulties and bruising.

The therapy of Cushing's syndrome is dependent on the etiology of the hypercortisolism and includes surgery, irradiation or chemotherapy.

Adrenocortical neoplasms or ectopic nonendocrine tumors should be removed surgically if possible. Radiation therapy is favored in Cushing's disease. Adrenocorticolytic and adrenocortical inhibitions generally are reserved for inoperable, refractory patients or those with metastatic lesions.

The prognosis is dependent on the etiology of the hypercortisolism. Cushing's disease and adrenocortical adenoma carry a favorable prognosis. On the other hand, adrenocortical carcinoma and the ectopic ACTH syndrome are related more closely to a poor prognosis.

REFERENCES

1. Cushing, H. C.: The basophil adenomas of the pituitary body and their clinical manifestations (pituitary basophilism). Johns Hopkins Med. J., 50: 137, 1932.
2. Liddle, G. W.: Tests of pituitary-adrenal suppressibility in the diagnosis of Cushing's syndrome. J. Clin. Endocrinol. Metab., 20: 1539, 1960.
3. Ross, E. J., Marshall-Jones, P., and Friedman, M.: Cushing's syndrome: diagnostic criteria. Q. J. Med., 35: 149, 1966.
4. Thomas, P.: The structure and synthesis of steroids. In Guide to Steroid Therapy, p. 3. J. B. Lippincott Co., Philadelphia, 1968.
5. Tucci, J. R., Espiner, E. A., Jagger, P. I., Pauk, G. L., and Lauler, D. P.: ACTH stimulation of aldosterone secrétion in normal subjects and in patients with chronic adrenocortical insufficiency. J. Clin. Endocrinol. Metab., 27: 568, 1967.
6. Perkoff, G. T., Eik-nes, K., Nugent, C. A., Fred, H. L., Nimer, R. A., Rush, L., Samuels, L. T., and Tyler, F. H.: Studies of the diurnal variation of plasma 17-hydroxycorticosteroids in man. J. Clin. Endocrinol. Metab., 19: 432, 1959.
7. Orth, D. N., Island D. P., and Liddle, G. W.: Experimental alteration of the circadian rhythm in plasma cortisol (17 OHCS) concentrations in man. J. Clin. Endocrinol. Metab., 27: 549, 1967.
8. Pincus, G., Nakao, T., and Tait, J. F. (editors): Symposium on the Dynamics of Steroid Hormones, p. 387. Academic Press, New York, 1965.
9. Cope, C. L., and Black, E. G.: The production rate of cortisol in man. Br. Med. J., 1: 1020, 1958.
10. Beisel, W. R., DiRaimondo, V. C., and Forsham, P. H.: Cortisol transport and disappearance. Ann. Intern. Med., 60: 641, 1964.
11. Conney, A. H.: Drug metabolism and therapeutics. N. Engl. J. Med., 280: 653, 1969.
12. Thomas, P.: Measurement of steroids. In Guide to Steroid Therapy p. 12, edited by P. Thomas. J. B. Lippincott Co., Philadelphia, 1968.
13. Orth, D. N., and Liddle, G. W.: Results of treatment in 108 patients with Cushing's sundrome. N. Engl. J. Med., 285: 244, 1971.
14. Lauler, D. P., Williams, G. H., and Thorn, G. W.: Diseases of the adrenal cortex. In Harrison's Principles of Internal Medicine, Ed. 6, p. 477, edited by G. W. Thorn, R. D. Adams, I. L. Bennett, E. Braunwald, K. J. Isselbacher and R. G. Petersdorf. McGraw-Hill, New York, 1970.
15. Graber, A. L., Ney, R. L., Nicholson, W. E., Island, D. P., and Liddle, G. W.: The natural history of pituitary-adrenal recovery following long term suppression with corticosteroids. J. Clin. Endocrinol. Metab., 25: 11, 1965.
16. Nelson, D. H., Sprunt, J. G., and Mimms, R. B.: Plasma ACTH determinations in 58 patients before or after adrenalectomy for Cushing's syndrome. J. Clin. Endocrinol. Metab., 26: 722, 1966.
17. Bledsoe, T., Island, D. P., and Liddle, G. W.: Studies of the mechanism through which sodium depletion increases aldosterone biosynthesis in man. J. Clin. Invest., 45: 524, 1964.
18. Hutter, A. M., and Kayoe, D. E.: Adrenal cortical carcinoma: clinical features of 138 patients. Am. J. Med., 41: 572, 1966.
19. Cope, C. L.: Cushing's syndrome. In Adrenal Steroids and Disease, Ed. 2, p. 313. J. B. Lippincott Co., Philadelphia, 1972.
20. Friedman, M., Marshall-Jones, P., and Ross, E. J.: Cushing's syndrome: adrenocortical hyperactivity secondary to neoplasms arising outside the pituitary adrenal system. J. Med., 35: 193, 1966.
21. Choi, Y., Werk., E. E., and Sholiton, L. J.: Cushing's syndrome with dual pituitary adrenal control. Arch. Intern. Med., 125: 1045, 1970.
22. Meador, C. K., Owen, W. C., and Farmer, T. A.: Primary adrenocortical nodular dysplasia: a rare cause of Cushing's syndrome. J. Clin. Endocrinol. Metab., 27: 1255, 1967.
23. Ross, E. J., Marshall-Jones, P., and Friedman, M.: Cushing's syndrome: diagnostic criteria. J. Med., 35: 193, 1966.
24. McArthur, R. G., Cloutier, M. D., Hayles, A. B., and Sprague, R. B.: Cushing's disease in children. Mayo Clin. Proc., 47: 318, 1972.
25. Relman, A. S., and Schwartz, W. B.: The metabolic effects of compound F. J. Clin. Invest., 31: 656, 1952.
26. Yrinis, S. L., Bercovitch, D. D., Stein, R. H.,

Levitt, M. F., and Goldstein, M. H.: Renal Tubular effects of hydrocortisone and aldosterone in normal hydropenic man: comment on sites of action. J. Clin. Invest., 43: 1668, 1964.

27. Bernick, S., and Ershoff, B. H.: Histochemical study of bone in cortisone-treated rats. Endocrinology, 72: 231, 1963.

28. Harter, J. G.: Corticosteroids. Their use in allergic disease. N. Y. State, J. Med., 66: 827, 1966.

29. Scoggins, R. B., and Gliman, B.: Percutaneous absorption of corticosteroids, systemic effects. N. Engl. J. Med., 273: 831, 1965.

30. Burch, P. G., and Migeon, C. J.: Systemic absorption of topical steroids. Arch. Ophthalmol., 79: 174, 1968.

31. Siegel, S. C., Heimlich, E. M., Richards, W., and Kelley, V. C.; Adrenal function in allergy. IV. effect of dexamethasone aerosols in asthmatic children. Pediatrics, 33: 245, 1964.

32. Farmer, R. G., and Shumacher, O. P.: Treatment of ulcerative colitis with hydrocortisone enemas: relationship of hydrocortisone absorption, adrenal suppression, and clinical response. Dis. Colon Rectum, 13: 355, 1970.

33. Weiss, E. R., Rayyis, S. S., Nelson, D. H., and Bethune, J. E.: Evaluation of stimulation and suppression tests in the etiological diagnosis of Cushing's syndrome. Ann. Intern. Med., 71: 941, 1969.

34. Migeon, C. J., Green, O. C., and Eckert, J. P.: Study of adrenocortical function in obesity. Metabolism., 12: 718, 1963.

35. Kenny, F. M., Jancayco, G. P., Heald, F. P., and Hung, W.: Cortisol production rate in adolescent males in different stages of sexual maturation. J. Clin. Endocrinol., Metab., 26: 1232, 1966.

36. Constatino, N. V., and Kabat, H. F.: Drug induced modifications of laboratory test values, revised 1973. Am. J. Hosp. Pharm., 30: 24, 1973.

37. Ekman, H., Hakansson, B., McCarthy, J. D., Lehman, J., and Sjogren, B.: Plasma 17-hydroxycorticosteroids in Cushing's syndrome. J. Clin. Endocrinol. Metab., 21: 684, 1961.

38. Laidlow, J. C., Reddy, W. J., Jenkins, D., Haydar, N. A., Renold, A. E., and Thorn, G. W.: Advances in the diagnosis of altered states of adrenocortical function. N. Engl. J. Med., 253: 747, 1955.

39. Liddle, G. W.: Cushing's syndrome. In The Adrenal Cortex, p. 523, edited by A. B. Einstein. Little, Brown and Co., Boston, 1967.

40. Pavlatos, F. C., Smilo, R. P., and Forsham, P. H.: A rapid screening test for Cushing's syndrome. J. A. M. A., 193: 720, 1965.

41. Nugent, C. A., Nichols, T., and Tyler, F. H.: Diagnosis of Cushing's syndrome: single dose dexamethasone suppression test. Arch. Intern. Med., 116: 172, 1965.

42. Liddle, G. W.: Tests of pituitary-adrenal suppressibility in the diagnosis of Cushing's syndrome. J. Clin. Endocrinol. Metab., 20: 1539, 1960.

43. Liddle, G. W., Estep, H. L., Kendall, J. W., Williams, W. C., and Townes, A. W.: Clinical application of a new test of pituitary reserve. J. Clin. Endocrinol. Metab., 19: 875, 1959.

44. Gold, E. M., Kent, J. R., and Forsham, P. H.: Clinical use of a new diagnostic agent, metopirone (SU 4885), in pituitary and adrenocortical disorders. Ann. Intern. Med., 54: 175, 1961.

45. Kaplan, H. M.: Methopyrapone test in primary hypothyroidism. J. Clin. Endocrinol. Metab., 25: 146, 1961.

46. Sutter, L. J., Geller, J., and Gabrilove, J. L.: Response of the plasma 17-hydroxycorticosteroid level to get ACTH in tumorous and nontumorous Cushing's syndrome. J. Clin. Endocrinol. Metab., 17: 878, 1957.

47. Scott, H. W., Jr., Foster, J. H., Liddle, G. W., Davidson, E. T.: Cushing's syndrome due to adrenocortical tumor: an eleven-year review of 15 patients. Ann. Surg., 162: 505, 1965.

48. Baxter, J. D., and Forsham, P. H.: Tissue effects of glucocorticoids, Am. J. Med., 53: 573, 1972.

49. Munck, A.: Glucocorticoid inhibition of glucose uptake by peripheral tissues: old and new evidence, molecular mechanism and physiologic significance. Perspect. Biol. Med., 14: 265, 1971.

50. Rudman, D., and Di Girolamo, M.: Effect of adrenal cortical steroids on lipid metabolism. In The Human Adrenal Cortex, Ed. 1, p. 241, edited by N. P. Christy. Harper and Row, New York, 1971.

51. Cahill, G. F.: Action of adrenal cortical steroids on carbohydrate metabolism. In The Human Adrenal Cortex, Ed. 1, p. 205, edited by N. P. Christy. Harper and Row, New York, 1971.

52. Frawley, T. F., Kistler, H., and Shelley, T.: Effects of anti-inflammatory steroids on carbohydrate metabolism with emphasis on hypoglycemia and diabetic states. Ann. N. Y. Acad. Sci., 82: 868, 1959.

53. Valance-Owne, J., and Lilley, M.: An insulin antagonist associated with human albumin. Biochem. J., 74: 18P, 1960.

54. Fajans, S. S.: Some metabolic actions of corticosteroids. Metabolism, 10: 957, 1961.

55. Thorn, G. W., Renold, A. E., and Winegrad, A. I.: Some effects of adrenal cortical steroids on intermediate metabolism. Br. Med. J., 2: 1009, 1957.

56. Muller, R., and Kugelberg, E.: Myopathy of Cushing's syndrome. J. Neurol. Neurosurg. Psychiatry, 22: 314, 1959.

57. Rosenberg, E. F.: Rheumatoid arthritis, osteoporosis and fractures related to steroid therapy. Acta Med. Scand., 162: Suppl. 341: 211, 1958.

58. Kimberg, D. V.: Effects of vitamin D and steroid hormones on the active transport of calcium by the intestines. N. Engl. J. Med., 280: 1369, 1969.

59. Regestein, Q. R., Rose, L. I., and Williams, G. H.: Psychopathology in Cushing's syndrome. Arch. Intern. Med., 130: 114, 1972.

60. David, D. S., Grieco, M. H., and Cushman, P. J.: Adrenal glucocorticoids after twenty years: a review of their clinically relevant consequences. J. Chronic Dis., 22: 637, 1970.

61. McArthur, T. G., Cloutier, M. D., Hayles, A. B., and Sprague, R. G.: Cushing's syndrome in children. Mayo Clin. Proc., 47: 318, 1972.

62. Anon: Cushing's syndrome in childhood (editorial). Lancet, 2: 267, 1972.

63. Kirsner, J. B., Kassreil, R. S., and Palmer, W. L.: Peptic ulcer, review of recent literature pertaining to etiology, pathogenesis and certain clinical aspects. Adv. Intern. Med., 8: 41, 1956.

64. Spiro, H. M., and Milles, S. S.: Clinical and physiologic implications of steroid induced peptic ulcer. N. Engl. J. Med., 263: 286, 1960.

65. Kirsner, J. B., Sklar, M., and Palmer, W. L.: The use of ACTH, cortisone, hydrocortisone and related compounds in the management of ulcerative colitis: experience in 180 patients. Am. J. Med., 22: 264, 1951.

66. Schwartz, E.: Prolonged therapy with adrenocortical steroids in allergic diseases. N. Y. State J. Med., 60: 3973, 1960.

67. Smyllie, H. C., and Connolly, C. K.: Incidence of serious complications of corticosteroid therapy in respiratory disease. Thorax, 23: 571, 1968.

68. Sanders, S. L., Brodey, M., Nelson, C. T.: Corticosteroid pemphigus. Arch. Dermatol. Syph., 82: 717, 1960.

69. Hutter, A. M., and Kayhoe, D. E.: Adrenal cortical carcinoma: results of treatment with o,p'DDD in 138 patients. Am. J. Med., 41: 581, 1966

70. Brown, J. H. U., Griffin, J. B., Smith, R. B., and Anason, A.: Physiologic activity of an adrenocorticolytic drug in the adult dog. Metabolism, 5: 594, 1956.

71. Cope, C. L.: Miscellaneous: o,p'DDD, the effects of triparanol, amino-glutethimide. In Adrenal Steroids and Disease, Ed. 2, p 697. J. B. Lippincott Co, Philadelphia, 1972.

72. Bledsoe, T., Istand, D. P., Ney, R. L., and Liddle, G. W.: An effect of o,p'DDD on the extra adrenal metabolism of cortisol in man. J. Clin. Endocrinol. Metab., 24: 1303, 1964.

73. Cash, R., Brough, A. J., Cohen, M. N. P., and Satoh, P. S.: Aminoglutethimide as an inhibitor of adrenal steroidogenesis: mechanism of action and therapeutic trial. J. Clin. Endocrinol. Metab., 27: 1239, 1967.

74. Camacho, A. M., Cash, R., Brough, A. J., and Wilroy, S. R.: Inhibition of adrenal steroidogenesis by aminoglutethimide and mechanism of action. J. A. M. A., 202: 20, 1967.

75. Schteingart, D. E., and Conn, J. W.: Effects of aminoglutethimidine upon adrenal function and cortisol metabolism in Cushing's syndrome. J. Clin. Endocrinol. Metab., 27: 1657, 1967.

chapter 22

DIABETES

Mary Anne Kimble, Pharm.D.

Diabetes is the seventh leading cause of death in America and one of the leading causes of blindness. An estimated 4 million Americans currently have this disease and only half of these are diagnosed. Although there is still no cure for diabetes, the relatively recent discovery of insulin and oral hypoglycemics has improved the quality and prolonged the duration of the diabetic's life.

The diabetic is somewhat unique in that he often serves as his own dietician, lab technician, nurse and physician. He must have a solid understanding of his complex disease so that he can adequately adjust his diet, exercise and dose of insulin. It becomes apparent that education of the patient with respect to his disease, medication, urine testing, diet and hygiene is a major component of diabetic management. Compliance studies have shown time and again that poor control of diabetes is often the result of medication error, misinterpretation of urine test results and ignorance of the disease.[1] Who educates the diabetic? Presumably the physician does; but insufficient time and the complexity of the disease limit his effectiveness. An interdisciplinary approach to education involving the physician, pharmacist, nurse, dietician and social worker would be an ideal one offering facts in small doses with repetition and reinforcement.

In order to serve in his role as a consultant to the physician and patient, the pharmacist must acquaint himself with the disease state and the drugs used in the treatment of that disease. Most pharmacists are familiar with or have access to the pharmacological facts but do not know how to select, initiate and individualize drug therapy. What urine tests and drugs are available? Which is the test or drug of choice for this patient and why? What are the advantages of this drug? What are the major complications of therapy? Can these be avoided? Are they worth the risk? Are they reversible? How should I initiate therapy? How shall I measure efficacy? These are the kinds of questions we must ask ourselves with the aim of promoting the safest, most rational therapy not for some obscure population, but for Mr. Jones, a patient with whom we are now confronted.

DEFINITION, PATHOPHYSIOLOGY AND SYMPTOMATOLOGY

There is no simple definition of diabetes. Although it is a disease which initially manifests itself as a carbohydrate intolerance due to an absolute or relative lack of insulin, investigators have found that it is a progressive, complex disease.

In order to understand the symptomatology of the disease, it is necessary to compare carbohydrate homeostasis of the normal and diabetic individual in the postprandial and fasting state.[2] Despite the fact that most symptoms may be related to hyperglycemia, the action of insulin is quite complex and its deficiency will result in disturbances of fat and protein as well as carbohydrate metabolism.

The homeostatic mechanisms in the body are aimed at maintaining a blood glucose level within a range of 40 to 160 mg/100 ml at all times. The minimal blood glucose level of 40 mg/100 ml is required to provide adequate fuel for the brain, which is able to use only glucose as fuel and is not dependent upon the presence of insulin for its utilization. Glucose spills into the urine resulting in energy and water loss when blood glucose levels exceed the reabsorptive capacity of the kidneys (180 mg/100 ml). Muscle and fat also use glucose as a major energy source but require the presence of insulin. If glucose is not available, these tissues are able to use other substrates such as amino acids and fatty acids for fuel. We need only concentrate on what happens to glucose in the liver, fat, muscle and brain to obtain a basic understanding of glucose metabolism in the normal, fed individual (Fig. 22.1).

Following the ingestion of food, blood glucose concentrations rise, stimulating the release of insulin. Insulin is the key to efficient glucose utilization. It promotes the uptake of glucose, fatty acids and amino acids and their conversion to storage forms in most tissues. It also decreases the blood sugar so that none will be unnecessarily wasted in the urine. In muscle, insulin promotes the uptake of glucose and the conversion to its storage form, glycogen [Fig. 22.1 (1)]. It also stimulates the uptake of amino acids and their conversion to protein [Fig. 22.1 (2)]. In adipose tissue, glucose is converted to free fatty acids, and it is stored as triglycerides [Fig. 22.1 (3)]. The presence of insulin also discourages the breakdown of these triglycerides to free fatty acids, a form which may be transported to other tissues for utilization. The liver does not require insulin for glucose transport, but the presence of insulin does encourage the conversion of glucose to glycogen [Fig. 22.1 (4)]. The breakdown of liver glycogen is the major source of glucose during the fasting state.

In the fasting individual (Fig. 22.2), hypoglycemia discourages the release of insulin. Additionally, a number of hormones (e.g., glucocorticoids, epinephrine, growth hormone and glucagon) are released which oppose the effect of insulin and promote an increase in blood sugar. As a result of this lack of insulin, several processes occur as the body attempts to maintain and conserve a minimal blood glucose level for the central nervous system. Glycogen in the liver is broken down to glucose [Fig. 22.2 (1)]; amino acids are converted to glucose by a process called gluconeogenesis [Fig. 22.2 (2)]; there is a diminished uptake of glucose by insulin-dependent tissues in an effort to conserve as much as possible for the brain; and, finally, triglycerides are broken down to free fatty acids which are used as fuel by those tissues (primarily muscle and fat) which are now unable to use glucose [Fig. 22.2 (3)].

It is easy to see, then, what happens in a

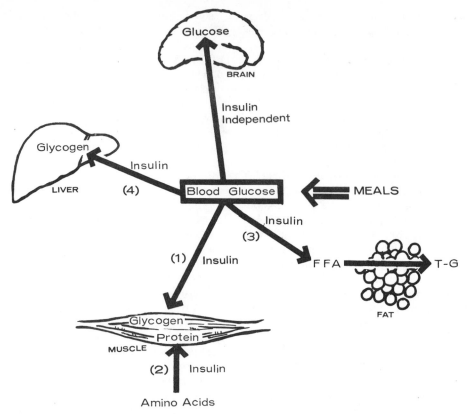

FIG. 22.1. Normal carbohydrate metabolism—post-prandial. High blood glucose → release of insulin → uptake of glucose and amino acids by peripheral tissues.

diabetic (Fig. 22.3). Following a meal, hyperglycemia occurs as usual. However, blood glucose remains high because the absence of insulin prevents its utilization by fat and muscle [Fig. 22.3 (1)]. Glucose then spills into the urine taking excess water with it by the process of osmosis, thus explaining the symptoms of polyuria and polydipsia [Fig. 22.3 (2)]. Excessive sugar in the urine provides an excellent medium for bacterial growth, predisposing the patient to urinary tract infections. Although the supply of glucose in the blood stream is bountiful, glucose can not get into the cells when the demand is there. Fasting metabolism answers the demand in an attempt to provide fuel for the cells. Free fatty acids are mobilized and metabolized to ketones [Fig. 22.3 (3)]; protein breaks down to amino acids to provide substrate for gluconeogenesis [Fig. 22.3 (4)] and liver glycogen is broken down to glucose [Fig. 22.3 (5)]. All of these processes result in symptoms of ketoacidosis, muscle wasting and

the perpetually elevated blood glucose level which we see in diabetes.

Because the disease is progressive in nature, its natural course has recently been divided into "stages" giving rise to new and confusing terminology with which we should become familiar.[3]

The disease is familial and, therefore, begins at conception. The time from conception to a demonstrable glucose intolerance is termed "prediabetes." In the next stage, "subclinical diabetes," fasting blood sugars and glucose tolerance tests are within normal limits except in times of stress, for example, in pregnancy. This is the basis for the cortisone tolerance test. Cortisone, a diabetogenic agent, can induce an abnormal glucose tolerance curve in a patient who is predisposed to diabetes. During "latent" or "chemical" diabetes, the patient has no symptoms of the disease but does have an abnormal fasting blood sugar or glucose tolerance curve. "Overt diabetes" is the full blown stage

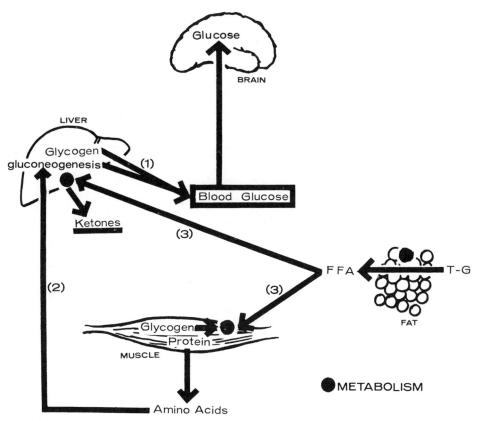

FIG. 22.2. Normal carbohydrate metabolism—fasting. Hypoglycemia → lack of insulin and release of hormones which increase blood glucose conservation of blood glucose levels for brain; other tissues use alternate substrates for fuel.

of the disease accompanied by symptoms of polyuria, polydipsia, muscle wasting, weight loss and infection, as well as an elevated fasting blood glucose and abnormal glucose tolerance test. Atherosclerosis, retinopathy, nephropathy and neuropathy are some of the long term complications of diabetes.

It is important for the pharmacist to be aware of these stages not only because of the need to keep abreast of current medical vocabulary but because the recognition of these stages has prompted investigators to ask whether treatment of a subclinical or latent diabetic would delay the natural progression of the diesease. Studies are currently in progress to determine whether such treatment is worthwhile.

Although all diabetics theoretically progress through the same stages of diabetes, some progress to the symptomatic stage more rapidly. Because the age at which symptoms appear can be correlated with the nature, severity and treatment of the disease, most clinicians prefer to classify diabetics as adult or juvenile in onset.

In general, 90% of all diabetics are adult onset and 80% are obese adult onset. Only 10% are of the juvenile onset type (onset of symptoms at less than 35 years of age).

The two forms of the overt stage of this disease differ in that the adult onset diabetics retain some pancreatic function and are, therefore, generally more stable and quite easily controlled with diet and oral hypoglycemics. Twenty to 30% may require insulin although they rarely become ketotic. Juvenile diabetics, on the other hand, have no pancreatic reserve, and for this reason they always require insulin for the management of their disease. Their blood sugars may fluctuate widely despite treatment, and they are more prone to ketosis than are the adult onset diabetics.

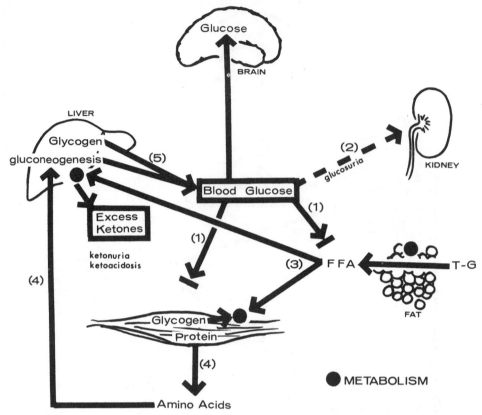

FIG. 22.3. Carbohydrate metabolism—diabetes. Meals → hyperglycemia. Lack of insulin → increased glucose production and decreased uptake of carbohydrate by peripheral tissues.

DIAGNOSTIC TESTS[3]

Several tests are currently used to diagnose diabetes and all measure an individual's ability to handle a glucose load.

The oral glucose tolerance test (OGTT) measures an individual's ability to handle a glucose load over a period of time and is the most reliable diagnostic test for diabetes. Following an overnight fast, a morning fasting blood sugar is drawn and a 100-g glucose load is then ingested by the patient. Thereafter, blood samples are drawn at half-hour intervals for 2 hr and at 3 hr following the ingestion of this glucose load. Urine samples are often taken simultaneously and tested for glucose in order to estimate the individual's renal threshold for glucose. In nondiabetics, the blood glucose returns to normal (less than 110 mg/100 ml) in less than 2 hr. In the diabetic, the glucose peak is higher and occurs much later than the normal curve; levels also decline at a slower rate.

Other tests which are used as diagnostic or screening tests for diabetes include the following.

Fasting Blood Glucose (FBS)

This blood sample is taken in the morning prior to breakfast. A normal value for venous blood is 60 to 100 mg/100 ml. Although a high value is fairly diagnostic of diabetes, a normal value is meaningless since a delay in glucose metabolism may be the only defect in early diabetes. It is therefore conceivable that a mild diabetic could handle the glucose provided by his dinner meal in 9½ hr, the required fasting time.

Two-Hour Postprandial (2HPP) Blood Glucose

This is used as a screening test for diabetes. A blood glucose level is drawn 2 hr following a 100-g glucose load. In nondiabetics, blood glucose levels return to normal in less than 2 hr following a glucose challenge whereas hyperglycemia persists in a diabetic. Values for this test are generally higher than the 2-hr oral glucose tolerance test values owing to less stringent diet preparation and the inconsistent use of the standard glucose dose.

Glucosuria (Urine Glucose Tests)

A positive test for glucose in the urine is not diagnostic for diabetes but is an indication for more definitive testing. It is important to realize that glucosuria is symptomatic of many other conditions (*e.g.*, pregnancy or faulty renal function), and that it is not a persistent finding in diabetes. Glucosuria generally occurs when the mean blood glucose level is 180 mg/100 ml or more, and it rarely occurs when this level is less than 130 mg/100 ml. There is an exception to this rule in that the renal threshold for glucose may increase with age so that older diabetics may "spill" no glucose at all despite a high blood glucose level.

The important role which urine glucose tests play in the regulation of the diabetic, however, cannot be overemphasized. There are two basic types of tests available. One is the glucose oxidase method (Testape, Clinistix and Ketodiastix) which is specific for glucose. The other is the copper reduction method (Clinitest) which is affected by any reducing substance in the urine.

Even though the glucose oxidase method is specific for glucose and the simplest to perform, it is not the test of choice for monitoring insulin therapy because of its qualitative nature. Despite the fact that "quantitative" figures appear on many of the product labels, glucose oxidase tests are quantitative only when the amount of glucose in the urine is less than 0.25%. Larger amounts (2, 3 and 4%) were interpreted as 0.5% or less in 502 out of 804 tests.[4] This high rate of interpretation error cannot be tolerated when hyperglycemia must be controlled. These tests are superior, however, to the copper reduction methods in the screening of patients for diabetes because of their simplicity, specificity and ability to detect such minute amounts of sugar in the urine. They are also the tests of choice for monitoring adult onset diabetes treated with oral hypoglycemics. Ascorbic acid in therapeutic amounts (1 to 2 g) will interfere with the glucose oxidase test resulting in a false negative reading.[5,6]

Schedules which are set up for the dosing of regular insulin on the basis of urine glucose readings are often referred to as the "rainbow schedule" or "sliding scale." Because there is no standard schedule, the physician must specify the number of units he desires for each reading. Generally, 5 units of regular insulin are administered for each "plus" recorded by the copper reduction method with provisions for supplemental insulin should the patient spill acetone in his urine as well. It is also important to emphasize that such dosing schedules always utilize the copper reduction method for reasons listed earlier, and that readings ascertained by the glucose oxidase method are not equivalent to those obtained by the copper reduction method (Table 22.1). Such a schedule is used for the hospitalized diabetic whose insulin requirements may vary owing to a variety of stresses (*e.g.*, infections, surgery or any acute illness) or for determination of the initial insulin requirements of a newly diagnosed diabetic. Generally the urine is tested every 4 hr and insulin administered accordingly. However, Bressler[7] recently recommended that this interval be increased to 6 hr since all diabetics who have been treated with insulin eventually develop antibodies which may delay the onset and prolong the action of regular insulin beyond that which is seen in nondiabetics.

Because of its importance, the urine test must be performed and interpreted correctly. A number of surveys[1] have shown that the diabetic's lack of understanding of his disease and the errors he makes in treating himself account for a good number of the "labile" or difficult-to-control diabetics. For this reason, some discussion of the basic points regarding the use of Clinitest should be pursued with each patient. The following parameters should be considered in such discussions.[8]

1. The frequency of testing varies with the degree of control. If the patient is labile, he may be requested to test his urine 3 to 4 times daily. If he has been controlled on one dose of insulin for some time, he may test his urine once daily or 2 to 3 times weekly. The urine should be tested more frequently at the first sign of infection or with the occurence of any change in activity, diet or emotional stress.[9]

2. The patient should be reminded to test a

TABLE 22.1

Comparative Readings for the Copper Reduction and Glucose Oxidase Methods (Urine Glucose Tests)

Urine Glucose Readings	Corresponding Percentage of Glucose in the Urine	
	Copper reduction method (*e.g.*, Clinitest)	Glucose oxidase method (*e.g.*, Testape)
	%	%
Negative	0	0
Trace	0.25	No such reading
One "plus" (+)	0.5	0.1
Two "plus" (++)	0.75	0.25
Three "plus" (+++)	1	0.5
Four "plus" (++++)	2	2
"Pass through" (see text)	Greatly exceeds 2	No such reading

double voided specimen. That is, the patient should void ½ hr prior to testing time (to eliminate the glucose that has accumulated since his previous voiding), drink a glass of water and test a freshly voided specimen. The second voiding will more accurately reflect the amount of sugar in the blood at the time of testing. This procedure is particularly important for the early morning test.[10]

3. Because the tablet generates its own heat and anaerobic environment with the production of foam, the tube should not be agitated during the reaction.

4. The patient should observe the reaction while it is occuring since a very high glucose content results in the so-called "pass through" phenomenon. This is demonstrated by a fleeting bright orange color which occurs during the "boiling" and which fades to a greenish brown once the reaction ceases. This color may be falsely interpreted as 0.75 to 1%, when there is actually more than 2% glucose in the urine.[8]

5. Because the color may fade with time, it must be read precisely 15 sec after the "boiling" has ceased.

6. A patient who spills 4+ (2%) or more glucose into his urine should also test his urine for acetone. Persistence of large amounts of glucose in the urine should be called to the physician's attention.

7. Several drugs may interfere with the test and cause a false positive reaction (Table 22.2). There is very little quantitative documentation in the literature with respect to these laboratory-drug interferences, but patients who take large amounts of salicylates or ascorbic acid should be warned of the possible effects. If unexpected positive readings occur, the patient may double check his urine by the glucose oxidase method to see if glucose was the reducing substance actually measured.

8. Because Clinitest tablets disintegrate rapidly in the presence of moisture and light, they should not be stored in the bathroom medicine cabinet (the most logical location from the patient's viewpoint). The disintegration is easily detected since the appearance of the tablet changes from the normal speckled robin's egg blue to white with splotches of dark blue.[16]

9. The tablets are poisonous and caustic. They should be manipulated with the lid of the container and kept out of the reach of small children. Should ingestion occur, do not induce vomiting.

TREATMENT OF THE JUVENILE ONSET DIABETIC

The treatment objectives for all diabetics are essentially the same. The physician attempts to attain a state which is free from symptoms and normal with regard to urine sugar and fasting blood glucose level. Dietary management always accompanies medical management and may be the determining factor of success.

TABLE 22.2

Substances Which May Cause a False Positive Glucosuria by the Copper Reduction Method[11,12]

p-Aminosalicylic acid
Ascorbic acid (large quantities)
Cephalothin[13]
Chloral hydrate
Isoniazid
Metaxalone
Nalidixic acid[14]
Penicillin (massive doses)[15]
Probenecid
Salicylates
Streptomycin
Uric acid

Insulin Dosing

As mentioned earlier, all juvenile diabetics require insulin for the treatment of their diabetes. There are many methods of insulin dosing and those which follow are only to give the reader an idea of how this may be done. Determination of a newly diagnosed diabetic's insulin requirements may be done on an outpatient or inpatient basis depending upon the severity of symptoms.

Ketotic diabetics are generally hospitalized so that insulin requirements are determined on the basis of frequent urine and blood glucose measurements. This process involves two basic steps. The first is to determine the total amount of insulin required in a 24-hr period. This is done by testing for urine glucose by the reduction method (Clinitest) every 4 hr (before meals and at bedtime) and administering 4 to 5 units of regular insulin 1/2 to 1 hr before meals for each "plus" which is measured. Additional doses may be given throughout the night if necessary (also refer to the earlier discussion on "rainbow schedule"). Blood glucose levels are drawn in the morning before breakfast and throughout the day as warranted. Once the 24-hr requirements of regular insulin are ascertained and the patient is under control, the multiple injections may be replaced by a single injection of intermediate acting insulin (NPH or lente). The dose of NPH is two-thirds to three-fourths of the 24-hr requirement and should be supplemented with regular insulin as indicated by the urine sugars. If the total requirement exceeds 40 units, the insulin may be given in 2 doses, generally two-thirds morning and one-third in the evening. Once the patient has been switched to an intermediate acting insulin, many physicians will order a blood sugar to be drawn at 4 p.m., the time at which insulin exerts its peak activity. This is done to assure the physician that there is no midafternoon hypoglycemia. Upon discharge, the dose is decreased by 4 to 6 units to compensate for increased activity which also has an insulin-like effect.[17,18]

Once the patient has left the hospital, changes in diet and activity make further adjustment of dose on an outpatient basis almost inevitable. Several problems may arise and a few of these will be discussed. The patient may experience midmorning hyperglcemia secondary to the slow onset of NPH. Supplementation of the morning dose of NPH with small amounts of regular insulin will generally correct this problem. If a patient experiences midafternoon hypoglycemia but nighttime and early morning hyperglycemia, the morning dose should be cut down and an additional dose added in the evening. This pattern occurs in patients who have a transient response to NPH. In other patients the activity of NPH may be delayed in onset so that they experience hyperglycemia throughout the day and hypoglycemia at night. Increasing the morning NPH would result in severe nighttime hypoglycemia so that this problem is managed by the addition of regular insulin to a lower dose of morning NPH. An evening snack may also help to alleviate the nighttime hypoglycemia.[7]

Dosing a mild, nonketotic diabetic on an outpatient basis is accomplished by giving an arbitrarily small dose of intermediate acting insulin and adjusting this dose on the basis of frequent (before meals and at bedtime) urine testing. The patient is given an initial dose of 10 to 20 units of NPH or lente insulin, instructed to test his urine 4 to 5 times daily and to increase or decrease his insulin dose according to a prescribed schedule. For example, if he spills 3+ to 4+ (*i.e.*, 1 to 2% glucose) in his urine all day, he is to increase his insulin dose the following morning by 4 units. If he spills 1+ to 2+ (0 to ¼% glucose) in his urine for the entire day, there is no change in the dose, and if he spills 0 to 1+ (0 to ¼% glucose), the insulin dose is decreased by 4 units. The patient returns weekly for a fasting blood glucose and re-evaluation of his therapy.[17]

The Use of Insulin

The pharmacist should be able to advise the patient and physician with respect to the particular properties and use of insulin. For the onset, duration and chemical-physical properties, the reader is referred to any basic pharmacology text.[5] Although the technique of insulin injection is most often taught by a nurse or physician, the pharmacist should be able to answer questions concerning injection technique, rotation of injection sites, sterilization procedures, proper use of the syringe and the types of syringes which are available for use. With the gradual replacement of U-40 and U-80 with U-100 insulin, it will be particularly important for the pharmacist to make certain the correct syringe is purchased and the patient is fully aware of which insulin he may use with the syringe. If small doses of U-100 must be measured (less than 35 units), the U-100 syringe which measures a maximum of 35 units should be dispensed. The caliber of the latter syringe is much smaller and permits greater accuracy. The importance of eliminating bubbles from these small caliber syringes cannot be overemphasized. Prior to the injection of a suspension (all insulins are suspensions except regular and globin), the vial should be gently roled

to assure withdrawal of a uniform suspension. Shaking results in excessive foaming.

If the patient is using a mixutre of two insulins, the compatibility of the mixture should be considered (Table 22.3). When using a mixture of PZI and regular insulin, the patient should be instructed to withdraw the regular insulin first so there will not be a contamination of this vial with the excess protamine contained in the diluent of PZI. Generally, all insulin mixtures are stable and retain the qualities of the individual preparations if they are mixed

TABLE 22.3
Stability of Various Insulin Mixtures[7,17]

Mixture	Proportion	Incompatibility	Stability
Neutral or acid regular-PZI	1:1 = PZI 2:1 = NPH 3:1 = NPH + Reg	Excess protamine in PZI combines with regular, prolonging its action; no advantages to any of these combinations	Mix just prior to injection.
Acid regular[a]-NPH	May be mixed in any proportion	Even though there is no excess protamine, physical changes may occur with time, presumably owing to pH differences	Mix just prior to injection
Neutral regular[b]-NPH	May be mixed in any proportion	No incompatibilities	May be mixed 2-3 months prior to injection
Acid regular-lente	Should not be mixed in a proportion greater than 1:1	Presumably physico-chemical changes may occur with the change in pH, resulting in an unpredictable time action curve	Mix just prior to injection
Neutral regular-lente	May be mixed in any proportion	No incompatibilities	May be mixed 2-3 months prior to injection
Lentes	May be mixed in any proportion	No incompatibilities	Stable indefinitely; may be premixed
Regular-normal saline	May be mixed in any proportion	pH change; dilution of buffer; exact incompatibility unknown	Use within 2-3 hr of mixing
Regular-insulin diluting fluid	May be mixed in any proportion	No incompatibilities	Stable indefinitely; may be premixed

[a]Acid regular insulin (ARI) = Squibb's U-40 and U-80 regular insulin.
[b]Neutral regular insulin (NRI) = Squibb's U-100 regular insulin; Lilly's U-40, U-80 and U-100 regular insulin.

just prior to injection. Problems arise only when insulins are mixed far in advance of the injection time as they may be in a unit-dose area. This situation may also occur when two insulins are premixed for a child who is incapable of accurately withdrawing his doses.

Once the disease is under control, the patients should always use insulin derived from the same animal source. For example, if a patient is stabilized on a beef/pork insulin, he should not switch to pure pork. Insulin from various species differs in its antigenicity and may not, therefore, substitute unit for unit. Clinically, this is not often a problem, although there are isolated case reports of hypoglycemia which have occurred following such inadvertent switches.[19]

In general, all insulins are stable at room temperature (75°F) for the life of the vial, which may be several weeks. Regular insulin may lose 10% of its activity at room temperature after 18 months. At temperatures greater than 75°F, the modified insulins will coagulate within a few days. Although there is not a total loss in potency, the ability to withdraw a uniform dose and to predict the onset of action and duration of response is significantly decreased.[17,20] This stability information has several implications. Vials of insulin which are dispensed to an inpatient area need not be refrigerated; patients generally prefer injecting solutions which have been brought to room temperature; injection of cold insulin has been implicated as a cause of lipodystrophy; and, finally, when traveling to relatively cool areas, patients should not require special paraphernalia for insulin storage. Insulation between several layers of clothing should suffice.

Adverse Effects of Insulin

It is important to be aware of the common adverse effects which can occur following the administration of insulin and to have an understanding of their clinical significance so that such situations can be handled appropriately.[17]

Hypoglycemia or Insulin Reaction.[21] This generally occurs when the blood sugar falls below 50 mg/100 ml. It is a problem which is often encountered in juvenile diabetics who have not yet learned to regulate their carbohydrate intake and exercise. With time, the patient will be able to identify a reaction at its onset and stop its progression with a concentrated source of sugar. Discontinuation of diabetogenic stress situations such as pregnancy, surgery, infection, emotional upset or weight reduction can also precipitate hypoglycemia. Some drugs also have hypoglycemic effects and may therefore potentiate the action of insulin.

Hypoglycemia commonly occurs in newly diagnosed juvenile diabetics within days to weeks of treatment owing to an apparent "remission" of the disease. Even though insulin requirements may fall to as little as 1 to 2 units daily, treatment should be continued since requirements will certainly increase in a few months and it would be unjustified to encourage false hopes in the youngster. It has also been said that intermittent insulin therapy is more frequently associated with antibody formation resulting in insulin resistance at a later date.

Severe renal disease can improve the diabetic state and decrease the requirements for insulin tremendously. Although the liver degrades 50% of the insulin, the kidney is the most important site of extrahepatic breakdown. In the face of renal failure, active insulin may be retained and only minute doses may be required. It should also be noted that patients with uremia may require increased amounts of insulin. The diabetogenic factor has not yet been isolated, but it is suspected that there is a diminished tissue responsiveness to insulin.[22,23]

In the above situations, dilution of insulin may be required to measure an accurate dose. Although saline is used to dilute insulin for desensitization procedures, it is recommended that such dilutions be used within 2 to 3 hr. Insulin diluting fluid, which may be obtained from Lilly Co. upon request, is recommended for the dilution of insulin which will be used over some period of time. These are simply the same diluents which are used for the various commercially available insulins and have the same pH and buffer components.[17]

Immunological Problems with Insulin. At least two types of antibodies to insulin are formed.[24] One is a blocking antibody, which occurs in the serum of all diabetics 6 weeks to 3 months after treatment is initiated. These antibodies may combine with and neutralize the activity of exogenous insulin, but in normal diabetics the binding capacity of these antibodies is fairly low (10 to 20 units). Insulin derived from various animal species differs in its affinity for these antibodies. Another antibody is responsible for the mediation of allergic reactions. Many adverse effects of insulin may be related to its antigenicity. It would be advisable for the reader to familiarize himself with the relative antigenicity of the various insulin preparations before proceeding further (Table 22.4).[18,25,26]

One of the claims made for the lente insulins is that they contain no foreign protein, that is, protamine or globin, and are therefore less antigenic than other modified insulins. Actually, there is little difference in the incidence of sensitivity between lente and NPH.[18] More local reactions are recorded with the use of modified insulins, but it is questionable whether this is due to their inherent antigenicity or their longer retention at the site, leading to greater antigenicity.

The relative antigenicity between insulins from various species generally correlates with their structural similarity to human insulin. For example, pork insulin, which differs in one amino acid, is less antigenic than beef insulin, which differs by three amino acids. Dealanated insulin and sulfated insulin are experimental modifications which are said to be less antigenic and less neutralizable than other insulins. Occasionally, a patient who is resistant to all mammalian sources of insulin will respond favorably to fish insulin.[28]

Within the near future, single peak insulin, a highly purified form of insulin, will be available. This insulin, which is purified chromatographically, is less antigenic and may be useful in the treatment of patients who are currently allergic to commercially available preparations. It is also anticipated that this form of insulin will be associated with fewer instances of allergic reactions and insulin resistance.[29,30]

Several adverse effects of insulin are directly related to its immunogenicity. The etiology, descriptions and therapy of these reactions are considered in Table 22.5.

Lipodystrophy.[9,17,35] This is due to insulin and can occur in two forms. Atrophy, which is a wasting of lipoid tissues, results in irregular concavities at the site of injection and occurs in 28 to 35% of the patients treated with insulin. The condition predominates in women and children and can be avoided by rotating the injection site. One site (2 cm) should not be used more than once every 3 to 4 weeks. The incidence is higher with the use of PZI and may be due to its long acting local effect. Injection of refrigerated material may also be a contributing factor.

Hypertrophy, or the occurrence of fat pads, usually appears on the thigh and is equally frequent in males and females. The patient generally gives a history of repeated injection at this site. Because the area becomes anesthetized, the process is self-perpetuating.

Both of these complications, which may remit spontaneously after many years, were initially thought to have only cosmetic significance. However, it has been shown that absorption of insulin from these areas may be delayed to a clinically significant extent. It has also been found that the half-life of disappearance from the injection site is much more prolonged from the thigh than the arm (310 versus 232 min), although the route of administration (subcutaneous versus intramuscular) makes no significant difference.[36] This is apparently a function of the ratio of fat to lean tissue in these areas. The greater vascularity of the lean tissue results in more rapid absorption of the drug.

TREATMENT OF THE ADULT ONSET DIABETIC

Several principles have always existed with respect to the treatment of adult onset diabetics. As with juvenile diabetes, an appropriate diet, one which gives the patient a balanced, well-distributed proportion of protein, carbohydrate and fat and which maintains the pa-

TABLE 22.4
Relative Antigenicity of Insulins[26,27]

Antigenicity increases with the duration of action and the presence of foreign protein. Therefore:

PZI > NPH > globin > lente > regular

Affinity for insulin-blocking antibody is influenced by structural similarity to human insulin and purity of the product.

Beef = sheep > pork > sulfated or > single peak> human
                           dealanated   insulin
                           pork

TABLE 22.5

Immunological Reactions to Insulin[7,17,31]

Reaction	Etiology, Description, Clinical Significance	Therapy
Local reactions[7]	Erythema, pain, swelling and urticaria may occur at the site of injection in 20-50% of patients initiated on insulin. They generally occur 20-40 min after injection and last 2-6 hr. The antigen is generally a noninsulin protein.	Suggested treatment is to complete the vial since spontaneous disensitization often occurs. if the patient continues to have reactions, consider changing to lentes or to insulin from another animal source.
Generalized allergic reactions[32]	These are rare but may be anaphylactic in nature. Antigen is probably insulin.	Treat acute reaction with antihistamines, epinephrine and glucocorticoids as indicated. Change insulin sources or desensitize with very dilute amounts injected in gradually increasing doses over 3 days. The patient may be covered with an antihistamine during this procedure.
Insulin resistance[26,33,34]	True insulin resistance is relatively rare. It is defined as a need for more than 200 units for 1 week or more in the absence of acidosis coma or infection. It generally occurs within the 1st year of treatment and is often associated with a history of intermittent insulin therapy.	Change animal sources; desensitize the patient; use purified forms; treat with sulfonylureas if patient is adult onset since antibodies may not bind endogenous insulin; prednisone 30-40 mg daily decreases antibody production and may alter binding characteristics—watch for dramatic fall in insulin requirements.
Insulin insensitivity[31]	Defined as an insulin requirement of more than 60 units daily, is far more common and may be caused by a variety of diabetogenic factors such as obesity, hyperthyroidism, infection, ketoacidosis, liver disease or diabetogenic drugs.	Treatment includes correction of diabetogenic conditions, use of concentrated forms of insulin, and as indicated for insulin resistance if all else fails.

tient at his ideal weight, is the bulwark of therapy. Drug therapy should never be considered in the mild, well tolerated form of the disease until the patient has been on a diet for an appropriate length of time (3 to 4 months). The importance of this principle was underlined with the publication of results of the University Group Diabetes Program (UGDP) in 1970.

The UGDP[37,38] was a prospective study initiated in 1961 to evaluate the effectiveness of antidiabetic therapy in preventing vascular and late complications of diabetes. Eight hundred patients from 12 different diabetic clinics were included. All of these were recently diagnosed maturity onset diabetics of the nonketotic type who had a life expectancy of 5 years or more and who could be maintained free of symptoms on diet alone. The patients were then assigned at random to one of five treatment programs: tolbutamide in fixed doses of 1.5 g, placebo or diet alone, insulin in a fixed dose (ISTD), insulin in variable doses (IVAR) and phenformin. Although the study was scheduled to continue, an unexpected finding of a higher incidence of cardiovascular deaths in the tolbutamide- and phenformin-treated groups resulted in its early termination. After 8 years, 26 cardiovascular deaths occurred in the tolbutamide group as opposed to 10 to 13 deaths in each of the other groups. Similar results were reported for the phenformin group.[39]

The study has given the medical profession cause for radical reappraisal of therapy. The controversy is not yet settled and bursts of anger sporadically appear in the literature. Nevertheless, the study has made us more critical of our drug therapy, not only in the area of diabetes, but in the treatment of other diseases as well where specific, traditionally used drugs are relied upon heavily. Most physicians have not discontinued oral hypoglycemics in patients who have been well controlled on these drugs. In new patients, however, diet is vigorously encouraged and insulin is seriously considered for therapy of relatively young, symptomatic patients who may have other cardiovascular problems. Oral hypoglycemics are still used, though with much more reserve, in patients who refuse to take insulin or are unable to care for themselves to a reliable degree. Additionally, the use of oral hypoglycemics in an attempt to delay the onset of the disease in patients with chemical or latent diabetes who have no overt symptoms has been abandoned.[9]

With the assumption that these criteria have been seriously considered, we may go on to define that group of patients who will most likely respond to the sulfonylureas. These agents stimulate the pancreas to produce more insulin. Therefore a minimum of pancreatic function is a prerequisite to sulfonylurea therapy. Since a normal pancreatectomized adult requires 40 to 60 units daily, an insulin requirement of less than 40 units would indicate that some pancreatic function remains. Patients who respond well to oral hypoglycemics have the following characteristics: they are not diagnosed as diabetics until after the age of 40, they are not overweight and their insulin requirements are less than 40 units daily (preferably 10 to 20 units daily).[18]

Once a firm diagnosis of diabetes (by the glucose tolerance test) has been made, diet has been given an adequate trial and the criteria for the use of oral hypoglycemics have been met, an appropriate drug must be selected.

Selection of an Oral Hypoglycemic Agent

Efficacy, potency and toxicity are major factors to consider in the selection of a drug. At present it is difficult to establish a variation in efficacy among the sulfonylureas. Tolbutamide and chlorpropamide are the oldest drugs and are therefore best studied. Long term studies (5 to 10 years' experience) for all sulfonylureas indicate a primary failure rate of 35 to 40% and a secondary failure rate of 3 to 30%. The final over-all success rate is 20%.[40] The efficacy of phenformin appears to be comparable to, if not better than, the sulfonylureas. The percentage of patients controlled initially ranges from 70 to 90%. Again, clinical trials have not been as abundant as for tolbutamide, and the high incidence of gastrointestinal side effects has discouraged the drug's widespread use. However, one study claims that 70% of those patients treated with phenformin were controlled initially, that 12% became secondary failures and that finally 56% were controlled.[41,42]

Some clinicians feel that the potency of a drug should be considered in the evaluation of its efficacy. In this case we are not referring to the milligram-for-milligram potency but to the maximal level of pharmacological activity which can be obtained from the drug. This information has been extrapolated from the abili-

TABLE 22.6
TABLE 22.6
Adverse Effects of the Oral Hypoglycemic Agents[41,43]

Adverse Effects	Comments
Gastrointestinal effects	Anorexia, nausea, vomiting and diarrhea may occasionally force withdrawal of drug treatment but are generally mild. Incidence ranges from 1-5% and occurs most commonly with acetohexamide (5%), then chlorpropamide (2%), and uncommonly with tolbutamide (1.4%). Local irritation is strongly suspected. Symptoms can often be alleviated by decreasing the dose.
Skin rash	Reported for all the sulfonylureas but occur in 3% of patients treated with chlorpropamide and in 1% of those treated with tolbutamide. Rarely, they can be severe.
Liver damage and cholestatic jaundice[44]	Rare. Reported for both tolbutamide and chlorpropamide. Seems to be more common with latter. Most cases appear within 1-3 months of therapy and are often accompanied by a skin rash indicating that they are most likely allergic in nature. The jaundice is generally reversible upon withdrawal of treatment, but severe hepatic damage and deaths have been reported. Although no cases of jaundice have been associated with acetohexamide, elevation of alkaline phosphatase has been reported.
Hematological disorders	All types have been reported but are rare. Of particular interest is a case of hemolytic anemia which occured in a patient with glucose 6-phosphatase deficiency, a metabolic disorder which occurs in 10% of the Negro population.
Hypersensitivity to alcohol[45,46]	An Antabuse type of effect appears to be a fairly common finding with the oral hypoglycemics (10-20%) but is most commonly associated with chlorpropamide. The onset of the reaction is 3-10 min after the ingestion of alcohol and may last for 1 hr. The reaction is characterized by flushing, nausea, shortness of breath and palpitations. Thought to be due to a noncompetitive inhibition of aldehyde dehydrogenase, a key enzyme in the metabolism of alcohol and serotonin.
Prolonged hypoglycemia[47-49]	Most common with the longer acting sulfonylureas. The incidence of 5-6% is high, but it is the exceptional case which is not surrounded by predisposing factors. Majority of cases reported in patients over 65 years of age who have renal or liver impairment and eat irregularly.
Effects on the fetus[50]	All sulfonylureas cross the placental barrier. Severe intractable neonatal hypoglycemia has been associated with the use of chlorpropamide and acetohexamide. Chlorpropamide may also increase the infant mortality rate. Kernicterus has also been considered as a potential side effect.
Hypothyroidism[51,52]	Three percent incidence of diminished thyroid function tests with no evidence of clinical thyroid disease. The effect is controversial. Incidences as high as 20% have been reported.
Hyponatremia[53,54]	Chlorpropamide in therapeutic doses may cause hyponatremia, hypo-osmolarity and water intoxication in approximately 4% of the patients taking this drug by potentiating the activity of antidiuretic hormone (ADH). Geriatric patients ingesting thiazides or large amounts of water and patients with congestive heart failure are particularly prone to these effects. Tolazamide does not induce an inappropriate ADH-like syndrome.
Phenformin	
Gastrointestinal effects[55]	Anorexia, metallic taste, nausea and vomiting. Dose-related and limits maximal useful dose of drug to 200 mg. Incidence decreased from 25-40% to 3-7% with the introduction of the time-disintegrated capsule. Centrally mediated. May be minimized by administration of DBI-TD, gradually increasing the dose, and by administration with food to slow absorption.

TABLE 22.6 Continued

Adverse Effects	Comments
Lactic acidosis[56,57]	A condition characterized by high lactate levels and an extremely high mortality rate. Numerous cases have been reported in patients who were taking the drug but all were very ill patients who had other conditions which cause lactic acidosis: hemorrhage, alcohol ingestion, septicemia, shock, heart failure, starvation, renal failure and pregnancy. The use of phenformin is contraindicated in the presence of any ischemic state.

ty of one sulfonylurea to control a patient in which another sulfonyurea has failed. On this basis, most authors agree that chlorpropamide is more potent than tolbutamide. The potency of phenformin, as judged by the same criteria, is similar to that of chlorpropamide, although its duration of action is much shorter.

The over-all incidence of adverse effects to the sulfonylureas is estimated to be less than 5%. This figure, however, is in direct conflict with that of researchers who report a 6% incidence of hypoglycemic attacks and a 10 to 20% incidence of alcohol intolerance. The obvious disagreement in these figures is indicative of the difficulty encountered in substantiating the true incidence of adverse effects. The side effects of the sulfonylureas and their clinical significance are tabulated (Table 22.6). In general, it can be said that the incidence of adverse effects reported for chlorpropamide is higher than that for tolbutamide (8% versus 1 to 3%). Acetohexamide has a 5 to 10% incidence of adverse effects, and most of these are gastrointestinal in nature (up to 5%).[43] Most of these adverse effects have been reported for all the sulfonylureas, but some are more frequently associated with a particular drug. The severity of many of these side effects can be correlated with the differences in the half-life, metabolism and excretion of the drugs, (Table 22.7). Note, for example, that although all of the drugs are dependent on the kidney for their ultimate excretion, only tolbutamide is excreted in an inactive form. In the presence of severe kidney dysfunction, one might consider the use of tolbutamide or insulin. In severe hepatic dysfunction, on the other hand, one may avoid the use of drugs which depend on the liver for metabolism. In general, the liver must be severely compromised before a dosage adjustment need be considered. Hepatic damage which may be induced by these agents must also be con-

sidered. In such cases insulin would most likely be the agent of choice. Note also that chlorpropamide which has the longest half-life also has a higher incidence of side effects of a serious nature.

In contrast to the sulfonylureas, the list of side effects for phenformin is relatively short. The majority of side effects are related to the gastrointestinal tract but lactic acidosis may occur in rare instances in the predisposed patient. It is important to note (Table 22.6) that phenformin is contraindicated in patients with decreased renal function or any other anoxic condition which may predispose to lactic acidosis, an often fatal side effect of the drug.[56,57]

Although one school of thought advocates using the most potent antidiabetic agent initially (chlorpropamide), most clinicians still favor tolbutamide because of its short half-life and lesser toxicity.[18] Acetohexamide and tolazamide offer no significant advantage over tolbutamide.

Phenformin is the drug of choice in the obese adult onset diabetic, primarily because it does not depend upon insulin for its action. It is said to increase the peripheral utilization of glucose by a mechanism different from that of insulin, to decrease the absorption of glucose and to decrease gluconeogenesis. It may, therefore, decrease the amount of insulin released by these patients in some indirect way thereby averting the lipogenic effects of insulin. The anorexic effect of the drug has also been an argument for its use in the obese adult onset diabetic, although the actual weight loss which can be expected from this drug is unpredictable and rarely profound.[62,63]

Initial Dosing of the Oral Hypoglycemic Agents

The patient is generally started on low doses of the selected drug which are increased weekly

Drug	Dose (g)	Maximum (g)	Half-life (hr)	Onset; Duration (hr)	Metabolism and Excretion	Comments
Tolbutamide (Orinase)	0.5-3.0 divided doses	2-3	5.6	6-12	Totally metabolized to inactive form. Inactive metabolite excreted in kidney.	Generally first drug of choice; most benign; least potent; short half-life. Especially useful in kidney disease.
Acetohexamide (Dymelor)	0.25-1.5 single or divided doses	1.5	5	8-10	Metabolite's activity equal to or greater than parent compound. Metabolite excreted via kidney.	Essentially no advantage over tolbutamide although few patients who fail on tolbutamide are controlled. Significant uricosuric effects.[58]
Tolazamide (Tolinase)	0.1-1.0 single or divided doses	0.75-1.0	7	1-2; 10-14	Absorbed slowly. Metabolite active but less potent than parent compound. Excreted via kidney.	Essentially no advantage over tolbutamide. Said to be equipotent with less severe side effects.
Chlorpropamide (Diabinese)	0.1-0.5 single dose	0.5	35	1; 72	Previously thought not to be metabolized but recently found that metabolism may be quite extensive. Activity of these unknown. Significant % excreted unchanged.[59,60]	More potent than tolbutamide. Caution in elderly patients and those with kidney disease.
Phenformin[61] (DBI)	0.05-0.2 in single or divided doses	Usually 200 mg (dose limited by GI effects)	3	Initial onset is 3-4 days; then onset is rapid; duration 12 hr for TD form	Metabolized but activity of metabolite unknown. 90% excreted via kidney in 24 hr.	Additive with sulfonylureas and insulin. Drug of choice for obese diabetics. Used to treat secondary failures and to stabilize brittle juvenile diabetics.

on the basis of blood glucose, urine glucose and symptomatology. This gradual method of dosing is particularly important for chlorpropamide and phenformin. Chlorpropamide should be started at very low doses in the elderly be-cause their poor eating habits and decreased renal function apparently predispose this group to hypoglycemic reactions.[57] The dose of phenformin should also be increased gradually since gastrointestinal effects may be averted by

TABLE 22.8
Drug-Induced Diabetes[66,67]

Drug	Comments
Asparaginase[68]	Can cause clinically significant hyperglycemia and glucosuria 2-4 days following a single therapeutic dose. Abnormal insulin response to glucose lasts from days to months but is eventually reversible. Occurrred in 5/39 patients in one series and in 3/5 patients in another. Proposed mechanism: inhibition of insulin synthesis or pancreatic destruction.
Birth control pills[69,70]	Diminished GTTs are most often reported in women with a family history of diabetes. Related to estrogen, although it may occur more often in women taking combination products. Generally reversible, but a few cases of irreversible diabetes have been reported in females with a history of gestational diabetes. Incidence approximately 53%.
Corticosteroids[71]	Promote gluconeogenesis and antagonize the effects of insulin. Incidence approximately 14% in diabetics. Reversible. Generally cause a mild hyperglycemia. Ketosis is rare but hyperosmolar, nonketotic coma has been reported.
Diuretics[72,73]	May decrease glucose tolerance in up to 50% of the patients with a history of diabetes. Can occur with usual therapeutic doses as soon as 3-7 days after therapy is begun. Increased insulin requirements rare. Effect reversible. Not contraindicated in diabetics as long as appropriate adjustments in therapy are made. Ethacrynic acid and furosemide are also diabetogenic. Spironolactone has no diabetogenic effects.
Glucagon[17]	Promotes breakdown of glycogen to glucose. Used in the treatment of hypoglycemia but works poorly in debilitated patients who have inadequate glycogen stores.
Diphenylhydantoin[74]	Impairs insulin release. Dose-related effect which may occur with therapeutic doses of the drug. Hyperglycemia requiring additional drug therapy occurred in a patient receiving 400 mg DPH daily.
Dextrothyroxine[75]	4-8 mg resulted in significantly increased FBG's 2 weeks after therapy was initiated. Further deterioration in 8/18 patients, requiring adjustment of diabetic therapy.
Diazoxide[76]	Produces a predictable, clinically significant hyperglycemia in therapeutic doses. Mechanism unknown but may decrease secretion of insulin in response to glucose. Effect is reversible by tolbutamide, although the latter does not interfere with the hypotensive effects of diazoxide.
Glycerol[77]	A 68-year-old patient who ingested higher than usual doses of glycerin (2.3 gm/kg for 3 days) for the treatment of acute glaucoma developed hyperglycemia. Mechanism: glycerol is metabolized to glucose.
Nicotinic acid[78]	Doses of 1.5-3.0 g caused glucosuria, ketonuria, hyperglycemia and increased insulin requirements. Reversible.
Sympathomimetics[79,80]	0.5 mg epinephrine S.Q. stimulates breakdown of glycogen to glucose.

dosing in this manner. Lower doses are given once daily before breakfast, while higher doses are split and given two or more times throughout the day, depending on the drug's half-life.[19,41]

Treatment of Primary or Secondary Failure[17,64,65]

How does one determine whether a patient has failed to respond to therapy and how does one make the decision to abandon treatment? There is, of course, no definitive answer to this question, and one must use his judgment and be rather arbitrary. Doses of any given agent should be pushed to maximal levels (Table 22.6) before a decision to abandon therapy is made. Increasing the doses above these maximums results in an increased incidence of adverse effects without producing any further decrease in the blood glucose. Most authors feel that treatment with any given agent should continue for 1 month before a change in therapy is made. Once diabetogenic factors have been eliminated and an adequate trial is completed,

TABLE 22.9
Drugs Which Cause Significant Hypoglycemia

Drug	Comments
Alcohol[81,82]	Impairs gluconeogenesis; may increase the amount of insulin which is excreted in response to glucose. Levels just high enough to cause mild intoxication can cause hypoglycemia in patients with no glycogen reserve. This is particularly applicable to alcoholics, who are notorious for neglecting their nutritional requirements.
Anabolic steroids[83]	Cause significant hypoglycemia in therapeutic doses which may require a decrease in the insulin dose. Reported with testosterone, Dianabol, Durabolin and methandrostenolone.
MAO inhibitors[84]	Block homeostatic response to hypoglycemia. May cause significant drop in blood sugar in therapeutic doses. Effect may be confined to hydrazine-type MAO inhibitors. INH, which has a hydrazine-type structure, has been reported to potentiate the hypoglycemic action of tolbutamide.
Pentamidine[85]	15/164 patients receiving therapeutic doses of pentamidine 4 mg/kg/day developed blood sugars of less than 60 mg/100 ml (normal = 100 mg/100 ml). No mechanism postulated.
Propranolol[86,87]	Blocks liver glycogenolysis which occurs in response to hypoglycemia. Usual doses of the drug taken over a short period of time (hours-days) have been reported to cause severe hypoglycemic reactions in diabetics.
Salicylates[88,89]	Doses of 5-6 g can decrease ketonuria and glycosuria in mild to moderate diabetics. Similar doses may potentiate insulin and sulfonylureas. May increase peripheral uptake of glucose, decrease gluconeogenesis and increase rate of glycolysis.
Theophylline[90]	Normals, prediabetics and overt diabetics were given a 200-mg intravenous bolus followed by a 200-mg infusion of theophylline prior to a glucose tolerance test. Theophylline improved the insulin response to glucose in prediabetics but failed to do so in diabetics. It is postulated that this drug causes an augmented release of insulin in response to glucose.
Drugs which potentiate sulfonylureas[66,67,91]	A number of drugs reportedly potentiate sulfonylureas by several proposed mechanisms: inhibition of metabolism, protein displacement or decreased excretion. In most cases, these interactions are poorly documented and are rarely corroborated by others. Drugs which *may* potentiate sulfonylureas in therapeutic doses include chloramphenicol, dicumarol, phenylbutazone, salicylates and sulfisoxazole. For further discussion of these interactions, see the cited references.

one of several alternatives may be contemplated. The patient may be switched to a more potent drug (*e.g.*, tolbutamide to chlorpropamide). Alternatively, 50 mg of phenformin, which has a different mechanism of action, may be added to a decreased dose of sulfonylurea. The sulfonylurea is then slowly increased to maximal doses, if necessary. If control is still unsatisfactory, the phenformin dose is increased by 50 mg each week. A definitive effect should occur within 7 to 14 days. If there is no effect at maximal doses in 14 days, it will be necessary to switch to insulin. If control is poor and symptoms are severe enough, the patient should be switched to insulin until control is achieved. Fifty percent of the patients can usually be successfully returned to oral therapy following control with insulin. Apparently, a yet-to-be-defined plasma factor present during uncontrolled diabetes makes the disease relatively resistant to any type of therapy. This resistance generally subsides in 1 to 2 weeks.[17]

FACTORS WHICH MAY ALTER DIABETIC CONTROL

Several abnormal physiological states and drugs may make alteration in the dose of insulin or oral hypoglycemic agents necessary (Table 22.7). The diabetogenic effects of drugs occur most frequently in patients who have a family history of diabetes mellitus. Other drugs may potentiate or inhibit the effects of the sulfonylureas and still others have a hypoglycemic effect of their own, thereby potentiating both insulin and the oral hypoglycemic agents. These have been enumerated in Tables 22.8 and 22.9.

PROGNOSIS

Although insulin and the oral hypoglycemics have definitely reduced the morbidity and mortality from the acute complications of the disease, their beneficial effect on the long term complications of the disease (neuropathy, nephropathy, blindness, infection, vascular insufficiency) is less certain. Certainly they have prolonged the diabetic's life span and improved the quality of his life. Because of lack of space,

this chapter did not cover the medical management of diabetic coma,[92,93] the pregnant diabetic,[50,94,95] or the patient in stress.[96] These areas are covered in detail elsewhere and references have been provided for further study.

REFERENCES

1. Watkins, J. D., Roberts, D. E., Williams, T. F., Martin, D. A., and Coyle, V.: Observation of medication errors made by diabetic patients at home. Diabetes, 16: 882, 1967.
2. Felig, P.: Pathophysiology of diabetes mellitus. Med. Clin. North Am., 55: 821, 1971.
3. Fajans, S. S.: What is diabetes? Definition, diagnosis and course. Med. Clin. North Am., 55: 793, 1971.
4. Leonards, J. R.: Evaluation of enzyme tests for urinary glucose. J.A.M.A., 163: 260, 1957.
5. Gifford, H., and Bergerman, J.: Falsely negative enzyme paper tests for urinary glucose. J.A.M.A., 178: 423, 1961.
6. Kristensen, K. A. B.: I.V. tetracycline and "dipstick" urine test. N. Engl. J. Med., 283: 660, 1970.
7. Bressler, R., and Galloway, J. A.: Insulin treatment of diabetes mellitus. Med. Clin. North Am., 55: 861, 1971.
8. Belmonte, M. M., Sarkozy, E., and Harpur, E. R.: Urine sugar determination by the two-drop clinitest method. Diabetes, 16: 557, 1967.
9. Knowles, H. C.: Diabetes mellitus in childhood and adolescense. Med. Clin. North Am., 55: 975, 1971.
10. Nunes, W. T.: A Manual of Diabetes for the House Officer, Ed. 1, p. 23. Charles C. Thomas, Springfield, Ill., 1963.
11. Ames Research Laboratory Literature, Elkhart, Ind. (available upon request).
12. Wirth, W. A., and Thompson, R. L.: The effect of various conditions and substances on the results of laboratory procedures. Am. J. Clin. Pathol., 43: 579, 1965.
13. Kostis, J., and Bergen, S. S.: Unusual color reaction in glycosiria testing during cephalothin administration (letter). J.A.M.A., 196: 805, 1966.
14. Klumpp, T. G.: Naldixic acid. False positive glycosuria and hyperglycemia. J.A.M.A., 193: 122, 1965.
15. Whipple, R. L., and Bloom, W. L.: The occurrences of false positive tests for albumin and glucose in the urine during the course of massive penicillin therapy. J. Lab. Clin. Med., 36: 635, 1950.
16. Clinitest Package Insert, Ames Drug Co., Elkhart, Ind.
17. Waife, S. D. (editor): Diabetes Mellitus, Ed. 7, p. 87. Lilly Research Laboratories, Indianapolis, 1967.
18. Donaldson, J. B.: Current concepts in the treatment of diabetes mellitus. Med. Clin. North

Am., 49: 1349, 1965.

19. Devlin, J. G.: Effect of alterations of species source of insulin on insulin antibody levels. Lancet, 2: 883, 1966.

20. Storvick, W., and Henry, H. J.: Effect of storage temperature on stability of commercial insulin preparations. Diabetes, 17: 499, 1968.

21. Arky, R. A., and Arons, D. L.: Hypoglycemia in diabetes mellitus. Med. Clin. North Am., 55: 919, 1971.

22. Rabkin, R., Simon, N. M., Steiner, S., and Colwell, J. A.: Effect of renal disease on renal uptake and excretion of insulin in man. N. Engl. J. Med., 282: 182, 1970.

23. Rubenstein, A. H., and Spitz, I.: Role of kidney in insulin metabolism and excretion diabetes. 17: 161, 1968.

24. Prout, T. E.: The antigenicity of insulin: a review. J. Chronic Dis., 15: 879, 1962.

25. Goldschmid, A., and Lavrian, L.: Sulfated insulin in resistant juvenile diabetes. Lancet, 2: 405, 1968.

26. Kreines, K.: The use of various insulins in insulin allergy. Arch. Intern. Med., 116: 165, 1965.

27. Williams, R. H.: Recent advances relative to diabetes mellitus. Ann. Intern. Med., 63: 512, 1965.

28. Yalow, R. S., and Berson, S. A.: Reaction of fish insulin antiserums: potential value in the treatment of insulin resistance. N. Engl. J. Med., 22: 1171, 1964.

29. Galloway, J. A., and Root, M. A.: New forms of insulin. Diabetes, 21: 637, 1972.

30. Root, M. A., Chance, R. E., and Galloway, J. A.: Immunogenicity of insulin. Diabetes, 21: 657, 1972.

31. Guthrie, R. A., Murphy, D. Y. N., and Womack, W.: Insulin resistance in diabetes in juveniles. Pediatrics, 40: 642, 1967.

32. Lieberman, P., Patterson, R., Metz, R., and Lucena, G.: Allergic reactions of insulin. J.A.M.A., 215: 1106, 1971.

33. Dolovich, J., Schnatz, J. D., Reisman, R. E., Yagt, Y., and Arbesman, C. E.: Insulin allergy and insulin resistance. J. Allergy, 46: 127, 1970.

34. Shipp, J. C., Cunningham, R. W., Russell, R. O., and Marble, A.: Insulin resistance: clinical features, natural course and effects of adrenal steroid treatment. Medicine, 44: 165, 1965.

35. Hadley, W. B.: Insulin treatment of diabetes mellitus. Med. Clin. North Am., 49: 921, 1965.

36. Nora, J. A., Smith, D. W., and Cameron, J. R.: The route of insulin administration in the management of diabetes mellitus. J. Pediatr., 64: 547, 1964.

37. Prout, T. E.: A prospective view of the treatment of adult onset diabetes. Med. Clin. North Am., 55: 1065, 1971.

38. The University Group Diabetes Program: A study of the effects of hypoglycemic agents on vascular complications in patients with adult onset diabetes. Diabetes, 19: Suppl. 2, 1970.

39. Knatterud, G. L., Meinert, C. L., Klimt, C. R., Osborne, R. K., and Martin, D. B.: Effects of hypoglycemic agents on vascular complica-

tions in patients with adult onset diabetes. IV: A preliminary report on phenformin results. J.A.M.A., 217: 777, 1971.

40. Singer, D. L., and Hurwitz, D.: Long term experience with sulfonylureas and placebo. N. Engl. J. Med., 277: 450, 1967.

41. Ferguson, B. D.: The oral hypoglycemic compounds. Med. Clin. North Am., 49: 929, 1965.

42. Hooper, M.: Diabetes mellitus treated with phenformin. Analysis of 94 cases with particular reference to weight changes. Br. J. Clin. Pract., 21: 389, 1967.

43. Pannekoek, J. H.: Side effects of drugs. In Oral Antidiabetic Drugs, Vol. 6, Chap. 28, p. 422, edited by L. Meyler and A. Herxheimer. Williams & Wilkins Co., Baltimore, 1968.

44. Hamff, H., Ferris, H. A., Evans, E. C., and Whiteman, H. W.: Effects of tolbutamide and chlorpropamide on patients exhibiting jaundice as a result of chlorpropamide therapy. Ann. N.Y. Acad. Sci., 74: 820, 1959.

45. Klink, D., Fritz, R., and Franke, G.: Disulfiramlike reaction to chlorpropamide. Wisc. Med. J., 68: 134, 1969.

46. Podgainy, H., and Bressler, R.: Biochemical basis of the sulfonylurea induced antabuse syndrome. Diabetes, 17: 679, 1968.

47. Bauer, H. G.: Severe and prolonged hypoglycemic shock during sulfonylurea treatment. Metabolism, 14: 220, 1965.

48. Kelley, D. B.: Diabetic emergencies: drug induced hypoglycemia. Med. Clin. North Am., 53: 465, 1965.

49. Seltzer, H. S.: Drug induced hypoglycemia. A review based on 473 cases. Diabetes, 21: 955, 1972.

50. Zucker, P., and Simon, G.: Prolonged symptomatic neonatal hypoglycemia associated with maternal chlorpropamide therapy. Pediatrics, 42: 824, 1968.

51. Hershman, J. M., Craane, T. J., and Colwell, J. A.: Effect of sulfonylurea drugs on the binding of tri-iodothyronine and thyroxine to thyronine binding globulin. J. Clin. Endocrinol. Metab., 28: 1065, 1968.

52. Portioli, I., and Rocchi, F.: Sulfonylureas and hypothyroidism. Lancet, 1: 681, 1969.

53. Early, L. E.: Chlorpropamide antidiuresis. N. Engl. J. Med., 284: 103, 1971.

54. Garcia, M., Miller, M., and Moses, A. M.: Chlorpropamide induced water retention in patients with diabetes mellitus. Ann. Intern. Med., 75: 549, 1971.

55. Goldner, M. G., Baldwin, R. S., Dobson, H. L., Krall, L. P., Lambert, T. H., Miller, E., Pomeranze, J., and Weller, C.: Phenformin in the management of diabetes, general clinical concepts. Diabetes, 9: 220, 1960.

56. Anon.: Phenformin and lactic acidosis. Calif. Med., 110: 348, 1969.

57. Williams, H. E.: Medical staff conference: lactic acidosis. Calif. Med., 110: 330, 1969.

58. Yu, T., Berger, L., and Gutman, A. B.: Hypoglycemic and uricosuric properties of aceto-

hexamide and hydroxyhexamide. Metabolism, 17: 309, 1968.

59. Brotherton, P. M., Grieveson, P., and McMartin, C.: A study of metabolic fate of chlorpropamide in man. Clin. Pharmacol. Ther., 10: 505, 1969.

60. Taylor, J. A.: Pharmacokinetics and biotransformation of chlorpropamide in man. Clin. Pharmacol. Ther., 13: 710, 1972.

61. Hamwi, G. J., and Seidensticker, J. F.: Therapy: oral hypoglycemic agents, Ed. 1, Vol. 2, Chap. 20, p. 109, edited by G. J. Hamwi and T. S. Danovski. In Diabetes Mellitus, Diagnosis and Treatment. American Diabetes Assoc., New York, 1967.

62. Ricketts, H. T.: Weight change with orally administered "antidiabetic" drugs. J.A.M.A., 213: 1676, 1970.

63. Abramson, E. A., and Arky, R. S.: Treatment of the obese diabetic. A comparative study of placebo, sulfonylurea and phenformin. Metabolism, 16: 204, 1967.

64. Anon.: Secondary failure to sulfonylureas in the treatment of diabetes. S. Afr. Med. J., 41: 453, 1967.

65. Beaser, S. B.: Oral treatment of diabetes mellitus. J.A.M.A., 187: 887, 1964.

66. Hussar, D. A.: The hypoglycemic agents – their interactions. J. Am. Pharm. Assoc., 10: 619, 1970.

67. Hansten, P.: Drug Interactions, Ed. 1, p. 57. Lea and Febiger, Philadelphia, 1971.

68. Gailani, S., Nussbaum, A., Ohnuma, T., and Freeman, A.: Diabetes in patients treated with asparaginase. Clin. Pharmacol. Ther., 12: 487, 1971.

69. Spellacy, W. N., Guhi, W. C., Spellacy, C. E., Moses, L. E., and Goldzieher, J. W.: Glucose, insulin and growth hormone studies, in long term users of oral contraceptives. Am. J. Obstet. Gynecol., 106: 173, 1970.

70. Szabo, A. J., Cole, H. S., and Grimaldi, R. S.: Glucose tolerance in gestational diabetic women during and after treatment with a combination type oral contraceptive. N. Engl. J. Med., 282: 646, 1970.

71. Gharib, H.: Steroid diabetes. Minn. Med., 52: 669, 1969.

72. Dollery, C. T.: Changes in carbohydrate metabolism after the use of diuretics. In Drug Induced Disease, Chap. 5, p. 95, edited by L. Meyler and H. M. Peck. Excerpta Medica Foundation, New York, 1968.

73. Rapoport, M. I., and Hurd, H. F.: Thiazide induced glucose intolerance treated with potassium. Arch. Intern. Med., 113: 405, 1964.

74. Fariss, B. L., and Lutcher, C. L.: Diphenylhydantoin induced hyperglycemia and impaired insulin release. Diabetes, 20: 177, 1971.

75. Zinn, W. J., and Schleissner, L. A.: The effect of dextrothyroxine in diabetes. Calif. Med., 101: 240, 1964.

76. Seltzer, H. S., and Allen, E. W.: Hyperglycemia and inhibition of insulin secretion during administration of diazoxide and trichloromethiazide in man. Diabetes, 18: 19, 1969.

77. D'Alena, P., and Ferguson, W.: Adverse effects after glycerol orally and mannitol parenterally. Arch. Ophthalmol., 75: 201, 1966.

78. Janovsky, R. C.: Diabetogenic effects of nicotinic acid. Ohio State Med. J., 64: 1137, 1968.

79. Inouye, S.: Effects of epinephrine on asthmatic children. J. Allergy, 40: 337, 1967.

80. Porte, D., Jr.: Sympathetic regulation of insulin secretion. Its relation to diabetes mellitus. Arch. Intern. Med., 123: 253, 1969.

81. Arky, R. A., Ververbrants, E., and Abramson, E. A.: Irreversible hypoglycemia. J.A.M.A., 206: 575, 1968.

82. Freinkel, N., and Arky, R. A.: Effects of alcohol on carbohydrate metabolism in man. Psychosom. Med., 28: 551, 1966.

83. Landin, J., Wynn, V., and Samols, E.: The effect of anabolic steroids on blood sugar and plasma insulin levels in man. Metabolism, 12: 924, 1963.

84. Cooper, A. J., and Ashcroft, G.: Modification of insulin and sulfonylurea hypoglycemia by monoamine oxidase inhibitor drugs. Diabetes, 16: 272, 1967.

85. Western, K. A., Perera, K. R., and Schultz, M. G.: Pentamidine isethionate in the treatment of pneumocystitis carinii pneumonia. Ann. Intern. Med., 73: 695, 1970.

86. Abramson, E. A., Arky, R. A., and Woeber, K. A.: Effects of propranolol on hormonal and metabolic responses to insulin induced hypoglycemia. Lancet, 2: 1386, 1966.

87. Reveno, W. S., and Rosenbaum, H.: Propranolol and hypoglycemia. Lancet, 1: 920, 1968.

88. Fang, V., Goye, W. O., and Robinson, S. M.: Hypoglycemic activity and chemical structure of the salicylates. J. Pharm. Sci., 57: 2111, 1968.

89. Hecht, A., and Goldner, M. G.: Reappraisal of the hypoglycemic action of ASA. Metabolism, 8: 418, 1959.

90. Cerasi, E., and Luft, R.: The effect of an adenosine 3', 5'-monophosphate diesterase inhibitor (aminophylline) on the insulin response to glucose infusion in prediabetic and diabetic subjects. Horm. Metab. Res., 1: 162, 1969.

91. Young, L., and Kimble, M. A. (editors): Applied Therapeutics for Clinical Pharmacists, Applied Therapeutics, Inc., San Francisco, 1975.

92. Winegrad, A. I., and Clements, R. S., Jr.: Diabetic ketoacidosis. Med. Clin. North Am., 55: 889, 1971.

93. Arieff, A. I.: Nonketotic hyperosmolar coma with hyperglycemia. Medicine, 51: 73, 1972.

94. Tyson, J. E.: Medical aspects of diabetes in pregnancy and the diabetogenic effects of oral contraceptives. Med. Clin. North Am., 55: 947, 1971.

95. Adam, P. A., and Schwartz, R.: Diagnosis and treatment: should oral hypoglycemic agents be used in pediatric and pregnant patients? Pediatrics, 42: 819, 1968.

96. Steinke, J.: Management of diabetes in the surgical patient. Med. Clin. North Am., 55: 939, 1971.

chapter 23

PARATHYROID DISORDERS

Marianne Ivey, B.S.

Parathyroid disorders involve aberrant calcium homeostasis mechanisms. The involvement of phosphorus, magnesium, potassium, acid-base balance, the kidney, bone metabolism and the compensatory system of the parathyroid glands makes the subject of calcium metabolism and parathyroid disorders highly complex (Fig. 23.1). To understand the treatment of the hypo-and hyperparathyroid states, the pharmacist must first understand the physiology of the parathyroid glands, the effects of parathormone and the manifestations of abnormal secretion or lack of end organ response.

The parathyroid glands are situated on the lateral lobes of the thyroid. There are usually four parathyroid glands; however, as few as one and as many as seven have been reported. The glands secrete parathormone in response to low serum calcium. Parathyroid hormone (PTH) increases the serum calcium levels by several mechanisms: it stimulates bone resorption, it may increase intestinal absorption of calcium and it may increase the reabsorption of calcium by the renal tubules. Furthermore, PTH acts on the kidney to decrease the tubular reabsorption of phosphate (TRP). Thus a reciprocal relationship between calcium and phosphorus exists. In hyperparathyroidism, serum calcium is elevated and serum phosphate is low; and in hypoparathyroidism, calcium in the serum is low and serum phosphate is elevated.

The compensatory mechanisms of the parathyroid gland are intact in the normal individ-

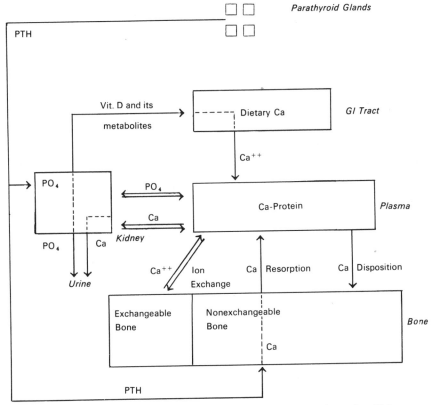

FIG. 23.1. A simplified diagram of some of the normal relationships of parathyroid hormone and calcium metabolism.

ual. A low serum calcium stimulates release of PTH which induces bone resorption and an increase in serum calcium. In contrast, an elevated serum calcium inhibits the secretion of PTH and therefore shuts off bone resorption and the source of nondietary calcium. Although the dietary intake of calcium can vary greatly from day to day, the fine regulator is the effect of PTH on the skeleton. Another homeostatic regulator of calcium is calcitonin. Calcitonin is produced in the ultimobranchial cells of the thyroid in the human and in separate glands in birds and fish. Calcitonin regulates calcium metabolism by inhibiting bone resorption, and thus it monitors the effect of PTH secretion by preventing an excess increase in the serum calcium. A more specific discussion of calcitonin will be presented under pharmacological management of hyperparathyroidism. Thus serum calcium is finely regulated between 8.5 and 10 mg/100 ml and phosphorous between 2.5 and 4.5 mg/100 ml (Table 23.1). In the individual with idiopathic or known causes of either

hypo- or hyperparathyroidism, the compensatory mechanisms of the gland either are not functional or are very sluggish.

In discussing parathyroid disease, it is necessary to understand bone metabolism and the roles played by calcium and phosphorous. Of the over 1,000 gm of calcium in the body, nearly all of it is in bone. Bone is composed of both stable and exchangeable calcium. The calcium in the exchangeable bone turns over many times a day with that in the fluid compartments of the body. Of the 500 gm of phosphorous in the body, over 80% is in the bone. The bone cells are very active. Some are osteoblastic, that is, in the process of bone formation; and some are osteoclastic, that is involved in the process of resorption.

HYPOPARATHYROIDISM

Etiology

In the past, the most common cause of hypoparathyroidism was thyroidectomy (Table 23.2). Furthermore, second and third successive operations for thyroid tumors are even more often associated with the loss of the parathyroid glands because the surgeon's operating field is made much more difficult by scar tissue. The second surgical cause for hypoparathyroidism is, of course, total parathyroidectomy due to adenomatous, hyperplastic or neoplastic glands. The third cause is idiopathic, and it is thought that an immune mechanism may be involved. A congenital form of hypoparathyroidism exists in children who are born without the parathyroid structures. Lastly, an iatrogenic cause is now being explored for a hypoparathyroid-like state. This is not an actual hypoparathyroid state but will be discussed because of its importance to pharmacists. (Table 23.3) It has been reported several times in the literature that long term use of diphenylhydantoin and phenobarbital in epileptic patients may cause hypocalcemia. It is thought that the mechanism of the anticonvulsants' hypocalcemic effect is the induction of enzymes which rapidly metabolize steroid hormone-like vitamin D to inactive metabolites.[1] Thus, vitamin D's effect in increasing calcium absorption from the gut is not present. The intensity of the hypocalcemia seen in epileptics also appears to be related to the amount of

TABLE 23.1
Laboratory Test Important in Evaluating Parathyroid Disease States.

Tests	Normal (adults)[a]
Screening tests	
Serum calcium	8.5-10 mg%
Serum phosphate	2.5-4.5 mg%
Serum alkaline	
phosphatase	30-85 milliunits/ml (I.U.)
Urine calcium	< 150 mg/24 hr with low Ca diet < 250 mg/24 hr with usual diet
Skeletal survey	Scans, biopsies
Total protein	6-9 g% (total)
and albumin	3.5-5.5 g% (albumin)
Specific supporting tests	
Urine hydroxyproline	10-30 mg/24°/m²
Calcitonin	
Parathyroid hormone	0-89 μlEq/ml
Tubular reabsorption	
of phosphate	85-95% reabsorption

[a]Different laboratories may have different normal values.

TABLE 23.2
Parathyroid Disorders with Cause and Effect Relationships.

isease	Cause	[Ca]	[P]	PTH
ypoparathyroidism	Idiopathic, thyroid surgery, parathyroid surgery, congenital	↓	↑	↓
seudohypoparathyroidism	Congenital	↓	↑	↑
seudopseudohypoparathyroidism	Congenital	nl	nl	nl
yperparathyroidism	Idiopathic, adenoma, hyperplasia, cancer, ectopic PTH production	↑	↓	↑
econdary hyperparathyroidism	Uremia	↓	↑	↑
econdary hyperparathyroidism[a] ith coincidental primary yperparathyroidism	Uremia and adenoma	↑	↓	↑ (postkidney transplant)

[a]This entity has also been called tertiary hyperparathyroidism.

calcium ingested in the diet and the amount of sunshine to which the patient is exposed. The hypoparathyroid-like state of anticonvulsant-induced hypocalcemia appears to occur in approximately 1/5 of patients on long term combined diphenylhydantoin-phenobarbital therapy. However, controlled studies are limited. Epileptic patients on either anticonvulsant drug alone show similar, however, less marked calcium responses. About 1/3 of the patients on combined anticonvulsant therapy, however, exibit other signs of vitamin D inhibition such as low serum concentrations of active vitamin D metabolites and bony changes which are seen by direct observation. In many of these patients, serum calcium and alkaline phosphatase levels are normal. The incidence of hypocalcemia appears to be more common in patients with combined anticonvulsant therapy and little sunlight exposure, in blacks because of greater resistance to the irradiating effects of sunlight and in persons whose diets are low in calcium. The hypocalcemia caused by anticonvulsants is obviously not entirely compensated for by the parathyroid glands, and the reason for this is not fully known. This last cause of hypocalcemia can lead to subnormal bone mineralization and osteomalacia, and it is of importance to pharmacists for it represents a drug induced abnormality. The pharmacist should thus review the epileptic's laboratory data for a low serum calcium level and serum alkaline phosphatase. The pharmacist in the community should realize the importance of complaints of bone and joint pains and, knowing the duration of anticonvulsant therapy, should not hesitate to consult with the patient's physician.

INCIDENCE

Idiopathic and congenital hypoparathyroidism appear to be extremely rare. Hypoparathyroidism because of thyroidectomy is also quite rare at this time owing to improved surgical techniques. Hypoparathyroidism after subtotal parathyroidectomy is usually transient and permanent hypoparathyroidism due to this cause is rare. This surgery, which is performed most frequently in uremic patients, will be discussed under secondary hyperparathyroidism. Obviously, total parathyroidectomy leads to hypoparathyroidism which must be treated. The incidence of this cause is directly related to the incidence of hyperparathyroidism responding only to surgical treatment.

PATHOGENESIS AND CLINICAL FINDINGS

In all cases of hypoparathyroidism discussed above (which does not include the anticonvulsant-induced hypocalcemia), there is

TABLE 23.3
Drugs Affecting Calcium and Phosphorus.

Drugs that increase calcium in the serum

    Vitamin D and metabolites
    Calcium salts
    Parathyroid extract
    Thiazides

Drugs that decrease serum phosphate

    Aluminum antacids
    Parathyroid extract
    Vitamin D

Drugs that decrease calcium in the serum

    Phosphates
    Calcitonin
    Sodium sulfate
    Furosemide
    Mithramycin
    Corticosteroids
    Anticonvulsants (diphenylhydantoin
       and phenobarbital)
    Magnesium
    Fluoride

Drugs that increase serum phosphate

    Phosphates

a decrease or absence of parathyroid hormone secretion.This leads to a decrease in bone resorption and thus a decrease in serum calcium concentration. In the absence of PTH, tubular reabsorption of phosphate (TRP) is not inhibited, and thus serum phosphorus levels are elevated. Both calcium and phosphorus are responsible for the clinical findings. The most common response to low serum calcium in increased neuromuscular irritability—low calcium tetany. This tetany is seen as carpopedal spasm in which the hand is hollowed, fingers rigid and all joints from the fingers to and including the elbows are flexed. Tonic and clonic convulsions may be seen. This may appear, to even medical observers, as epileptic seizures. The most intense form of tetany progresses to opisthotonos. Another form of muscular irritability masquerades as asthma due to laryngeal stridor. This can be a severe complication of parathyroidectomy. Spasms of other systems such as the gastrointestinal tract, genito urinary tract and the musculature of the eye can also occur. Psychiatric symptoms are present in all or nearly all hypoparathyroid individuals. These can range from anxiety to schizophrenia.

The high levels of phosphate also contribute to the clinical findings of hypoparathyroidism. In spite of the hypocalcemia, hyperphosphatemia may cause an increase in calcium-phosphorous solubility product. Thus there is an increased density of the bone. There may be ectopic calcifications in blood vessels, brain, subcutaneous tissues, muscles and the cartilage of the ear. The brain calcifications can lead to loss of mental capacity.

Other complications of hypoparathyroidism include lenticular cataracts, impaired dental structures, sparse or prematurely gray hair, dry scaly skin with a predisposition of monilial infection and ECG changes.

DIAGNOSIS

Usually hypoparathyroidism is suspected first by either manifestaions of tetany or the detection of low serum calcium levels during routine laboratory testing. Patients presenting with hypocalcemia do not all have hypoparathyroidism. Tetany may not always be related to hypocalcemia, but it may be related to alkalosis or hypomagnesemia. Obviously, the physician must differentiate the causes of the tetany if this is the first presenting symptom. If the tetany is caused by hypocalcemia, he must then decide the cause of it.

The tetany of alkalosis is usually produced because of prolonged vomiting, excessive alkali ingestion of hyperventilation. Because alkalosis due to hyperventilation and vomiting may be a metabolic response after any type of surgery, a transient hypocalcemia may develop postoperatively. If tetany develops for this reason, it is obviously treated but for only a short period.

Another body constituent of importance in hypocalcemia is the total serum protein correlation. Since approximately 50% of serum calcium is bound to protein, hypoproteinemia (hypoalbuminemia) will also cause hypocalcemia. Thus part of the hypocalcemic workup should include measurement of total serum protein levels and protein electrophoresis.

Hypocalcemia also occurs in renal disease, intestinal malabsorption, osteomalacia and rickets. Initially these are non parathyroid diseases and are related to problems in vitamin D absorption or metabolism. The differentiating factors of these diseases with hypoparathyroidism involve unexpected relationships of other body chemistries such as serum phosphate, alkaline phosphate and blood urea nitrogen (BUN).

Hypoparathyroidism is differentiated from pseudohypoparathyroidism by the Ellsworth-Howard test. This test determines whether the kidney is responsive to PTH. In pseudohypoparathyroidism the PTH levels are elevated, but because of a lack of adenyl cylase in the kidney, TRP is not inhibited. After parathyroid extract is given to a patient with pseudohypoparathyroidism, phosphate concentrations in the urine will not increase to the extent that would be encountered in the hypoparathyroid individual. The specifics of this test will be covered in the diagnostic section on pseudohypoparathyroidism.

A form of hypoparathyroidism has been described in which the serum calcium is normal. However, a general feeling of malaise is present with mental depression. It is assumed that parathyroid reserve is decreased or that the tissue calcium pool is decreased and thus normal compensatory mechanisms are depressed. A diagnostic test for this type of hypoparathyroidism is administration of ethylenediaminetetraacetic acid. Given by the intravenous route, this compound, which complexes calcium into an unabsorbable molecule, will deprive the serum of calcium. In normal patients, compensatory mechanisms will increase the serum calcium to 8.5 mg/100 ml in 24 hr. In the patient with this particular hypoparathyroid disease, the compensatory mechanisms are much more sluggish.

Lastly, two tests for latent tetany are the Chvostek's sign and Trousseau's sign. A tap to the facial nerve in front of the ear usually causes a grimace or contraction of the facial muscles in a hypoparathyroid patient. This is a positive Chvostek's sign. Trousseau's sign is positive if the application of a blood pressure cuff and occlusion of blood supply to the arm cause carpopedal spasm. These signs are helpful, but they may be positive in a few normal individuals.

The most important test to determine the exact cause of many of the disease states above is the radioimmunoassay for PTH. At this time, however, the test has been perfected in only a few hospital laboratories.

TREATMENT

The treatment of hypocalcemic tetany is, of course, the intravenous infusion of a calcium salt. Calcium chloride and calcium gluconate are most frequently used. Based on blood level of calcium, it is not possible to predict the exact amount of the calcium salt needed and this must be determined on the basis of resultant serum calcium levels. However, usually 5 to 20 ml of 10% solution of either of the salts is an effective dose. The effects of both salts are rapid but of short duration, and they may need to be given frequently to maintain the correct blood level. A continuous effect may be obtained by administering 100 ml of the 10% calcium gluconate in 1 liter of saline or dextrose solution infused over 12 to 24 hr. When the acute phase of hypocalcemia is past, calcium levels may be maintained by oral calcium salts. Calcium lactate, 10 to 20 g daily, is the salt most commonly seen to be successful by this author. It is available in 300, 500 and 600-mg oral dosage forms.

Important to the pharmacist are some inherent characteristics of calcium and some differences of the salts. Calcium in high doses is constipating, and often a patient requiring such dosages may also need a stool softener such as dioctylsodiumsuccinate. Calcium also may potentiate the toxicity of digoxin, and even without digoxin, high concentration calcium infusions can cause syncope. The calcium gluconate and calcium chloride solutions provide different percentages of calcium. Ten milliliters of a 10% solution of calcium chloride contain 270 mg of calcium while 10 ml of 10% calcium gluconate solution contain only 90 mg of calcium. The chloride salt, however, is extremely irritating and must be infused slowly. It must never be given by the I.M. route since it can cause tissue sloughing. Extravasation and irritation are limitations to its intravenous I.V. administration. This author recommends calcium gluconate for the acute hypocalcemic episode.

In the past, long term treatment of hypocalcemia usually involved a low phosphate diet, phosphate-binding antacids such as aluminum hydroxide or aluminum carbonate and vitamin D_2 or dihydrotachysterol and calcium salt supplements. In the initial therapy, the aluminum antacids decrease the phosphate and make it safe to increase the serum calcium. It is now thought that the use of an effective preparation of vitamin D is adequate for treatment of hypocalcemia and will prevent the toxicities which are sometimes seen with the use of vitamin D and calcium supplements in combination.[2] The claimed refractoriness to vitamin D of the past may have been because of poor vitamin D preparations. In fact, assay of some lots of dihydrotachysterol in the past have found no activity at all. A crystalline form of dihydrotachysterol is of uniform quality. Dihydrotachysterol is preferred now because of its more rapid onset and shorter duration of action. Vitamin D_2 (ergocalciferol) is much less expensive than dihydrotachysterol and, therefore, is to be recommended unless its delayed onset, which is 4 to 12 weeks and its long duration of effect, which is 3 to 6 months or more, is contraindicated. The dose of vitamin D is not effectively based on the patient's serum calcium level. Initial doses of vitamin D should begin at 50,000 units daily and should be increased only after approximately 6 weeks when a response should have been seen. The usual dose of vitamin D_2 which is effective is 100,000 units. Greater than 150,000 units are seldom needed. If more than one capsule of vitamin D is required to achieve the dosage necessary, they may all be taken in one daily dose. Because of the long half-life of vitamin D, multiple daily dosing is unnecessary and will only add to the problem of patient noncompliance. As mentioned before, the combination of anticonvulsants, diphenylhydantoin and phenobarbital may necessitate increased intake of vitamin D, as may corticosteroids, since they also have an inhibitory action on vitamin D.

Many medical texts still contain instructions to be conveyed to the patient using the Sulkowitch test to determine calcium in the urine, and its value as a guide to the amount of vitamin D to be used is recommended. However, it is now known that vitamin D may increase urinary excretion of calcium even before serum calcium levels have reached renal threshold concentrations. Thus the hypoparathyroid patient must have serum calcium level determinations as a guide to vitamin D therapy. A Sulkowitch test may be of value for another reason, however, and that is that hypercalciuria in the presence or absence of high serum calcium levels may lead to kidney stones. Also, it is for this reason

that hypoparathyroid patients should maintain a good fluid intake.

Treatment of hypoparathyroidism does not presently include chronic parathormone. The bovine parathyroid extract available is used primarily in the early control of tetany of hypoparathyroidism. The patient is given 50 to 150 units of the extract by the subcutaneous, intramuscular or intravenous route. Since the onset of action is in hours, parenteral calcium is given for the immediate relief of the tetany. For chronic control, the extract must be injected every 1 or 2 days. It can not be given orally because it is destroyed by proteolytic enzymes. There may be antigenicity in a few patients using the drug on a long term basis. Until very recently, chronic administration of PTH was not advised because of the desirability of having the patient in the hospital and because of side effects. In 1972 the active portion of human PTH was elucidated and synthesized.[3] The synthesis of human PTH should improve chronic treatment, diagnostic PTH assays and the study of the hormone's role in metabolism.

Prognosis

If the dose of vitamin D is adequate to prevent hypocalcemia and if hypercalcemia due to vitamin D is prevented, the hypoparathyroid patient can be well controlled. Thus, the adequate dosing of vitamin D is crucial to the hypoparathyroid patient's welfare. Some patients, even with seemingly adequate vitamin D and calcium, do not feel well. Common complaints are of perioral numbness and tingling in the extemities. Better control may be gained with the use of the recently synthesized human PTH.

PSEUDOHYPOPARATHYROIDISM

Etiology

Pseudohypoparathyroidism is a congenital disease in which body structure abnormalities exist in conjunction with mineral level abnormalities. The condition is termed "pseudo" because parathyroid function is actually intact. However, the kidney is unable to respond to PTH, and as a result, calcium and phosphate abnormalities are very similar to hypoparathyroidism.

Incidence

Pseudohypoparathyroidism is rare and was first described in 1942. In 4½ years of clinical experience in both referral and nonreferral hospitals, this author has seen only two patients with the disease—one a 6-year-old female who showed many of the structural abnormalities described in the clinical findings and the other, a 48-year-old male in whom the diagnosis was questioned because of the absence of the structural abnormalities. Both patients were diagnosed on the basis of their response to the Ellsworth-Howard test.

Pathogenesis and Clinical Findings

It is now known that pseudohypoparathyroidism is due to the lack of end organ response by the kidney to parathyroid hormone. In the normal individual, PTH administration inhibits the tubular reabsorption of phosphate (TRP) by stimulating adenyl cyclases which convert adenosine triphosphate (ATP) to adenosine monophosphate (AMP). AMP is responsible for the cellular responses of PTH, *i.e.,* for inhibition of TRP[4] (Fig. 23.2 and Fig. 23.1). The failure of this inhibition of phosphate reabsorption in the pseudohypoparathyroid patient is due to a lack of renal adenyl cyclase.[5] Because of the effect on the TRP, serum phosphate levels are high and calcium levels are low. The parathyroid glands react appropriately by secreting PTH. Because the serum calcium remains low in spite of the compensatory attempt, the glands become hyperplastic and radioimmunoassays have shown high PTH serum concentrations. The other part of the disease that is extremely interesting and of genetic origin is the round face, short, blocky body, short, wide neck and stubby fingers. Other signs and symptoms of hypocalcemia may also be present, such as tetany, neurosis and psychosis, sparse hair, bone changes, abnormal dentition, poor eyesight and skin and nail involvement including moniliasis are seen.

Diagnosis

For the most part, the hypocalcemia of pseudohypoparathyroidism is discovered on the basis of the signs and symptoms mentioned above. As in the hypocalcemia of hypoparathy-

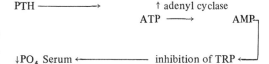

FIG. 23.2. Parathyroid hormone increases the formation of AMP from ATP. AMP provides the energy source for the inhibition of tubular reabsorption of phosphate resulting in increased phosphate in the urine.

roidism, the disease may masquerade as asthma or epilepsy due to muscle spasms. A similar diagnostic workup must be undertaken to rule out other causes of hypocalcemia. If both hypocalcemia and the body stature abnormalities exist, pseudohypoparathyroidism is highly suspect. The Ellsworth-Howard test has been used for years to diagnose the disease. It is based on the kidney's inability to respond to PTH. Parathyroid extract is given in a dose of 200 units by slow intravenous injection. Three hours before and 3 hr after the test, urine phosphate levels are measured. After the inhibition of TRP due to the injected extract, normal persons have approximately a 5-fold increase in urinary phosphate, hypoparathyroid patients a 10-fold increase and pseudohypoparathyroid patients only a 2-fold, or less, increase. A confirming test which may, when it becomes widely available, alleviate the need for the Ellsworth-Howard test, is the radioimmunoassay for serum parathormone concentration. After other forms of hypocalcemia are ruled out, a high serum PTH level should indicate pseudohypoparathyroidism if there is no history of uremia. Levels of cyclic AMP in the urine can also be measured and will be low in the pseudohypoparathyroid patient.

Treatment

The treatment of pseudohypoparathyroidism is essentially the same as for hypoparathyroidism. Acute hypocalcemia leading to tetany is treated with intravenous calcium chloride or calcium gluconate. After the acute phase, the patient may receive an oral calcium preparation. The same precautions regarding calcium and its effect on the cardiac system, gastrointestinal tract and infused veins exist as described under treatment of hypoparathyroidism. After the acute stages of hypocalcemia are corrected by calcium, the patient may be given vitamin D without other medications. Again the dosage of vitamin D can not be determined from the patient's serum calcium level. The initial dosage is 50,000 units and is regulated according to the response of the patient. The Sulkowich test is unreliable as a guide to serum calcium levels since vitamin D inhibits the tubular reabsorption of calcium.[6] Thus calcium may appear in the urine before serum levels have increased significantly. The Sulkowitch test may provide information regarding the potential for nephrolithiasis since high calciuria can lead to calcifications in the urinary tract. Patients with high urine calcium should be advised to increase their fluid intake to 2 to 3 liters daily. The reader is referred to the section on the treatment of hypoparathyroidism for a more complete discussion of drugs and their appropriate dosages.

It is of interest to the pharmacist that parathyroid extract is capable of producing anaphylactic reactions. When the Ellsworth-Howard test is carried out, the pharmacist should provide the physician with the drugs to reverse anaphylaxis—that is, aqueous epinephrine and parenteral antihistamines such as diphenhydramine. The pharmacist should also be concerned with the availability of adequate emergency equipment in the nursing unit such as the presence of various sizes of endotracheal tubes.

As with other parathyroid disorders, the difficulty of pseudohypoparathyroidism rests with the diagnosis. After that is made, the treatment is relatively simple.

Prognosis

As with hypoparathyroidism, if the patient with pseudohypoparathyroidism understands his disease, including the necessity to take vitamin D along with regular visits for serum calcium measurements, the prognosis is good. It is felt that compliance by the patient with medication directions is facilitated by providing him adequate information and instructions regarding the drug. In this respect, the pharmacist can be a significant participant. He can also monitor the patient to see that he is getting serum calcium determinations and can also be alert to reports of colicky renal pains which may mean nephrolithiasis. In such even, the patient should be referred to his physician immediately.

PSEUDOPSEUDOHYPOPARATHYROIDISM

To be complete, pseudopseudohypoparathy- will be mentioned briefly.

In pseudopseudohypoparathyroidism, the patient's appearance includes the short stature of pseudohypoparathyroidism. The round shaped skull and short metacarpals are also seen, and obviously abnormal bone formation is involved. However, the parathyroid glands are not involved. The cause is probably a separate gene. The calcium, phosphate and PTH levels in the serum are normal. Thus the name, pseudopseudohypoparathyroidism.

HYPERPARATHYROIDISM

Etiology

Primary hyperparathyroidism is a disease resulting from hypersecretion of the parathyroid glands. The most common cause is an adenoma of one or more glands. Less frequently it is caused by parathyroid hyperplasia or parathyroid carcinoma. Carcinomata of other organ systems, especially lung and kidney,[8] which produce PTH or a PTH-like hormone may produce clinical and laboratory findings identical to primary hyperparathyroid disease.

Incidence

The reports of the incidence of hyperparathyroid disease have been changing over the recent years owing to wide scale mass screening. Although still thought to be a very rare disease occuring in 0.1% of the population, Drs. Goldman and Gordon[2] reported that 50% of the patients screened at the University of California San Francisco Medical Center had hyperparathyroidism.* Others also report that the frequency of serendipitous finding of hyperpara-

---

*It was not reported whether the patients screened were representative of a random selection. It is obvious that in such a screening program a high calcium is being specifically checked for a parathyroid cause, and that some of the patients reported as having the disease, have it in a very mild, nonsymptomatic form. However, this does not change the value of the statistic. Wide scale screening for hypercalcemia represents preventative medicine in that many of these patients can be treated before there is severe bone and renal system involvement.

thyroidism indicates a disease less rare than is generally appreciated.[9]

Pathogenesis

Hypersecretion of the parathyroids causes an elevated serum calcium due to PTH's stimulation of bone resorption. It causes an elevated urine phosphate level due to PTH's inhibition of TRP. In many patients, the serum phosphate level is decreased. Thus the reciprocal relationship of serum calcium and phosphate mentioned in the introduction is again present. Because PTH stimulates bone resorption and because phosphorus, as well as calcium, is a constituent of bone, untreated hyperparathyroidism involves bone malformation. When the calcium in the serum surpasses the renal threshold, the calcium in the urine is also increased. Nephrolithiasis may be the result of high urine calcium, and severe irreversible renal malfunction can be a consequence.

Diagnosis and Clinical Findings

The various degrees of involvement which occur in this disease can lead to different symptoms in patients with hyperparathyroidism. If not diagnosed on the basis of a chemical screen, a patient may present to a physician in several ways. High urine calcium may have caused kidney stones, and the patient may present with symptoms attributable to this factor or the patient may present with symptoms resulting from high serum calcium. Calcium's effect on the gastrointestinal tract may include nausea, vomiting or constipation. It may cause an EKG change reflecting a change in cardiac conduction. Since high calcium levels can effect the urine-concentrating ability of the kidney, symptoms may include polyuria. Other severe symptoms of hypercalcemia include paralytic ileus, muscular weakness and sometimes psychosis. If long term hyperparathyroid secretion has occurred, bone disease may be present. Bone pain and fractures may occur if bone resorption has occurred at a rate in excess of bone formation.

The diagnosis involves many laboratory studies, the first of which is serum calcium determinations. If hypercalcemia exists, causes other than hyperparathyroidism must be ruled out. Carcinomata are the most frequent cause of hypercalcemia. Carcinoma of the breast produces very high calcium levels. This is not because the breast carcinoma is producing a PTH-like hormone. In fact, in breast carcinoma, the PTH in the serum is decreased due to a feedback mechanism caused by the high calcium. Thus the phosphate level in the serum may be normal or high and urinary phosphate low. This is unlike the chemical profile seen in hyperparathyroidism. Carcinomas of the lung and kidneys are the ones which most frequently produce a PTH-like hormone. Other causes of hypercalcemia include sarcoid disease, vitamin D intoxication, milk-alkali syndrome, immobility, laboratory error and dirty-glassware, hyperthyroidism and multiple myeloma.

Calcium balance studies may be done. This involves a calcium infusion test, and a low phosphate diet. Appropriate response of the serum calcium and phosphorous are determined. In the low phosphate diet test, the response of serum calcium, serum phosphate and TRP are measured. In the normal patient after 3 days of a low phosphate diet, the TRP would increase in an attempt to maintain a normal serum phosphate. In the hyperparathyroid patient there is a greater than expected fall in serum phosphate and rise in serum calcium. In the calcium infusion test, 15 mg per kg of calcium are given intravenously over a 4 hr period. In the normal patient, 1/3 to 1/2 of the calcium is excreted within 12 hr. The serum phosphate also increases with an increase in the TRP. In the hyperparathyroid patient, there is retention of the calcium and a smaller increase in the TRP. A high phosphate diet was part of balance tests in the past; however, in the presence of high serum calcium, this now is considered to be dangerous because the calcium phosphate produced may be deposited in soft tissues such as the brain, blood vessels, etc.

If the patient is diagnosed as having a renal stone, the location of the stone(s) is followed meticulously. Urine is screened in an attempt to recover the stone for analysis. Renal stones may be composed of uric acid, another common constituent of stones. Calcium stones may be due to the milk-alkali syndrome. This syndrome occurs when patients with peptic ulcer disease ingest large amounts of milk and antacids such as calcium carbonate over long periods of time. This must be ruled out as the cause of any existing renal stones. However, renal stones are found in approximately 75% of hyperparathyroid patients, and 2.5 to 12.5% of those patients with recurrent stones have hyperparathyroidism.[10]

The existence of bone disease is determined and measured by several diagnostic tests which include measurements of serum alkaline phosphatase and urine hydroxyproline. Both will be elevated when bone resorption is in excess of normal bone turnover. X-rays can detect resorption of bone in the fingers. In some hospitals, bone biopsies are done to determine the metabolic status of bone cells.

The important studies are, of course, serum calcium and urine phosphate. Although the serum calcium level is elevated in hyperparathyroid disease, serum phosphate is not always low. This may be due to increased ingestion of phosphate via the diet. Therefore, studies to determine the TRP have been developed (Fig. 23.3). Presently the radioimmunoassay for PTH is being developed. As mentioned before, the test is done in only a few medical centers because of the inherent problems in the test. Where it is available, however, an elevated PTH concurrent with hypercalcemia is positive for hyperparathyroidism.

Complications

Pancreatitis may be a rare complication of hyperparathyroidism. Several theories exist to explain the etiology of the pancreatitis. It has been suggested that the high calcium causes calcification within the pancreatic ducts or, alternatively, that high serum calcium levels speed the transformation of trypsinogen to the active trypsin.

Peptic ulcer disease has also been reported to be a complication of hyperparathyroid disease, although the association continues to be de-

$$TRP = \left[1 - \frac{(\text{urine phosphorus excretion} \times \text{serum creatinine})}{(\text{serum phosphorus} \times \text{urine creatinine excretion})} \right]$$
$$\times 100$$

FIG. 23.3. The tubular reabsorption of phosphate may be calculated from this equation. Normal persons have a TRP of 80 to 90% while patients with hyperparathyroidism and other hypercalcemic states usually have a TRP of a lower value.

bated. It is felt by some that most cases of peptic ulcer disease associated with hyperparathyroidism may be due to the Zollinger-Ellison syndrome.[2] This syndrome is peptic ulcer disease related to a gastrin-secreting tumor of the pancreas. If this syndrome exists concurrently with hyperparathyroid disease, there is the possibility of multiple endocrine gland involvement, namely the parathyroid and the pancreas. Other endocrine glands may also be involved. Other authors feel that there may be a definite relationship between peptic ulcer disease and hyperparathyroidism which involves the ability of calcium to stimulate gastric acid secretion.[11] They point out the danger of treating the peptic ulcer when hyperparathyroidism is also present. Since such treatment frequently includes the administration of calcium antacids, a hypercalcemic state with deposition of renal calculi can ensue. Still other authors feel, on a statistical basis, that there is a relationship between hyperparathyroidism and peptic ulcer disease. They note that the occurrence of peptic ulcer disease in the general population is significantly lower than in those patients with hyperparathyroidism.[12] Whatever view finally may prove to be correct, it seems prudent to screen for hyperparathyroidism before ulcer treatment is begun.

Treatment

Primary hyperparathyroidism is a surgical disease although there is medical management involved both before and after surgery.

Before surgery, attempts to lower the serum calcium by medical means may be carried out. Several pharmacological agents have been used. Steroids are often used in the management of hypercalcemia because the glucocorticoids antagonize the vitamin D-induced intestinal absorption of calcium and also increase calcium excretion in the kidneys. Approximately 100 mg of hydrocortisone are given daily. This is obviously not meant to be long term therapy. In fact, steroids in hypercalcemia may be more diagnostic than therapeutic. Some causes of hypercalcemia such as vitamin D intoxication respond to steroids more frequently than in primary hyperparathyroidism.

Oral and intravenous phosphate solutions have been given in the past to decrease the serum calcium. This is no longer recommended. It was found that when phosphates are given, the serum calcium does decrease but that there is not a proportional increase in urine calcium. It is now known that increased phosphate administration during hypercalcemia increases the calcium-phosphorous solubility product. The calcium-phosphate complex is driven into soft tissues such as the brain and there is also perivascular disposition. Because of this, giving phosphate in the face of hypercalcemia is now considered to be a dangerous procedure and is contraindicated.

In acute hypercalcemia, levels of calcium may be 16 to 17 mg% or greater. Solutions of sodium sulfate may be given in the emergency management of hypercalcemia. Unlike phosphate solutions, sodium sulfate does increase calcium excretion in the urine. Isotonic solutions containing 38.9 g of sodium sulfate decahydrate per liter are given fairly rapidly by the intravenous route (3 liters over 9 hr).[13] In 9 hr, the serum calcium should return to normal. The problems with treatment are due to the sodium and fluid given. If the patient has congestive heart failure or renal disease, intravenous sodium sulfate may be contraindicated. Normal saline is equally effective in lowering serum calcium.

Furosemide is now being used by many physicians to treat hypercalcemia. If the patient is adequately hydrated before therapy and hydration is maintained during therapy, furosemide is said to be relatively free of side effects. The diuresis of calcium is proportional to sodium diuresis in the treatment of hypercalcemia by furosemide. Intravenous doses of 80 to 100 mg of furosemide for a total of from 160 to 3,200 mg per day are given.[14] Furosemide's effect is unlike the thiazides in hypercalcemia. Thiazides increase serum calcium and do so on an apparently extrarenal basis. Patients with no kidney function given thiazides show an increase in the calcium level. It is thought that thiazides may potentiate PTH.[15]

Calcitonin is a newly purified substance secreted by the thyroid, parathyroids and thymus. Recently, clinical studies evaluating this drug as a replacement for surgery in hyperparathyroidism have been carried on. Synthetic salmon calcitonin is more potent than pork or human calcitonin and also appears to have a longer duration of action. In some patients with active bone disease such as ostetis deformans (Paget's disease of bone) or high turnover osteoporosis, calcitonin administered subcutaneously appears to decrease bone resorption.[16] In these patients treated with calcitonin, serum alkaline phosphatase decreases and urinary hydroxyproline decreases along with urinary excretion of calcium and phosphorus. Its use may be limited by an induction of secondary hyperparathyroidism. A finely regulated dose may solve this problem. Additional clinical studies are needed to establish its clinical usage.

In preparation for surgery, diagnostic procedures are often done which normally would call for the patient to be NPO (receive nothing by the oral route). Preparation for surgery itself also usually requires that the patient be NPO. However, for the hypercalcemic patient a decrease in the intravascular volume may lead to acute hypercalcemia. An intravenous solution must therefore be infused if the NPO order includes fluids. Directly after surgery, the patient should have 2 or 3 ampuls of 10% calcium gluconate, or the equivalent as calcium chloride, available at the bedside for intravenous administration in event of emergency. It is felt that calcium need not be given prophylactically after surgery; however, any signs of hypocalcemia should be treated promptly in order to prevent more severe complications such as laryngeal stridor. Oral calcium salts can be given if postoperative hypocalcemia persists. If a total parathyroidectomy has been done, the patient will need long term vitamin D therapy with a dose similar to that mentioned previously for the treatment of hypoparathyroidism.

Prognosis

After parathyroidectomy, long term follow-up should be carried on. Patients with subtotal removal of the glands may again become hyperparathyroid. However, in most cases, without significant renal damage at the time of the operation, the prognosis is good. Usually, hypertension decreases resulting from a decreased serum calcium and improved renal function. Renal stones may disappear without operation. Mental depression as a result of hyperparathyroidism usually disappears after surgery.

SECONDARY HYPERPARATHYROIDISM

Secondary hyperparathyroidism is most commonly the result of uremia. It is interesting that the management of secondary hyperparathyroidism due to uremia has changed greatly since the development of hemodialysis and kidney transplantation. In the past, individuals with renal disease severe enough to cause parathyroid disorders eventually died due to complete renal failure. Since the advent of dialysis and transplantation, the problems of calcium and vitamin D metabolism have been of much greater concern to the physician.

Etiology

It has recently been demonstrated that vitamin D is also active in the form of its metabolites.[17] 25-Hydroxycholecalciferol and, most recently, 1,25-dihydroxycholecalciferol have been found to be active metabolites of vitamin D_3. The transformation of 25-hydroxycholecalciferol to 1,25-dihydroxycholecalciferol occurs in the kidney. This last metabolite appears to be the most important in stimulating intestinal absorption of calcium. Thus when a patient has little or no renal function, the lack of this metabolite is part of the reason for hypocalcemia and bone disease. Another factor leading to calcium and phosphate imbalance is the kidney's decreased ability to filter. Initially the diseased kidney excretes a greater percentage of the filtered load of phosphorous, but as the renal function decreases to a glomerular filtration rate of 25 to 30 ml per min. the ability to excrete phosphorus decreases. Eventually hyperphosphatemia results. Renal osteodystrophy is the term used for this disease.

Incidence

Secondary hyperplasia of the parathyroid glands is a common complication of long term glomerulonephritis or pyelonephritis.

Pathogenesis

In severe, long standing renal disease, there is decreased production of an active vitamin D metabolite. Because of vitamin D activity in stimulating intestinal absorption of calcium and in stimulating bone resorption to provide for the appropriate serum calcium, the uremic patient may have hypocalcemia. The hypocalcemia engages the feedback mechanism and the parathyroid glands are stimulated. Because of the importance of vitamin D in regulating calcium, however, PTH is not initially effective in increasing the serum calcium. As a result, the parathyroids continue to be stimulated and become hyperplastic. The parathyroids are also stimulated by hyperphosphatemia since, owing to poor kidney function, phosphate is not adequately filtered and the blood level of phosphate is high. In spite of the low serum calcium, the increased amounts of phosphate bind with the calcium and soft tissue calcifications may occur.

Clinical Findings and Diagnosis

The diagnosis of secondary hyperparathyroidism is generally based on a history of renal disease existing with a reciprocal relationship of hypocalcemia and hyperphosphatemia. If a direct PTH assay is available, the level is considerably increased. There is usually also an increase in fecal calcium. An increase in soft tissue calcium deposits may occur and may lead to severe itching. Generally, the same bone changes are seen in secondary hyperparathyroidism as are seen in hypoparathyroidism. It is known that the serum calcium levels in secondary hyperparathyroidism may be normal. In fact, if a patient remains on hemodialysis for extended periods, low serum calcium levels often stimulate the parathyroid glands to produce huge amounts of PTH. Resorption of the bone follows, serum calcium increases, alkaline phosphatase increases and bone pain occurs in the patient. That is, the serum calcium increases at the expense of the bone. This condition resembles primary hyperparathyroidism. If this exists, the treatment is parathyroidectomy. The patient can be managed medically in the initial uremic state so that excess parathyroid gland stimulation and bone resorption can be prevented.

Treatment

Treatment of secondary hyperparathyroidism prior to a kidney transplant generally involves an attempt to decrease the serum phosphate and to increase the serum calcium. Such patients are usually placed on hemodialysis, and some calcium regulation can be achieved by adjusting the amount of calcium in the dialysate. The hyperphosphatemia should be controlled before administration of vitamin D or calcium replacement is carried out. Increasing the calcium when high levels of phosphate are present can lead to metastatic soft tissue calcifications. Besides the obvious ill effects calcifications have if they deposit in the heart or brain, they can become infected. Calcifications in blood vessel walls make shunt revision very difficult when this is required to maintain the patient on hemodialysis. Serum phosphate can be lowered by administering nonabsorbable, low phosphate-containing aluminum antacids. Aluminum antacids bind the phosphate in the gastrointestinal tract. This seemingly simple treatment can become difficult if the patient has trouble tolerating the antacid. There is a choice of antacids including aluminum hydroxide or aluminum carbonate allowing the patient some selection, if he is nauseated by the flavor or consistency of one of them. The dosage is about 30 ml 4 times daily with meals.

Vitamin D is given in an attempt to increase the intestinal absorption of calcium. Dihydrotachysterol is given is small doses initially. Approximately 0.125 mg to 0.25 mg is given per day. If calcium levels do not respond to 2 to 4 weeks, the dose is increased. In order to prevent calcium resorption from the bone, calcium supplements are administered with vitamin D. Usually 5 to 8 g of calcium carbonate or an equivalent calcium salt are given per day. Dihydrotachysterol is the vitamin D product given because of its shorter half-life. The active metabolite of vitamin D_3 1,25-dihydroxycholecalciferol, is available investigationally. It may afford better control of calcium levels and studies are being carried out to assess this possibility.

Prognosis

The prognosis of secondary hyperparathyroidism is mixed. To a great extent, this is related to the patient's response to vitamin D and other therapies employed for the uremic patient as well as his success in getting a functioning kidney transplant. The problems of vitamin D intoxication may be overcome when the more active metabolites of vitamin D become available. The kidney transplant often causes additional problems for the patient with secondary hyperparathyroidism.

Hyperparathyroidism after Kidney Transplant

As discussed in the preceding section, the uremic patient has hypocalcemia because his kidneys are not able to produce the active vitamin D metabolite. The parathyroids respond to the hypocalcemia by becoming hyperplastic. After a kidney transplant, however, the functioning kidney can again produce the dihydroxy vitamin D metabolite and the hypersecreting, hyperplastic parathyroids cause an increase in serum calcium. The calcium often remains high. In the past this was explained by saying that the hyperplastic glands became autonomous and thus led to a primary hyperparathyroidism-like state which was called tertiary hyperparathyroidism. The treatment was surgery.

This theory has now been challenged, and it is felt that in most kidney transplant patients the hyperplastic glands will respond to the corrected calcium level.[2] In some patients, this occurs fairly rapidly (in several weeks to a few months). In other patients, the parathyroid glands respond very sluggishly and some physicians feel that this lag and difficulty in controlling the hypercalcemia justify surgery. There are a very few patients who have developed a coincidental adenoma along with their hyperplasia. This adenoma is the so-called tertiary hyperparathyroidism and is thought by some experts as being the only reason for parathyroidectomy after renal transplantation.

Treatment

The treatment of post-transplantation hypercalcemia is a combination of hydration, mobilization and a low calcium diet. Calcium antacids should not be used. If these measures fail to correct the hypercalcemia, furosemide or dialysis may be employed.

In the case of a coincidental adenoma, the treatment is subtotal parathyroid surgery. This possesses the same inherent risks as in parathyroidectomy from primary hyperparathyroidism, such as inadvertent total parathyroidectomy with a need for lifetime vitamin D therapy, injury to the recurrent laryngeal nerve and infection. The immunologically suppressed post-transplant patient will be at a greater risk of infection after surgery. Post operative precautions for treatment of tetany must again be observed.

CONCLUSIONS

Parathyroid disorders are very complex. Texts may be misleading by virtue of making the various froms of the disease seem quite clear-cut. Until the diagnostic and management problems of patients are actually observed, it is not appreciated how often several aspects of all the variables overlap in the same patient. Patients with any form of the disease are almost always referred to clinicians who are very familiar with the diagnostic and management procedures. Much in the way of the appropriate perspectives of therapy has only recently been appreciated. With a good understanding of the basic diseases processes and the drugs to treat them, the pharmacist can be of assistance to the physician and nurse in the appropriate care of the patient.

REFERENCES

1. Hahn, T.A., Hendlin, B. A., Scharp, C. R., and Haddad, J. G., Jr.: Effect of anticonvulsant therapy on serum 25-hydroxycalciferol. N. Engl. J. Med., 287: 900, 1972.
2. Goldman, L., Gordon, G. S., and Roof, B. S.: The parathyroids: progress, problems and practice. Curr. Probl. Surg., 8: 1, 1971.
3. Brewer, H. B., Fairwell, T., Ronan, R., Sizemore, G. W., and Arnaud, C. D.: Human parathyroid hormone: amino-acid sequence of the amino-terminal residues 1-34. Proc. Natl. Acad. Sci. U. S. A., 69: 3585, 1972.
4. Chase, L. E., and Aurback, G. D.: Renal adenyl cylase: anatomically separate sites for parathyroid hormone and vasopressin. Science, 159: 545, 1968.
5. Chase, L. R., Mason, G. L., and Aurback, G. D.: Pseudohypoparathyrcidism: defective excretion of 3'5' AMP in response to parathyroid hormone, J. Clin. Invest., 48: 1832, 1969.
6. Goodman, L. S., and Gilman, A.: The Pharmacological Basis of Therapeutics Ed. 4. The Macmillan Co., New York, 1970.
7. Wintrobe, M. M., Thorn, G. W., Adams, R. D., Bennett, I. L., Jr., Braunwald, E., Isselbacher, K. J., and Petersdorf, R. G.: Harrison's Principles of Internal Medicine, Ed. 6, p. 470. McGraw-Hill Book Co., New York, 1970.
8. Schwartz, S. I.: Principles of Surgery, Ed. 1, p. 1328. McGraw-Hill Book Co., New York, 1969.
9. Kearing, F. R., Jr.: The clinical problem of primary hyperparathyroidism. Med. Clin. North Am., 54: 515, 1970.
10. Schwartz, S. I.: Principles of Surgery, Ed. 1, p. 1331. McGraw-Hill Book Co., New York, 1969.
11. Black, B. M.: Primary hyperparathyroidism and peptic ulcer. Surg. Clin. North Am., 51: 955, 1971.
12. Schwartz, S. I.: Principles of Surgery, Ed. 1, p. 1334. McGraw-Hill Book Co., New York, 1969.
13. Chakmakjian, Z. H., and Bethune, J. E.: Sodium sulfate treatment of hypercalcemia. N. Engl. J. Med., 275: 862, 1966.
14. Suki, W. N., Yium, J. J., Von Minden, M., Saller-Hebert, C., Eknoyan, G., and Martinez-Maldonado, M.: Acute treatment of hypercalcemia with furosemide. N. Engl. Med., 283: 836, 1970.
15. Koppel, M. H., Massry, S. G., Shinaberger, J. H., Hartenbower, D. L., and Coburn, J. W.: Thiazide-induced rise in serum calcium and magnesium in patients on maintenance hemodialysis. Ann. Intern. Med., 72: 895, 1970.
16. Goldfield, E. G., Braiker, B. M., Prendergast, J. J., and Kolb, F. O.: Synthetic salmon calcitonin. J.A.M.A., 221: 1127, 1972.
17. Brickman, A. S., Coburn, J. W., and Norman, A. W.: Use of 1,,25-dihydroxycholecalciferol in uremic man. N. Engl. J. Med., 287: 891, 1972.

Rheumatic diseases

chapter **24**

RHEUMATOID ARTHRITIS

Brian S. Katcher, Pharm.D.

The history of medicine is replete with nostra for rheumatism—the generic term for pain stiffness or deformity of the joints, muscles and related structures. Although there are many rheumatoid diseases, rheumatoid arthritis is the most common. Table 24.1 gives a representative list of the most frequently encountered rheumatoid diseases. Rheumatoid arthritis is a systemic chronic progressive disease of unknown etiology for which there is no known cure. It belongs to the complex and interesting group of autoimmune diseases. Although it is a systemic disease, it manifests itself primarily in the joints and related structures. Therapy is aimed at making the symptoms more bearable and preserving the function of the affected joints.[1] Patients who carefully follow a well thought out program of rest, exercise, heat treatment and drug therapy find their desease significantly less disabling than do untreated patients.

EPIDEMIOLOGY

Rheumatoid arthritis is distributed uniformly throughout the population. Although the incidence and course of the disease are not influenced significantly by climate or latitude, patients tend to feel better in warm, dry climates. Surveys indicate an incidence of about 1% definite rheumatoid arthritis and 3% probable rheumatoid arthritis in the United States. The disease may occur at any age from infancy throughout life, although the prevalence increases with age. Females are affected more often than males and there is no preference for race.[2] A recent review of the literature on the influence of heredity and environment makes it clear that heredity plays little part in the etiology of seronegative disease, but is important in the more severe seropositive disease.[3] The effect of environment can be evaluated best by comparison of monozygous twins living in different environments. A few such studies have been carried out with negative results. There is some evidence that psychic trauma may exacerbate the disease.[3]

PATHOGENESIS

A great deal of research is being directed toward clarification of autoimmune disorders, the results of which will be of importance in the treatment of this disease and a number of others. The immune process involves production of antigen-antibody complexes which fix complement and induce phagocytosis and lysosomal release, with subsequent inflammation of the synovial membrane. The destructive process continues with expansion of a layer of granulation tissue called panus, which expands to invade and destroy cartilage. Although inflammation and destruction of joints is by far the most common feature, it must be remembered that rheumatoid arthritis is a systemic disease and related processes may occur in other connective tissues. Thus, fibrotic lesions may be seen in the lung, in cardiac tissue, in the eye or in other tissues.[2]

CLINICAL FEATURES

Affected joints are warm and red, and generally there is symmetry of joint involvement. Soft tissue swelling and osteoporosis are seen radiologically. Joint involvement is frequently preceded by nonrheumatic complaints of fatigability, anorexia, weight loss and occasional fever. Muscle aches and prolonged morning stiffness are common. The disease is characterized by spontaneous exacerbations and remissions, but affected joints become progressively worse.

TABLE 24.1
Rheumatic Diseases

Rheumatoid arthritis
Ankylosing spondylitis
Psoriasis
Reiter's syndrome
Systemic lupus erythematosis
Polyarteritis nodosa
Rheumatic fever
Degenerative joint disease (osteoarthritis)
Arthritis associated with inflammatory
    intestinal disease
Acute bacterial arthritis
Gonococcal arthritis
Arthritis due to tuberculosis
Gout
Serum sickness and drug reactions

Subcutaneous nodules varying from 2 mm to 2 cm in diameter are seen in as many as 1/3 of the patients with rheumatoid arthritis. These nodules are not attached to the skin and tend to occur over pressure points near joints, such as below the elbow. Patients with nodules usually have severe, active disease.

Laboratory findings include elevated erythrocyte-sedimentation rate during active disease, a hyperglobulinemia and a positive serological test for rheumatoid factor (RA factor is a high molecular weight macroglobulin) in about 75% of the patients with definite rheumatoid arthritis. Patients with consistently positive RA factors generally have more severe disease. The serological test for RA factor involves agglutination with serial dilutions of sensitized red blood cells, latex or bentonite. A moderate normocytic, hypochromic anemia is often seen during the active phase of the disease.[2]

TREATMENT

Treatment is aimed at reducing pain and inflammation and preventing deformity.[1] Adequate diet is important because the accompanying anorexia may lead to poor nutrition and subsequent dietary deficiencies. Rest is important to minimize excessive strain on the already inflamed joints. A cane may be of considerable value in relieving stress to an inflamed knee or hip. A regular program of exercise will prevent muscle atrophy and help maintain function of the joint. Splints are useful, especially at night, to minimize flexion contractures. Joint pain is relieved by the application of heat to the affected area; hot compresses, heating pads or heat lamps are useful for this purpose. Recently, orthopedic surgeons have investigated the surgical removal of diseased synovium and successful results have established orthopedic surgery as an important treatment modality.[4]

DRUG THERAPY

The drug therapy of rheumatoid arthritis has received an extraordinary amount of attention (Table 24.2). The chronic discomforting and disabling nature of this disease, which afflicts more than 6,000,000 Americans, has created a tremendous demand for an effective treatment. This demand, coupled with the prevailing attitude of our society, which expects a chemical solution to every possible human problem, has created a busy and highly competitive marketplace for arthritis medications. Nevertheless, aspirin is still the drug of choice. Other drugs may be used in conjunction with aspirin, but the rational approach is to weigh carefully expected benefits against predictable toxicities. Unfortunately, most patients with this disease are the recipients of too many drugs, and often their drug-induced disease is far worse than their rheumatoid arthritis. Drug therapy should consist of maximally tolerated doses of salicylate with the addition of other drugs reserved for extremely advanced cases. It should be remembered that none of the drugs currently used alters the basic course of the disease. They are not curative.

ASPIRIN

When used in adequate doses, aspirin has anti-inflammatory activity and is the single most important drug used in the treatment of rheumatoid arthritis.[5] Patients are dosed often to the point of tinnitus and then the dose is cut back slightly. Adults should take a minimum of 3.6 g per day.[6] A dosage regimen of 2 or 3 300-mg tablets every 4 hr should be initiated, along with an explanation and considerable encouragement. Aspirin is continued indefinitely on a regular basis. Patients have to be educated to the fact that at these doses aspirin is anti-inflammatory and thus has a different effect than the occasional 1 or 2 tablets taken for headache. With encouragement, patients can

TABLE 24.2

Drugs Used In Rheumatoid Arthritis

Drug	Dose	Comments
Aspirin	4-6 g/day	Mainstay of therapy
Gold salts	See text	Use early in disease; for patients with postive rheumatoid factor
Phenylbutazone oxyphenbutazone	Variable, not more than 600 mg/day	Highly protein-bound, therefore many drug interactions; significant sodium retention; see text for other side effects; discontinue if no improvement within a week
Indomethacin	Variable	Poor patient acceptance due to side effects; more effective in other rheumatoid diseases; see effects within a few weeks, if at all
Chloroquin hydroxychloroquin	200-250 mg **BID** for several months, followed by 200-250 mg/day with meals	Three to 6 months required for effect; regular opthalmological evaluation required
Steroids	Variable, use the lowest dose for shortest period of time	Dramatic effects, but many serious side effects; see text

tolerate considerably more aspirin than they accept early in therapy. Patients with active disease and young adults can tolerate much larger doses.[33] Heavier patients require higher doses for effective blood levels. Adults must take at least a dozen tablets per day; some patients can tolerate twice this dosage. The doses should be taken with meals or antacids to minimize gastric distress.[7]

Probably the most important component of salicylate therapy is patient education. A regular regimen must be followed if blood levels are to be maintained. With any drug therapy, patient compliance with the prescribed regimen should be considered. Studies of patients on various chronic medications show that the incidence of noncompliance with the prescribed therapy is about 30 to 50%.[8,9] Thus, a continuing treatment program involving the regular and frequent ingestion of many tablets of a common drug that many lay people do not even consider to be a drug may be expected to have a high rate of failure unless it is thoroughly explained and actively promoted to the patient.

Aspirin USP is the salicylate of choice. Generic tablets are available for 1/3 to 1/4 of the cost of the leading proprietary brand. Aspirin tableted with buffering agents is needlessly expensive. The main consideration in choosing a brand of aspirin is that it be fresh; the sour odor coming from a freshly opened bottle of aspirin is a qualitative indication of the degree to which the aspirin has hydrolyzed to the highly irritating and toxic salicylic and acetic acids. Enteric coated aspirin may be of value in providing prolonged blood levels, although some enteric coats do not allow enough aspirin to be absorbed to provide measurable blood levels.[10,11] Other mild analgesics such as acetaminophen, phenacetin and propoxyphene do not have any anti-inflammatory activity; therefore, they should not be used except for additional pain relief.[7]

Aspirin at these doses is ulcerogenic. Administration with meals, antacids or large amounts of fluid will minimize this effect. Although some gastrointestinal (GI) blood loss can be expected, the patient should be cautioned to report black or tarry stools and indication of active bleeding. Patients may worry over frequent episodes of tinnitus, but there is no danger of permanent hearing damage.[12]

Remission of active disease, tapering of steroids or decreases in fluid intake may result in increased salicylate levels and tinnitus from a dose of aspirin previously well tolerated. In the latter case, increasing fluid intake without decreasing the dose of aspirin will reverse this tinnitus.

Once therapy with aspirin is begun, it should be continued indefinitely on a regular basis.[1,3] If it is decided that further drug therapy should be added to the aspirin, the next least toxic drug should be added. Although there is some disagreement as to the next choice beyond aspirin, many rheumatologists would now consider gold salts as a very likely possibility.

Gold Salts

Gold therapy in the form of intramuscular injections of solubilized gold is a highly effective symptomatic treatment for rheumatoid arthritis.[13-16] Gold should be used only in patients with positive RA factor, and it must be used fairly early in the course of the disease, since it is of no value to severely damaged joints. This is necessarily a clinic or office procedure, since gold is not absorbed after oral administration. There are two preparations available—autothioglucose and gold sodium thiomalate. The dosage of both preparations is somewhat variable, but it is generally given in a schedule of 25 mg per week for 2 or 3 weeks, then 50 mg per week for a period of about 20 weeks or until signs of toxicity occur. Doses are given less frequently once improvement is noted (usually 2 or 3 months after therapy has started). Frequent first indications of gold salt toxicity are pruritis, usually of the oral mucosa and metallic taste. Patients should be monitored for stomatitis, pharyngitis, tracheitis, gastritis, colitis or vaginitis. Patients should receive weekly or biweekly urinalysis and complete blood count.[17] Gold is concentrated preferentially in inflamed joints, and patients who benefit from therapy are less likely to show toxicity. Severe toxicity includes blood dyscrasias, renal and hepatic damage and exfoliative dermatitis. When used appropriately by rheumatologists well aware of its potential toxicities, gold therapy is one of the more effective, although difficult to administer, adjuncts to salicylate therapy for the symptomatic treatment of rheumatoid arthritis.

Phenylbutazone

Although more often effective in the treatment of the symptoms of gouty arthritis and ankylosing spondylitis, many patients with rheumatoid arthritis show good response to phenylbutazone. The anti-inflammatory effect should be noted within a week. If no effect is seen within that time, the drug should be discontinued.

It must be emphasized that phenylbutazone is a very toxic drug. It should be used only for short term therapy, preferably for less than a week. Phenylbutazone causes a significant degree of sodium and water retention and must be considered contraindicated in patients with congestive heart failure or hypertension. Like most of the other drugs used in the treatment of rheumatoid arthritis, it is ulcerogenic. Additionally, phenylbutazone can cause blood dyscrasias. The brief review by Brownlie,[18] of seven cases of blood dyscrasias, three of them fatal, provided graphic evidence of how sudden and drastic these blood changes can be. Patients should be cautioned to report immediately any prodromal symptoms, such as fever, rash or sore throat. Oxyphenbutazone, one of the principal metabolites of phenylbutazone, has similar therapeutic and toxic actions. Both drugs are highly protein-bound and compete for plasma binding sites with sulfonamides, warfarin, tolbutamide, indomethacin and glucocorticoids; thus, a number of drug interactions are possible.

Indomethacin

Patients with other rheumatoid diseases such as gout, anklyosing spondylitis or osteoarthritis show greater benefit from this drug than do patients with rheumatoid arthritis. Most of the patients who take this drug complain of at least one of its many side effects. About 20% of patients cannot tolerate indomethacin because of GI pain, nausea, dizziness, severe frontal headaches or psychiatric disturbances. Although this drug may benefit some patients, a recent well controlled study and extensive review revealed the very limited value of indomethacin in rheumatoid arthritis.[19]

Antimalarials

Hydroxychloroquine and chloroquin administered in doses of 200 to 250 mg twice a day for several months followed by 200 to 250 mg a day will provide some symptomatic relief for many patients.[20] The drug should be taken with meals to minimize gastric distress. Three to 6 months of therapy are required before beneficial effect is seen. For this reason the patient must be counseled not to expect dramatic effects; otherwise, compliance to therapy will be difficult to attain. Minor side effects include skin rashes, frequent upper GI distress, headaches and psychiatric disturbances. Infrequent bone marrow depression and ocular abnormalities are more serious. Every patient on antimalarial therapy should receive thorough ophthalmological evaluations every 3 months to monitor for the rare but serious retinopathies which are irreversible and progressive for 1 or 2 years after discontinuing the drug.[20,21] Fortunately, most ocular lesions seen are the less serious, reversible corneal opacities. These drugs should not be given to patients with psoriasis because of the high frequency of skin reactions in this group of patients. Likewise, patients receiving gold therapy should not be given these drugs, since the occurrence of a skin rash would lead to diagnostic difficulties.

Steroids

Of all the various modes of therapy for rheumatoid arthritis, glucocorticoid therapy is by far the most readily accepted by patients. In fact, the avidity with which patients will take these drugs has no doubt caused many clinicians to be somewhat shortsighted in weighing their significant and often predictable toxicities against their dramatic and immediate effects. Nonetheless, steroids do occupy a place in the symptomatic treatment of the late stages of rheumatoid arthritis where intensive therapy with rest, physical therapy and salicylates is not enough.

The toxicities of the steroids are related to the dose and duration of therapy. Once therapy is begun, it is often difficult to stop. Thus steroids should be avoided in younger patients, and they should never be given to anyone who can tolerate his disease with more conservative therapy.

Once the decision to use steroids has been made, therapeutic goals should be carefully set. The goal is to provide enough relief to allow for functional use of the most seriously affected joints. Complete relief should not be the goal since this would require higher doses.[22] Doses should start at a level of 5 to 10 mg of prednisone each morning. Small increments in dosage may be made until the desired response is seen. Once an effective dose is found, frequent attempts should be made to cut back, since spontaneous exacerbations and remissions are characteristic of the disease. Alternate day dosing, such as 10 mg every other day rather than 5 mg daily, causes less adrenal suppression and fewer side effects.[23] Although most compliance studies show that 1/3 to 1/2 of patients fail to take an adequate amount of their prescribed drugs, it has been shown that patients taking steroids do not follow this typical pattern. In the case of steroids, many patients actually take more than their prescribed dosage.[24] This fact, along with the well known euphoria produced by steroids must be kept in mind when evaluating steroid therapy and attempting to taper steroid dosage.

Some of the side effects of steroids are additive to symptoms which may already be present in patients with rheumatoid arthritis. For example, osteoporosis is a frequent and serious complication of steroid therapy, while it is also part of the basic disease process in rheumatoid arthritis. Osteoporosis is, in addition, a common pathology in old age and after menopause. Any patient begun on steroids would already be taking aspirin and perhaps other ulcerogenic drugs. Thus, the chances of drug-induced peptic ulcer are increased. Muscle weakness caused by steroids may be confused with that caused by rheumatoid arthritis. If steroid dosage is tapered too abruptly, the characteristic withdrawal syndrome of fever, joint and muscle pain and malaise may be mistaken for an exacerbation of the rheumatoid arthritis.

Some other steroid toxicities include increased susceptibility to infection, aggravation of diabetes mellitus, cosmetic disfiguration characteristic of Cushing's syndrome, sodium and water retention, potassium depletion, cataracts, potential adrenal insufficiency and mental disturbances. Mental disturbance is seen in about 1/4 of patients receiving steroids chronically.[25] These drugs should also be considered as being potentially habit forming.[26]

Intra-articular injections may be used if a single large joint is affected. Relief may last for a few days to a number of weeks. Hazards include danger of infecting the joint with bacteria and danger of painless degeneration of the joint after repeated injections.

In summary, steroids should be used with considerable caution. In most cases, their hazards outweigh their potential benefits. Ready patient acceptance, failure of clinicians to evaluate their patients with due consideration for chronic toxicities and promotion of these drugs by the drug industry have led to their widespread overuse in rheumatoid arthritis.

Immunosupressive Drugs

Antineoplastic drugs, most notably cyclophosphamide, have been tried with some success in rheumatoid arthritis.[27,29] Their side effects are many and their use is still investigational. As more is learned abut immunology, new drugs with specific effect on the basic disease process of rheumatoid arthritis may be developed.

SEDATIVES AND TRANQUILIZERS

A few patients with rheumatoid arthritis may have use for these drugs, but their need should be carefully evaluated.[30] There is a tendency to give minor tranquilizers and antidepressants to all patients who complain. Rheumatoid arthritis is a painful and debilitating disease. Patients should be counseled and made to understand their disease and its treatment. Drug treatment aimed at the psychosocial aspect of the disease should be discouraged unless counseling without psychoactive drugs has failed.

IRON

Iron therapy does not relieve the moderate normocytic, hypochromic anemia seen in the active phase of the disease; however, it may be of benefit for the chronic blood loss which occurs secondary to salicylate therapy.

Drug Combinations

A number of fixed dose drug combinations are promoted for rheumatoid arthritis. All are irrational and some are dangerous. Butazolidin

Alka employs a subtherapeutic dose of antacid with each dose of phenylbutazone. Decagesic, Medaprin and Sigmagen are all combinations of a steroid, salicylate and ascorbic acid or a subtherapeutic dose of antacid. Pabalate includes aminobenzoic acid and ascorbic acid with a salicylate, even though there is no clinical evidence that inclusion of these ingredients will enhance the anti-inflammatory activity of the salicylate. Sterazolidin is a combination of steroid, phenylbutazone and a subtherapeutic dose of antacid.

External Analgesics

Over-the-counter products such as Banalg, Ben Gay, Heet, Sloan's Liniment and others employ counterirritants for the relief of muscle and joint pain. Methyl salicylate, menthol and camphor are typical ingredients. These preparations are available in both liquid and ointment form. The effectiveness of these products is difficult to evaluate, but they are safe to use on intact skin, and some patients may benefit from their use. They are reviewed in detail in the *Handbook of Non-Prescription Drugs.*[31]

Historical Treatments

A number of historical remedies for rheumatism are still employed in the treatment of rheumatoid arthritis.[32] Their value is questionable, but they are of enough general interest to warrant mention.

Bee venom has been used in medicine since antiquity. Its use in arthritis is based on the theory that bee keepers do not suffer from rheumatism. Since 1928 an injectable bee venom has been available, displacing the traditional live bee sting method. Reliable clinical evidence is lacking, although several books have been published on the subject. Allergy to bee venom can result in anaphylaxis.

A preparation of apple cider vinegar, honey and water is traditionally employed in New England folk medicine cures for arthritis.

Copper bracelets are also employed in arthritis. Although evidence of their efficacy is lacking, they are safe, the only side effect being superficial green discoloration of the wrist on which the bracelet is worn.

CONCLUSION

Rheumatoid arthritis is a chronic, progressive disease for which there is no known cure.

Therapy provides symptomatic relief only and has no effect on the basic course of the disease. Aspirin in large doses is the drug of choice, and other drugs should be used only when their need outweighs their risks. Patients with rheumatoid arthritis require a great deal of counseling by health professionals to insure maximally effective therapy.

In addition to being acquainted with the pathophysiology and clinical features of rheumatoid arthritis, pharmacists should have a thorough understanding of the drugs used so they can become actively involved in therapy by promoting adequate utilization of salicylates and monitoring all drug therapy.

REFERENCES

1. Engleman, E. P.: Conservative management of rheumatoid arthritis. Med. Clin. N. Am., 52: 699, 1968.
2. Shulman, L. E.: Rheumatoid arthritis. In Harrison's Principles of Internal Medicine, Ed. 6, p. 1944, edited by Wintrobe, Thorn, Adams, Bennett, Braunwald, Isselbacher, and Petersdorf. McGraw-Hill Book Co., New York, 1970.
3. Lawrence, J. S.: Heberden oration, 1969, rheumatoid arthritis—nature or nurture? Ann. Rheum. Dis., 29: 357, 1970.
4. Davis, P. H.: Orthopedic surgery in the management of rheumatoid arthritis. Med. Clin. N. Am., 52: 717, 1968.
5. Bayles, T. B.: Salicylate therapy in rheumatoid arthritis. Med. Clin. N. Am., 52: 703, 1968.
6. American, Rheumatism Association: Primer on the rheumatic diseases. J. A. M. A., 224: Suppl., 1973.
7. Woodbury, D. M.: Analgesics, antipyretics, anti-inflammatory agents, and inhibitors of uric acid synthesis. In The Pharmacological Basis of Therapeutics, Ed. 4, edited by L. S. Goodman and A. Gilman. McMillan Co., New York, 1970.
8. Maddock, R. K.: Patient cooperation in taking medicine. J. A. M. A., 199: 169, 1967.
9. Wilcox, D., Gillan, R., and Hare, E.: Do psychiatric outpatients take their drugs? Br. Med. J., 2: 790, 1965.
10. Hollister, L. E., and Kanter, S. L.: Studies of delayed action medication. IV. Salicylates. Clin. Pharmacol. Therap., 6: 5, 1965.
11. Lasagna, L., and Clark, R.: How reliable are enteric-coated aspirin preparations? Clin. Pharmacol. Therap., 6: 568, 1965.
12. Meyers, E. N., Bernstein, J. M., and Fostiropolous, G.: Salicylate ototoxicity; a clinical study. N. Engl. J. Med., 273: 587, 1965.
13. Empire Rheumatism Council: Gold therapy in rheumatoid arthritis: report of a multi-centre controlled trial. Ann. Rheum. Dis., 19: 95, 1960.

14. Empire Rheumatism Council: Gold therapy in rheumatoid arthritis: final report of a multi-centre controlled trial. Ann. Rheum. Dis., 20: 315, 1961.
15. Hill, D.: Gold therapy for rheumatoid arthritis. Med. Clin. N. Am., 52: 733, 1968.
16. Jessop, J. D.: The present status of chryso-therapy. Practitioner, 208: 28, 1972.
17. Manufacturer's recommendations.
18. Brownlie and Stang: Oxyphenbutazone and blood dyscrasias. N. Z. Med. J., 69: 77, 1969.
19. Cooperating Clinics of the American Rheumatism Association: A three month trial of indo-methacin in rheumatoid arthritis with special reference to analyst interference. Clin. Pharmacol. Therap., 8: 11, 1967.
20. Mackenzie, A. H.: An appraisal of chloroquine. Arthritis Rheum., 13: 280, 1970.
21. Giles, C., and Henderson, J.: The ocular toxicity of chloroquine therapy. Am. J. Med. Sci., 249: 230, 1965.
22. American Rheumatism Association: Primer on the rheumatic diseases. J. A. M. A., 190: 127, 1964.
23. Harter, J., Reddy, W., and Thorn, G.: Studies on an intermittent corticosteroid dosage regimen. N. Engl. J. Med., 269: 591, 1963.
24. Nugent, C., Ward, J., MacDiarmid, W., McCall, J., Baukol, J., and Tyler, F.: Glucocorticoid toxicity. J. Chronic Dis., 18: 323, 1965.
25. Sayers, G., and Travis, R.: Adrenocorticotropic hormone; adrenocortical steroids and their synthetic analogs. In The Pharmacologic Basis of Therapeutics, Ed. 4, p. 1604, edited by L. S. Goodman and A. Gilman. The MacMillan Co., New York, 1970.
26. Kimball, C. P.: Psychological dependence on steroids? Ann. Intern. Med., 75: 111, 1971.
27. Alepa, F. P., Zviafler, N. J., and Sliwinsi, J. A.: Immunologic effects of cyclophosphamide in rheumatoid arthritis. Arthritis Rheum., 13: 754, 1970.
28. Fosdick, W., Parsons, J., and Hill, D.: Long-term cyclophosphamide therapy in rheumatoid arthritis. Arthritis Rheum., 11: 151, 1968.
29. Cooperating Clinics of the American Rheumatism Association: A controlled trial of cyclophosphamide in rheumatoid arthritis. N. Engl. J. Med., 283: 883, 1970.
30. Lennard. H.: Mystification and Drug Misuse; Hazards in Using Psychoactive Drugs. Jossey-Bass, San Francisco, 1971.
31. Griffenhagen, G., and Hawkins, L.: Handbook of Non-Prescription Drugs. Amer. Pharm. Assoc., Washington, D.C., 1973.
32. Jarvis, D. C.: Arthritis and Folk Medicine. Holt, Rinehart, and Winston, New York, 1960.

chapter 25

HYPERURICEMIA AND GOUT

Lloyd Y. Young, Pharm.D.

The word "gout" is derived from the Latin "gutta," abbreviated "gtt," which is a term pharmacists readily translate as "drop." This term reflects the early concept that gout was caused by a noxious poison that drops consistently into joints. Gout is an ancient affliction of man and descriptions are found in the literature of every century. In early descriptions, gout was associated with vagaries of the wealthy and with excesses of food, wine and sex. Even now, myths continue. Recent studies have tried to correlate intelligence or social status with the occurrence of gout and this, no doubt, relates to the fact that many distinguished historical figures such as Martin Luther, Michaelangelo, Leonardo da Vinci, John Milton, Benjamin Franklin, Isaac Newton and Charles Darwin had the gout.

It was not until the 18th Century that uric acid was found to be an integral part of the gouty arthritic picture; and as science and biochemistry progressed, so did knowledge regarding gout and uric acid. Now, primary gout is considered to be an inborn error of uric acid metabolism that is manifested by hyperuricemia, acute or chronic recurrent arthritis and deposits of monosodium urates.

PREVALENCE AND INCIDENCE

Gout occurs in about 0.3% of the United States' population with a higher frequency reported in other countries. Exceptionally high frequencies of gout have been noted in the male Maori of New Zealand, in the natives of the Mariana Islands, and in American Filipinos.[1]

Gout is primarily a disease of middle-aged men. It seldom occurs during childhood or prior to the onset of puberty, and women rarely manifest this disease before menopause. It is also thought that inheritance plays a major role in the development of gout because hyperuricemia can be found in about 25% of close relatives of patients with clinical gout. In many cases, however, genetic factors are not involved. One rare form of gout is caused by a deficiency of the enzyme, hypoxanthine-guanine phosphoribosyltransferase, which is known to be transmitted as a sex-linked recessive trait. It is very clear, however, that an enzyme deficiency is only one of the many variables which influence the heterogenous disorder known as gout. If a mode of genetic transmission is ultimately discovered, the gouty trait will probably involve several genes.

PATHOGENESIS

In essence, gout is caused by the precipitation of excess uric acid from saturated body fluids. These excesses usually result from either an increase in uric acid production or a decrease of uric acid excretion. In some instances, it is a combination of these two factors.

The pathophysiological components of an acute gouty attack are not known, although the following is the most widely accepted postulate. First, monosodium urate crystals precipitate from hyperuricemic body fluids and an inflammatory response ensues with polymorphonuclear leukocyte infiltration and release of vasoactive humoral agents. These leukocytes then phagocytize the urate crystals. Local environmental changes resulting from the phagocytosis and the generalized inflammatory reaction cause a local increase in acidity which further decreases uric acid solubility. More urate crystals precipitate, and this vicious cycle is continued.

CHEMISTRY AND PHYSIOLOGY
OF URIC ACID

Uric acid is derived from purines which are primarily formed from the normal breakdown of body tissue and secondarily from dietary sources. In body fluids at pH 7.4, it exists almost entirely in the salt form and deposits in tophi as monosodium urate monohydrate. At lower pH levels such as those encountered in the urinary tract, tophaceous deposits are in the form of undissociated uric acid.

Uric acid is poorly soluble in water, but a pKa of 5.75 allows for a greater solubility of the ionized form in alkaline environments. At a urine pH of 5, only 6 to 8 mg of uric acid are soluble per 100 ml of urine; however, when the urine is alkalized to pH 7, the solubility of uric acid increases to 120 to 160 mg/100 ml. When we consider that the prevalence of uric acid urolithiasis among the gouty is 1,000 times greater than in the nongouty, and that urinary calculi occur in 10 to 20% of gouty patients, we can appreciate the importance of alkalinization of urine as a treatment modality.

In normal subjects, plasma becomes saturated with sodium urate at concentration of 7 mg/100 ml. However, supersaturated solutions of sodium urate readily form, and serum urate concentrations as high as 40 to 60 mg/100 mg are not uncommon in untreated, nongouty patients with myeloproliferative disorders. It is not clear why uric acid can stay in a supersaturated solution and then, suddenly, under appropriate conditions begin to precipitate out. However, it is known that plasma urate-binding protein deficiency, urate affinity for chondroitin sulfate, local pH changes, cold, trauma and stress can cause seeding of urate crystals.

Uric acid is not metabolized in man and serves no biochemical function. It is simply the end product of purine metabolism. This is the consequence of a genetic mutation error which occurred in the course of evolution that resulted in the loss of uricase, an enzyme that degrades uric acid into more soluble products.

The miscible pool of uric acid, in normal man, is approximately 1,200 mg with a daily turnover of about 700 to 800 mg per day. While approximately 1/3 of the daily excretion of uric acid can be accounted for by secretion into the gastrointestinal (GI) tract where it is degraded by bacteria, this route does not appear to be of significance in the production of hyperuricemia. Of greater magnitude and significance is the renal excretion which accounts for the other two-thirds.

A familiarity with the complexities of uric acid excretion is essential since drugs can alter these processes. Uric acid is completely filtered by the glomerulus only to have 99% of it reabsorbed in the proximal renal tubule. Approximately 86% of uric acid appearing in the final urine is accounted for by tubular secretion at the distal end of the proximal tubule. This dual handling of urate in the renal tubule logically accounts for the fact that some drugs may either increase or decrease urinary urate excretion depending on the dose. For example, salicylates have this dose-related effect on the renal excretion of uric acid.

Salicylates decrease urate excretion and elevate plasma urate at low oral doses of 1 to 2 g per day. Larger doses of 5 to 6 g per day of salicylate cause marked uricosuria and thereby lower serum urate levels.[2] Intermediate doses have little or no effect. This paradoxical dose-dependent action of salicylate is due to the fact that small doses of salicylate inhibit the tubular secretion of uric acid, and larger doses inhibit the tubular reabsorption of uric acid. The thiazide diuretics also are handled by the kidneys in a similar manner. Large intravenous doses cause an initial uricosuria, but small daily oral doses inhibit the tubular secretion of uric acid.[3]

Actually, all diuretics capable of producing a relative depletion of plasma volume will indirectly cause hyperuricemia. Several studies have indicated that if urinary salt and water losses were replenished, diuretic-induced hyperuricemia would be prevented. Thus the more potent diuretics such as furosemide, ethacrynic acid and the thiazides are much more commonly associated with drug-induced hyperuricemia than the milder diuretics such as spironolactone and triamterene.

CLINICAL FEATURES

Clinically, gout is characterized by urate tophaceous deposits and periodic attacks of acute joint pain. When severe attacks occur, systemic manifestations such as fever, leukocytosis and an increase in the erythrocyte sedimentation rate may appear in conjunction with inflammatory changes in the muscles and skin surrounding the affected joint. Sometimes these acute attacks are preceded with an aura of subjective changes such as malaise, pruritis, mood changes and joint discomfort. Early attacks are characteristically monoarticular but, suprisingly, tophi do not predispose the affected joint to attacks. When attacks occur, they can be accompanied not only by severe inflammation in the joint itself but also in periarticular tissues and skin.

The best description of an acute gouty attack is that of Thomas Sydenham in the 17th century, a description that still applies today. "The victim goes to bed and sleeps in good health. About two o'clock in the morning he is awakened by a severe pain in the great toe; more rarely in the heel, ankle or instep. The pain is like that of a dislocation, and yet the parts feel as if cold water were poured over them. Then follow chills and shivers, and a little fever. The pain, which was at first moderate, becomes more intense. With its intensity the chills and fevers increase . . . . Now it is a violent stretching and tearing of the ligaments—now, it is a gnawing pain, and now a pressure and tightening. So exquisite and lively meanwhile is the feeling of the part affected, that it cannot bear the weight of the bedclothes nor the jar of a person walking in the room. The night is spent in torture."[1]

TREATMENT OF ACUTE GOUT

The basic chemotherapy of an acute attack of gout has not changed dramatically since the above 17th Century observation, and colchicine continues as the cornerstone of therapy. Nevertheless, very little is known about colchicine pharmacology, metabolism and mechanisms of action. Indeed, the entire phenomenon of acute inflammatory gouty attacks remains to be elucidated, with the result that treatment continues to be mostly empirical.

Colchicine is the drug of choice for an acute attack of gout and provides relief to 80 to 95% of patients when properly administered. The best results are obtained if acute attacks are treated early. The relief provided by colchicine in acute gouty attacks is very specific, and if no relief is obtained, the diagnosis of acute gout should be questioned. For the fully developed acute attack, the traditional dosage of colchicine has been 1 or 2 0.5-mg to 0.6-mg tablets initially, followed by 0.5 to 0.6 mg hourly until joint pain relief is produced or until GI toxicity intervenes. A maximum of 12 to 15 tablets is generally recommended[4,5] because as little as 7 mg has been fatal.[5] The hourly colchicine regimen is not based on improving therapeutic results, but rather on minimizing colchicine GI toxicity since patients vary considerably in the amount of colchicine which they can tolerate.

Patients generally obtain relief from colchicine within 8 to 12 hr, although some patients begin to get relief about 6 hr after initiation of therapy. This delay in onset is very troublesome and narcotic analgesics should be administered during the interim. Salicylates (as found in Empirin compound, Percodan, etc.)

should be avoided because they decrease urate tubular secretion[2] as well as decrease urate solubility.[6] Recovery with resolution of swelling and redness is complete within 48 to 72 hr.[5] To prevent a relapse, prophylactic colchicine 0.5 to 0.6 mg twice daily should be administered for a few days after the acute attack.[7] In the few patients who do not experience relief of symptoms after a full course of colchicine treatment, additional therapy with an agent such as phenylbutazone is in order.

Intravenous colchicine can also be used for acute attacks and is preferred by some clinicians because it is less apt to cause GI distress. The entire dose of 2 to 3 mg should be dissolved in 30 cc of normal saline and administered over a 5-min span. A repeat intravenous dose may be necessary if no response is observed after 8 hr. Hourly administration of smaller intravenous doses is not necessary since toxicity is already diminished by this route of administration. Furthermore, intravenous colchicine solutions are extremely irritating, and phlebitis[8] is more common with repeated intravenous doses.

Although colchicine has been in clinical usage for over a 100 years, little is known of its specific mechanism of action. Some investigators believe colchicine interferes in some manner with the ability of leukocytes to perpetuate gouty attacks. In experimental studies, colchicine is known to interfere with kinin release, leukocyte motility, phagocytosis, leukocyte adhesiveness, leukocyte chemotaxis and a host of other biochemical effects. Wallace[9] measured the plasma levels of colchicine and concluded that colchicine at normal therapeutic doses most likely interferes with leukocyte motility or chemotaxis.

Nonspecific anti-inflammatory agents, such as phenylbutazone, are also effective alternatives to colchicine for chemotherapy of acute gouty attacks. Phenylbutazone 200 mg 4 times daily for the 1st day, followed by 200 mg 3 times daily for 2 days and then rapidly tapered to discontinuation over the next 2 days, is equally as effective as colchicine.[5] In fact, many clinicians consider phenylbutazone to be the agent of choice. Unlike that of colchicine, the GI distress induced by this drug is not as predictable, and patients need not be wakened hourly for drug administration. The hematological toxicities of phenylbutazone are extremely rare

in short term therapy of acute gout, but these adverse reactions are severe enough to warrant the continued use of colchicine as the first agent of choice. Other common phenylbutazone side effects include sodium and fluid retention, mild uricosuria, peptic ulceration, nausea, vomiting and skin rashes.

Indomethacin, a general anti-inflammatory drug, is yet another alternative, effective in the treatment of acute gouty attacks when administered at 150 to 200 mg per day in divided doses. Adrenalcorticotropin (ACTH) or glucocorticoids also occasionally are valuable in treating severe attacks resistant to other forms of therapy.

It should be noted that probenecid, sulfinpyrazone and allopurinol are ineffective in the treatment of acute gout and actually may precipitate acute attacks.[10] Thus, these drugs should not be used during an acute attack to achieve a reduction in serum urate levels.

MANAGEMENT OF INTERCRITICAL AND CHRONIC GOUTY ARTHRITIS

During the intercritical phase, patients with early gout are again asymptomatic and free of physical findings. The diagnosis at this time is dependent on both the history of a typical attack and the presence of hyperuricemia. The duration of the symptom-free period between the first and second gouty attack varies with individuals from several hours to several years. Eventually, however, these gouty attacks occur with increased frequency, greater severity and often in several joints simultaneously. If the serum uric acid concentration remains elevated, urate tophaceous deposits will occur in approximately 50 to 60% of gouty patients. These tophi classically occur in the cartilage of the ear pinna and in the first metatarsophalangeal joint of the big toe; although urate deposits can be found in any cartilagenous or soft tissue areas such as the kidney, heart, tendons and skin.

Secondary gouty tophaceous deposits may develop as a complication of diseases, such as myeloproliferative disorders where accelerated production and catabolism of nucleic acids cause greater production of uric acid. This same problem of accelerated nucleic acid catabolism also is seen during cancer chemotherapy or radiotherapy. However, whether gout is primary or secondary, the common metabolic abnormality responsible for its clinical manifestations continues to be hyperuricemia.

ASYMPTOMATIC HYPERURICEMIA

Although hyperuricemia is defined as being an excess of uric acid in the blood, the level at which serum uric acid becomes abnormal is not clearly established. An analysis of the Framingham Heart Study population and the results of a 12-year follow-up period[11] indicated that when maximal serum uric acid values were used, gouty arthritis occurred in 11.8% of those with levels between 7.0 to 7.9 mg/100 ml, and in 36% of those with uric acid levels above 8 mg/100 ml. On the other hand, of the men who had actually developed gouty arthritis, 15% did not have a value above 6.9 mg/100 ml, and 81% of the subjects with serum uric acid values of greater than 7.0 mg/100 ml did not develop gouty arthritis. Therefore, increased serum uric acid levels will predispose individuals to greater risks of developing gouty arthritis although no clear correlation or definition of an upper limit of normal for serum uric acid exists.

The treatment of mild to moderate asymtomatic hyperurcemia should be conservatively approached by increasing fluid intake, gradual weight reduction if indicated and periodic patient follow-ups. An evaluation of possible underlying disorders also should be undertaken. Since a high percentage of patients never experience an acute attack of gout, they should not be exposed unnecessarily to adverse drug reactions, although drugs can decrease the incidence of gouty arthritis by decreasing serum uric acid. If patients have already suffered an acute attack of gout or if serum uric acid concentrations are elevated consistently in the range of 9 to 10 mg/100 ml, drug therapy is indicated regardless of the underlying cause. The Framingham Study showed that in populations with serum uric acid levels greater than 9 mg/100 ml, approximately 83% were likely to develop gouty arthritis. These patients should be treated not to prevent tophaceous joint deposits, which can be resolved with therapy, but hopefully to prevent uric acid renal deposits. Uric acid nephrolithiasis in hyperuricemic subjects occasionally may be the only overt expression of primary gout. Moreover, the onset of uric acid nephrolithiasis often precedes acute gouty arthritis by several years in a large percentage of patients with uric acid stones.[12]

Therapy for asymptomatic hyperuricemia, however should not be initiated before determining the actual clinical significance of the abnormal laboratory test. Pharmacists should be aware that there are several methods for the analysis of serum uric acid and that each method and laboratory has different standard normal values for the same sample. The phosphotungstic acid cyanide colorimetric method, commonly utilized in automated laboratory screening panels (e.g., SMA 12 to 60), is not as specific as the uricase method of analysis and generally provides values approximately 1 mg/100 ml higher.

After substantiating the high laboratory results for serum uric acid, the clinician should determine if medications could have interfered with the laboratory test. We also know that methyldopa, levodopa, salicylates and aminophylline can cause false rises in serum uric acid by interfering with the phosphotungstic acid colorimetric test. Other agents such as diuretics, ethambutol and asprin can also interfere with laboratory testing by causing actual physiological increases in serum uric acid.

URICOSURIC THERAPY

Uricosuric drugs such as probenecid and sulfinpyrazone increase uric acid excretion by inhibiting the renal tubular reabsorption of uric acid. When these drugs are properly used, they will: decrease the plasma level of uric acid; prevent the formation of tophi; and mobilize already existing tophaceous deposits. However, these agents must be used consistently as the plasma urate levels will rise to initially high levels within a day or two upon cessation of these drugs.[13] Probenecid is well absorbed orally. Peak plasma concentrations occur within 2 to 4 hr, and the plasma half-life of the drug is approximately 6 to 12 hr. When therapy is begun, a prompt fall in plasma urate concentration usually is seen and is accompanied by rapid urinary excretion of uric acid.[5] After the 1st day or 2, the urinary uric acid excess disappears in a normal man, but in hyperuricemic individuals, excess uric acid is mobilized continually until the body pool of urate is reduced to normal levels.[13]

A potential risk of renal uric acid stones exists with the excretion of large amounts of uric acid. These stones then are treated as foreign bodies and a connective tissue reaction ensues with subsequent renal damage. However, this risk can be minimized by starting with small doses of uricosurics so as not to overwhelm the kidney with a flood of uric acid, by alkalinizing the urine in order to increase uric acid solubility and by maintaining a high fluid intake in order to maintain urine flow of at least 2 liters per day. With few exceptions it is not necessary to alkalinize the urine provided a high fluid intake is assured.

Since uricosuric drugs such as probenecid do not affect the production of uric acid but merely increase urate excretion, these drugs have certain limitations. Probenecid can not be used in patients with renal insufficiency with a glomerular filtration rate less than 30 ml per min or a blood urea nitrogen (BUN) greater than 40 mg/100 ml. Patients with a history of frequent renal stones and patients who are gross overexcretors of uric acid (greater than 1,200 mg/24 hr) also should not be treated with uricosourics.

Probenecid is a safe and well tolerated drug, as indeed it should be, since therapy must be continued for a long period of time. Serious side effects such as nephrotic syndrome, bone marrow suppression and hepatic necrosis are extremely rare. Common complaints generally involve GI distress (2 to 8% and drug hypersensitivity reactions (5%). Probenecid therapy should be initiated at 250 mg twice daily for 1 week and increased by weekly increments of 250 mg until a daily dose of 2 g per day is achieved.[10]

Sulfinpyrazone is a phenylbutazone analogue that is also a very effective uricosuric agent. Like all uricosurics, it inhibits tubular secretion of uric acid at low doses, but at normal therapeutic doses it inhibits reabsorption of uric acid. Therapy should be initiated at a dosage of 50 mg twice daily and gradually increased by 100-mg weekly increments to the daily maintenance dosage range of 200 to 400 mg to be given in divided doses. Untoward reactions and precautions are similar to that of probenecid with GI distress and hypersensitivity skin rashes being the most common. Hematological reactions rarely have been associated with the administration of sulfinpyrazone, but there is the potential for blood dyscrasias since this drug is a congener of phenylbutazone.

Therapy with all uricosuric agents should be initiated at a low dosage, then slowly increased not only to prevent the renal precipitation of uric acid stones as previously discussed but also to prevent the possibility of precipitating an acute gouty attack. Additionally many clinicians feel that colchicine should be administered prophylactically when initiating therapy with hypouricemic agents and, indeed, the manufacturers package inserts for allopurinol, probenecid and sulfinpyrazone include this suggestion. It is somewhat controversial, however, whether prophylactic colchicine indeed does decrease the incidence of acute gouty attacks when used either chronically or during the first 6 weeks of hypouricemic therapy.

Although the ideal double blind, long term study evaluating the efficacy of colchicine prophylaxis has yet to be done, reputable clinicians are of the opinion that colchicine prophylaxis clearly decreases the frequency and severity of acute gouty attacks. Thus, major texts state that colchicine is generally effective in reducing recurrences of acute attacks and usually recommend a dosage of 0.5 mg of colchicine twice daily.

The only detailed reports available on colchicine prophylaxis were done by Yu and Gutman[14,15] who reported that gouty attacks increased in frequency and severity in 80% of 734 patients before treatment; however, this trend was clearly reversed in about 75% by prophylactic colchicine with or without concomitant uricosuric therapy. While Gutman removed as many variables as possible in setting up these evaluations of colchicine, these studies were not controlled and were dependent on subjective evaluations. Nevertheless, Gutman's data were very impressive and in the low dosages used prophylactically, untoward reactions to colchicine were extremely rare. However, the controversy continues because of the lack of controlled trials.

This author is of the opinion that colchicine prophylaxis is not always necessary when initiating allopurinol or uricosuric therapy, except in patients with a history of frequent acute gouty attacks. The decision to use colchicine prophylaxis should be based on the clinical circumstances of the individual patient.

Other than probenecid and sulfinpyrazone, a large number of diverse pharmacological agents possess varying degrees of uricosuric properties. Although most of these drugs are organic acids, they do not seem to share any other similarities either in chemical structure or in pharmacological properties. A list of such drugs includes acetohexamide, ethyl biscoumacetate, chlorprothixene, clofibrate, phenosulfonphthalein and various diuretics.[13] Recent studies[16,17] indicated that radiocontrast agents such as iopanoic acid should also be added to this list. A standard 3 g dose of iopanoic acid increases 24-hr urate excretion by 68%, which is similar to the 60% obtainable with probenecid. Further comparisons show that iopanoic acid has a plasma half-life of 12 to 20 hr and increases the excretion of uric acid for 5 to 6 days. In contrast, probenecid has a plasma half-life of only 6 to 12 hr and has a duration of activity of approximately 2 days.[18]

DRUG INTERACTIONS

Whenever pharmacists either recommend or monitor drug therapy, they also should be alert for the possibility of clinically significant drug interactions. Uricosuric agents affect not only the tubular secretion of uric acid but also the tubular secretion of other organic acids. For example, in adequate doses, probenecid can block the tubular secretion of penicillin, cephalothin, aminosalicylic acid, dapsone, indomethacin, pyrazinamide and phenosulfonphthalein.[19] Of even greater importance is the competition of the salicylates with probenecid for tubular transport. It has been shown that 2 5-grain aspirin tablets every 6 hr completely antagonize the uricosuric effect of probenecid. Even one dose of aspirin will antagonize some of probenecid's uricosuric effects.[20] Acetaminophen does not interfere and is a viable alternative for antipyresis and mild analgesia in patients treated with probenecid.

XANTHINE OXIDASE INHIBITOR

Xanthine oxidase is an essential enzyme that converts the more soluble uric acid precursors, hypoxanthine and xanthine, to uric acid. Allopourinol and its metabolite, oxypurinol, prevent the formation of uric acid by nature of their potent xanthine oxidase-inhibiting properties. This ability of allopurinol to inhibit xanthine oxidase and to lower serum uric acid is a dose-related phenomenon. The higher the dose of allopurinol used, the greater the fall in serum uric acid levels. Generally, the dose required to normalize hyperuricemia in patients with mild disease is 200 to 300 mg per day and in those

with moderate or severe disease, 400 to 600 mg per day. Higher dosages may be used, but most clinicians prefer to add a uricosuric to the allopurinol.

Approximately 80% of an oral dose of allopurinol is rapidly absorbed; once absorbed (30 min to 2 hr), allopurinol is rapidly cleared from plasma with a probable plasma half-life of less than 2 hr.[21] A small part of allopurinol is excreted in the urine unchanged, but the remainder is oxidized rapidly to alloxanthine (oxypurinol). Oxypurinol slowly is eliminated from the blood by renal excretion and has a prolonged plasma half-life of 18 to 30 hr in man.[21] Thus, smaller doses should be used in patients with renal failure. Oxypurinol is also a potent inhibitor of xanthine oxidase, but it is only 1/5 to 1/10 as potent *in vitro* as allopurinol.[22] However, *in vivo*, it probably accounts for much of allopurinol's xanthine oxidase-inhibitor effects. Furthermore, allopurinol's oxidation to its metabolite, oxypurinol, is regulated by xanthine oxidase. Therefore, allopurinol by nature of xanthine oxidase inhibition slows its own metabolism in patients on long term therapy. Because of these reasons, allopurinol can be administered on a once daily basis in some individuals.

Serum uric acid levels usually begin to fall within 1 to 2 days after initiating allopurinol therapy with maximal uric acid suppression usually requiring about 7 to 10 days. Clinical improvement takes longer, but after approximately 6 months one should be able to see a gradual decrease in the size of established tophi and the absence of new tophaceous deposits.

Allopurinol is especially useful in:

1. patients with severe tophaceous gout.

2. patients who are allergic or exhibit an intolerance to both uricosuric agents.

3. gouty patients not controlled by uricosuric agents.

4. patients who already have kidney stones or who show a marked predisposition to renal calculus formation.

5. patients with advanced renal failure.

6. patients with neoplastic or myeloproliferative disorders whose nucleic acid turnover is very high and who excrete very high levels of urinary uric acid especially when cytotoxic therapy is initiated.

7. patients with high urate excretion (*i.e.,* greater than 1,200 mg/24 hr) since further

uricosuric therapy could lead to renal lithiasis.

Rational drug therapy of hyperuricemia would be to inhibit the formation of unwanted uric acid with allopurinol rather than to hasten uric acid excretion after it is formed with a uricosuric. When one considers the possibility of uric acid precipitation and uric acid nephrolithiasis, one must conclude that allopurinol represents a better choice than uricosuric drugs if it is equally safe and efficacious.

Allopurinol and probenecid are both capable of effectively lowering serum uric acid and serious adverse reactions to the agents are very rare. Even commonly encountered side effects such as hypersensitivity and GI distress are of a relatively low order of magnitude with these drugs. Nevertheless, probenecid is this author's choice for the treatment of uncomplicated gout simply because it has been used for over 22 years as compared to 7 years for allopurinol and much more clinical experience has accrued with its usage. Reports are still filtering in regarding recently discovered allopurinol effects. In the last 2 years, significant allopurinol drug interactions have been reported with bishydroxycoumarin[23] and ampicillin.[24] Also, it has been demonstrated that allopurinol ribonucleotide forms *in vivo* and functions as an inhibitor of enzymes other than xanthine oxidase. This nucleotide could, theoretically, be incorporated into nucleic acids. Other recent reports include fatal allopurinol allergic vasculitis[25] and xanthine nephropathy.[26] Because of the deaths associated with severe allopurinol hypersensitivity reactions and because new effects of allopurinol are still being uncovered, uricosuric therapy, whenever possible, is the therapy of choice for uncomplicated treatment of gout.

Allopurinol drug interactions to be considered are those with 6-mercaptopurine, azathioprine, iron salts, bishydroxycoumarin and ampicillin.

Clinicians should be aware that 6-mercaptopurine, and azathioprine are metabolized by xanthine oxidase and that the dosage of these drugs should be decreased to 1/3 to 1/4 of the usual dosage when allopurinol is administered concomitantly.

Animal studies have indicated that xanthine oxidase also plays an important role in the reduction of ferric ferritin to ferrous ferritin. Thus, allopurinol, by preventing this first step in the mobilization of iron from the liver, theoretically, can cause hemosiderosis. However, evidence is lacking in man that the ferritin-xanthine oxidase system is important in iron transport or mobilization. Since allopurinol has been used extensively without reports of hemosiderosis occurring in humans, this drug interaction is not clinically significant at this time. Clinicians, however, should be aware that such a reaction theoretically could occur, and the necessity of the administration of these two agents in conjunction should be re-evaluated carefully.

Allopurinol has also been demonstrated to increase by 3-fold the mean bishydroxycoumarin half-life supposedly by slowing the biotransformation of bishydroxycoumarin in liver microsomes.[23]

An excess of ampicillin[24] rashes have also been associated with concomitant allopurinol administration. In one series of patients, 22.4% on both allopurinol and ampicillin developed an ampicillin rash as compared to 7.5% of patients on ampicillin alone.

GOUTY NEPHROPATHY

When urate crystals precipitate into renal tissue, a local inflammatory reaction occurs followed by possible fibrosis and loss of renal function. Approximately 15% of gouty patients have urate nephrolithiasis and approximately 30 to 50% die of renal disease. Moreover, in one series of 305 patients, the onset of uric acid nephrolithiasis preceded acute gouty arthritis by more than 5 years in 40% of the patients with uric acid stones.[12]

Therapy of gouty nephropathy should be aimed at increasing the solubility of urate stones and at decreasing the uric acid presented to the kidneys. Maintaining a urinary output of at least 2 liters per day and alkalinizing the urine will increase uric acid solubility. Decreasing the urinary excretion of uric acid will be achieved by the xanthine oxidase inhibitor, allopurinol.

Since uric acid solubility can be increased 20-fold by increasing urine pH from 5.0 to 7.0, alkalinization of urine is often attempted. Sodium or potassium bicarbonate can be used as the alkalinating agent as an initial 4-g dose followed by 1 to 2 g every 4 hr. The urine pH should be tested (*e.g.*,nitrazine paper) at intervals throughout the day and the dose of bicarbonate adjusted accordingly. Potassium (or sodium) citrate also can be used in doses of 1 g 3 to 6 times daily. The citrate molecule apparently enters the Krebs citric acid cycle and is excreted as bicarbonate. Therefore, the citrates have the urine-alkalinizing properties of sodium bicarbonate without neutralizing gastric secretions and without promoting a dumping syndrome. When using either the bicarbonates or citrates, it is important to divide the doses evenly throughout the day and night. It is during the night that urine becomes the most concentrated and acidic. Although acetazolamide produces an alkaline urine, the effects are self-limiting after a few days.

While urine alkalinity is desirable in order to increase the solubility of uric acid, it is often difficult to achieve clinically without affecting other organ systems. In patients with congestive heart failure, sodium intake must be considered. Furthermore, the ability of the kidneys to excrete potassium is of critical importance in patients with gouty nephropathy. The cation content of the common alkalinizing agents are as follows: Sodium bicarbonate has 11.90 m Eq Na^+ per g. Sodium citrate .2 H_2O has 10.19 m Eq Na^+ per g. Sodium citrate .5 H_2O has 8.40 m Eq Na^+ per g. Potassium bicarbonate has 9.99 m Eq K^+ per g. Potassium citrate .H_2O has 9.25 m Eq K^+ per g. Because of the difficulty in maintaining an alkaline urine in gouty arthritic patients, this treatment modality rarely is used except in some hospitalized patients with nephrolithiasis.

The use of allopurinol in patients with gouty nephropathy is not without risks. There is a slight increased susceptibility to the hepatotoxic effects of allopurinol as well as slight increased frequency of severe hypersensitivity allopurinol reactions in patients with renal impairment. However, poor renal function does not contraindicate the use of allopurinol, especially since uricosurics cannot be used.

Since allopurinol and its metabolite, oxypurinol, are slowly eliminated from the blood by renal excretion, care should be taken to decrease the dose in renal failure. Fortunately, allopurinol's toxicities usually are not dose-related and because of the relatively large safety margin, adjustments need not be exactly calculated. In patients with severe renal impairment (creatinine clearance $\leq$ 10 ml per min), the allopurinol-dosing interval should be increased by about 1.5 to 3.0 times normal.

CONCLUSION

Gout is a metabolic disease caused by excessive amounts of uric acid. Modern pharmacology has created uricosuric drugs which hasten the excretion of uric acid and a drug which can inhibit uric acid formation by blocking the enzyme xanthine oxidase. Hopefully, even better and safer drugs will be produced in the future. Until that time, pharmacists should acquaint themselves with all aspects of the available drugs used in the therapy of gout.

REFERENCES

1. Wyngaarden, J. B.: Gout and other disorders of uric acid metabolism. In Harrison's Principles of Internal Medicine, Ed. 6, p. 597. McGraw-Hill Book Co., San Francisco, 1970.
2. Yu, T. F., and Gutman, A. B.: Study of the paradoxical effects of salicylate in low, intermediate and high dosage on the renal mechanisms for excretion of urate in man. J. Clin. Invest., 38: 1298, 1959.
3. DeMartini, F. E.: Effect of chlorothiazide on the renal excretion of uric acid. Am. J. Med., 32: 572, 1962.
4. Calkins, E.: The treatment of gout. Ration. Drug Ther., 5: 1, 1971.
5. Woodbury, D. M.: Analgesics, antipyretics, anti-inflammatory agents, and inhibitors of uric acid synthesis. In the Pharmacological Basis of Therapeutics, Ed. 4, edited by L. S. Goodman and A. Gilman. MacMillan Co., New York, 1970.
6. Klinenberg, J. R., Bluestone, R., Schlosstein, L., Waismann, J., and Whitehouse, M. W.: Urate deposition disease. Ann. Intern. Med., 78: 99, 1973.
7. Yu, T. F., and Gutman, A. B.: Principles of current management of primary gout. Am. J. Med. Sci., 144: 893, 1967.
8. Wallace, S.: Colchicine—clinical pharmacology in acute gouty arthritis. Am. J. Med., 30: 439, 1961.
9. Wallace, S., Omokoku, B., and Ertel, N.: Colchicine plasma levels: implications as to pharmacology and mechanism of action. Am. J. Med., 48: 443, 1970.
10. Young, L. Y.: Gout and hyperuricemia. In Manual of Clinical Pharmacy, edited by L. Young, M. A. Kimble, B. Katcher, and T. Tong. Williams and Wilkins Co., Baltimore, in press.
11. Hall, A. P., Barry, P. E., Dawber, T. R., and McNamara, P. M.: Epidemiology of gout and hyperuricemia. Am. J. Med., 42: 27, 1967.
12. Gutman, A. B., and Tu, T. F.: Uric acid nephrolithiasis in gout. Ann. Intern. Med., 67: 1133, 1967.
13. Gutman, A. B.: Uricosuric drugs with special reference to probenecid and sulfinpyrazone. Adv. Pharmacol. Chemother., 4: 91, 1966.
14. Yu, T. F., and Gutman, A. B.: Efficacy of colchi-

cine prophylaxis in gout. Ann. Intern. Med., 55: 179, 1961.

15. Gutman, A. B.: Treatment of primary gout: the present status. Arthritis Rheum., 8: 911, 1965.

16. Mudge, G. H.: Uricosuric action of cholecystographic agents. N. Engl. J. Med., 284: 931, 1971.

17. Postlewaite, H. E., and Kelley, W. N.: Uricosuric effects of radio-contrast agents.

18. Mikkelsen, W., and Robinson, W. D.: Physiological and biochemical basis for the treatment of gout and hyperuricemia. Med. Clin. North Am., 53: 1331, 1969.

19. Hansten, P.: Drug Interactions. Lea and Febiger, Philadelphia, 1972.

20. Pascale, L. R., Dubin, A., and Hoffman, W. S.: Therapeutic value of probenecit in gout. J.A.M.A., 149: 1188, 1952.

21. Elion, G. B., Yu, T. F., Gutman, A. B., and Hitchings, G. H.: Renal clearance of oxypurinol, the chief metabolite of allopurinol. Am. J. Med., 45: 69, 1968.

22. Elion, G. B.: Enzymatic and metabolic studies with allopurinol. Ann. Rheum. Dis., 25: 608, 1966.

23. Vesell, E. S., Passananti, T., and Greene, F. E.: Impairment of drug metabolism in man by allopurinol and nortryptyline. N. Engl. J. Med., 283: 1484, 1970.

24. Boston Collaborative Drug Surveillance Program: Excess of ampicillin rashes associated with allopurinol or hyperuricemia. N. Engl. J. Med., 286: 505, 1972.

25. Jarzobski, J., Ferry, J., Wombolt, D., Fitch, D. M., and Egan, J. D.: Vasculitis with allopurinol therapy. Am. Heart J., 79: 116, 1970.

26. Band, P. R., Silverberg, D. S., Henderson, J. F., Ulan, R. A., Wensel, R. H., Banerjee, T. K., and Little, A. S.: Xanthine nephropathy in a patient with lymphosarcoma treated with allopurinol. N. Engl. J. Med., 283: 354, 1970.

section 8
Diseases of the blood

chapter **26**

IRON DEFICIENCY ANEMIA IN THE PEDIATRIC PATIENT

Robert H. Levin, Pharm.D.

The practicing pharmacist will be exposed to and called upon to recommend treatment for many childhood dietary deficiency states. One can appreciate the problem by considering the huge amount of special pediatric formulas, enriched children's foods and vitamin and mineral supplements the average mother will purchase for her growing child. The majority of added supplements are unnecessary for the average American child except one—iron. Iron deficiency anemia, the most prevalent nutritional deficiency in this country,[1] is as common now in our affluent society as it was 30 years ago.[2] The increased use of enriched foods and improved diets has done little to decrease the incidence of this easily curable disease.

PHYSIOLOGY OF IRON METABOLISM

Before considering the etiology of iron deficiency anemia, it is helpful to review the mechanism of body iron homeostasis. Virtually every cell in the human body contains some iron, but the bulk of stored iron is concentrated in only a few sites. After iron is absorbed, it is utilized either by the body (as functional iron) or stored for future use. The functional iron is incorporated predominately into hemoglobin by the erythrocytes of the bone marrow. This accounts for about 75 to 85% of total body iron in infants. There are other functional iron-containing heme proteins located in muscles as myoglobin and in the reticuloendothelial system as part of the cytochrome oxidase system. The remaining iron is found in storage sites as ferritin, hemosiderin and transferrin.

With adequate iron stores, iron is absorbed and stored as an organic protein complex, never as free iron, which is highly toxic. Ferritin and hemosiderin are functionally indistinguishable, but there are small molecular differences. There are three types of ferritin molecules, differing only in their protein moiety.[3] Ferritin is found in four separate storage organs—the liver, spleen, reticulocytes and epithelial cells. When 1 molecule of ferritin is saturated fully, it can furnish iron for 1,200 hemoglobin molecules. There are 5 chemically different hemosiderin molecules found in separate areas of the body, but, again, all are functionally identical.[3] The last storage protein, transferrin, is contained in the circulating blood. Transferrin participates in iron utilization by conveying iron from its absorption sites in the gastrointestinal (GI) tract to its utilization sites in the bone marrow and its storage sites in the liver, spleen and reticulocytes. Iron also can be stored in circulating transferrin which normally remains approximately one-third saturated with iron.

The principal factors influencing absorption are those operating in the lumen of the intestine.[4] Together they constitute the homeostatic functions which regulate the transit of iron across the intestinal mucosa by a feedback mechanism.

Iron is absorbed throughout the GI tract. Over 90% of this absorption normally occurs in the duodenum and upper jejunum.[5] In cases of iron deficiency anemia, increased absorption occurs further along the GI tract.[3] The process of absorption is a complex active absorption requiring oxidative metabolism and generation of biochemical phosphate energy.[6] Inorganic ferrous ion is converted to ferric ion which is complexed by a gastric iron-binding protein which recently has been elucidated and named gastroferrin.[4,7] This mucopolysaccharide forms a macromolecule which acts as a carrier of iron and allows it to remain in solution in the jejunum. If iron remained as the free ion in the high pH of the jejunum, it would quickly precipitate out as the insoluble phosphate, phytate, or as insoluble bases and be unavailable for absorption. On the contrary, organically bound iron in heme (from blood contained in meat) is readily absorbed unchanged through the gut wall into the epithelial cell where it is broken down into ionizable iron. About 20 to 40% of most food iron is released as ionizable inorganic iron by peptic digestion.[4]

The complex process of iron absorption is undergoing considerable research and is still largely unsettled. It is evident that the body can quantitatively control the amount of iron absorbed from the gastrointestinal tract by at least two processes. The epithelium of the small intestine can pick up iron directly and convert it to its storage form of ferritin through an intermediary, apoferritin.[6] The ferritin in the cell is largely unavailable to the body for heme utilization and subsequently is sloughed off into the intestine. A large percentage of this cellular iron plus any transferrin that has exuded into the GI tract is reabsorbed by other epithelial cells.[4] The second controlling process is the active absorption of iron through the mucous cells utilizing transferrin, with conveyance to the bone marrow or storage sites for incorporation directly into heme or storage depots. These two pathways allow for precise control of the amount of iron absorbed. As little as 5% to as much as 30 to 40% of food and medicinal iron will be absorbed in the GI tract.[3] In normal individuals, approximately 10% of iron presented to the GI tract will be absorbed. High levels of body iron (hemochromatosis) are largely prevented by the mucosal cells by preferential absorption of iron as ferritin. Conversely, in iron deficiency states, the intestine, via the transferrin route, can readily assimilate 30 to 40% of presented iron to increase lost body stores.[8]

Normal iron homeostasis depends completely upon this absorption process, because there is no significant excretion of iron. It is estimated the average loss of iron in adult males is between 0.5 to 1 mg per day. Red blood cells are catabolized by the liver and the liberated iron either is utilized for further hemoglobin production or stored by the body. Epithelial shedding, sweating, urination and blood loss are the routes through which iron is eliminated

from the body. An increased turnover rate of iron by the body will cause a concomitant increase in absorption.[4] This turnover rate will be increased in cases of anemia, anoxia, increased erythropoiesis, pregnancy, decreased iron stores and increased iron ingestion. Paradoxically, with diseases like sickle cell anemia and thalassemia, increased amounts of iron are absorbed even when high total body iron stores exist owing to hemolytic anemia and intermittent blood transfusions.[4] In contrast, absorption normally will be decreased with increased body iron stores, decreased erythropoiesis and generalized malabsorption.

ETIOLOGY

Iron deficiency anemia in infants may be present at birth or develop later in infancy. The finding of anemia at birth is dependent upon a number of interrelated factors. The majority of hemoglobin synthesis, with concomitant accumulation of iron stores, occurs during the 3rd trimester of pregnancy with 50% of this synthesis occurring during the last month. A number of conditions during the last trimester of fetal life can cause a newborn to be deficient in iron; e.g., 1 month prematurity will leave the infant with only 1/2 of his normal hemoglobin stores.

As a pregnancy progresses, iron crosses the placenta in increasing amounts to the fetus regardless of maternal iron stores. The fetus is extremely efficient in accumulating iron even in the face of maternal iron deficiency. A full term, 3-kg newborn will have 78 mg per kg of iron of which 60 mg per kg is hemoglobin, for a total body store of about 240 mg iron.[3] In contrast, a 1-month premature baby will only have approximately 120 mg of iron. In both cases, the fetal hemoglobin is slowly hemolyzed and the iron is stored for the initiation of erythropoiesis.

The etiology of iron deficiency anemia in the growing child depends on a number of parameters, including: the amount of the newborn's iron stores at birth; the iron requirements for an expanding body mass; the amount of iron absorbed from the diet; and the loss of iron, either physiologically or pathologically.

The premature infant may initially grow 2 to 3 times as fast as a newborn and, without iron supplements, will become iron deficient in 6 to

12 weeks and symptomatic in about 12 to 16 weeks. The full term infant, without iron supplementation, may become deficient in 4 to 5 months but will not show symptoms until after 6 months.[9] It can readily be appreciated from the above that decreased birth weight with attendant decreased hemoglobin and iron stores makes the premature infant a considerably higher anemia risk than the full term infant.

However, all infants after birth develop decreasing hemoglobin levels until a "physiological anemia of the newborn" occurs. This self-limiting anemia is "normal" and should not be treated with iron or confused with iron deficiency anemia.[10] The reduced hemoglobin levels and expanded plasma volume of the growing infant stimulate the dormant erythropoietic system to commence production of red cells and adult hemoglobin. At birth, the infant has 90% fetal hemoglobin and 10% adult hemoglobin. The two forms are slightly different chemically but identical in function. The fetal hemoglobin and red cells have a shorter life of approximately 60 to 70 days, compared to a normal red blood cell life of approximately 120 days.[11] This would account for the physiological anemia occurring at about 8 to 12 weeks of life. When hemoglobin production commences, adult hemoglobin is synthesized and eventually accounts for 98% of the hemoglobin of a 1-year old.

Besides prematurity, there are other causes of low iron stores at birth: blood loss due to perinatal hemorrhage; intrauterine exchange transfusions; fetomaternal transfusions; or cord hemorrhage secondary to accidents or malformation of the cord or placenta.[12] In utero, twin-to-twin transfusions occur, leaving one twin with excess hemoglobin and the other very anemic. Blood loss may also occur after birth and could account for a significant percentage of iron deficiency anemia.[9,12]

Milk-induced enteric blood loss may account for the unchanging incidence of iron deficiency anemia over the past 30 years even though the population is more affluent and has an improved diet.[2] Pasteurized whole cows' milk is extensively utilized for feeding infants and has been implicated as the causative agent of occult bleeding and decreased absorption of nutrients, including iron. This blood loss possibly may account for 50% of the cases of iron deficiency anemia.[13] Milk-induced iron deficiency anemia should be suspected if the infant consumes a quart or more of whole cows' milk per day (typically the child is fat and healthy looking and the mother is proud of his well being); iron deficiency anemia cannot be explained by prematurity, poor iron intake or excessively rapid growth; iron deficiency anemia recurs, having once been adequately corrected with iron; an iron-deficient child is said to be "unresponsive to iron therapy"; finally, the anemia is associated with hypoproteinemia and hypocupremia.[14]

With the cessation of whole milk intake, intestinal function returns to normal in a few days. This milk-induced anemia does not occur with breast-fed babies or babies fed formula, e.g., Similac or Enfamil.[13,15] Blood loss due to external hemorrhage, other internal hemorrhages, exchange transfusions or hookworms and other parasites also can account for decreased iron stores. Additionally, recurrent infections, renal disease, gastroenteritis, and malabsorption, e.g., celiac disease, will eventually lead to iron deficiency anemia.[16]

Inadequate dietary intake of iron in relation to the child's growth rate accounts for a considerable number of cases of iron deficiency anemia. Poorly planned meals, feeding problems and behavior disturbances can result in poor dietary intake of iron. Steatorrhea, chronic diarrhea and colitis can cause diminished absorption of essential nutrients. By age one, a full term infant must have a total of 155 mg of iron from exogenous sources for normal growth and development.[17] A premature infant needs about 240 mg during this same period.[17] It takes 3.4 mg of iron to produce 1 g of hemoglobin and 1 mg of iron to produce 1 ml of packed red blood cells.

The amounts of iron needed by different age groups are listed in Table 26.1. A large majority of this iron is supplied by foods (Table 26.2). A differential absorption occurs depending on the needs of the body. Younger infants will absorb more iron from some foods than older children, e.g., 3-year olds will absorb more iron from eggs than 3- to 10-year olds.

INCIDENCE AND OCCURRENCE

The highest incidence of iron deficiency anemia occurs in the age group of 6 months to

TABLE 26.1
Iron Requirements

Age	Requirements per Day mg
Full term infants (with poor stores)	0.73 after 3 months old
Premature infants (with poor stores)	0.8 after 2 months old
Average full term infants	0.5
Infants (with severe deprivation)	2
Children	0.5-1.5
Adult men, postmenopausal women	0.5-1
Menstruating women	1-1.5
Pregnancy, lactation, delivery	2-3

3 years of age, especially in the 1- to 2-year olds.[3] It is uncommon to find this deficiency in infants younger than 6 months, and in children from 4 years of age to adolescence. Adolescents, especially menstruating females, because of increasing growth and development and inadequate dietary intake, have a high incidence of iron deficiency anemia. It is estimated that in some areas of this country as much as 65% of menstruating girls suffer decreased hemoglobin levels with concomitant findings of anemia.[13]

In the 6-month to 3-year-old age group, there is no preferential incidence of anemia related solely to sex or race alone; however, socioeconomic factors are important.[3] Multiparity and low socioeconomic status are commonly linked to iron deficiency anemia. Anemia is frequently seen in low birth weight infants who receive inadequate postnatal iron intake.

Studies done in different parts of the country show the incidence of anemia in 1-year olds in impoverished areas to average about 50%,[18] with a range of 25 to 75%.[1] By contrast, middle class areas have incidence levels of 5 to 15%.[1] Studies done with well fed babies still report an incidence of 4 to 8% of anemia in 1-year olds.[1] As the child grows older (3 to 5 years old), his diet will generally supply an adequate amount of iron.[13]

PATHOGENESIS

There are progressive stages of iron depletion leading to a state of iron deficiency anemia.[12] The areas first affected are the storage sites for iron, particularly the bone marrow. Ferritin and hemosiderin, the storage protein molecules, are progressively depleted and finally disappear. The second stage involves the circulating serum. The level of serum iron decreases and the serum iron-binding capacity (unsaturation of transferrin) increases, which leads to a decreased percentage of iron saturation of transferrin. The third stage is a decreasing level of circulating red cell mass. The fourth stage affects the morphology of red blood cells. The erythrocytes become microcytic and hypochromic, and they assume abnormal, unequal shapes and sizes (poikilocytosis and anisocytosis, respectively). In the fifth stage, an anemia of a progressive degree of severity supervenes. Ultimately, in the last stage of development, the iron content of intracellular enzymes is progressively depleted.

DIAGNOSIS AND CLINICAL FINDINGS

Iron deficiency anemia is not likely to be confused with other anemias and rarely coexists with megaloblastic anemias of infancy, *e.g.,* vitamin B_{12} and folic acid deficiencies.[19] Appropriate hematological standards of hemoglobin, hematocrit and other parameters based on age must be used to evaluate laboratory results. Erroneous values can be expected if general rather than specific norms are used, especially in the first 18 months of life.[12] The hemoglobin and hematocrit normally fluctuate widely in this age group with levels generally lower than adults.

The blood smear is the most common test for anemia but is only useful after iron stores are depleted and the patient is usually symptomatic.[3,5] The usual hematological tests are normal until iron stores are depleted and are not useful for diagnosing early anemia. Only bone marrow aspirates are effective in diagnosing early occult anemia; however, these are rarely necessary in infants—as anemia, if present, always is well established. In children, changes in erythrocytes begin to be noticeable at hemoglobin levels of 10 to 11 g% and increase in severity as the hemoglobin level decreases.[3] As the hemoglobin level decreases to less than 7 g%, an increased reticulocyte response of 4 to 6% is noticed. If this response is more than 6%, the patient probably is bleeding internally.

In most cases, a simple inspection of a peripheral blood smear will be enough to confirm the suspected diagnosis. The smear will show hypochromic, microcytic cells with marked variation in size and shape.[5,19] Other laboratory values used for diagnosis would be a hemoglobin level of less than 10 g% and a hematocrit level of less than 30%.[1,20] Reticulocytes, platelets or white blood cells are usually of little use in diagnosis. Their levels may be normal, slightly elevated or slightly decreased. Decreased values of mean corpuscular volume, mean corpuscular hemoglobin and mean corpuscular hemoglobin concentration indicates anemia.[19]

Additional laboratory tests seldom are needed but others may be used, such as the percent of serum iron (PI), total iron-binding capacity (TIBC), iron saturation of transferrin and free erythrocyte protoporphyrin. The most sensitive measure of iron deficiency anemia is measurement of stainable marrow iron; however, bone marrow measurement rarely is needed in infants to document iron deficiency anemia. It must be remembered that absence of stainable marrow and liver iron is almost universal in the 6-month to 2-year-old child.[3]

There are other useful tests that can be employed. A stool guaiac or benzidine test should be performed to detect occult blood. The ingestion of iron does not affect these tests even though the stools are black. The guaiac test is only sensitive enough to pick up more than 5 ml of occult blood.[9] A 2-ml blood loss per day probably will go undetected. This amounts to a loss of 1 mg of iron per day which is more than normally is absorbed by infants under the age of one. Benzidine is so sensitive that it will react with the blood in an ingested meat meal. A one plus reaction (four plus maximum) is considered normal and not indicative of occult blood. Since there is a high incidence (approximately 60%) of occult blood loss in iron-deficient infants, this factor is significant.[13] Serum protein should be tested

when indicated, because hypoproteinemia associated with severe microcytic anemia is not uncommon and may indicate a concomitant copper deficiency.[3,21]

In surveys of individuals with low hemoglobin who are otherwise healthy, symptoms such as fatigue, weakness and pallor (symptoms commonly ascribed to iron deficiency anemia) have been shown to be unrelated to levels of hemoglobin and hematocrit.[4,12] It is possible that the clinical symptoms could be related to the cytochrome oxidase system.[5] These catabolic enzymes, which use endogenous and exogenous compounds as substrates have been shown to increase in activity 24 to 36 hr after starting iron therapy.[1,13] The symptomatic relief individuals achieve with iron before there is any evidence of hematological change makes this thesis seem reasonable, but the entire question of tissue effects of iron depletion remains unsettled.[12]

Adults exibit lethargy and lassitude with minimal decreases in serum iron. In contrast, infants usually do not have any clinical symptoms even with low hemoglobin values of 5 to 7 g%.[3] A significant quantity of iron deficiency anemia in 6-month to 3-year olds is found by blood smear during a routine office visit. The mother is usually unaware of the problem because the child is usually well and happy. The pediatrician undoubtedly will notice the occurrence of pallor (usually his only clue) in the ears, conjunctivae and mucous membranes of the mouth.[3] When symptoms do occur in later stages of anemia, they consist of irritability, decreased exercise tolerance, apparent weakness and listlessness. Spoon nail (koilonychia), glossitis, stomatitis and dysphagia are symptoms that occur in adults but rarely in children. Children will, however, develop abnormal GI tract function. The mucosa becomes abnormal, causing an impairment in the absorption of fats and fat-soluble vitamins. Increased permeability of blood vessels occurs with exuding of red cells and plasma proteins into the lumen of the intestine.

Infants with iron deficiency anemia do not have any decrease in either weight gain or linear growth when compared to normal infants.[1,18] Weight loss and decreased growth, because of a decreased caloric intake, occur only in severe iron anemic infants who exhibit anorexia.[1,13]

Some of these infants with iron deficiency anemia also have pica (abnormal eating habits), although it is not clear which occurs first.[3] Pica, due to poor environmental conditions, probably leads to an inadequate dietary intake and, thus, anemia.[19] There is also no difference in the I.Q. of normal and anemic children even though the anemic children have decreased attentiveness and decreased learning.[1,13] These symptoms are readily cured when the child is given therapeutic iron.[1] There is also no convincing evidence that iron-deficient infants have an increased incidence of infections.[13]

COMPLICATIONS

With progressive untreated states, hepatomegaly, splenomegaly and heart murmurs may occur. Rarely, cardiorespiratory distress in severe cases may terminate in cardiac failure. Severe dysphagia (Plummer-Vinson syndrome) possibly could develop in older children.

PREVENTION

The primary concern in treating the problem of iron deficiency anemia should be with the nutritional implications rather than the anemia. The crucial matter is the education of parents concerning the importance of nutritional balance. Dietary sources of iron (Table 26.2) are accessible and economically feasible.

Good food sources are eggs and meat, but these are rather expensive staples. Ready-to-use and concentrated infant formulas will cost somewhat less, with pasteurized whole cows' milk, evaporated cows' milk and powdered milk costing even less. Cereals have anywhere from 14 to 28 mg of added iron per dry ounce (10 to 12 tablespoons).[22] This iron is in the form of the phytate or sodium pyrophosphate salts which allow a very limited amoung of absorption.[1,13] Fortified cereals are more expensive and less convenient than regular cereals, so most mothers do not use them after the infant is 6 months old and is eating table food.

Bread could be fortified, but using large quantities of bread as an iron source would supply excessive carbohydrate. Cows' milk appears to be a logical choice for supplementation because it is both economical and practical. In fact, in the past, iron fortified milk was commercially available. Mothers found it

TABLE 26.2
Iron Content of Foods[a]

Food	Normal Absorption %	Elemental Iron Content
Breast milk	10 (4-12)	1-1.5 mg/liter
Cows' milk	9.1 (4-12)	0.5 mg/liter
Iron enriched milk	10.6	10-15 mg/liter
Beef liver (raw)	20	6.6 mg/100 g
Iron supplemented cereals (mixed), oatmeal, rice	12 (0-25)	2.5-5 (1.2-17 mg/30 g)
Chicken liver	8	7.4 mg/100 g
Chicken muscle	10	1.8 mg/100 g
Green and yellow vegetables		0.05-.28 mg/15 cc
Strained meats	10	0.23-.56 mg/15 cc
Fruits		0.1-.32 mg/15 cc
Egg yolk	11	1 mg/egg
Egg (scrambled)	5-17	1 mg/egg
Ferrous sulfate	12-15	20%

[a]Average infant diet at six months of age = 1.1 mg iron per kg weight.

objectionable because it turned dark when heated and it also turned rancid sooner than regular milk.[18] In approximately 25% of infants, as mentioned before, the milk causes occult blood loss due to GI inflammation and iron loss frequently was greater than the intake.[1,13] The small amount of phosphate in milk does not significantly alter iron absorption.[1] Anemic infants given fortified milk have shown increased hemoglobin levels. Iron-supplemented whole cows' milk should be used initially and continued in those infants who tolerate it.

The American Academy of Pediatrics, realizing that the fortified foods available for the past 30 years have done little to alter the incidence of anemia, have recommended the addition of iron to infant feedings.[12] The Academy states that iron supplements should be given in infant formulas throughout the first year of life.[12] The recommended dose of iron for full term infants is 1 mg per kg per day. For low birth weight and premature infants, the dose is 2 mg per kg per day with a maximal of 15 mg per day for both groups. The fortified formulas such as Similac with Iron and Enfamil with Iron, contain between 10 to 15 mg per liter. The use of these formulas or evaporated milk would eliminate the problem caused in some infants by whole cows' milk.

If the anemia has progressed, dietary sources of iron will prove to be inadequate for treatment. Specific iron therapy must be used in these cases.

TREATMENT

The treatment for iron deficiency anemia is specific and generally produces excellent results. Pierre Blaud in Paris recommended the first treatment for iron deficiency anemia around 1830. His pills contained a combination of ferrous sulfate and potassium carbonate with a recommended adult dose of 12 pills per day which gave a total of 800 mg of iron. Oral iron (Tables 26.3 and 26.4) is preferred in the therapeutic doses of 4 to 6 mg per kg per day in three divided doses. The divided doses allow for full utilization of the iron for hemoglobin synthesis.[8] Regeneration of hemoglobin proceeds at a maximal rate of 0.3 g of hemoglobin/100 ml of blood per day.[23] Hemoglobin contains 0.34% iron (1 g of hemoglobin contains 3.4 mg of iron) and a 10-pound infant with 500 cc of blood could optimally produce 1.5 g of hemoglobin per day. He would need just over 5 mg of body iron to do this. With anemia, the absorption of iron is increased from a normal of 10% ingested iron to over 20%. This means the infant should ingest about 25 mg of iron per day to obtain the required 5 mg of iron.

Most of the problems associated with iron ingestion can be easily overcome. Gastric irritation can be circumvented by initiating treatment with low doses and slowly increasing the dose.[5,23] Taking the iron preparation after meals is also helpful in reducing gastric irritation.[19] Tooth staining from liquid preparations can be avoided by either brushing the child's teeth,[19] rinsing his mouth or utilizing a straw. Taste problems can be overcome by incorporating the preparation in fruit juices or milk. Chewable tablets, which are well accepted by children, are available and can be utilized effectively.

Satisfactory response may be heralded by an increase in appetite and disposition days before there is any evidence of hemoglobin regeneration.[13,23] Hemoglobin and hematocrit changes may occur as early as 4 days after commencement of treatment, depending on the severity of anemia. Reticulocyte levels may rise in 4 to 6 days with a peak effect at 9 to 12 days[5,19]; this increase is inversely proportional to the severity of the anemia.[5] By the end of 3 weeks, there should be an increase in hemoglobin of approximately 2 g/100 ml of blood.[5,23] Adequate treatment allows the return of blood values to normal and the replenishment of iron stores. This requires about 2 months each or a total treatment time of

TABLE 26.4
Common Oral Iron Liquids

Proprietary Name	Active Ingredient	Elemental Iron mg/cc
Mol-Iron Liquid	Ferrous sulfate	10
Mol-Iron Drops	Ferrous sulfate	25
Feosol Elixir	Ferrous sulfate	8
Fer-In-Sol Syrup	Ferrous sulfate	6
Fer-In-Sol Drops	Ferrous sulfate	25
Fergon Elixir	Ferrous gluconate	7
Chel-Iron Liquid	Ferro cholinate	10
Chel-Iron Drops	Ferro cholinate	25
Ferrolip Pediatric Syrup	Ferro cholinate	4
Ferrolip Pediatric Drops	Ferro cholinate	25
Ferro Drops	Ferrous lactate	25

TABLE 26.3
Common Oral Iron Tablets

Proprietary Name	Active Ingredient	Elemental Iron per Tablet	Iron %
Ferrous sulfate, U.S.P. (generic)	Ferrous sulfate heptahydrate	60 mg/300 mg	20
Feosol (initial formulation)	Ferrous sulfate dried	60 mg/200 mg	30
Fergon	Ferrous gluconate	39 mg/325 mg	11.5
Ircon	Ferrous fumarate	66 mg/200 mg	33
Chel-Iron	Ferrocholinate	39 mg/333 mg	12

around 4 months. Interestingly enough, iron does not stimulate erythropoiesis but plays only a passive role in red cell production and hemoglobin synthesis.[24] A failure to increase hemoglobin levels by 2 g/100 ml in 3 weeks indicates treatment failure due to one of the following factors:

1. Use of inadequate dosages.
2. Failure of the parents or guardian to administer the preparations correctly.
3. Coexistent disease which interferes with absorption or utilization of the iron, e.g., infections, inflammation or malignant disease.
4. Continued uncompensated, active blood loss.
5. An error in diagnosis.

The first two factors are the most common reasons for failure in children. If there is no response and no reason for failure found after 6 weeks, treatment should be discontinued and more definitive diagnosis sought.[23]

Ferrous sulfate, ferrous fumarate and ferrous gluconate are the preferred preparations because of low cost and palatability. The decreased incidence of side effects claimed for other products is due to the fact that they contain less iron per dose. The combination hematinic products add nothing to the therapy of iron deficiency anemia except cost. Folic acid, vitamin B_{12}, and vitamin B_6 may even mask an underlying disease state.[16] Trace elements, liver extract, surface-active agents and bile acids have no rational basis for use.[23] Cobalt is contraindicated because of the possible deleterious effect on thyroid function (hypothyroidism and goiter).[23] The sustained release iron preparations can not be recommended because of decreased and unreliable absorption and increased cost.[16] Other agents used with iron may increase or decrease iron absorption. Ascorbic acid in 500 to 1000-mg doses has been shown to increase iron absorption by approximately 10% (a 20% absorption is increased to 22%).[3,23] However, added ascorbic acid is unnecessary because of increased cost and limited enhancement of absorption of iron.[23] Phosphorous will decrease iron absorption by forming insoluble precipitates.[25] Calcium will increase iron absorption by precipitating phosphorous.[25] Dietary protein may decrease absorption if it induces inflammation,[1,13] but amino acids alone will combine with iron to increase iron absorption.[3] Antacids and stool softeners may decrease absorption, but the clinical significance of this is not known. Hydrochloric acid, by lowering the pH in the stomach, will increase iron absorption by preventing the formation of insoluble gels. Iron absorption can occur even with achlorhydria, so this effect may not be as important as once thought.[26] Fructose will increase iron absorption, probably owing to its metabolism to furnish energy for utilization in iron absorption.[3] Glucose and galactose have no effect on iron absorption.[3] Finally, a partial or complete gastrectomy will decrease iron absorption.

There are indications for the use of parenteral products in lieu of the preferred oral route:

1. A failure to absorb oral preparations.
2. Inability to tolerate adequate oral iron intake.
3. Recurrent GI blood loss exacerbated by the iron.
4. GI disease states which contraindicate iron use (ulcers, colitis).
5. Uncomplicated, well documented iron deficiency anemia unresponsive to prolonged adequate oral iron therapy.
6. An unreliable patient.

However, parenteral iron should not be used unless there is no doubt that one of the above indications truly exists. The risk of allergic reactions, the increased incidence of side effects and the possibility of permanently stained skin are obvious reasons to avoid these preparations. For children, iron dextran, preferably given intramuscularly, is the only recommended product (Table 26.5). Side effects associated with this product include local pain, headache, fever, urticaria, angioneurotic edema, arthralgias, systemic illness with fever and inguinal lymphadenopathy. Fatal anaphylaxis has also occurred.[27]

The regeneration of hemoglobin with parenteral perparations is no more rapid than with oral products, but the parenteral products have the advantage of a smaller number of administrations instead of months of oral consumption.[28] A general dosing regimen and formulas used for computing iron replacements are depicted in Table 26.6.[21] The dose is given intramuscularly by a special method in daily aliquots of 50 to 100 mg. Twenty to 40% of the dose may still be found in the injection area

TABLE 26.5
Common Iron Injectables

Proprietary Name	Active Ingredient	Elemental Iron mg/cc	Average Recommended Dosage	Comments
Jectofer	Iron sorbitol-citric acid complex	50	1.5 mg/kg/day I.M. only (adult)	Not recommended for pediatric use
Imferon	Iron dextran complex	50	25 mg/day I.M. or I.V. (empirical pediatric); may be given once a week or at other suitable intervals, *e.g.,* every other day; maximal dosage per injection should not exceed 100 mg for children	Acceptable for pediatric use; use special I.M. administration technique to avoid staining skin

40 to 50 days after an injection. A second course of therapy is indicated only if there is a recurrence of anemia or a treatment failure occurs. Where an immediate need to raise hemoglobin values exists, an infusion of whole blood or packed cells is indicated. Severe blood loss, severe infection and high fever are reasons for blood infusions.[16] It should be noted, however, that the indiscriminate use of iron can cause hemochromatosis and siderosis.

Iron preparations must be kept out of the reach of children. Serious toxicities have occurred from accidental ingestions of oral preparations with ensuing severe bleeding and, occasionally, death. As little as 15 tablets of ferrous sulfate 200 mg have caused shock due to massive GI hemorrhage and death in a few hours.[29] Deferoxamine, a specific iron chelater, can effectively reduce tissue iron levels and has been successfully used to treat acute iron toxicity in children.[4]

PROGNOSIS

If simple iron deficiency exists, the prognosis with adequate iron treatment is excellent.

All physiological parameters will soon return to normal, restoring the individual to his prior health. If there are attendant abnormal conditions, such as continued blood loss, other deficiency states, congenital malformations or infection, the outcome of treatment with iron therapy alone may prove to be unrewarding. Succesful treatment of underlying disease combined with iron therapy will achieve optimal results.

CONCLUSION

The high incidence of iron deficiency anemia in this country obligates the health care team to actively treat affected individuals and provide prophylactic iron supplementation to prevent the development of anemia. Careful investigation must be carried out to find the most efficacious means for doing this. For the present, all infants prone to developing anemia because of poor diet, low birth weight or prematurity must be supplemented with iron. The American Academy of Pediatrics' recommendation for medicinal iron of 1 to 2 mg per kg per day should be followed. The supplemen-

TABLE 26.6

Computation of Parenteral Iron Replacement

$$\text{Dose} = \frac{\text{B.V. } (12.5\text{-H}) \times 3.4 \times 1.5}{100}$$

or

$$\text{Dose} = \frac{(12.5\text{-H})\ 80\text{W} \times 3.4 \times 1.5}{100}$$

B.V. = blood volume
H = observed hemoglobin
3.4 = 3.4 mg fe/1g hgb
1.5 = for replacing iron stores
w = weight/kg

For calculating iron requirements in children, the above formulas can be utilized or the empiric doses listed below can be given.

Dose =   100 mg iron in less than 6-months olds
         200 mg iron in less than 12-month olds
         300 mg iron in 12-24 month olds
         400 mg iron in older than 24-month olds

tation or fortification of foods with iron is attractive but presents problems. The foods now fortified have been relatively ineffective in reducing the incidence of anemia. This may be due to a number of reasons, including the lack of parent education in their optimal usage, the unavailability of the iron in these preparations or the prohibitive cost for routine use. What quantity of iron should be added to dietary sources? If food provides 1 mg per kg, it will be insufficient for the minority of infants who most need iron. If 2 mg per kg is used for dietary fortification, the majority of infants would receive twice their need. Until a satisfactory answer to dietary supplementation is found, iron drops, at a cost of about 1¢ per day, should be added to the infant's diet.

REFERENCES

1. Filer, L. J., Jr.: The case for iron supplements in infant feeding regimens. Hosp. Practice, 6: 79, 1971.
2. Lahey, M. E., and Wilson, J. F.: The etiology of iron deficiency anemia in infants—a reappraisal. J. Pediatr., 69: 339, 1966.
3. Maurer, A. M.: Pediatric Hematology, Ed. 1, p. 195. McGraw-Hill Book Co., New York, 1969.
4. Jacobs, A.: Iron balance and its disorders. Proc. R. Soc. Med., 63: 1215, 1970.
5. Brown, E. B.: Clinical pharmacology of drugs used in the treatment of iron deficiency anemia. Pharmacol. Physicians, 2: 1, 1968.
6. Crichton, R.: Ferritin: structure, synthesis and function. N. Engl. J. Med., 284: 1413, 1971.
7. Luke, C. G., Davis, P. S., and Deller, D. J.: Change in gastric iron-binding protein (Gastroferrin) during iron-deficiency anemia. Lancet, 1: 926, 1967.
8. Woodruff, C.: The utilization of iron administered orally. Pediatrics, 27: 194, 1961.
9. Hoag, M. S., Wallerstein, R. O., and Pollycove, M.: Occult blood loss in iron deficiency anemia of infancy. Pediatrics, 27: 199, 1961.
10. O'Brien, R., and Pearson, H. A.: Physiologic anemia of the newborn infant. J. Pediatr., 79: 132, 1971.
11. Pearson, H. A.: Life-span of the fetal red blood cell. J. Pediatr., 70: 166, 1967.
12. Committee on Nutrition: Iron balance and requirements in infancy. Pediatrics, 43: 134, 1969.
13. Anon: Iron Nutrition in Infancy, Report of the 62nd Ross Conference. Ross Laboratories, Columbus, Ohio, 1970.
14. Woodruff, C. W., and Clark, J. L.: The role of fresh cow's milk in iron deficiency. I. Albumin turnover in infants with iron deficiency anemia. Am. J. Dis. Chil., 124: 18, 1972.
15. Woodruff, C. W., Wright, S. W., and Wright, R. P.: The role of fresh cows' milk in iron deficiency. II. Comparison of fresh cows' milk with a prepared formula. Am. J. Dis. Child., 124: 26, 1972.
16. Gellis, S. S., and Kagan, B. M.: Current Pediatric Therapy, Ed. 5, p. 252. W. B. Saunders Co., Philadelphia, 1971.
17. Schulman, I.: Iron requirements in infancy. J.A.M.A., 175: 118, 1961.
18. Anon: Iron-fortified formulas for infants. Med. Lett. Drugs Ther., 13: 65, 1971.
19. Nelson, W. E., Vaughan, V., and McKay, R. J.: Textbook of Pediatrics, Ed. 9. W. B. Saunders Co., Philadelphia, 1969.
20. Hunter, R. E., and Smith, N. J.: Hemoglobin and hematocrit values in iron deficiency in infancy. J. Pediatr., 81: 710, 1972.
21. Ross, J. D.: Treatment and prevention of iron deficiency of infancy. N. Engl. J. Med., 266: 1372, 1962.
22. Anderson, T. A., and Fomon, S. J.: Commercially prepared infant cereals: nutritional considerations. J. Pediatr., 78: 788, 1971.
23. Shirkey, H. E. (editor): Pediatric Therapy, Ed. 4, p. 668. C. V. Mosby Co., St. Louis, 1972.
24. Bothwell, T. H., and Finch, C.: Iron Metabolism, Ed. 1. Little Brown and Co., Boston, 1962.
25. Anderson, H. D., McDonough, K. G., and Elvehjem, C. A.: Relation of the dietary calcium-phosphorous ratio to iron assimilation. J. Lab. Clin. Med., 25: 464, 1960.
26. Jacobs, P., Bothwell, T., and Charlton, R. N.: Role of hydrochloric acid in iron absorption. J. Appl. Physiol., 19: 187, 1964.
27. Becker, C. E., MacGregor, R. R., Walker, K. S., and Mandl, J. S.: Fatal anaphylaxis after intramuscular iron dextran. Ann. Int. Med., 65: 745, 1966.

28. McCurdy, P. R.: Oral and parenteral iron therapy. J. A. M. A., 191: 859, 1965.
29. Gleason, M. N., Gosselin, R. E., Hodge, H. C., and Smith, R. P.. Clinical Toxicology of Commercial Products, Ed. 3, p. 107, Williams and Wilkins Co., Baltimore, 1969.

chapter 27

APLASTIC ANEMIA

Larry E. Patterson, Pharm.D.
Perry G. Rigby, M.D.

The term "aplastic anemia," has been applied to diverse clinical syndromes that have similarities in peripheral blood manifestations but with a variety of etiologies and accompanying bone marrow abnormalities. The term is generally used, however, to indicate a severe anemia and hyporegenerative bone marrow manifested by pancytopenia.[1] In this discussion, aplastic anemia will be used in this context.

CLASSIFICATION

Patients with aplastic anemia are arranged by etiology and by age. The patients with hereditary and acquired types may manifest only anemia with a hypoplastic marrow or pancytopenia with a marked depression of marrow cellularity and function. The genetic abnormalities include a hypoplastic anemia of Blackfan and Diamond, a hypoplastic anemia associated with pancytopenia, some conditions with congenital deformity such as Fanconi's anemia and some hypoplastic anemias without congenital deformities such as those described by Estren and Dameshek.[2]

When an underlying disorder cannot be identified, the possibility that a cytotoxic agent is involved should be considered. For example, the antimetabolites regularly produce aplastic anemia in patients with malignant disorders such as leukemia, lymphoma and solid tumors and sometimes in patients with autoimmune and other disorders requiring these agents. Such drug-induced aplastic anemias may be either primary or idiosyncratic. However, it is difficult to prove that medications are the causative agents unless the patient is exposed to the medication a second time with equivalent results. Obviously, this is not a feasible diagnostic approach. Therefore, to arrive at a drug etiology, the patient should be removed from all possible agents and the bone marrow examined. The marrow of patients with drug-induced aplastic anemia is identical to the marrow of patients with idiopathic aplastic anemia. It is also characteristic of the former to be associated with pancytopenia. Thus, a definitive diagnosis can not be made until all nondrug causes are ruled out.

Some medications produce aplastic anemia as a side effect presumably from an idiosyncratic reaction. Chloramphenicol is certainly the leading drug in this category. This liability must be considered carefully and placed in perspective when contemplating the use of this drug. Medications other than chloramphenicol have also been shown to have a marrow-toxic effect. These include phenylbutazone, the gold compounds, quinacrine, sulfonamides, oral hypoglycemic agents, chlorpromazine, mepazine and the sulfones.[3]

Some chemical agents such as insecticides, hair sprays, benzene and benzol,[4] fertilizers and a host of other pollutants have been implicated as well. Other causes of aplastic anemia include infection, although it is often transient in this circumstance, but infectious hepatitis has been implicated as a cause of prolonged aplastic anemia. Other viral infections also have been suspected from time to time.

The myeloproliferative disorders deserve special consideration in aplastic anemia. Aplasia, after a period of time, may continue to shift to erythroleukemia, acute granulocytic leukemia or some other myeloproliferative change. Although the preleukemic state occasionally is recognized by careful inspection of the bone marrow, even when the usual manifestations of leukemia are not present, more often it can not be ascertained that it will indeed progress to a myeloproliferative disorder. Patients with paroxysmal nocturnal hemoglobinuria also can show aplastic marrows at times, and these marrows have been shown to transform into acute granulocytic leukemia. Also, aplasia is a sequela of malignancy itself.

A hypoplastic bone marrow may include only red cells, only platelets or only white blood cells, but usually combinations of these are seen and, on occasion, all three are depressed in the peripheral blood. While we are concerned here only with those elements associated with anemia, it should be mentioned that the complications of drug therapy can involve any of the peripheral blood elements to some degree.

INCIDENCE

The incidence of aplastic anemia in the general population is very low; the mortality rate is about two deaths per 1,000,000 people per year. However, this statistic does not include the risk of death from aplastic anemia as a result of exposure to chloramphenicol. The risk of fatal aplastic anemia seems to be 13 times higher after the use of this drug.[5]

SYMPTOMATOLOGY

The severity of symptoms is related to the relative absence of normal cells. There are no symptoms that are primarily attributable to the aplastic process in the marrow so the severity of the anemia and the resulting complications are responsible for the patient's symptoms. Christian, Cornelius and Fortner[6] in their article on the acute leukemias discussed the general kinds of symptoms that occur in the patient with a reduction in the number of normal cells. These symptoms fall into two general classifications: the manifestation of infection because of a reduced white blood cell count and the occurrence of bleeding due to thrombocytopenia. In addition, the severity of the anemia itself can contribute to the symptomatology and eventually may result in congestive heart failure and hypoxemia.

PATHOPHYSIOLOGY AND DIAGNOSIS

Since aplastic anemia includes a number of syndromes with various etiologies, the pathophysiology must be understood. The basic pathological process is a defect in the production of normal blood cells which may lead to an adverse change in the cellular environment of the marrow. Studies by Crosby[7] and others indicated that with specific damage to the bone marrow cells, regrowth of the marrow cells following hypoplasia eventually may be complicated by a lack of normal cells when the marrow environment has damaged specifically. Examination of the bone marrow is thus the most important clinical step for a differential diagnosis and for an assessment of the degree of damage and possible recovery from the disease. Attention to iron stores[8] is also appropriate, since this pattern can give clues to the extent and degree of damage and the time sequence involved.

Dr. Frederick Stohlman[1] described the following pathophysiological abnormalities as being the functional disorders of aplastic anemia. These include changes of the marrow cells, changes in the marrow environment, failure of regulatory mechanisms such as erythropoietin feedback control arrangements and the presence of inhibitors or antibodies to a specific regulatory mechanism. Also an abnormal clone of cells, such as those found in the myeloproliferative disorders, is always a consideration, even in those patients who appear to have a drug etiology.

Perhaps the best studied cause of drug-induced aplastic anemia is that of chloramphenicol.[9] It has been postulated that chloramphenicol bears a structural similarity to the pyrimidine nucleotides, specifically uridine 5'-phosphate and competes with messenger ribonucleic acid (RNA) for the ribosomal binding site. Chloramphenicol may also stimulate the specific transfer RNA for phenylalanine. This false molecule may interfere with the translational step at the messenger RNA ribosomal level.[10] As a result of these biochemical interferences, chloramphenicol is an inhibitor of protein synthesis. This effect, while responsible for its antibiotic activity, also adversely affects the human bone marrow. Clinically, these are noted as leukopenia, anemia, decreased hematopoiesis and thrombocytopenia. All patients who receive chloramphenicol will exhibit these effects on RNA-protein synthesis if the dosage and duration of administration is sufficient. For example, decreased hematopoiesis can be demonstrated in most patients with dosages above 4 g per day. However, the aplastic anemia is not a normal response but rather an idiosyncratic reaction. While presumably based on the RNA-protein synthesis effects of the drug, there is something present in the susceptible individual that allows the toxicity to progress to aplasia, while in others, it never goes beyond leukopenia despite high dosages and long duration of therapy.

This idiosyncratic reaction perhaps is due to certain genetic variables. It has been shown by Weisberger[11] that clearance of chloramphenicol from the blood stream is diminished in some patients who have experienced aplasia secondary to chloramphenicol exposure.

Chloramphenicol toxicity such as leukopenia but not aplasia usually is related to the dosage received and the duration of time that the drug is administered.[12,13] However, some patients may show signs of toxicity after a few doses of chloramphenicol, while other patients may have received sizable dosages of the drug and show no signs of toxicity. Even though aplastic anemia resulting from chloramphenicol toxicity may not be reversible, signs of aplasia nevertheless should be monitored since the damage may occasionally be reversible in nature. Bone marrow in the early stages of chloramphenicol toxicity shows a lack of normal cells without stromal involvement or destruction. Such biopsy of the bone marrow is the only effective monitoring device to differentiate the underlying processes.

THERAPY

The therapy of aplastic anemia is generally nonspecific and supportive. The most important principle is to discontinue the suspected offending agent, whether it be a drug, chemical, hair dyes, sprays or other environmental hazard. Most patient die of bone marrow failure, but some patients will recover with time, and a few will do just as well without the addition of medications. Prednisone has shown some benefit, mainly in those patients who are severely anemic and have either a shortened red cell survival time or severe thrombocytopenia. Prednisone has a positive effect on capillaries if it is administered in the early stages of the disease. It strengthens capillaries and make them less fragile. The effect may benefit some patients by decreasing the chances of bleeding due to thrombocytopenia.

Androgens have an effect on the red cell mass.[14-16] It may take up to 6 months to see this effect, although usually some change will be seen in 2 months. Macrocytosis tends to occur with an increase in erythropoiesis.[17] Reticulocytosis generally accompanies a rise and a stabilization of hemoglobin concentration. This rise in hemoglobin occurs in perhaps 50% of the patients treated whose cause of anemia does not involve severe hemolysis or blood loss. Androgens also may have an effect by increasing the amount of erythropoietin present; however, this contention has been disputed. The effects of androgens on leukopenia and thrombocytopenia are not so well documented. These drugs also carry some risk of liver damage whenever they are used. Jaundice with increases in serum glutamic oxalacetic transaminase (SGOT), serum glutamic pyruvic transaminase (SGPT) and bilirubin may occur.

The addition of prednisone to the androgen therapy has little bearing on the outcome of aplastic anemia in some patients. The over-all results of prednisone-androgen-treated patients has not been good. The mean survival time is about 6 months[18]; however, some patients have lived a year and other patients have done quite well postdiagnosis. The remission rate of treated patients is less than 50%. Patients tend to succumb because of infections and hemorrhage.

Supportive therapy has improved with the use of blood products over the years. The use of packed cells is obvious for patients with severe anemia and can be typed and given on a chronic basis to many patients.

If there is a constant transfusion requirement, it is often better to space it at weekly or biweekly intervals, instead of giving massive transfusions on one occasion and waiting until the patient becomes severely anemic before doing so again. The possible reactions from transfusions should be considered, including the hazards of infectious hepatitis, sensitivity to antigens with fever, circulation overload, iron accumulation and infections.

The transfusion of platelets in large numbers is a more recent undertaking and is used successfully in those patients who have a relatively normal platelet lifespan with an aplastic marrow. Platelets can be typed by the human leukocyte antigen (HLA) typing mechanism and specifically identified for infusion. Often this procedure requires donation from relatives on a continuing basis with platelet-phoresis.

The transfusion of white cells has been attempted on a number of occasions. This type of transfusion is more difficult because more blood has to be processed to obtain a significant number of white cells. A donor with chronic granulocytic leukemia with a very high white count can be identified for utilization. A centrifuge to concentrate white cells has been used experimentally in an attempt to improve the concentration process and to obtain normal white cells for patients who are in need of them because of very low leukocyte count and infections. The transplantation of bone marrow has been attempted on numerous occasions but with minimal success. Overcoming the transplant barriers by HLA matching and improving the environment with reverse isolation and life islands has been undertaken.

The use of splenectomy in patients who have a shortened red cell survival time may be appropriate, especially in those patients with splenomegaly who have received considerable amounts of blood. While the splenectomy may not totally correct the red cell survival time and increase platelet lifespan, it may decrease the need for transfusions and may improve the situation considerably in combination with other therapy. The use of antibiotics is appropriate in those patients who have infections, especially when the specific organisms can be identified and the appropriate antibiotics chosen. Some patients in the hospital may need reverse isolation to prevent the onset of infections.

Therapy with numerous other agents has been tried. The use of vitamins such as folic acid, vitamin B_{12}, and pyridoxine has generally shown no benefit in patients with true aplastic anemia. If patients have other syndromes with hypocellular marrow, such as primary refractory anemia, or if they lack specific vitamins, these agents may be beneficial. The specific deficiency should be identified with appropriate testing, although a trial of these medications generally is not harmful.

The use of iron in aplastic anemia generally is not indicated since these patients usually have markedly increased iron stores. Phenylalanine has been used specifically in those patients who have toxicity with chloramphenicol. The literature is somewhat conflicting, although some patients do appear to improve when large doses of phenylalanine are administered orally.[19]

There has been an attempt to treat patients with phytohemagglutinin (PHA), a known stimulant of normal lymphocytes identified as T or thymus-derived cells. This stimulant causes fever and produces toxicity in patients, but several have shown apparent improvement after the use of PHA. PHA generally is not used, however, since it is postulated that such patients properly supported would regain a functional marrow. Early lymphocytes, thought to be stem cells, are present if PHA works.[20]

Antimetabolites have been used in patients thought to be suffering from preleukemic myeloproliferative syndromes or possibly autoimmune disorders. If an autoimmune disorder directed against the precursor erythrocytic cells can be identified, then prednisone and other antimetabolites might be successful. The use of erythropoietin has been postulated as an aid in aplastic anemia, although no controlled therapeutic trials have been performed at this time.

PROGNOSIS AND FOLLOW-UP

Recovery from aplastic anemia depends on the underlying etiology and severity of this disorder as well as considerations for treatment. The deletion of specific causative agents may allow recovery to proceed without therapy. Recovery may be in terms of a total, partial or minimal remission, or death may ensue. The recovery varies with the blood elements involved, namely erythrocytes, granulocytes and thrombocytes.

It is difficult to predict the outcome of aplastic anemia, although generally those patients with the most marrow damage, specifically to the stromal portion of the marrow, are the most difficult to treat and have the worst prognosis. Those patients who have severe depletion of normal cells from the peripheral blood, with counts at minimal levels, also have the most difficulty in survival. Follow-up includes visits for monitoring the blood count which should include examination of all the elements. Family counseling should be considered regarding both the patient's problem and possible genetic abnormalities.

CONCLUSION

Aplastic anemia is a term used to describe a wide range of clinical disorders characterized by hypoplasia of the bone marrow and the reduction of normal cell counts in the peripheral blood. Its causes include idiopathic, genetic abnormalities, cytotoxic agents, medications, infections, chemicals, myeloproliferative disorders and others. The symptomatology is the result of an absence of normal cells. The complications of the anemia contribute to the patient's condition. The manifestations include various infections with granulocytopenia and/or bleeding from a reduction in thrombocytes.

The pathophysiology is related to the extent of damage to the stromal area of the bone marrow. A biopsy is important to differentiate the degree of damage and to predict the extent of recovery. The hematopoietic system may be suppressed to the extent that the patient's hypoplastic bone marrow will have difficulty in recovering. Supportive therapy generally is needed and employed. Transfusions and antibiotics can improve the patient with severe anemia or infections, respectively. Recovery depends upon the etiology of the aplastic anemia and the amount of damage that has been done.

REFERENCES

1. Stohlman, F. J. L.: Aplastic anemia. Blood, 40: 282, 1972.
2. Leavell, B. S., and Thorup, O. A.: Fundamentals of Clinical Hematology, Ed. 3, p. 157. W. B. Saunders Co., Philadelphia, 1971.
3. Leavell, B. S., and Thorup, O. A.: Fundamentals of Clinical Hematology, Ed. 3, p. 159. W. B. Saunders Co., Philadelphia, 1971.
4. Bowditch, M., and Elkins, H. B.: Chronic exposure to benzene (Benzol). I. The industrial aspects. J. Indust. Hyg. Toxicol., 21: 321, 1939.
5. Wallerstein, R. O., Condit, P. K., Kasper, C. K., Brown, J. W., and Morrison, F. R.: Statewide study of chloramphenicol therapy and fatal aplastic anemia. J.A.M.A., 208: 2045, 1969.
6. Christian, D. G., Cornelis, W. A., and Fortner, C. L.: The acute leukemias. J. Am. Pharm. Ass., NS 12: 476, 1972.
7. Crosby, W. H.: Experience with injured and implanted bone marrow; relation of function of structure. In Hemopoietic Cellular Proliferation, Ed. 1, p. 87, edited by F. J. Stohlman. Grune and Stratton, New York, 1970.
8. Armitage, J. O. and Rigby, P. G.: Why look at marrow iron stores? Current Med. Dialog, 655, 1971.
9. Bithell, T. C., and Wintrobe, M. M.: Drug-induced aplastic anemia. Semin. Hematol., 4: 194, 1967.
10. Weisberger, A. S., Wolfe, S., and Armentrout, S.: Inhibition of protein synthesis in mammalian cell free systems by chloramphenicol, J. Exp. Med., 120: 161, 1964.
11. Weisberger, A. S.: Mechanisms of action of chloramphenicol. J.A.M.A., 209: 97, 1969.
12. Saidi, P., Wallerstein, R. O., and Aggeler, P. M.: Effect of chloramphenicol on erythropoiesis. J. Lab. Clin. Med., 57: 247, 1961.
13. Yunis, A. A., and Bloomberg, G. R.: Chloramphenicol toxicity; clinical features and pathogenesis. Prog. Hematol., 4: 138, 1964.
14. McGuire, L. B.: Aplastic anemia in an adult with two remissions on androgen. Va. Med. Mon., 91: 207, 1964.
15. Silinik, S. J., and Firkin, B. G.: An analysis of hypoplastic anemia with special reference to the use of oxymetholone ("Adroyd") in its therapy. Aust. Ann. Med., 17: 224, 1968.
16. Gardner, F. H., and Pringle, J. C., Jr.: Androgens and erythropoiesis. I. Preliminary clinical observations. Arch. Intern. Med., 107: 846, 1961.
17. Gordon, A. S., Mirand, E. A., Wenig, J., Katz, R., and Zajani, E.: Androgen actions on erythropoiesis. Ann. N.Y. Acad. Sci., 149: 318, 1968.
18. Li, F. P., Alter, B. P., and Nathan, D. G.: The mortality of acquired aplastic anemia in children. Blood, 40: 153, 1972.
19. Ingall, D., Sherman, J. D., Cockburn, F., and Klein, R.: Amelioration by ingestion of phenylalanine of toxic effects of chloramphenicol on bone marrow. N. Engl. J. Med., 272: 180, 1965.
20. Humble, J. G.: The treatment of aplastic anaemia with phytohaemagglutinin. Lancet, 1: 1345, 1964.

Neurological and Psychological Disorders

chapter **28**

EPILEPSY

Ronald R. Conte, Pharm.D.

Through the ages the word "epilepsy" has taken on very diverse connotations. In the absence of real knowledge of the disease, man's imagination has been allowed to wander freely creating bizarre concepts about the epileptic state. Even today, unfortunately, relatively little is known about the disease.

It was not treated as a medical disorder until the beginning of the 19th Century. Before that time, it was described as the "sacred disease" or the "falling sickness." Long before the days of Hippocrates, around 2,000 B.C., the Egyptians noted strange mannerisms in certain offspring, very similar to the peculiar behavior of their parents. The Greeks observed the foul works of the gods upon individuals who seemed to have been "seized." During this time the "sacred disease" was surrounded by a great many mystical and magical beliefs that prevailed until the time of modern therapeutics. It was apparent to the Romans that epilepsy was due to the forces of evil spirits and so it was common practice to spit on the patient to ward off the evil. Hippocrates ridiculed the fraudulent practices of the magician's work that nurtured the concept of the "sacred disease" and claimed that "the sacred disease appears to be no more divine, no more sacred than other diseases . . ." However, the mysticism which surrounded epilepsy continued to spread through the dark ages and up to the 17th Century.

The Christians believed that the epileptic was possessed by the devil. If the usual treatment of enemas, purges, plasters and sweatings failed, exorcism was deemed necessary. Scientists of the time believed that unusual attacks of certain individuals were due to the forces of the moon, similar to the effects it had on the tides. Certain physicians believed that epilepsy was due to some sort of sexual instability or masturbation. One medical practitioner even published clinical findings that showed promising improvement in one of two male epileptics who were castrated. The only side effects recorded were some "personality" problems.

In the early 1800's, medical evidence connecting epilepsy with brain dysfunction was established. Doctor Hughlings Jackson, for whom one type of focal epilepsy was named, was the greatest contributor of his time. There have been great accomplishments since the time of Dr. Jackson. However, some false notions have persisted in the minds of a large proportion of the lay public. For example, it is not true that epilepsy can cause insanity, and it is not disfiguring or painful. It does not shorten one's life. The intelligence of an epileptic is equal to the intelligence of the majority of people: Socrates, Julius Caesar, Dostoevski, Napoleon and Van Gogh are just a few of the figures in history who have suffered from epilepsy.

The use of the electroencephalogram (EEG) has been a great asset in the diagnosis of seizures. However, it does have shortcomings. It will record impulses due to external stimuli and produce abnormal readings. The EEG also has shown abnormal brain dysfunction in 10% of the normal subjects tested. Though these problems add to the question of the electroencephalogram's validity, in the hands of an expert technician it can be accurately interpreted.

Many factors must be considered in the proper therapy of epileptics. The first error usually made is an inaccurate accounting of the predisposing events which may lead to an attack. This is one area in which a pharmacist can contribute significantly. Many chemicals, drugs and metabolic disorders can cause convulsions, but they are overlooked in the patient's history and therapy is prolonged or misdirected.

ETIOLOGY

Epilepsy consists of a complex set of symptoms, including altered states of consciousness, changes in behavior and perception and convulsions, and it is due to the activation or inactivation of neurons which exhibit an abnormal degree of electrical discharge.

Epilepsies are divided into two groups: generalized and focal, depending on the site of origin of abnormal discharge in the brain. In most cases, unfortunately, the site of discharge can not be pinpointed. Grand mal and petit mal are considered generalized seizures. All other seizures, including infantile spasms, psychomotor, myoclonic and sensory type, are grouped under focal epilepsies.

A number of factors can precipitate convulsions (Table 28.1). However, to the clinician's dismay, these factors are responsible for only a small proportion of seizures in patients. As a consequence, there is a tendency to treat all epilepsies as being idiopathic in origin since most physicians seldom see or find secondary seizure activity. Thus, in some patients the underlying cause may be overlooked, and they

TABLE 28.1
Examples of Causative Factors in Epilepsy[a]

---

1. Increase in intracranial pressure
2. Metabolic disorders (alkalosis, hypocalcemia, hypoglycemia, hypomagnesia, porphyria)
3. Infections (meningitis, encephalitis)
4. Trauma (50% of penetrating skull wounds produce at least one seizure)
5. Vascular accidents (hemorrhage, thrombosis, hypertension, systemic lupus erythematosis)
6. Tumors and cysts
7. Aneurysms
8. Chemicals (lead, carbon monoxide, iron tetrachlorethane, methyl bromide)
9. Drugs (atropine, abrupt barbiturate withdrawal, chlorpromazine, cycloserine, isoniazid, amphetamines, metrazol, cocaine, ergot, epinephrine, nitrous oxide, ether, chloroform, tricyclic antidepressants)

---

[a] Reprinted with permission from Ref. 1.

may be treated with anticonvulsants on the assumption that their disease is primary.

There are many precipitating factors which do not directly cause but which can trigger abnormal electrical discharges in susceptible individuals. Grand mal attacks can be precipitated by excessive hydration. Looking at a flickering, poorly adjusted television image also can hasten such a seizure. This has been documented in 4% of the child and 2% of the adult epileptics. In petit mal, the precipitating factor can be hyperventilation. This fact is taken advantage of in the clinical diagnosis of petit mal. A patient undergoing an electroencephalogram is asked to hyperventilate in order to record seizure activity.

In grand mal and focal epilepsies, convulsant drugs are common precipitating agents. The use of central stimulants, such as pentylenetetrazol or a strobe light, can foment grand mal or petit mal seizures. In addition to the above elements, other conditions, such as emotional stress, fatigue and febrile illnesses, may precipitate an attack in susceptible individuals. However, the most prevalent cause is the patient's irregular use of anticonvulsant medication. Pharmacist-assisted patient compliance could eliminate much of this latter problem.

PATHOPHYSIOLOGY

In the normal brain, propagation of nerve impulses is largely asynchronous; electrical charges fire sporadically and the electrical potential is close to zero. In an epileptic, a large number of brain impulses fire synchronously. The reason for this phenomenon is not yet known. The result of synchronous firing is a summation of activity resulting in an electrical potential which can be measured in microvolts. The abnormal synchrony of nerve impulses in the brain, increased amplitude and altered rate of discharge are termed paroxysmal cerebral dysrhythmia.

The seizure threshold is a function of the excitability of the neurons as well as the electrical instability of tissue. Interestingly enough, in studies where acetylcholine was applied directly to the brain, there was an increase in the brain's susceptibility to seizures.[2] These findings offer no conclusive evidence as to the extent of chemical involvement in the pathophysiology of epilepsy since, as yet, no laboratory abnormalities of acetylcholine levels can be detected in epileptics.

Other studies concerning brain lesions provide evidence that the focus of discharge is located not in the necrotic tissue but in the surrounding normal brain cells.

INCIDENCE

There are approximately 1,000,000 epileptics in the United States today, 90% of whom suffer grand mal seizures. Many epileptics suffer from multiple forms of the disease. The incidence of epilepsy is higher in males than females, but the ratio varies according to age at onset. The highest incidence of onset of convulsive disorders occurs in the preschool age group, and the lowest occurs in the 20- to 70-year-old group. Around 80 to 90% of the patients with epilepsy experience their first attack by the age of 20. If the first seizure begins after this age, it is usually due to a brain lesion.

There seems to be a genetic trait involved with grand mal and possibly petit mal epilepsy. In other seizure types, heredity has not been proven to be a factor. There is 1 in 40 chances of an epileptic being born to parents, one of whom is an epileptic.[3] If both parents are epileptics, the incidence increases.

DIAGNOSIS

All epilepsies are diagnosed on the basis of tests, such as an electroencephalogram; but probably the most useful information is the description of an attack noted by a witness to the event. The witness' report of the events which took place, their duration, the loss or retention of consciousness and the possible predisposing factors which may have led to the attack are of special interest in the diagnosis.

Laboratory values of blood, urine and cerebral spinal fluid are rarely abnormal in the true epileptic. Of importance to the pharmacist is the possibility of ingestion of various chemicals and drugs, such as lead and amphetamines, which can precipitate seizures. Before diagnosis of true epilepsy is made and treatment with anticonvulsants is begun, the possible etiological factors (discussed previously) must be ruled out.

The Electroencephalogram

In order to gain a proper understanding of a disease state, it is important to have some familiarity with the instruments used in diagnosing the disease. In epilepsy, the EEG is the most important diagnostic tool. It measures the electrical activity of the brain with the aid of electrodes applied to the scalp. No electrical current is applied to the brain. The electrical charges of the brain are multiplied by a factor of 100,000 by the instrument, which then produces a graphic recording of the impulses on paper.

The electrical impulses (measured in cycles per sec) are classified according to frequency, amplitude and wave form into five classes: alpha, beta, theta, delta and gamma. In the normal brain, alpha (α) rhythm (8 to 13 cycles per sec) is predominant. It can be recorded easily when the eyes are closed, but not when they are open, or when the patient is asleep. Beta (β) activity also is seen, and it is especially prevalent in normal individuals taking anticonvulsant drugs. The frequency of β rhythm is between 14 and 30 cycles per sec. Occasionally, theta (θ) activity (4 to 7 cycles per sec) may be seen, usually in persons in a drowsy state. Theta waves are more common in children. When seen consistently in an adult, they usually indicate the presence of disease. The wave forms with extremely high or low frequencies, gamma (γ), measuring 30 to 50 cycles per sec and delta (δ), with a frequency of 3 to 5 cycles per sec, are not seen with ordinary equipment and thus are not of diagnostic significance. See Figure 28.1 for different types of normal and abnormal EEG activity. The beta and theta activities are difficult to record using electrodes on the intact skull. On exposing the cortex of the brain, however, better recordings are obtained. It should be pointed out that the presence of a focus in one area of the cortex does not indicate specifically that the lesion originates in that area.

There are various ways in which a more ideal situation can be set up in order to record a more accurate EEG. One method involves deep breathing by the patient for 3 to 5 min. This will create a respiratory alkalosis which can activate abnormal activity not usually seen at rest in a susceptible individual. Other special recordings involve the use of barbiturates to

Alpha (normal)

Beta (normal)

Theta (seen more commonly in adult epileptics, but found in normal children)

Delta (observed primarily in disease)

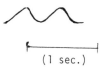

(1 sec.)

FIG. 28.1. Some examples of normal and abnormal EEG activity.

induce sleep. Focal necrosis, especially if temporal lobe epilepsy is suspected, can be detected easily during sleep. In establishing the existence of focal lesions of either the motor or sensory cortex, small amounts of analeptic drugs, such as pentylenetetrazol, can be used.

The scalp electroencephalogram is more complex to read than the electrocardiogram of the heart. Inaccuracy, usually due to electrical potentials produced by eye twitching and sweating, is always a problem with the EEG. Chemical impurities in the paste used to affix the wire plate to the scalp may also cause abnormal readings. Aside from the shortcomings mentioned, the EEG has proven to be an indispensable tool in the diagnosis of epilepsy.

CLINICAL FEATURES

Grand Mal Epilepsy

Grand mal is by far the most common form of epilepsy, occurring in around 90% of all epileptics (Table 28.2). The course and severity of this seizure type vary greatly from epileptic to epileptic. It may be so unimpressive as to be unnoticed by onlookers. In around 50% of these fits, there is an aura or warning signal telling the patient that an attack is beginning. Most epileptics do not have time to seek safety since the aura occurs only a brief moment before the full blown attack takes hold. Auras differ from patient to patient; they may consist of a strange smell, a tingling sensation or even a change in mood.

The aura leads to the tonic or muscular contraction phase. Air being forced up the larynx produces an audible cry-like sound which is not, however, an indication of pain. The epileptic may fall to the ground and lie rigid or tremble, usually for a period of 30 sec to a minute. Breathing ceases with only a slight amount of oxygen entering the lungs. The clonic movements that usually follow are slight at onset and gradually become more violent involving the whole body musculature. There may be some tongue biting and, because of the violent contractions, some involuntary urination or defecation. During this clonic phase, the patient is still cyanotic and comatose.

As the clonic phase dies away, the next stage—flaccid paralysis—begins. This actually is a resting phase involving the return of ventilation and color to the face. If the breathing becomes labored, foam and saliva which have collected during the clonic phase can be dislodged.

The epileptic will then pass into a deep sleep. After a period varying from a few minutes to hours, the patient will awaken and have no recollection of the preceding events. The severity and duration of seizures are highly variable: an attack can last from 1 to 30 min. Attacks may occur at a rate of one a day or as infrequently as one in every 10 years.

The grand mal fit may be centrocephalic in origin or the result of an abnormal impulse stemming from some cortical area. The type of aura is suggestive of the place of origin of the cortical impulse. For example, an aura of blurred vision suggests that the occipital lobe is

TABLE 28.2
Major Epilepsies

Type		Features	Duration
I.	Generalized		
	A. Grand mal	Aura (50% of the patients)	1-30 min
		Tonic phase—muscular contractions, cry-like sound, may fall to ground (rigid or tremble), cyanotic and comatose	
		Clonic phase—jerking which gradually worsens, involuntary urination, comatose, cyanotic	
		Flaccid paralysis—return of ventilation and facial color	
		Sleep, if not, then cerebral headaches always present	
	B. Petit mal	Triad of events:	90 sec
		1st—myoclonic jerks (involve all muscles)	
		2nd—akinetic phase (may fall to floor)	
		3rd—unawareness	
II.	Focal		
	A. Psychomotor (temporal lobe epilepsy)	Involves memory and familiarity problems, always conscious, automatism present, sometimes fugue states, sleep	30 sec to 2 min
	B. Jacksonian seizures	Sensory and muscle, usually unilateral; if bilateral, grand mal may result	3 min
	C. Other	"Involuntary" antisocial acts; infantile spasms (rapid akinetic and myoclonic convulsions)	Variable
III.	Status epilepticus	Continuous series of seizures without regaining consciousness	Variable

the origin of impulse. The abnormal brain discharges of grand mal usually occur in the thalamus and putamen areas of the brain.[5] The EEG pattern during a grand mal attack is very characteristic (Fig. 28.2A).

Petit Mal Epilepsy

The most common form of epilepsy in children and adolescents is petit mal. Some studies indicate as much as 6% of the general child population may suffer from this disease. The onset is usually at 4 to 8 years of age and rarely before 3 or after 15 years of age. It is possible for an epileptic to experience over 100 uncontrolled petit mal attacks a day.

Brain damage from petit mal is not significant. Unless the patient suffers from frequent and very violent attacks, the seizures are benign. However, if anticonvulsant therapy is only partially successful, grand mal epilepsy may develop around the age of puberty. In one study, only 31% of petit mal epileptics taking major anticonvulsants developed grand mal compared to 81% of those not taking these drugs.[6]

The petit mal attack usually occurs without warning. The fit may pass unnoticed. There may be a brief lapse of consciousness, a flickering of the eyelids or merely a faltering in speech. The attack lasts for about 3 or 4 sec. In a full blown attack, a triad of events has been described. First, there are myoclonic jerks

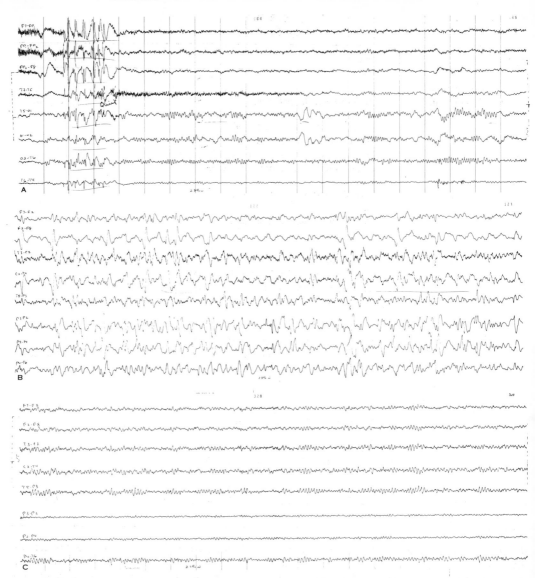

FIG. 28.2. A, Typical EEG pattern of grand mal epilepsy (16-year-old male); B, common EEG pattern of petit mal epilepsy (6½-year-old male); C, typical adult normal EEG pattern (20-year-old female).

involving muscles of the arms, legs and trunk. The patient may then lose his balance and fall to the floor and exhibit no movement; this is the second phase, or akinetic state. The third part consists of a transient loss of contact with the environment. The three phases may last up to 90 sec.

Myoclonic seizures exhibiting brief muscle contractions are considered a special subgroup of petit mal. The most common form of these attacks is experienced at night as the patient enters the threshold of sleep; the limbs give a sudden convulsive jerk which annoyingly awakens the individual. Normal people may also experience these contractions. However, in an epileptic, these symptoms may be related to some sort of organic brain disease.

The characteristic spike and wave EEG of petit mal (3 cycles per sec) is shown in Figure 28.2B. The slow wave is due to an abnormal discharge from the medial part of the putamen, and the spike is from the anterior part.

Psychomotor Epilepsy

Psychomotor epilepsy is often referred to as temporal lobe epilepsy. The onset of psychomotor attacks is from 11 to 15 years of age. The duration is from 30 sec to 2 min. The focus of abnormal discharge is usually found in the anterior part of the temporal lobe. The temporal lobe stores memory and complex events which may be suddenly relived in the mind of the epileptic. Problems of familiarity and unfamiliarity have also been revealed. This type of attack has been compounded by the occurrence of supervening grand mal seizures.

Because so many diverse things happen during a psychomotor attack, an onlooker may not recognize it as such. The patient may turn his head for a moment in one direction or another as if some other individual is speaking to him. He may stretch his fingers to grasp an invisible object. He may even complete complex tasks. Although his outward appearance may be normal and he is conscious throughout, he is in a type of dream state. This phenomenon is known as automatism.

This attack, like others, customarily ends in sleep or with a clouding of the senses. The epileptic resumes normal behavior almost immediately upon recovery and remembers little of what occurred during the seizure.

The EEG of psychomotor epilepsy characteristically shows squared topped waves varying from 2 to 4 cycles per sec.

Jacksonian Epilepsy

Jacksonian epilepsy, which involves sensations or movements along a limb, is the least common of all epilepsies. It may begin with a local twitch on the lip, then spread to the rest of the face and then down the neck to the arm and leg on the same side from which the twitch began. If both sides of the body are involved, grand mal epilepsy may result. The frontal motor cortex is the suspected focal point of Jacksonian epilepsy.

Other Focal Epilepsies

There is a kind of epilepsy in which the seizures involve involuntary antisocial acts, such as the epileptic stripping off his clothes. A form of epilepsy which occurs in infants with gener-alized brain disease is called "infantile spasms" or West's syndrome, and is characterized by lightning fast akinetic and myoclonic convulsions. When the child's body bends forward he is unable to speak. This disorder is usually associated with phenylketonuria or hypoglycemia which, if untreated, may result in mental retardation.

Status Epilepticus

Status epilepticus differs from other epilepsies; it consists of a continuous series of seizures without recovery of consciousness between attacks. From 1 to 10% of the epileptic population suffers from this form of seizure once a year or more. Of these, 10% will die from the uncontrolled attack. In those afflicted, irreversible cortical, cerebellar, frontal and temporal lobe damage which can possibly be attributed to anoxia may be found. The known causes of status epilepticus are the same as for other epilepsies. It can be due to infections, septicemia, alcohol, electroshock, rapid withdrawal from barbiturates and other drugs, cerebral edema and so forth. Historically, the treatment of this disorder consisted of warm baths, dilation of the anus, intravenous 50% glucose, lumbar puncture and many other semisuccessful treatments.

DRUG THERAPY

Barbiturates

More modern drug therapy has included the use of phenobarbital and shorter acting barbiturates (Table 28.3). However, in effective intravenous dosages, respiratory depression is a problem, and an adequate airway must always be maintained.

Paraldehyde has been used with some success in adult doses of 8 to 10 ml intramuscularly, followed by 5 ml every 30 min if seizures continue. The dose in infants is 1 to 2 ml intramuscularly, and in children, 2 to 3 ml.

Diphenylhydantoin has been used in a large number of patients, but on a neurophysiological basis, phenobarbital elevates the stimulation threshold and decreases the duration of the after discharge. It is still quite obscure how the long acting barbiturates, as a class, minimize seizures. Mephobarbital and metharbital are

TABLE 28.3
Major Anticonvulsant Drugs

	Drug	Oral Dose	Side Effects
I.	Long acting barbiturates		
	Phenobarbital	Adult: 120-200 mg/day Child: 6 mg/kg/day	Sedation and inhibition
	Mephobarbital	Adult: 600 mg/day Child: 65-300 mg/day	See above
	Metharbital	Adult: 250-300 mg/day Child: 5-15 mg/kg/day	See above
	Primidone (oxidized in body to phenobarbital	Adult: 250 mg—2.0 g/day Child: under 8 yrs. old, ½ adult dose	Dizziness & sedation
II.	Hydantoins		
	Diphenylhydantoin	Adult: 300-600 mg/day Child: 3-8 mg/kg/day	If oral intake of 300 mg/day—nystagmus; if oral intake of 400 mg/day—ataxia; if 500 mg/day—mental confusion; gingival hyperplasia (20%); hirsutism; morbilliform rash; megaloblastic & macrocytic anemia
	Mephenytoin	Adult: 50-100 mg/day, increase until 100- 600 mg/day Child: 100-400 mg/day	Sedation, rashes, bone marrow depression, some gingival hyperplasia
	Ethotoin	Adult: 1 g initially, then 1-3 g/day Child: 0.5-1 g/day	Little gingival hyperplasia & hirsutism; least toxic of the group

two other long acting barbiturates which have been used in grand mal as well as other epilepsies.

Rapid withdrawal of these drugs can produce hyperexcitability. The first signs of phenobarbital toxicity usually occur in excess of 200 mg a day, and most patients can not tolerate doses of phenobarbital that exceed 400 mg daily. At this point, additional anticonvulsants should be used to reduce the dose of each drug and thereby reduce side effects.

Refractory cases of epilepsy are usually due to a structural lesion, such as an angioma or glioma. Primidone, which is structurally related to the barbiturates, has been used with good results.

There may be some dizziness and sedation at the onset of therapy in 20% of the patients, but the side effects usually subside after a few days of treatment.

If phenobarbital has proven to be ineffective, primidone should be tried while gradually withdrawing the barbiturate. One primidone dose of 0.125 g is given orally in the morning. After 1 month, primidone is increased to a dose of 0.250 g and one dose of phenobarbital is withdrawn. After a 2nd month, primidone, 0.25 g is given twice daily, and another phenobarbital dose is withdrawn. At the end of the 3rd month, the primidone dosage should be 0.25g, 3 times daily, with no phenobarbital being given.

The Hydantoins

The hydantoins have been found to be very effective, especially when used in conjunction with phenobarbital, in suppressing all but petit mal epilepsies. Diphenylhydantoin (DPH) is the hydantoin of choice. This drug has been very successful in reducing the number of convulsive attacks. The major activity of DPH is its ability to suppress transmission of discharge away from the focus.[9] According to one theory, suppression is achieved by reduction of post-tetanic potentiation which limits the spread of abnormal discharges in the brain stem and cortex where numerous multisynaptic connections exist.

Though DPH is usually prescribed in divided doses of 300 mg orally a day, in many cases in combination with phenobarbital, the dosage should be individually titrated for each patient. By "loading" a patient with DPH, therapeutic blood levels can be reached in 3 to 10 hr. This is achieved by giving a single oral loading dose of 1,000 mg at one time or in divided doses a few hours apart. In the 2nd 24 hr, a dose of 500 mg will complete loading. The maintenance dose should be 300 to 400 mg daily thereafter.[10]

Two other hydantoins, mephenytoin and ethotoin, have been used in certain epileptics with some success. Ethotoin is the least toxic of the three hydantoins. However, it is also the least effective.

Oxazolidinediones

It is still unclear how oxazolidinediones effectively can reduce the number of petit mal and myoclonic seizures. The beneficial effectiveness of this class of drugs is limited owing to the severity of side effects and is usually reserved for refractory cases. Paramethadione is somewhat safer than trimethadione. Metabolites of these drugs also have been found effective. The two oxazolidinediones may be used in combination with phenobarbital. If this combination fails, DPH can be tried.

Of the many side effects seen with this class of drugs, sedation and headache are most common. Trimethadione may cause some alopecia and hiccups. Hemeralopia, resulting from direct action of these drugs on the retina, is also seen.

Eighty percent of the patients on these drugs show a reduction in neutrophils. The agranulocytosis which may appear slowly in the course of a few months, especially with trimethadione, disappears in 3 to 6 weeks after the drug has been discontinued. Initially, there is a drop of polymorphonuclear leukocytes to 3,000 cells

per mm.[3] If the level drops to 1,500 cells per mm,[3] the drug should be discontinued and not tried again.[11] Trimethadione and mephenytoin should never be used in combination because they greatly increase the incidence of aplastic anemia.

Succinimides

Ethosuximide is the drug of choice in petit mal epilepsy though the incidence of agranulocytosis and pancytopenia is high with this drug. Photophobia is seen only with the two other succinimides, methosuximide and phensuximide. In some cases, the use of trimethadione and ethosuximide together has successfully controlled petit mal attacks. In psychomotor epilepsy, methosuximide may be tried as a second or third drug. Phensuximide is less toxic than the other two in this class, but it is also less effective.

Phenacemide

Although phenacemide has inhibited all epileptic forms, it is so toxic that it is used only as a last resort when all other forms of therapy have failed. There may be some anorexia, nausea and vomiting; but the more toxic effects are proteinuria, exfoliative dermatitis and aplastic anemia. Acute psychotic manifestations have developed in 20% of the patients.[12] The patient may become depressed and paranoid, revealing suicidal tendencies.

Miscellaneous Agents

In some epilepsies in children, water retention may precipitate attacks. This is also true in epileptic females with premenstrual tension. The effectiveness of diuretics has been demonstrated to a limited extent. Acetazolamide is the most commonly used diuretic. This carbonic anhydrase inhibitor produces a systemic acidosis aside from its diuretic effect. Whether or not reduction in the number of attacks is due to the diuresis or the acidosis is still not certain. The effectiveness of this drug lasts for only a couple of days. Acetazolamide has also been used with primidone to treat infantile spasms.[13]

Oral contraceptives have been tried as alternatives to diuretics in cases where there is an increase in frequency of seizures during periods of premenstrual tension. Production of an anovular cycle does lessen the amount of water retention. However, the beneficial effects of these drugs in epileptics rarely outweigh the risk involved with oral contraceptives.

Amphetamines have been used in adults who have shown extreme lethargy from using major anticonvulsants. However, the effectiveness of the amphetamines is quite questionable since they can induce seizures of their own. The amphetamines are no longer used in epilepsy unless an epileptic child also exhibits a hyperkinetic syndrome.

Sodium salicylate has been used to a limited extent in infantile forms of epilepsy. The mechanism is obscure and dosages used are quite high. Because of the high degree of toxicity of the salicylates in large doses, the use of these drugs is limited to refractory cases.

Carbamazepine, which has been used in trigeminal neuralgia, also exhibits antiepileptic activity. Though its place in the management of the epilepsies is not clear, it is effective in all forms of epilepsy except petit mal. Side effects consisting of ataxia, diplopia, skin rashes and jaundice are rare and can be minimized by starting with very small doses. There has been a disturbing incidence of adverse hematological effects including at least eight cases of aplastic anemia. The oral dose of carbamazepine is usually 400 to 1,800 mg a day.

Meprobamate may be helpful in petit mal when used in conjunction with other major anticonvulsants. Its effectiveness may be based on its so-called muscle relaxant effect and nothing else.

Quinacrine may be used in petit mal only if other drugs have failed. The severe side effects which limit its use include diarrhea, central nervous system (CNS) stimulation and psychosis. In infantile spasms, adrenocorticotropic hormone has been shown to have some effect. Though evidence is limited, the hormone, as well as steroids, should be tried if other drugs have failed.

The bromides were the first medicinals used in the treatment of epilepsy. Because of the high incidence of side effects (*e.g.*, acneiform rash, ataxia, urinary incontinence and toxic psychosis), the bromides no longer are used.

Shifting the acid-base balance to the acid side will prevent seizures. A so-called ketogenic diet consisting of excessive amounts of fats will facilitate this shift by establishing ketosis. Adherence to such a diet is quite unlikely because of the unbearable taste and consistency of the food involved. The diet is rarely considered as a part of the therapy in epilepsy.

ANTICONVULSANT DRUG INTERACTIONS

The most studied drug interaction has been that of phenobarbital and diphenylhydantoin because they are the two most commonly used anticonvulsants. Drug interactions involving DPH are extensive. Various drugs decrease its effect by enzyme induction while other drugs increase its anticonvulsant effect by inhibiting enzymatic degradation. See Table 28.4 for these DPH drug interactions. Other drug interactions involving diphenylhydantoin are of some clinical value. For example, there are a few studies showing a delay of intestinal absorption of DPH due to racemic amphetamine. Studies also show that anticoagulants can be displaced from binding sites by DPH. In high doses, DPH can displace tricyclic antidepressants from secondary binding sites precipitating seizures. Barbiturates may be potentiated by competitive inhibition with DPH. Digoxin and digitoxin effects may be increased initially by DPH; but on continued use, their effects may be decreased. It has been shown that methotrexate toxicity is increased owing to displacement by diphenylhydantoin.

TABLE 28.4
Diphenylhydantoin Drug Interactions[a]

Enzyme Inducers	Enzyme Inhibitors
Alcohol	Coumarins
Chlorpheniramine	Chloramphenicol
(and other antihistamines)	(more studies needed)
Barbiturates	PAS
(especially phenobarbital)	
Corticosteroids	Cycloserine
Glutethimide	Disulfuram
	Estrogens
	Isoniazid
	Methylphenidate
	Phenyramidol
	Propranolol
	Quinidine
	Sulfisoxasole

[a] Reprinted with permission from Ref. 14.

A couple of drug interactions involving ethotoin have proven to be of some clinical significance. In combination with phenacemide, extreme paranoid symptoms develop and disulfiram has been found to increase ethotoin effects, just as it does for diphenylhydantoin.

An increase in libido has been found in a number of patients using ethosuximide in combination with other anticonvulsants. Primidone usage has caused an increase in the CNS depressant effects of anticholinergics. Methylphenidate has been implicated in potentiating the anticonvulsant activity of primidone.

SURGERY

Only after all drug therapy at maximal doses has failed should surgery be considered. Surgical intervention is contemplated if a lesion exists only when the lesion is focal and removal of the lesion will not create a neurological deficiency. An aura, if it is part of a seizure, usually indicates the site of the focal lesion. Temporal lobe lesions are more accurately located through the use of the depth EEG in which the brain is exposed and the electrodes are placed directly on the cerebrum. If characteristic spikes of one lobe are recorded on the depth EEG, surgery can be performed.

One complication of surgery occurring in 5% of the patients is hemiplegia. Hemispherectomy in these patients usually improves mental ability by 70%.[15] After surgery, patients should continue to take anticonvulsant medication. If there is no seizure in the month following the operation, the dose of the drug may be decreased gradually.

PROGNOSIS

For most epileptics, the effectiveness of drug therapy is the only basis for prognostic predictions. If lesions are present in the brain, anticonvulsants can bring about only a therapeutic cure. Complete remission in epilepsy is rare. Remission for up to 5 years has been seen in 23% of epileptics. Only 6% have had complete remission beyond 5 years.[16] There is effective control of grand mal attacks in ½ of the patients. In another 35%, the frequency of seizures has been decreased. Thirty-three percent of the cases of petit mal and 28% of the psychomotor epilepsies are controlled.

Mental deterioration has been seen in epileptics with frequent seizures over a period of years. Petit mal has been indicated in more cases than grand mal.

For the most part, relatively little is known about epilepsy. A more concrete understanding of the pathophysiology involved would help immensely in arriving at a sound therapeutic approach to the problem.

CONCLUSION

In most cases of epilepsy, only drug therapy is of value in reducing the severity and number of seizures. Epileptics who are adequately controlled through the use of anticonvulsants can, for the most part, lead normal lives. However, some exogenous factors, such as certain diseases, drugs, and chemicals and drug interactions with anticonvulsants, can be extremely dangerous to the epileptic because they may lower seizure thresholds. It is the responsibility of the pharmacist, through the monitoring of the drug therapy of the epileptic, to prevent these potential problems from arising.

REFERENCES

1. Merritt, H. H.: Textbook of Neurology, Ed. 4, p. 753. Lea and Febiger, Philadelphia, 1968.
2. Vercelletto, P., and Courjon, J.: Heredity and generalized epilepsy. Epilepsia, 10: 7, 1969.
3. Rodin, E., and Gonzalez, S.: Hereditary components in epileptic patients. J.A.M.A., 198: 221, 1966.
4. Pryse-Phillips, W.: Epilepsy, Ed. 1, p. 37. John Wright and Sons, Ltd., Bristol, England, 1969.
5. Takenbayashi, H., Komai, N., and Imamura, D.: Depth EEG, analysis of the epilepsies. Confin. Neurol., 27: 144, 1966.
6. Livingston, S., Torres, I., Pauli, L., and Rider, R.: Petit mal epilepsy. J.A.M.A., 194: 227, 1965.
7. Sawyer, G. T., Webster, D. D., and Schut, L. J.: Treatment of uncontrolled seizure activity with diazepam. J.A.M.A., 203: 115, 1968.
8. Kelly, R.: Treatment of epilepsy. Curr. Med. Drugs, 5: 25, 1965.
9. Lipp, J. A.: Epilepsy. II. Basic neurophysiological aspects of anticonvulsant drugs. Appl. Ther., 8: 438, 1966.
10. Kutt, H., and Fletcher, M.: Management of epilepsy with diphenylhydantoin sodium. J.A.M.A., 203: 168, 1968.
11. Kelly, R.: Treatment of epilepsy. Curr. Med. Drugs, 5: 23, 1965.
12. Way, E.: Antiepileptic drugs. Pharmacology-136 lecture, University of California-San Francisco Medical Center, February 2, 1968.
13. Millicap, J. B.: Anticonvulsant drugs: clinical and

electroencephalographic indications, efficacy and toxicity. Postgrad. Med., 37: 22, 1965.

14. Hartshorn, E. A.: Drug interactions, central nervous system drugs: anticonvulsants. Drug Intell. Clin. Pharmacol, 6: 130, 1972.

15. Rhoton, A. L., Jr., and Groover, R. V.: The surgical treatment of epilepsy. Surg. Clin. North Am., 49: 1028, 1969.

16. Rodin, E. A.: Medical and social prognosis in epilepsy. Epilepsia, 13: 121, 1972.

chapter 29

PARKINSONISM

Sam K. Shimomura, Pharm.D.

Over 150 years ago a general practitioner in London, Dr. James Parkinson, first described a disease he called the "shaking palsy" or "paralysis agitans." It has since become known as Parkinson's disease, parkinsonism or Parkinson's syndrome.

His initial observations were so accurate and succinct that even today very little can be added to the description of the symptomatology of this disease. A brief excerpt from "An Essay on the Shaking Palsy" published in 1817 adequately characterizes this disease as follows:

Involuntary tremulous motion, with lessened muscular power, in parts not in action and even when supported; with a propensity to bend the trunk forwards, and to pass from a walking to a running pace: the senses and the intellects being uninjured.[1]

Historically, anticholinergics have been the mainstay of treatment for Parkinson's disease. Surgical treatment has benefited a few patients in recent years, but it has not been proven to ameliorate the symptoms of the vast majority of patients. The introduction of levodopa has been hailed by a recent editorial in the *New England Journal of Medicine* as "... the most important contribution to medical therapy of a neurological disease in the past 50 years because of its usefulness in one of the more prevalent and disabling neurologic illnesses of

man."[2] Parkinson's disease is of special interest to pharmacists because of its biochemical pathogenesis and the unique pharmacological treatments available that are based on these biochemical aberrations. By understanding the rationale for the use of levodopa in parkinsonism, the pharmacist can contribute significantly to the medical treatment of this neurological disease by monitoring patients for adverse reactions, drug interactions and laboratory test interferences. The pharmacist also can contribute to the education of the patient regarding his drug therapy and its relationship to his disease.

BIOCHEMICAL BASIS OF PARKINSONISM

In recent years, much has been elucidated about the biochemical basis of parkinsonism but, as yet, not all the information is in. A cholinergic component appears to be involved since anticholinergics have been employed in treatment for over 100 years. This cholinergic overactivity has been confirmed by studies that show that centrally acting cholinesterase inhibitors such as physostigmine aggravate parkinsonism while centrally acting anticholinergics such as benztropine will reverse the effect. The finding that reserpine produced a parkinson-like syndrome by depleting the brain of dopamine gave tremendous insight into the biochemical basis of idiopathic parkinsonism. Treatment of parkinsonism with levodopa is predicated on the findings that there is a depletion of dopamine in the brain (Fig. 29.1). Based on these observations and more complicated studies, parkinsonism can be thought of as an imbalance of cholinergic and dopaminergic activity. Parkinsonism may be caused by any degenerative, toxic, infective, traumatic, neoplastic or vascular pathology altering the balance between acetylcholine and dopamine in favor of cholinergic overactivity. Therefore, based on this simplistic hypothesis, anticholinergics are given to decrease central cholinergic activity and dopamine, as its precursor, levodopa, is given to increase dopaminergic activity.

INCIDENCE

At least 200,000[4] and perhaps more than 1,000,000[5] patients in the United States are estimated to suffer from the major manifesta-

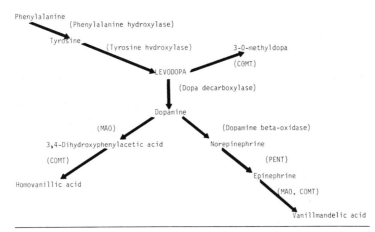

FIG. 29.1. Synthesis and metabolism of levodopa. COMT, Catechol-O-methyltransferase; MAO, mono- amine oxidase; PENT, phenylethanolamine- N-methyltransferase.

tions of parkinsonism, namely akinesia, rigidity and tremor. The risk of developing parkinson- ism sometimes during one's lifetime is 2 to 3%. Most patients, at least 66% of all those afflicted, have onset of symptoms between 50 and 69 years of age. The age of onset is the same in men and women. It is slightly more common in males (55 to 60%) than in fe- males.[6,7]

ETIOLOGY

The signs and symptoms of parkinsonism are produced by many different causes. Before a diagnosis of primary parkinsonism is estab- lished, secondary causes of parkinsonism must be ruled out. Unlike idiopathic parkinsonism, many of the secondary parkinson-like states can be cured.

Idiopathic Parkinsonism

The term "idiopathic" denotes a disease of unknown cause. Many theories have been pro- posed and each in succession either has been refuted or has been abandoned owing to lack of supporting evidence. A few of the etiologies that have been considered from time to time are head injuries, viruses and allergic reaction to unidentified agents. Although little is known about precipitating factors in this disease, much has been elucidated in the past 10 to 15 years about the biochemical basis for this dis- ease.

Trauma-induced Parkinsonism

Severe injuries to the head very rarely pro- duce tremor and extrapyramidal rigidity similar to that seen in primary parkinsonism.[8] Usually this occurs soon after the injury and recovery is the general rule.

Chemical-induced Parkinsonism

Many chemicals produce parkinson-like symptoms upon acute ingestion of large amounts or occasionally upon chronic exposure. Acute carbon monoxide poisoning can be a cause of secondary parkinsonism. It is not a common sequela of carbon monoxide intoxica- tion but when it does occur, recovery may be slow.[8,9] Chronic exposure to heavy metals such as lead, manganese and mercury may cause symptoms of parkinsonism. Other chemicals which have been reported to produce some or all of the signs of parkinsonism are carbon disulfide, cyanide, methylchloride and some photographic dyes.[10] In most cases of chemi- cal-induced parkinsonism, recovery is complete if the patient survives the acute exposure to the chemical.

Drug-induced Parkinsonism

Phenothiazines (e.g., chlorpromazine) commonly produce extrapyramidal side effects which ultimately may manifest themselves as a parkinson-like syndrome (Table 29.1). Early in the treatment with phenothiazine derivatives, a dystonic syndrome may develop. This side effect consists of torsional movements involving most muscles of the body, especially those of the tongue and face. Stiff neck (torticollis), facial grimacing and retrocollis are often seen. Dystonic reactions occur twice as frequently in males and most often between 5 and 45 years of age. The parenteral administration of diphenhydramine 50 mg or benztropine 2 mg will produce dramatic response within 10 to 30 min. Akathisia may occur after a few weeks of phenothiazine therapy. Patients with akathisia are often "jittery" and appear very anxious. They may pace the floor, tap their fingers and generally give the impression of restlessness. This occurs twice as often in females as in males and usually in patients between 12 and 65 years of age. The true parkinson-like syndrome usually becomes apparent 2 to 3 months after initiation of drug therapy. It consists of the usual symptoms associated with idiopathic parkinsonism, namely rigidity, tremor, bradykinesia, salivation, slurred speech, mask-like facies, festinating gait and seborrhea; and it occurs most frequently in patients over 50 years of age.[11] This condition responds well to conventional anticholinergic therapy but, unlike idiopathic parkinsonism, does not usually respond to levodopa therapy. This is not totally unexpected since phenothiazine presumably produces the extrapyramidal side effects by its ability to block dopamine.

The extrapyramidal side effects are dose-related so that benztropine, trihexyphenidyl or another centrally acting anticholinergic is usually added to high dosage phenothiazine regimens. In general, phenothiazines should be avoided in Parkinson's disease although there are a few phenothiazines such as ethopropazine that are used to treat this disease. Thioridazine has the fewest extrapyramidal side effects so that it is the tranquilizer of choice in cases of psychotic reactions in parkinsonism patients.

Other drugs besides the phenothiazines have the potential for producing a parkinson-like syndrome (Table 29.2)). Haloperidol and other butyrophenones produce pharmacological effects similar to that of the phenothiazines, and the same precautions should be observed. Reserpine depletes the brain of dopamine and in high doses can produce a parkinson-like syndrome. Methyldopa is a decarboxylase inhibitor which can also produce parkinson-like symptoms when given in large doses. As will be discussed later, methyldopa may prove to be useful in the treatment of parkinsonism when used in combination with levodopa.

Other drugs which have been reported to produce extrapyramidal symptoms are carbamazepine, thiothixene and chlorprothixene.

Postencephalic Parkinsonism (Encephalitis Lethargical)

Between 1917 and 1925 there was an epidemic of encephalitis lethargica (von Economo's disease).[12] A sequela of this viral infection was an onset of symptoms similar to parkinsonism which include seborrhea of the face, sialorrhea, oculogyric crisis and a respiratory tic. Although new cases are rare, it is currently one of the major causes of secondary parkinsonism. Because of its viral origin, investigators have been trying to establish a viral basis for primary parkinsonism. At present there is not evidence to support this hypothesis.

Atherosclerotic Parkinsonism

With advancing age, atherosclerosis may produce some of the symptoms of parkinsonism.[6] The clinical picture is atypical with patients showing merely rigidity, some tremor and spas-

TABLE 29.1
Examples of Phenothiazines That Produce Extrapyramidal Effects

Drug	Relative Degree
Trifluoroperazine	High
Perphenazine	High
Fluphenazine	High
Prochloperazine	High
Promazine	Moderate
Chlorpromazine	Moderate
Thioridazine	Low

TABLE 29.2
Drugs Which May Produce a Parkinson-like Syndrome

Amitriptyline and other tricyclic antidepressants
Carbamazepine
Chlorpromazine and other phenothiazines
Chlorprothixene
Haloperidol and other butyrophenones
Reserpine
Thiothixene

ticity without the resting tremor or cogwheel rigidity typical of true parkinsonism. There is some controversy about the validity of this diagnosis, and perhaps this term should be abandoned and more specific terms adopted, describing the type of stroke, the vessels involved and the actual clinical picture.

Infection-induced Parkinsonism

Besides the viral etiology of postencephalic parkinsonism, a number of other infectious diseases mimic parkinsonism as an occasional complication. A few examples are syphilis, polio, malaria, typhoid, herpes zoster and coxsackie.[8]

Tumor-induced Parkinsonism

Another rare cause of parkinson-like symptoms are intracranial tumors. The symptoms are usually unilateral and very rarely produce a mask-like facies.

DIAGNOSIS AND CLINICAL FINDINGS

The symptoms of advanced parkinsonism are so striking and unique that it hardly ever poses a diagnostic challenge.[13] The patient presents with rigidity, bradykinesia, seborrhea, festinating gait, flexed posture, increased salivation and a characteristic "pill rolling" tremor. With further observation, the clinician notices a "reptilian stare" consisting of a frozen, mask-like facie, infrequent blinking of the eyes and the tendency to sit for long periods of time in a stationary position. The voice initially may be hoarse and harsh which with time decreases in volume and resonance into a low monotone.

Most of the clinical features of parkinsonism fall into three general categories: bradykinesia, rigidity and tremor. Bradykinesia and akinesia are a slowing down of voluntary actions with apparent difficulty in initiating movement. This is often severe enough to cause the patient to "freeze" into immobility. This can be tested for by assessing the ability of the patient to perform rapid, alternating movements. Rigidity is the tendency to move "en bloc." There is an increased hypertonicity with resistance to passive and active movements of muscles. Muscle control and normal associated movements are hampered. Cogwheel rigidity is seen upon apply-

ing force to bend the limbs; the muscles yield jerkily giving the impression of cogwheels moving one upon another. It has a higher frequency and may not be related to resting tremor. The tremor of parkinsonism is generally coarser, slower and of wider amplitude than that associated with alcoholism, hyperthyroidism or nervousness. Resting tremor is seen in a relaxed patient and is a slow, rhythmical tremor.

Although moderately advanced to advanced parkinsonism is easily diagnosed, early features and findings of the disease frequently can be confused with many other diseases. The early presenting signs and symptoms vary from patient to patient so that there is no set presenting pattern.

The masking of facial expression is often an early feature of parkinsonism appearing long before more overt symptoms such as the festinating gait. A friendly, outgoing and smiling individual may slowly appear to become more restrained, emotionless and depressed. There is a subtle restraint of smile, a drawing down of the lips and lower face into an unchanging and worried expression. A slight bulging of the eyes and the barely noticeable tremulousness of early parkinsonism easily can mislead the physician into a diagnosis of an anxiety state, nervousness or depression. Not only can this diagnosis destroy the confidence and self-esteem of the patient but it sets in motion a self-fulfilling prophecy wherein the patient actually becomes depressed, anxious and nervous. The patient may be referred to a psychiatric clinic where treatment with a phenothiazine may exacerbate the extrapyramidal symptoms of the disease. Many cases of irreversible phenothiazine-induced Parkinson's disease may, in reality, be due to misdiagnosis and mistreatment of idiopathic parkinsonism.

Another patient may present with weakness and stiffness of one hand. There may be no tremor or other symptoms of parkinsonism. He also may complain of "stiff joints" and difficulty in turning over in bed or getting up out of a chair. His wife may complain of his slowness of movement and inability to button the top button of his shirt or to put on his cuff links. These presenting symptoms can often be misdiagnosed as arthritis or when unilateral involvement is apparent, the possibility of a stroke may be raised.

Early symptoms of parkinsonism frequently involve only one of the three cardinal symptoms of rigidity, bradykinesia and tremor. Symptoms often are unilateral and almost imperceptible at first and slowly progress in severity and spread from one area of involvement such as one finger, hand or shoulder to the whole body. The upper part of the body is usually affected first with involvement of the lower part of the body *e.g.,* shuffling gait, a later finding.

TREATMENT

Treatment is aimed primarily at providing maximal symptomatic relief of symptoms and maintaining the independence and movement of the patient. At present there is no cure for this disease, but dramatic improvement in drug therapy in the form of levodopa has greatly improved the prognosis of parkinsonism. Successful treatment involves a total program consisting of drug therapy, physical therapy, psychological support and, occasionally, surgical intervention.

Drug Treatment

Anticholinergics. Drugs with anticholinergic properties have been the mainstay of Parkinson therapy for over a century (Table 29.3). The mechanism of action involves the suppression of cholinergic overactivity in the brain. Anticholinergics that do not cross the blood-brain barrier, *e.g.,* quarternary ammonium compounds such as propantheline, are ineffective. These drugs produce moderate symptomatic improvement in tremor and rigidity with some improvement in akinesia in 1/2 to 2/3 of the patients.

The belladonna alkaloids such as atropine and scopolamine have largely been replaced in therapy by the synthetic anticholinergics. Although the synthetic agents are not more effective, they produce somewhat fewer side effects.

Of the synthetic anticholinergics, trihexyphenidyl is currently the most popular. A number of cogeners such as procyclidine, cycrimine and biperiden are also available. There is no clinically apparent difference between these agents, and the only reason trihexyphenidyl enjoys greater usage is that it was developed first and, therefore, more extensive clinical trials are available. Any one of this group is suitable for initial therapy. One should begin with low doses and gradually increase the dose, weighing satisfactory response against undesirable side effects.

Benztropine is used widely because of its long duration of action. It has antihistaminic as well as anticholinergic action. One to 2 mg at bedtime will allow most patients mobility upon arising during the night or getting up out of bed in the morning.

All of the anticholinergics share these common side effects: blurred vision, dry mouth, drowsiness, mild confusion, constipation and urinary retention. In toxic doses, they may produce hallucinations, agitation and elevation of body temperature.[14]

Antihistamines. Diphenhydramine is the most popular agent in this group and provides mild anticholinergic and antiparkinson effects. The other drugs in this class, orphenadrine and chlorphenoxamine,. are similar in action.[14] These agents are useful in initiating therapy in very mild cases. Diphenhydramine is also useful as a hypnotic in Parkinson patients who have difficulty going to sleep or staying asleep. Orphenadrine and propoxyphene have been reported to produce anxiety, mental confusion and tremors when given together. In reality, there appears to be no interaction between these two drugs.[15] This interaction is based on a few case reports to the manufacturers when in fact each of these agents alone can produce these symptoms as side effects. The author has observed a number of patients who have received this combination without apparent adverse effects.

Phenothiazines. Oddly enough, certain phenothiazines such as ethopropazine have mild antiparkinson effects while the majority of the phenothiazines may induce parkinson-like symptoms. Its antiparkinson effects are probably related to its anticholinergic properties. There is very little indication for using this agent since it is less effective than the synthetic anticholinergics and may produce serious adverse reactions such as agranulocytosis.[14]

Amantadine. Amantadine is an antiviral agent that produces moderate improvement in parkinsonism.[16, 19] Presently, the mechanism of action is unknown, although it is postulated that amantadine may inhibit the reuptake of

TABLE 29.3
Antiparkinson Drugs

Drug	Dose	Side Effects
Anticholinergics		
Trihexylphenidyl	1-5 mg 3 times daily; start with low doses; doses over 20 mg a day rarely tolerated	Blurred vision, dry mouth, vertigo, drowsiness, muscle weakness, mild confusion; in toxic doses tachycardia, hallucinations, agitation, elevation of body temperature; contraindicated in narrow angle glaucoma
Biperiden	2 mg 3-4 times a day	See above
Cycrimine	Initially 1.25 mg 2-3 times a day; usual range 3.75-15 mg daily in divided doses	See above
Procyclidine	Initially 2.5 mg 2 or 3 times a day; usual dosage range 10-20 mg daily in 3 or 4 doses	See above
Benztropine	Initially 0.5-1 mg daily with slow increase to 1-2 mg per day; maximal dose 8 mg in divided doses	See above
Antihistamines		
Diphenhydramine	Initially 25 mg at bedtime and 75 mg daily in divided doses; usual range 75-150 mg daily with 300 mg day maximum	Drowsiness, confusion, dizziness, atropine-like effects
Chlorphenoxamine	Initially 50 mg 3 times a day; may increase to 100 mg 4 times a day	See above
Orphenadrine	Initially 50 mg 3 times a day with adjustment upwards as required	Same as diphenhydramine but sedation less; does *not* interact with propoxyphene as previously reported
Phenothiazine		
Ethopropazine	Initially 10 mg 2-4 times daily; may be increased to 25 mg 3 or 4 times a day; some patients may tolerate up to 1 g	Drowsiness, dizziness, dry mouth, blurred vision, rash, ataxia and rarely agranulocytosis
Miscellaneous agents		
Levodopa	Initially 300-500 mg a day with slow increase to 2-8 g per day	Nausea, vomiting, hypotension, abnormal movements, behavioral changes
Amantadine	100 mg with breakfast for 5-7 days then 100 mg with breakfast and lunch	Hyperexcitabiltiy, tremor, slurred speech, ataxia, depression, hallucinations, insomnia, livido reticularis

dopamine and other catecholamines from neuronal storage sites.[17, 20] Side effects include slurred speech, ataxia, depression, hyperexcitability, insomnia, dizziness, livido reticularis and in extremely large doses, convulsions and blurred vision. The usual dose is 100 mg a day with breakfast for the 1st week and then 100 mg with breakfast and lunch thereafter. Tachphylaxis occurs after 4 to 8 weeks in about ½ of patients. Amantadine is not a first line drug, but it may be useful as an adjunct to therapy with anticholinergics and levodopa.

Levodopa. Cotzias first demonstrated the efficacy of levodopa in parkinsonism in 1967.[21] Although small doses of dopa were tried as early as 1961 in parkinsonism, most investigators reported transient or no improvement.[22] By switching to the levo isomer of dopa and gradually increasing the dose of the drug, Cotzias was able to push the dose high enough to achieve therapeutic results while keeping the gastrointestinal (GI) side effects at a tolerable level.[23]

Initial improvement usually is noted after 2 weeks of therapy as a subjective increase in well being. Facial expressions appear more lively and the drooling disappears. It takes about 5 weeks before measurable objective improvement occurs. Akinesia is generally the first symptom to improve, followed by improvements in rigidity and tremors. Over-all, therapy with levodopa can be expected to produce 50 % or greater improvement in about 2/3 of patients. Levodopa is approximately 3 1/2 times more effective in treating parkinsonism when compared to traditional anticholinergic therapy.

The rationale for the use of levodopa is based on the findings that parkinsonism may be caused by the depletion of dopamine in the basal ganglia. Dopamine seems to act as a specific transmitter at certain dopaminergic synapses. Dopamine itself was tried in the treatment of parkinsonism, but it does not cross the blood-brain barrier to any appreciable extent. However, the immediate precursor of dopamine, levodopa, does so easily, and it is therefore effective in restoring dopamine levels in the brain.

Dosage and Administration. The slow careful titration of dosage for each individual patient is of the utmost importance in achieving successful therapy. The usual effective dose of levodopa is 2 to 8 g per day in divided doses given with meals or food. Therapy begins with low doses of 300 to 500 mg and then is increased by 100 to 500 mg every 3 to 4 days as tolerated by the patient. The doses are divided into four and sometimes more doses to decrease side effects and to produce a more even response. Full dosage is usually achieved in 5 to 7 weeks. If patients have difficulty swallowing the tablet or capsules, the tasteless powder can be removed from the capsule and sprinkled on food.

Improvement is not always immediate so that a 4- to 6-month trial is warranted before abandoning therapy as ineffective. There are also day-to-day variations in response to levodopa, and alteration of dose may be required even after the patient has been apparently stabilized for several months on the same dose. Tolerance does not appear to occur and it may even be necessary to reduce the dosage in some patients on long term therapy.

Absorption, Metabolism and Excretion.[24,26] Approximately 80 % of orally administered levodopa is absorbed, primarily in the small intestine. Peak levels occur 1/2 to 2 hr after an oral dose is given in a fasting state. Although food delays absorption, generally it is administered with meals to decrease nausea and vomiting. Even before absorption begins, some levodopa is metabolized in the gut. Once it reaches the general circulation, metabolism is fairly rapid with detectable levels present for only 4 to 6 hr. Levodopa is converted to dopamine in the stomach, liver and kidneys as well as in the brain. The metabolic transformation is very complex (Fig. 29.1). Initially it is decarboxylated to dopamine and then it is further metabolized to norepinephrine, epinephrine and a host of other metabolites. Most of these metabolites are excreted in the urine within 6 hr with very little excreted unchanged.

Side Effects. Gastrointestinal—Nausea and vomiting are seen at one time or another in almost all patients taking levodopa.[22] Anorexia may also occur in conjunction with the nausea and vomiting but occasionally may occur alone. The nausea and vomiting are probably a result of both the local and central effects of levodopa. In order to prevent the GI side effects, levodopa should be initiated with low doses and then slowly increased as tolerated by the patient. Administering the drug with food or antacid will decrease the nausea. If nausea and vomiting become severe enough to limit the dosage despite slow increases in dose and administration with food, symptomatic treatment may be required. Phenothiazine derivatives such as prochlorperazine should be avoided since they may counteract the therapeutic effects of levodopa. Also, pyridoxine-containing antinauseants may antagonize levodopa's therapeutic effects. Antihistamine-type antinauseants such as cyclizine, while less effective than the phenothiazine antiemetics, are preferred for levodopa-induced nausea. Other GI side effects include abdominal pain, diarrhea, constipation, peptic ulcer and GI bleeding.

Cardiovascular—Cardiac arrhythmias, most commonly sinus tachycardia, and premature ventricular contractions occur in a small number of patients.[27] This side effect can be attributed to the stimulation of beta-adrenergic receptors in the heart by dopamine and its metabolites, such as norepinephrine. Treatment consists of discontinuing the levodopa and starting an antiarrhythmic agent. Propranolol is the logical agent since it has primarily beta-blocking actions.

The orthostatic hypotension frequently found in patients with parkinsonism can be aggravated by levodopa. Several different mechanisms have been proposed including direct beta effects of dopamine on blood vessels producing vasodilation, alpha blockade of the peripheral vascular system and depletion of norepinephrine from adrenergic nerve endings by dopamine. Whatever the mechanism, it occurs in excess of 25 to 35% of patients early in treatment but, fortunately, the blood pressure usually returns to normal within 2 to 3 months after initiation of therapy. If symptoms are severe, treatment with elastic stockings, increased salt intake or sympathomimetic drugs, such as ephedrine, is indicated.

Central Nervous System—Levodopa causes behavioral changes manifested as hallucinations, depression, paranoia, agitation, delusions and loss of judgement.[22] The magnitude of these behavioral changes is difficult to determine since parkinsonism occurs primarily in older patients who may develop impairment of memory, dementia and other personality changes independent of levodopa therapy. When these reactions occur, levodopa should be discontinued for several days and, depending upon the type and severity of the reaction, treatment with a tricyclic antidepressant or a phenothiazine with low extrapyramidal side effects may be warranted. Levodopa can usually be reinstituted at a lower dose after the reaction has subsided.

Abnormal involuntary movements are related to high doses and prolonged therapy with levodopa. After 6 months or more of therapy, over half the patients show symptoms of grimacing, chewing, active tongue movement, bobbing of the head and neck and rocking movements of the trunk. These symptoms respond to lowering of the dose of levodopa. Pyridoxine 10 to 25 mg will also inhibit abnormal movement, but it is only indicated when the symptoms are violent or cause great discomfort to the patient.[28] In these instances, this vitamin will produce prompt relief of the abnormal involuntary movements while reversing the beneficial actions of levodopa as well.

Other Adverse Effects—Many unusual adverse reactions have been attributed to levodopa. For instance, many patients report an aversion to coffee because of a nauseating aroma and a bitter taste. It apparently is unrelated to its caffeine content since cola beverages and other caffeine-containing products are well tolerated. Perhaps this strange reaction is due to the volatile oils in the coffee. Another unique reaction is an increase in the number of dental caries. Patients should be aware of this side effect so they can be followed by a dentist. Probably the best publicized reaction in the lay press has been levodopa's aphrodisiac property. In reality, the awakening of sexual activity is probably secondary to its beneficial effects on rigidity and movement. Unfortunately for mankind, no true aphrodisiac effects have been established to date.[29,30]

Levodopa Drug Interactions. Table 29.4 illustrates examples of drugs that may be used with impunity in patients receiving levodopa. However, a number of drugs have a potential for interacting with levodopa. The clinical significance of these interactions is largely unknown because most reports of the interactions are either theoretical in nature or only anecdotal.

Pyridoxine (vitamin B_6) — Even small amounts of pyridoxine can antagonize the beneficial effects of levodopa.[31,32] The mechanism of this interaction is not entirely clear, but

TABLE 29.4
*Common Drugs That Can Be Safely
Given to Patients on Levodopa*

Acetaminophen	Oral hypoglycemics
Amphetamines	Penicillins
Antacids	Phenindione
Corticosteroids	Sulfonamides
Digitalis alkaloids	Thiazide diuretics
Insulin	Thyroid

it may be due to an enhancement of peripheral metabolism of levodopa. A pyridoxine-dependent enzyme catalyzes the conversion of levodopa to dopamine. For this reason, pyridoxine was initially administered to potentiate the effect of levodopa but instead completely reversed them. By enhancing the conversion of levodopa to dopamine in the gut, liver and kidneys, pyridoxine decreases the amount of levodopa available to cross the blood-brain barrier. Although even 5 to 10 mg may antagonize the therapeutic effects of levodopa, in some patients such doses may be given to overcome the torsion dystonia produced by levodopa.[28] However, reducing the dose slowly usually will produce the same effects and is the preferred method for treating this side effect. Small doses of pyridoxine may be given to overcome pyridoxine deficiency resulting from the large amount utilized in levodopa metabolism or to prevent the peripheral neuropathy associated with isoniazid or hydralazine therapy. Pyridoxine generally is contraindicated in patients on levodopa therapy. As a consequence, pyridoxine-containing drugs such as multiple vitamins, or antinauseants such as Benedectin should be avoided. A multivitamin without pyridoxine such as Larobec can be recommended to patients requiring vitamins.

Decarboxylase Inhibitors—High doses of levodopa, 4 to 8 g per day, are generally needed because much of the levodopa is "wasted" through extracerebral metabolism (Fig. 29.1). Decarboxylase inhibitors which do not cross the blood-brain barrier would theoretically be useful in preventing the conversion of levodopa to dopamine outside of the brain. This would enable the dose of levodopa to be reduced to 1/8 to 1/5 of the original dose with a concomitant decrease in nausea and other peripheral side effects.[22] Several investigational drugs as well as methyldopa are now being tested for their general usefulness in combination with levodopa. Methyldopa appears to block aromatic amino acid decarboxylase, the enzyme that is responsible for converting levodopa to dopamine. This produces higher serum levels and subsequently higher brain levels. Even though there is blockade of decarboxylase in the brain as well, it appears to be greater in the periphery. When methyldopa is used in conjunction with levodopa, the dose has to be re-titrated. Since the dose of levodopa usually can be reduced by 1/2 to 2/3, it is sometimes advantageous to use this interaction as a means of reducing the side effects and cost of levodopa therapy. There appears to be no concomitant hazardous reduction of blood pressure.[33] Methyldopa given alone can exacerbate parkinsonism and in high doses can produce a parkinson-like syndrome in normal patients by interfering with decarboxylation of dopa to dopamine in the brain.

Phenothiazines and Butyrophenones—It is well known that phenothiazines in large doses cause extrapyramidal side effects. Phenothiazines apparently produce extrapyramidal symptoms by their ability to block dopamine receptors in the brain.[25] Although low doses of phenothiazines for short periods of time do not significantly reverse levodopa effects, it is best to avoid this combination if possible. An additive hypotensive effect may also complicate therapy with this combination.[8] Clinicians unaware of this interaction may try to treat the nausea and vomiting produced by levodopa with prochlorperazine or one of the other phenothiazine antiemetics. Levodopa may also cause psychic manifestations which may prompt the use of chlorpromazine or similar tranquilizers. If a phenothiazine tranquilizer is required, thioridazine is the drug of choice since it appears to have the fewest extrapyramidal side effects. Haloperidol, a butyrophenone, has actions similar to those of the phenothiazines and produce considerable extrapyramidal side ef-

TABLE 29.5
Foods High in Pyridoxine Content

Avocados	Oatmeal
Bacon	Pork
Beans and peas	Salmon, fresh
Bread, vitamin-enriched	Sweet potatoes
Breakfast cereals,	Tuna
vitamin-enriched	Wheat bran
Milk, dry skim	Wheat germ
Milk, malted	Yams
Nuts	Yeast

fects. Thus, haloperidol and its congeners should also be avoided in parkinsonism patients.

Reserpine—Reserpine can also antagonize the "dopa effect."[23, 25] In fact, the discovery that it depletes the brain of dopamine and produces a parkinson-like syndrome was an important clue in determining the biochemical defect in parkinsonism. Reserpine should be avoided in parkinsonism patients whether or not they are on levodopa.

Food—Early reports suggested that certain foods such as Chianti wine, old cheese, and chocolate antagonize the effects of levodopa,[34] but subsequent reports indicate there is no antagonism from these foods.[35] In general, food tends to decrease levodopa absorption by delaying gastric emptying time. Absorption is inversely proportional to gastric emptying time because some metabolism of levodopa occurs in the stomach. It should also be kept in mind that certain foods contain large amounts of pyridoxine (Table 29.5). However, restriction of foods containing pyridoxine is normally unnecessary[36, 37] and may be reserved for those patients who are unresponsive to levodopa therapy alone or require abnormally large doses of the drug.

Monomamine Oxidase Inhibitors—Monoamine oxidase inhibitors (MAOI) prevent the inactivation of catecholamines such as dopamine and norepinephrine, and they may interact with many other drugs. MAOIs have been tried in combination with levodopa to decrease the metabolism of dopamine and thereby potentiate its action.[25] Although they appear to increase the effectiveness of levodopa, they also can produce a hypertensive reaction.[38] This is probably due to a buildup of dopa metabolites such as norepinephrine which have vasopressor activity. The combination of levodopa and MAOI is potentially dangerous and should be avoided.

Antacids—Preliminary studies indicate that raising the pH of the stomach will increase the absorption of levodopa.[22, 39] Absorption occurs mainly in the small intestine, but alkalinization may enhance direct gastric absorption. The significance of this interaction is, as yet, unknown.

Tricyclic Antidepressants—Tricyclic antidepressants block the amine uptake mechanism and may potentiate the vasopressor effects of norepinephrine. These agents also can produce extrapyramidal symptoms in high doses. In clinical practice, this interaction is insignificant, and a number of patients have been treated successfully with combined therapy without untoward reaction. Both levodopa and the tricyclic antidepressants can produce cardiac arrhythmias so that patients taking this combination should be closely monitored for cardiac irregularities.[22, 25]

Guanethidine—The dosage requirements of guanethidine may be reduced in hypertensive patients on levodopa.[22, 38] Guanethidine does not significantly cross the blood-brain barrier so it has little effect on levodopa's antiparkinson actions.

Benzodiazepines—The benzodiazepines, chlordiazepoxide and diazepam, occasionally may antagonize the beneficial effect of levodopa.[8, 38] Only a handful of cases have been reported thus far, and the reversal of levodopa effects may have been just coincidental. Many patients take benzodiazepine derivatives and levodopa without apparent untoward reaction. The mechanism and clinical significance are unknown. Drugs of this class are not contraindicated in parkinsonism, but if patients do not respond as expected to levodopa while on benzodiazepines, it may be prudent to discontinue the benzodiazepine and observe the results.

Anticholinergics—The combination of an anticholinergic and levodopa appears to be more beneficial than either drug used alone.[25] The dose of the anticholinergic can be reduced to 1/2 to 2/3 of the original dose when levodopa is added. Although current information suggests that the effect is merely additive since the two drugs work by different mechanisms, further study may reveal other mechanisms.

Levodopa Laboratory Test Interference. Very few laboratory abnormalities have been noted thus far with levodopa therapy. There is no significant interference with the hematological system, renal function, endocrine function or liver function.[40] There have been reports of slight, transient elevations of serum glutamic oxaloacetic transaminase (SGOT) and serum glutamic pyruvic transaminase (SGPT), and interference with the determination of serum uric acid by the colorimetric method but not by the more specific uricase test.[41, 42] Levodopa also produces an excess excretion of catecholamine metabolites in the urine. Certain metabolites of levodopa cause false positive reactions for ketoacidosis by the dip-stick method. The urine, saliva and sweat may turn reddish and then black owing to levodopa metabolites. Positive Coomb's test without frank hemolysis may also be noted. Phenistix, used to test for phenylketonuria, is relatively sensitive to levodopa. In fact, it can be used as a screening test for consumption of levodopa in patients who may not respond to levodopa therapy as expected.

General Comfort Medications. Many of the minor symptoms of parkinsonism can be corrected easily with simple over-the-counter medications. For example, constipation is a common symptom of parkinsonism. It is frequently aggravated by the anticholinergic drugs and levodopa. A stool softener such as dioctyl sodium sulfosuccinate or a mild laxative like milk of magnesia is usually effective. Another common complaint of parkinsonism is blurred vision, especially while watching television or movies. This can be attributed to the infrequent blinking of the eyes in parkinsonism. The lubricating action of 1/2 to 1% methylcellulose eye drops or an equivalent solution of "artificial tears" often gives relief. The blurred vision may also be due to therapy with anticholinergic drugs and a reduction of dosage may be beneficial in this case.[43] Parkinson patients often have difficulty falling asleep and staying asleep. After initiation of therapy with levodopa, more patients may begin to complain about insomnia even though studies indicate that levodopa neither improved or worsened sleeping difficulties.[44] This may be explained by the observation that prior to levodopa therapy, daytime symptomatology may be so severe that sleeping difficulties at night are overlooked. As their condition improves, patients may become more aware of their sleeping difficulties and report them to the physician. The drug of choice in this situation is diphenhydramine because not only is it an effective hypnotic, but it possesses significant antiparkinson effects as well. Flurazepam and diazepam have been recommended for insomnia in parkinsonism, but benzodiazepine derivatives have been reported to antagonize the beneficial actions of levodopa.

Supportive Psychotherapy

The symptoms of parkinsonism frequently can be aggravated by psychic factors. The patient usually has suffered much humiliation from the readily obvious symptoms of his disease and often becomes defensive, uncommunicative and introverted. Since the patient's outlook and motivation can seriously influence his disease, it is important for all members of the health care team to provide reassurance, sympathetic understanding and encouragement. Keep in mind that behind the "fixed facies" and slowed slurred speech exists a person whose intelligence is unaffected by the disease and who craves intellectual stimulation and acceptance. To add to the problem, many drugs used in the treatment of parkinsonism produce hallucinations, paranoid delusions and changes in mood and behavior.

Physical Therapy

The purely neurological symptoms such as tremor and rigidity do not respond to physical therapy. However, certain secondary disabling manifestations such as bradykinesia, festinating gait and freezing of motion can be lessened, although sometimes only temporarily. The goal is to turn a normally unconscious, automatic voluntary movement such as walking into a conscious voluntary movement where the patient attempts to place undivided attention on the performance of a series of small sequential acts. Activities such as getting up from a chair and walking are broken down into prearranged units so that the patients can practice performing these acts in a flowing, coordinated motion.[45]

Heat and massage are also helpful in alleviating painful muscle cramps, and exercise can be useful in preventing flexion contractions. A program of physical therapy may slow down the progression of the disabling symptoms of parkinsonism and allow the patients many added years of independence.

Surgical Treatment

In carefully selected patients, surgery may relieve the tremor and rigidity of a parkinsonism patient in over 70% of cases for periods up to 5 years or longer. Surgical intervention is primarily directed to the interruption of one or more neural pathways in the globus pallidus or the ventrolateral nucleus of the thalamus. While tremor and rigidity may be effectively reduced, the akinesia and disturbances in gait, posture and voice are not significantly improved. For this reason, surgery has not been a wholly satisfactory treatment since the akinesia rather than the rigidity or the tremor is the disabling factor in parkinsonism.

Those patients most likely to benefit from surgery are those with primarily unilateral tremor and rigidity rather than akinesia; reasonably good health, *i.e.,* no hypertension, mental deterioration or extreme old age; sufficient motivation to carry out the postoperative physical rehabilitation program; and inadequate response to medical treatment. Thus far, surgical treatment has been carried out in over 25,000 patients with parkinsonism and other involuntary disorders. The mortality rate of an unilateral operation is probably less than 2%. The most common cause of postoperative death is due to hemorrhage and edema of the brain. Nonfatal complications include hemiplegia, hyperkinetic movements, transient inability to open the eyes and changes in mentation.

At present, thalamotomy appears to be beneficial only in a few well selected patients with primarily unilateral rigidity and tremor. Probably less than 10% of Parkinson patients will derive any significant improvement with this form of therapy.[4 5]

PROGNOSIS

Parkinsonism is a slow, progressive disease. Surgery has cured, or at least decreased, the tremor and rigidity in some cases, but very few patients are suitable candidates for this form of treatment. Drugs may relieve many of the symptoms of the disease with levodopa producing very encouraging results. However, drug therapy does not appear to alter the progression of the disease. All of the long term effects of levodopa therapy are not known yet.

Parkinsonism significantly shortens life with mortality being 3 times that of the general population of the same age, sex and race. The average patient dies about 9 years after onset of symptoms, but some have survived for 30 years or more. The commonest cause of death is not the disease itself but vascular complications, bronchopneumonia and cancer.[6, 7]

The dramatic breakthrough of levodopa in the treatment of Parkinson's disease has spurred new interest and greater research in this area which will undoubtedly produce further major advances in the treatment of this disease.

CONCLUSION

The Parkinson patient is an ideal candidate for monitoring of drug therapy by the pharmacist on an outpatient basis. The diagnosis is known (the symptoms of parkinsonism are unmistakable) and the disease is chronic, so that the pharmacist will be in a position to know the patient and his problems from frequent contacts over many years. The drug therapy has a high potential for adverse drug reactions and drug interactions so that a knowledgeable and sympathetic pharmacist can significantly contribute to the long term success of any treatment plan.

REFERENCES

1. Parkinson, J.: An essay on the shaking palsy. Arch. Neurol., 120: 141, 1969.
2. Poskanzer, D. C.: Editorials. N. Engl. J. Med., 280: 383, 1969.
3. Duvoisin, R. C.: Cholinergic-anticholinergic antagonism in parkinsonism. Arch. Neurol., 17: 124, 1967.
4. McDowell, F. H., and Markham, C. H. (editors): Recent Advances in Parkinson's Disease. F. A. Davis Co., Philadelphia, 1971.
5. Anon.: AMA Drug Evaluations, Ed. 1. American Medical Association, Chicago, 1971.
6. Calne, D. B.: Parkinsonism: Physiology, Pharmacology and Treatment. Edward Arnold, Ltd., London, 1970.
7. Hoehn, M. M., and Yahr, M. D.: Parkinsonism: onset, progression and mortality. Neurology, 17: 427, 1967.
8. Schwarz, G. A., and Fahn, S.: Newer medical treatments in parkinsonism. Med. Clin. North Am., 54: 773, 1970.
9. Gleason, M. N.: Clinical Toxicology of Commercial Products, Ed. 3. Williams and Wilkins Co., Baltimore, 1969.
10. McMasters, R. E.: The shaking patient and advances in the therapy of parkinsonism. Mod. Treat., 8: 245, 1971.
11. North, R. R.: Drug-induced movement disorders. Postgrad. Med., 50: 180, 1971.
12. Duvoisin, R. C. and Yahr, M. D.: Encephalitis and parkinsonism. Arch. Neurol., 12: 227, 1965.
13. Webster, D. D.: Critical analysis of the disability in parkinson's disease. Mod. Treat., 5: 257, 1968.
14. Yahr, M. D., and Duvoisin, R. C.: Drug therapy of parkinsonism. N. Engl. J. Med., 287: 20, 1972.
15. Pearson, R. E., and Salter, F. J.: Drug interaction?—orphenadrine with propoxphene. N. Engl. J. Med., 282: 1215, 1970.
16. Schwab, R. J., Poskanzer, D. C., England, A. C., and Young, R. R.: Amantadine in parkinson's disease. J.A.M.A., 222: 792, 1972.
17. Barbeau, A., Mars, H., Botez, M. I., and Joubert,

M.: Amantadine-HC1 (symmetrel) in the management of parkinson's disease: a double-blind cross-over study. Can. Med. Assoc. J., 105: 42, 1971.

18. Schwab, R. J., England, A. C., Poskanzer, D. C., and Young, R. R.: Amantadine in the treatment of parkinson's disease. J.A.M.A., 208: 1168, 1969.

19. Mowdsley, C.: Treatment of parkinsonism by amantadine and levodopa. Clin. Pharmacol. Ther., 13: 575, 1972.

20. Anon: Levodopa and related drugs. Med. Lett. Drugs Ther., 15: 21, 1973.

21. Cotzias, G. C., Van Woert, M. H., and Schiffer, L. M.: Aromatic amino acids and modification of parkinsonism. N. Engl. J. Med., 276: 374, 1967.

22. Brogden, R. N., Speight, T. M., and Avery, G. S.: Levodopa: a review of its pharmacological properties and therapeutic uses with particular reference to parkinsonism. Drugs, 2: 262, 1971.

23. Gotzias, G. C., Papavasilou, P. S., and Gellene, R.: Modification of parkinsonism—chronic treatment with L-Dopa. N. Engl. J. Med., 280: 337, 1969.

24. Morgan, J. P., Bianchine, J. R., Spiegel, H. E., Nutley, N. J., Rivera-Calimlin, L., and Hasey, R. M.: Metabolism of levodopa in patients with parkinson's disease. Arch. Neurol., 25: 39, 1971.

25. Morgan, J. P., and Bianchine, J. R.: The clinical pharmacology of levodopa. Ration. Drug Ther., 5: 1, 1971.

26. Abrams, W. B., Coutinero, L. B., Leon, A. S., and Spiegel, H. E.: Absorption and metabolism of levodopa. J.A.M.A., 218: 1912, 1971.

27. Goldberg, L. I., and Whitsett, T. L.: Cardiovascular effects of levodopa. J.A.M.A., 218: 1921, 1971.

28. Jameson, H. D.: Pyridoxine for levodopa-induced dystonia. J.A.M.A., 211: 1700, 1970.

29. Shapiro, S. K.: Hypersexual behavior complicating levodopa therapy. Minn. Med., 56: 58, 1973.

30. O'Brien, C. P., DiGacomo, J. N., Fahn, S., and Schwarz, G. A.: Mental effects of high dosage levodopa. Arch. Gen. Psychiatr., 24: 61, 1971.

31. Duvoisin, R. C., Yahr, M. D., Coté, L. D., Spiegel, H. E., Thomas, G., and Abrams, W. B.: Pyridoxine reversal of L-Dopa effects in parkinsonism. Trans. Am. Neurol. Assoc., 94: 81, 1969.

32. Leon, A. S.: Pyridoxine antagonism of levodopa in parkinsonism. J.A.M.A., 218: 1924, 1971.

33. Sweet, R. D., Lee, J. E., and McDowell, F. H.: Methyldopa as an adjunct to levodopa treatment of parkinson's disease. Clin. Pharmacol. Ther., 13: 23, 1972.

34. Fangman, A., and O'Malley, W. E.: L-Dopa and the patient with parkinson's disease. Am. J. Nurs., 69: 1455, 1969.

35. Jenkins, R. B., and Groh, R. H.: Psychic effects in patients treated with levodopa. J.A.M.A., 212: 13, 1970.

36. Van Woert, M. H.: Low pyridoxine diet in parkinsonism. J.A.M.A., 219: 1211, 1972.

37. Yahr, M. D., and Duvoisin, R.: Pyridoxine and levodopa in the treatment of parkinsonism, J.A.M.A., 220: 861, 1972.

38. Hunter, K. R., Stern, G. M., and Lawrence, D. R.: Use of levodopa with other drugs. Lancet, 2: 1283, 1970.

39. Rivera-Calimlin, L., Dujovire, C. A., Morgan, J. P., Lasagna, L., and Bianchine, J. R.: L-Dopa treatment failure: explanation and correction. Br. Med. J., 4: 93, 1970.

40. McDowell, F.: Clinical laboratory abnormalities. Clin. Pharmacol. Ther., 12: 335, 1971.

41. Cawein, M. J.: False rise in serum uric acid. N. Engl. J. Med., 281: 1489, 1969.

42. Honda, H., and Gindin, R. A.: Gout while receiving levodopa for parkinsonism. J.A.M.A., 219: 55, 1972.

43. Smith, J. L.: The eye in parkinsonism. Mod. Treat. 5: 316, 1968.

44. Kales, A.: Sleep in patients with parkinson's disease and normal subjects prior to the following levodopa administration. Clin. Pharmacol. Ther., 12: 397, 1971.

45. Wagner, S. L.: The management of parkinson's syndrome. Med. Clin. North Am., 56: 693, 1972.

46. Nashold, B. S.: Surgical treatment of parkinsonism and related disorders. Mod. Treat., 5: 301, 1968.

chapter 30

SCHIZOPHRENIA

Glen L. Stimmel, Pharm.D.

Schizophrenia is not a definite nosological entity, but rather a group of syndromes with some common features. Of the functional psychoses, the schizophrenias constitute the largest class, with affective disorders the other large class. Separate from the functional psychoses are the organic psychoses, such as acute and chronic brain syndromes.

The diversity of schizophrenic manifestations makes a comprehensive orientation extremely difficult, if not impossible. There are passing schizophrenic episodes in persons apparently well before and after; and there are severe psychoses that end in permanent dementia.[1]

The clinical picture we now know as schizophrenia has long been recognized. The term "dementia praecox" was first used by Morel in 1860. His classification also included mental deficiency and organic brain disease, all thought to be hereditary. It was Eugen Bleuler in 1911 who introduced the term "schizophrenia" and separated it from mental deficiency and organic brain disease. Bleuler believed that the schizophrenic syndrome was not one of dementia, but rather a disharmony of the mind with coexistence of contradictory throughts.[3]

In general, schizophrenia is a group of syndromes characterized by disordered content and form of thoughts, bizarre behavior, regressive intellectual functioning, inappropriate affective expression and often hallucinations and delusions. It is when several of these manifestations form a constellation of related symptoms that schizophrenia is diagnosable.[3]

EPIDEMIOLOGY

At the present time, schizophrenia is the most prevalent of the major psychoses. It is estimated that in the United States, 1% of the population will experience a schizophrenic illness sometime in his or her lifetime, and in a significant percentage of these people it will take the form of an incapacitating chronic illness.

Schizophrenia is not a cultural phenomenon, for it has been found in all cultures. The cultural forces appear only to modify the clinical symptomatology.[2]

ETIOLOGY

There is no clear etiological explanation for the functional psychoses. Schizophrenia, as mentioned earlier, should be considered a group of syndromes with some common features. A schizophrenic illness represents a complex interaction of biological and many social factors. There seems to be a definite genetic basis for schizophrenia, but of equal importance are the family and social experiences and stresses during the many phases of development.[4] The current opinion is that there is a genetic predisposition to schizophrenia which requires

environmental stresses to become manifest. An analogy can be made to the disease of acute intermittent porphyria. It is a hereditary, biochemical abnormality in which the patient may remain completely asymptomatic. It is only upon exposure to external stresses such as barbiturates, alcohol, infections or pregnancy that the disorder becomes clinically manifest. Identification of environmental stresses responsible in schizophrenia is more difficult, however. These involve more complex factors such as qualitative deficiencies in the mother-infant relationship and the nature of family and social experiences and stresses during successive periods of development.[2] In summary, schizophrenia seems to be a result of genetic predisposition which, by interaction with environmental factors, can lead to a phenotype of varying intensity of illness.[5]

DIAGNOSIS AND CLINICAL FINDINGS

Since a psychiatric diagnostic formulation differs so much from a medical one, it is important to first describe the psychiatric work-up. Of major importance is the history, with particular attention given to personal and family history of neurological and psychiatric disorders. The other major part of the work-up is the mental status examination, which is homologous with the physical examination in a medical work-up. It is an assessment of the patient's mental function based on behavior sampled during a psychiatric interview. Verbal and nonverbal behavior are evaluated. Appearance and general behavior, speech, mood, thought content and intellectual functions are specific areas evaluated. From all this information, a case formulation is made.

The history of a schizophrenic patient can be very important. In a majority of cases, the family will report a long standing inability of the patient to form warm and satisfactory contacts with other people, a tendency to avoid outgoing type activities and involvement largely in solitary pursuits and daydreaming.[6]

Mental status examination of a schizophrenic patient will reveal certain abnormalities of thinking and affect. The most classic description of the primary symptoms was that by Bleuler, the four A's: association, affect, ambivalence and autism.[7]

Primary Symptoms

Association. Disturbance in association is manifest as illogical, tangential, irrelevant or inappropriate ideas or responses. There is looseness, lack of sequence and absence of organization in thinking. Logical links between ideas are lost, producing interruption of one idea with others.

Affect. Affect, the outer expression of emotion, is frequently flat, rigid, indifferent and inappropriate. Events such as death of a parent are discussed with the same lack of emotion as is a discussion of the weather. The patient may smile or giggle about a situation where he should be concerned or anxious.

Ambivalance. A schizophrenic patient has extreme difficulty in dealing with coexistent positive and negative feelings or thoughts. Making a commitment one way or another is a difficult task, so the resultant behavior is ambivalence.

Autism. Autism refers to an excessive focusing of attention on the internal mental life. There is a detachment from reality and thus a lack of awareness and attention paid to the external life. An interviewer frequently may feel that he is competing with the internal life for the patient's attention.

Accessory Symptoms

In addition to the four primary symptoms above, there are several symptoms that are important in formulating a diagnosis of schizophrenia.

Hallucinations. These are false perceptions in the absence of external sensory stimuli. They are usually auditory, meaning the patient will report hearing voices. Visual, olfactory or tactile hallucinations are rare. The voices are usually hostile or threatening, but they can be pleasurable.

Delusions. Delusions are false, fixed beliefs which are not shared culturally. Delusions of persecution are the most common. Delusions of self-reference are also common, such as when a patient believes the radio or television is talking directly to him. Other common delusions involve religion, sin and sex. The content of delusions frequently reflects the wishes and fears of the patient.

Catatonic Behavior. This refers to peculiar-ities of motor activity and other voluntary muscular activity. This includes alterations in posture, gait, speech and mannerisms. Also included are states of stupor and excitement.

Memory Disturbance. Memory disturbance can be present, especially when a delusion or hallucination intrudes into the consciousness of the patient. After recovery, amnesia for the acute episode is common.

Although these accessory symptoms are not unique to schizophrenia, they are important because they can dominate the clinical picture. If a diagnosis of schizophrenia is made predominately upon the presence of these accessory symptoms, it is extremely important to differentiate from organic psychoses such as hallucinogenic drug intoxication, Korsakoff's psychosis and neurosyphilis. Delusions and memory disturbance are also common in severe psychotic depressions.[7]

Physical Changes

Physical findings in schizophrenia are conspicuously absent. Some patients may show an imbalance of the autonomic nervous system, manifest by cold extremities and mydriasis. Many patients lose weight during acute schizophrenic episodes and gain weight during convalescence. All of these physical findings can be obscured, however, because of the autonomic and endocrine effects of the antipsychotic drugs.

SCHIZOPHRENIC SUBTYPES

Many different diagnostic subtypes of schizophrenia have been proposed, usually serving to confuse rather than to clarify understanding of the disorder. Kraeplin's classification into simple, hebephrenic, catatonic and paranoid types is the most widely known. Since many other classification schemes are at least based upon this traditional system, it is important to define these subtypes.[2, 8]

Simple. This subtype is characterized by marked disturbances in emotion, interest and activity. Delusions and hallucinations are less common. There are rarely any spectacular or bizarre symptoms. These patients seem to just slide quietly into an autistic world, losing interest in school, job and family. Premorbid personality is usually asocial and eccentric.

Scholastic difficulty is prominent. The onset is usually very slow and insidious. These patients are more often fearful rather than depressed or angry. In milder cases, the simple schizophrenic patient may never come to psychiatric attention but be considered the neighborhood eccentric. The poor performance in school or job is an important diagnostic distinction from schizoid personality.

Hebephrenic. The hebephrenic schizophrenic is characterized by shallow, inappropriate affect, silliness, giggling and inappropriate laughter. It generally begins in early adolescence and is slow in onset. Regressive features are prominent, such as bed wetting and childish behavior. The hebephrenic leads a highly autistic life and is greatly introverted and withdrawn.

Catatonic. This subtype consists of two phases: stupor and excitement. It is generally more acute in onset and sometimes is traceable to a precipitating event. In a stuporous phase, a patient may be mute and immobile, and catalepsy, either flexible or rigid, may be present. Catatonic excitement is characterized by purposeless, stereotyped and sometime aggressive motor activity.

Paranoid. This subtype is characterized by more clear-cut delusions, ideas of reference and prominent auditory hallucinations. The onset is usually later in life, most frequently after age 30. Intellectual function, except for the delusional thinking, is usually well preserved.

Although the four subtypes listed above are the most widely known, the diagnostic subtypes in current use are somewhat different. Simple and hebephrenic schizophrenia are rare, and catatonic schizophrenia is uncommon. Paranoid and undifferentiated schizophrenia are most common. Undifferentiated schizophrenia can be classified as a fifth subtype, which describes the patients who show signs and symptoms of a thought disorder but do not show distinct characteristics of one of the first four subtypes.

Klein and Davis have proposed a subclassification that incorporates the patient's affective state and degree of premorbid social defect.[6] These two features have been shown to be of utmost prognostic importance and have a clear-cut relationship to drug effect. The reader is referred to Klein and Davis' textbook for details of their classification, but several points

deserve mention here. Generally, patients with a highly asocial childhood with the schizophrenic process beginning early and slow in onset are the most treatment refractory and have the poorest over-all prognosis. The fearful paranoid schizophrenics have a poor long term prognosis but do benefit somewhat from drug treatment. Schizoaffective patients, who show evidence of schizophrenia as well as an affective disorder, benefit the most from drug treatment and have the best long term prognosis.

ONSET AND COURSE

The age of onset of schizophrenia generally is considered to be from adolescence to early adult life, with some exceptions in childhood schizophrenias. There are distinct differences in the age of onset of the various subtypes as mentioned earlier. Although there is a striking contrast between a normal well integrated person and a grossly schizophrenic person, there is usually a transition period of a year or years between the schizoid personality and the prepsychotic state. So often the mode of onset is a gradual process requiring a long time period of a prepsychotic or incipient phase. The natural course of the illness varies widely. Before discussing the treatment of schizophrenia, it is useful to first identify four stages: incipient, acute, resolving and residual.[2, 9]

Incipient. This is the prodromal phase preceding the acute schizophrenic stage. It can be thought of either as the symptomatology preceding an acute episode, or as the stage in early teens where social functioning progressively and insidiously deteriorates. The differential diagnosis of this stage from the psychiatric symptomatology produced by psychotogenic agents like LSD and amphetamines has become very difficult. Intervention with antipsychotic medication in an incipient psychosis can block its further development.

Acute. The acute stage consists of gross overt psychosis and poor ability to function in the community. Hospitalization is frequently necessary, either for crisis intervention or longer. Initiation of drug therapy is most frequent during the acute stage. Dosage may be very high in an attempt to control the psychosis.

Resolving. This is the phase of transition from acute to residual. The outstanding findings include massive denial of the illness and periods of depression as the patient faces the realization that he has been "crazy." Psychosocial treatments are of extreme importance during this time, including individual or group psychotherapy. Drug therapy during the resolving phase is most difficult. It is necessary to decrease the dosage of medication used during the acute episode, while still maintaining an adequate effective dosage. Thus, dosage becomes a matter of trial and error for an individual patient. The depression of this phase seems to respond well to the tricyclic antidepressants.

Residual. The residual stage consists of a patient's defects and disabilities that are chronic. Since many patients have a recurring pattern to their psychoses, attention should be directed toward monitoring for signs and symptoms that may be indicative of the beginning of another psychotic episode. The use of long term, low dose antipsychotic medication has been shown to be of value in decreasing the rate of rehospitalization. During this phase of long term medication, it is especially important to monitor the many side effects of the drugs to make the patient most comfortable and compliant.

Another way to describe the course of schizophrenia is to look at the natural, untreated course in terms of outcome. If one considers those patients who present with their first schizophrenic reaction, less than 10% will recover and never have another acute reaction. About 15 to 20% will recover but will have recurrences of acute episodes. All the rest, about 75%, will go on to chronic states for the remainder of their lives. In terms of the benefit of drug treatment, it has been said that 1/3 of the patients will recover and do well in spite of medication, 1/3 will get worse regardless of medication and 1/3 will benefit, at least to some degree, from medication.[2]

TREATMENT

The treatment of schizophrenia consists primarily of antipsychotic medication and various psychosocial therapies. Drug therapy is by far the major treatment modality, regardless of the subtype or phase of schizophrenia. The psychosocial approaches have variable influences upon the schizophrenic patient, and their contribution to the total treatment program depends much upon the subtype and stage. These approaches include individual psycho-therapy, family therapy, group psychotherapy and a variety of alternative methods to traditional therapies.

DRUG TREATMENT OF SCHIZOPHRENIA

The drugs used for treating schizophrenia are generally classified as antipsychotics. Other terms describing these drugs include neuroleptic, major tranquilizer and ataractic. The easiest and most convenient classification is based upon the clinical use of the drug. So for this chapter, the term "antipsychotic" will be used. Under this classification, drugs used in psychiatry would be classified as antipsychotic, antidepressant, antimanic and antianxiety agents.

Antipsychotic agents have two unique properties in addition to their many other properties. The first is their ability to ameliorate psychotic symptomatology of the schizophrenic patient, and the second is their ability to cause extrapyramidal reactions. These two properties are found in all the various antipsychotic classes, including reserpine, the butyrophenones, thioxanthenes and phenothiazines. The mechanism for both these effects has been suggested to be the same, which is diminished postsynaptic dopaminergic activity within the brain. However, the efficacy of antipsychotic agents does not depend upon the appearance of extrapyramidal effects.[10, 11]

Classes of Antipsychotic Agents

There are at present three classes of antipsychotic agents in use in the United States—phenothiazines thioxanthenes and butyrophenones. Chemically, the phenothiazines and thioxanthenes are very similar, while the butyrophenones are quite different. Representatives of each class have been shown to be effective antipsychotics. There are, however, many differences among the various drugs that allow one to choose the best agent for a particular patient. These differences will be emphasized as each class is discussed separately below.[11, 12]

Phenothiazines. Of the three classes of antipsychotics, the phenothiazines are the best known and most used clinically. Their introduction in the early 1950's was revolutionary in changing mental health care in the United States. The emphasis changed from restraint or custodial care to amelioration of psychotic symptomatology and social rehabilitation.

Since the introduction of chlorpromazine as the first phenothiazine, massive programs by drug companies to develop new and better phenothiazines began and continue still. The result is that there are now over a dozen phenothiazines on the market.[13] Since the phenothiazines are more similar than they are different, it is useful to separate three major subgroups of phenothiazines whose differences may be utilized clinically. The subgroups are based upon chemical differences in the side chain. These are the aliphatic, piperidine and piperazine subgroups.

The aliphatic group includes chlorpromazine, trifluopromazine and promazine. It is the least potent group, meaning only that more milligrams of these agents are necessary compared to doses of other phenothiazines. Sedative effects are prominent, while the incidence of extrapyramidal symptoms is moderate.

The piperidine group includes thioridazine, mesoridazine and piperacetazine. Thioridazine and mesoridazine are low in potency, have prominent sedative effects and have the lowest incidence of extrapyramidal effects. Piperacetazine, although chemically a piperidine compound, has pharmacological properties more like the piperazines. Over-all, the piperidines are the most pharmacologically distinct group of phenothiazines.

The piperazine group includes the largest number of available phenothiazines. It includes trifluoperazine, fluphenazine, perphenazine, acetophenazine, prochlorperazine, carphenazine, butaperazine and thiopropazate. This group is the most potent of the phenothiazines, the least sedating and has the highest incidence of extrapyramidal effects.

Thioxanthenes. The thioxanthene group resulted from chemical modification of phenothiazine compounds. The difference is that the nitrogen of the phenothiazine nucleus is replaced by a carbon atom. Nearly 70 thioxanthene compounds have been investigated, yielding two agents available for use in the United States. The first introduced was chlorprothixene, which is the thioxanthene analogue of chlorpromazine. The second agent is thiothixene. Clincally the thioxanthenes should be considered as equivalent to phenothiazines. In terms of efficacy as antipsychotic agents, studies show the thioxanthenes to be either inferior or equal to various phenothiazines, but not superior.[11,14] In terms of side effects, there is lack of clinical evidence to allow comparison with phenothiazines. Statements are made that side effects are reported least often with thioxanthene compounds than any other antipsychotic. Such a statement is due to the fact that the thioxanthenes are prescribed less frequently and lack sufficient clinical usage.[14] Side effects reported with phenothiazines are identical to those reported with thioxanthenes. Chlorprothixene is the most sedating, while thiothixene is the least. Extrapyramidal effects are most frequent with thiothixene, less frequent with chlorprothixene. Over-all, thioxanthenes constitute another group of antipsychotic agents that may be a useful alternative in previously treatment-resistant patients.

Butyrophenones. The butyrophenone group in the United States is represented by haloperidol. As an antipsychotic agent, haloperidol offers the most useful alternative to the phenothiazine agents. Its antipsychotic efficacy is at least equal to that of the phenothiazines. For acute psychiatric disorders, haloperidol appears to be more efficacious than many phenothiazines.[15] Additionally, many patients who do not respond to phenothiazines will respond to haloperidol. It is also the antipsychotic of choice for patients who are phenothiazine-intolerant or-allergic or who suffers from the long term toxicities of phenothiazines such as ocular pigmentation.

The butyrophenones are chemically very distinct from the phenothiazines and thus have many differences in terms of pharmacological effects and adverse effects. The incidence of extrapyramidal effects is reported to be high. This seems to be related more to neurologically susceptible patients than to dosage, although a definite answer is not yet clear.[11,15] Haloperidol is nonsedating and, in fact, sometimes delays onset of sleep. In these cases, the daily dose should be taken in the morning. Hypotension seldom is encountered, and haloperidol does not cause any EKG changes.[16,17] For these reasons, it may be preferred over a phenothiazine in elderly patients or those with coronary or cerebrovascular disease.[17]

As suggested by Hollister, the many available antipsychotic agents can be reduced down to one representative of each class. This allows the prescriber the whole range of differences in side effects that may be useful or avoided for a particular patient, while still keeping the number of agents used within reasonable limits. Based upon the evidence presented above and this author's experience, chlorpromazine, thioridazine, trifluoperazine, fluphenazine, thiothixene and haloperidol would provide the widest flexibility in effects while still being limited in number. Fluphenazine is included as a second piperazine compound because it is the only antipsychotic available as a long acting parenteral preparation. Table 30.1 gives the approximate equivalent doses for the major antipsychotic agents in current use.

Antipsychotic of Choice

Many clinical studies have attempted to differentiate the antipsychotic agents in terms of efficacy. In general, when antipsychotic agents are used in adequate dosages, they are equal in therapeutic efficacy to chlorpromazine. The only exception is promazine, which has been shown to be clearly inferior in efficacy as an antipsychotic agent.[11],[19] A review of the many studies of efficacy shows no phenothiazine to be superior to chlorpromazine, but all of the major phenothiazines equal to chlorpromazine.[11]

There have been numerous attempts to correlate a particular phenothiazine as most efficacious for certain types of schizophrenic symptomatology. The most notable attempt was the prediction that the agitated patient would respond best to a sedating phenothiazine like chlorpromazine, while a withdrawn, apathetic patient would respond best to a "stimulant" phenothiazine like trifluoperazine or perphenazine. Other studies have attempted to correlate a particular phenothiazine as most efficacious for certain schizophrenic symptom complexes. Such information would allow a prescriber to predict and choose a particular drug for a patient with a particular symptomatology. Unfortunately, at the present time, there exists no consistent information which allows such a prediction. Chlorpromazine can be just as efficacious in a withdrawn apathetic patient as trifluoperazine or perphenazine. Several National Institute of Mental Health cooperative studies supported with evidence the concept that the initial choosing of a phenothiazine for a patient is largely empirical.[20] Despite manufacturer's claims, there is, as yet, no basis for claiming superiority of one phenothiazine over another or that a particular type of patient will benefit most from a particular phenothiazine.

The preceding statements are probably counter to most prescriber's clinical impression, which tells them a particular patient will not respond to one phenothiazine but will respond to another. This impression is a valid one, for it is commonly observed that a given patient will do well on one phenothiazine but do poorly on another. An important distinction is that it is not presently possible to predict ahead of time which antipsychotic will be most effective for a patient. It is only after some trial and error or review of past psychiatric history that it becomes known that a patient responds best to one particular antipsychotic agent.

Since it has been shown that schizophrenic symptomatology and efficacy differences offer no guide to choosing a drug for a patient, the obvious problem is how to choose a drug. The major determinant initially is the difference in side effects and toxicity of the various antipsychotic agents. If sedation is a desirable side effect, then a logical choice would be chlorpromazine or thioridazine. If sedation is undesirable, trifluoperazine or haloperidol is an appropriate choice. When extrapyramidal effects are particularly serious in a patient, thioridazine would be best while the piperazine phenothiazines should be avoided. When high dose long term therapy is necessary, the more

TABLE 30.1
Equivalent Doses of Antipsychotic Agents

Drug	Dosage
Phenothiazines	*mg*
Chlorpromazine (Thorazine)	100
Thioridazine (Mellaril)	100
Trifluoperazine (Stelazine)	5
Fluphenazine (Prolixin)	2
Perphenazine (Trilafon)	8
Piperacetazine (Quide)	10
Prochlorperazine (Compazine)	15
Thioxanthenes	
Chlorprothixene (Taractan)	100
Thiothixene (Navane)	2
Butyrophenones	
Haloperidol (Haldol)	2

potent piperazines and haloperidol are the best choices. Chlorpromazine and thioridazine should be avoided in this situation owing to skin and eye pigmentation. For the patient who is unreliable in taking his medication, the long acting fluphenazine enanthate or decanoate is most appropriate.

Dosage and Administration

There is no standard dosage for antipsychotics when treating schizophrenia. This author has seen chronic schizophrenic patients effectively maintained on as low as 25 mg daily of chlorpromazine, while other schizophrenic patients are only partially controlled on 3,000 mg daily of chlorpromazine or a combination of fluphenazine enanthate 200 mg IM weekly plus trifluoperazine 100 mg daily. It is useful, however, to consider separately the various schizophrenic phases as outlined earlier as they pertain to dosage.

The higher doses of antipsychotics are frequently necessary during acute schizophrenic reactions. Several grams of chlorpromazine daily, 60 to 120 mg of trifluoperazine daily or up to 150 mg daily of haloperidol are not uncommon. During the resolving phase, attempts are made to decrease the dose and find an effective maintenance dose. The doses commonly encountered are in the range of 500 to 1,000 mg daily of chlorpromazine or its equivalent. Finding the appropriate dose is mostly by trial and error, and the most frequent error is reducing the dosage too quickly. During the residual phase, the lowest possible dose is sought since this level will be long term. The dosage for chronic maintenance varies from extremely low to moderate levels, depending upon the schizophrenic residual of the patient.[9]

High dose antipsychotic therapy currently is being studied to determine which patients may benefit. In general, chronic schizophrenic patients who have been hospitalized less than 10 years and are under 40 years of age will benefit most from high dose therapy. High dose in these studies was defined as 2,000 mg of chlorpromazine daily and 80 mg of trifluoperazine daily.[21, 22] Similar observations have been made with high dose haloperidol. Doses ranging from 30 to 200 mg and higher have proven to be more effective than low doses in patients who are physically fit and who have had schizo-

phrenia for less than 10 years.[15]

A practice becoming increasingly common is dosing the antipsychotics once daily rather than using divided doses. Recent studies have clearly shown once daily dosing is equal in efficacy to a divided dosing schedule.[23, 24] Once daily dosing is best done after several weeks of a divided dosing schedule to allow accumulation of the drug in the tissues. There are several distinct advantages to using once daily dosing. The primary advantage is better patient compliance, since the patient must remember to take only one dose per day. Another advantage is that the sedative properties of many antipsychotic drugs can be utilized to promote a better night's sleep, and the patient is not drowsy during the daytime. A third advantage is that the peak blood levels are reached while the patient sleeps, so the many side effects that are related to blood level occur while the patient sleeps. These include sedation, extrapyramidal, and some anticholinergic effects.[23]

Differences in routes of administration are an important consideration with the antipsychotic drugs. In general, the most reliable route is the IM injection, which is at least several times more potent than the oral route.[25, 26] When chlorpromazine is given IM, a peak level of about 5% of the administered dose is reached in the blood. This contrasts with about 0.5% when chlorpromazine is given orally.[27] Of the oral forms, the liquid concentrate is most reliable, followed by tablets and, lastly, followed by spansules. Because of the ability to dose the tablets once daily, there is no justification for using the more expensive spansules.[10, 26, 28]

Side Effects and Toxicity

Table 30.2 lists side effects and toxicities of the antipsychotic agents in common use today. Although the list is lengthy, there are several that deserve special comment. The most common of these effects include the extrapyramidal effects, dry mouth, blurry vision, constipation and sedation. These are the effects that are a constant annoyance to the patient, and ones that can be minimized or eliminated by proper monitoring and judicious use of other medications. The pharmacist can be of great value to the prescriber in providing information on management of these side effects once he be-

TABLE 30.2
Side Effects and Toxicities of Antipsychotic Agents

Extrapyramidal
Parkinsonian tremor, gait, rigidity; akinesia, dystonia; dyskinesia; akathisia; tardive dyskinesia
Central nervous system
Drowsiness, fatigue, toxic confusion, increased dreaming, seizures, depression
Autonomic
Dry mouth, constipation, blurred vision, nasal stuffiness, urinary retention, tachycardia, orthostatic hypotension, hypotensive episodes, inhibition of ejaculation
Skin
Pruritis, erythema, urticaria, photosensitivity, pigmentation
Gastrointestinal
Anorexia, nausea, vomiting
Endocrine
Weight change, menstrual irregularity, galactorrhea, gynecomastia, peripheral edema
Hematological
Agranulocytosis, leukopenia, eosinophilia, thrombocytopenia purpura
Hepatic
Abnormal liver function tests, cholestatic jaundice
Eye
Corneal and lens pigmentation, pigmentary retinopathy (thioridazine)

comes familiar with their manifestations.

The extrapyramidal effects of the antipsychotic agents are by far the most troublesome common complaint. The term "extrapyramidal effect" is a general one that describes a variety of specific symptoms. These include Parkinson symptoms (tremor, rigidity, and akinesia), dystonias and akathisia. The Parkinson symptoms seem to be more prevalent with chlorpromazine, while dystonias occur most often with prochlorperazine and perphenazine. Pediatricians have become very aware of the acute dystonias sometimes seen in children given prochlorperazine suppositories for nausea and vomiting. Akathisia seems to be more prevalent with the use of fluphenazine and trifluoperazine.[9]

Tardive dyskinesia is a side effect of antipsychotic drugs presently causing considerable concern. It is a drug-induced neurological disorder that appears to be irreversible and resistant to drug treatment. It is characterized by involuntary movement of the lips, tongue or jaw, most common in the form of smacking of the lips, rhythmical movement of the tongue or facial grimaces. Prolonged use of antipsychotic drugs plays a major role in the development of the syndrome, although cases now are being seen in patients on fluphenazine enanthate after only several years of therapy. The incidence of tardive dyskinesia in the more recent and better controlled studies consistently falls in the range of 15 to 25%. The incidence seems to be higher in patients taking both an antipsychotic and antiparkinson agent as compared to an antipsychotic drug alone. The best pharmacological mechanism thus far proposed is that of hypersensitivity of the dopaminergic receptors to endogenous dopamine after long term blockade by antipsychotic drugs. This explains why antiparkinson agents tend to aggravate tardive dyskinesia, while increasing the dose of the antipsychotic may be of temporary value.[29, 31]

The endocrine effects of phenothiazines deserve comment since patients frequently do not spontaneously relate their occurrence. Simple reassurance that menstrual irregularity or galactorrhea is of no medical significance can allay a patient's fears and anxiety.

Management of Side Effects

In patients on chronic antipsychotic medication, management of side effects can become as important as management of the antipsychotic medication itself. Most patients are constantly annoyed by bothersome side effects, many of which can be minimized or eliminated. Table 30.3 lists some common side effects and their preferred treatment.

Extrapyramidal effects can be minimized and sometimes eliminated by using antiparkinson agents. Those in current use include benztropine mesylate, trihexyphenidyl, procyclidine and biperidin. Benztropine seems to have the clear advantage over the other agents, primarily owing to its longer duration of effect. Although benztropine has a biological half-life of about 6 to 8 hr, the therapeutic effect may last for 24 hr allowing once daily dosage.[32] A recent study by Neu supported the therapeutic efficacy of daily dosing of benzotropine when compared to a divided dosage.[33] The other three antiparkinson agents usually require dosing of 3 or 4 times daily. In terms of over-all efficacy, there is no evidence to show consistent differences in the four drugs. However, it is often clinically observed that patients do better on one agent than another. Diphenhydramine is a useful adjunct to the antiparkinson agents listed

TABLE 30.3
Preferred Treatment of Side Effects

Autonomic		
	Dry mouth	Sugarless hard candy as needed daily; if severe, oral pilocarpine
	Constipation	Dioctyl sodium sulfosuccinate; if severe, occasional bisacodyl
	Blurry vision	Pilocarpine 1% or physostigmine 0.25% eye drops only if severe
Extrapyramidal		Benztropine mesylate preferred, diphenhydramine as adjunct as needed
Central nervous system		
	Drowsiness, fatigue	tolerance will usually develop; if persistent, dosing once daily at bedtime of the antipsychotic drug

above. Alone it is a relatively poor drug for nonacute extrapyramidal effects. But whenever the antiparkinson agents are pushed to maximal levels without response, diphenhydramine can be a very helpful adjunct. Its beneficial effect in treating extrapyramidal effects appears to be unrelated to its antihistaminic activity.[34] Table 30.4 provides estimated equivalent doses of the drugs used to treat extrapyramidal effects.[34, 35]

Attention currently is being given to the advisability of using antiparkinson agents prophylactically. Such practice is very common as an attempt to prevent the occurrence of extrapyramidal effects. It is becoming clear that many patients receive antiparkinson agents unnecessarily when used prophylactically. Klett reported that of 403 patients withdrawn from antiparkinson agents under double blind conditions, 82% got along quite well without them, 11% were judged to be worse, and 7% were withdrawn from the study because of appearance of extrapyramidal effects.[35] Other similar studies show some variety in the incidence of symptom recurrence, but all very clearly show that the majority of patients do not need antiparkinson drugs.[36, 37] In addition to the evidence that antiparkinson agents are frequently unnecessary, there are several distinct disadvantages to their prophylactic use. As was mentioned earlier, there appears to be an increased incidence of tardive dyskinesia in patients taking both antipsychotic and antiparkinson drugs as compared to antipsychotic agents alone. The other disadvantage is the additive anticholinergic effects. Discontinuing the unnecessary antiparkinson agent may provide significant relief from the anticholinergic effects being caused by the antipsychotic and antiparkinson agents.

The other side of the controversy is that even though patients may not exhibit extrapyramidal effects, prophylactic antiparkinson drugs are indicated. Without them, patients show a lack of spontaneity and complain about feelings of lifelessness and drowsiness.[9] In looking at the total picture and on both sides of the controversy, the present evidence suggests that prophylactic antiparkinson drugs are beneficial for the first few months of antipsychotic therapy. This is when extrapyramidal effects occur if they will at all, and antiparkinson agents will prevent their occurrence which may promote patient compliance with the antipsychotic drug. After the first few months, however, the antiparkinson agent should be tapered and discontinued, whenever possible. There is no justification for long term antiparkinson agents in the absence of any extrapyramidal effects.

Dry mouth and throat is probably the most common side effect and the most frequent complaint. Although not a major side effect when compared to others, it should be of significant concern to the prescriber. When severe, dry mouth can be of sufficient concern to the patient and compliance may be affected. Dental

TABLE 30.4
Estimated Equivalent Doses of Antiparkinson Drugs

Drug	Dose
	mg
Benztropine mesylate (Cogentin)	2
Trihexyphenidyl (Artane, Tremin)	5
Procyclidine (Kemadrin)	5
Biperiden (Akineton)	4

hygiene may suffer, and patients who wear dentures may particularly suffer from this effect.[38] The dry mouth can be treated by several methods. For most cases, having the patient suck on sugarless hard candy several times daily can be of significant benefit. The candy should not contain sugar, since cases of oral moniliasis have been reported with candy containing sugar.[39, 40] If the dry mouth persists or is severe, oral pilocarpine can be useful for symptomatic relief.[41] Dry mouth usually disappears within 30 min of administration, and returns in 6 to 8 hr. Patients sometimes report that their constipation is less while taking pilocarpine. This author has found that 5 mg of pilocarpine orally several times daily can benefit a significant number of patients, without any other side effects from the pilocarpine.

Constipation is another very common complaint. It is usually a constant annoyance to patients and can lead to serious problems. A report of three fatal cases and five severe cases of adynamic ileus caused by various psychotropic drugs emphasizes the necessity of monitoring complaints of constipation.[42] In all eight cases, there was a period of chronic constipation. Occurrence of any abdominal pain in such a patient should be promptly evaluated. When discovered and treated early, fecal impaction, abdominal distention, ileus and the resultant complications can be avoided. Since the most frequent complaint of patients is hard, dry stools, the most logical drug treatment of constipation should begin with a stool softener. It is infrequent when dioctyl sodium sulfosuccinate (DOSS), in doses up to 1,500 mg daily, will not correct the constipation. Maximal utilization of a very safe agent like DOSS obviates the need to use laxatives with their potential for overuse and dependence.

Visual disturbance is a third very common autonomic effect of the antipsychotic agents. Blurred near vision is a result of mydriasis and cycloplegia. Use of pilocarpine or physostigmine eye drops is seldom of clinical benefit.[9] A trial of eye drops indicated only when the blurred vision constitutes a threat to patient compliance or in patients whose job or hobby require much reading.

Drug Interactions

If it is remembered that antipsychotic agents can generally be considered central nervous system (CNS) depressants, then most of the clinically significant interactions are predictable. As expected, combination of antipsychotic agents with alcohol, barbiturates, other sedative hypnotics, narcotics, antihistamines and antianxiety agents will result in additive CNS depression. This effect is of critical importance in drug overdoses. Successful suicides with antipsychotic drug overdoses are extremely rare, but when combined with more toxic CNS depressants like barbiturates, the overdose becomes extremely dangerous.

A second group of interactions, also very predictable, is the additive anticholinergic effects seen when antipsychotic agents are used with drugs with anticholinergic effects. These drugs include antihistamines, tricyclic antidepressants and the various anticholinergic agents used to treat peptic ulcer, Parkinson's disease, and over-the-counter sleep and cold preparations.

Phenothiazines have been reported to elevate blood glucose levels, presumably because of activation of adrenergic responses. This effect seems to be of clinical significance only in diabetic or prediabetic patients and when large doses are used.[43, 45] Haloperidol, however, has been implicated in a case of hypoglycemic coma.[46]

Both phenothiazines and haloperidol have been reported to potentiate the effect of some oral anticoagulants. The significance of this effect in humans is not well established and the mechanism is not known.[15, 47, 49]

PROGNOSIS

Since schizophrenia was defined earlier as a group of syndromes rather than a definite nosological entity, the prognosis of schizophrenia necessarily depends upon many factors. These include acuteness, the diagnostic subtype and many social variables. In general, the acute schizophrenic reactions are more hopeful than chronic cases that are slow and insidious in onset. Of major importance is the prepsychotic personality. If the psychosis represents the end result of a long period of maladaption and is preceded by a schizoid personality, the prognosis is unfavorable. A better prognosis is predicted when the onset is sudden, an external precipitating event is easily identifiable and there is much affect associated with the episode.[2]

In terms of the diagnostic subtypes, a few generalizations can be made. In the simple type of schizophrenia, the prognosis is poor owing to its insidious onset and absence of external precipitating causes. In the hebephrenic schizophrenia, the prognosis is generally poor since the course tends to be one of regression and ultimate personality disorganization. In catatonic schizophrenia, the prognosis is many times more favorable when the episodes are acute. Relapse is usually certain but in the intervals between episodes the personality can be near to the prepsychotic level. Paranoid schizophrenia can have a variable prognosis. When reality testing remains intact and the patient still doubts the reality of his paranoid ideation, the prognosis is more favorable. The prognosis is poor when the patient accepts the paranoia and loses reality testing. The schizoaffective subtype generally has the best prognosis.[2, 6, 8]

Schizophrenia, no matter what the type, often becomes a chronic illness requiring long term treatment. The advent of antipsychotic agents has played a major role in allowing patients to leave state hospitals and become members of their community. The commitment to seek the best treatment methods for a particular patient is best emphasized by the conclusion of Bleuler:[2]

Although a certain number of patients become deteriorated with every treatment, and others improve even in apparently severe cases, the treatment will decide in more than one-third of schizophrenic cases whether they can become social men again or not.

CONCLUSION

Schizophrenia is a chronic psychiatric disorder whose therapy depends to a major extent on drug treatment. The efficacy of the antipsychotic agents has been well proven. Of any commonly used class of drugs in current use, the antipsychotic agents cause the highest incidence of adverse effects and toxicity. Most patients on these drugs are constantly beset by annoying side effects, and many experience a variety of their many toxicities. Thus, the pharmacist who becomes knowledgeable and sympathetic can do much to facilitate a successful treatment program by working closely with the prescriber and the patient.

REFERENCES

1. Fenichel, O.: The Psychoanalytic Theory of Neurosis, Ed. 1, p. 415. W. W. Norton and Co., Inc., New York, 1945.
2. Kolb, L. C.: Noyes' Modern Clinical Psychiatry, Ed. 7, p. 355. W. B. Saunders Co., Philadelphia, 1968.
3. Colby, K. M.: A Primer for Psychotherapists, Ed. 1, p. 143. Ronald Press Co., New York, 1951.
4. Kallmann, F. J.: Heredity in Health and Mental Disorder, Ed. 1, p. 121. W. W. Norton and Co., Inc., New York, 1953.
5. Wintrobe, M. M., Thorn, G. W., Adams, R. D., Bennett, I. L., Braunwald, E., Isselbacher, K. J., and Petersdorf, R. G.: Harrison's Principles of Internal Medicine, Ed. 6, p. 1878. McGraw-Hill Book Co., New York, 1970.
6. Klein, D. F., and Davis, J. M.: Diagnosis and Drug Treatment of Psychiatric Disorders, Ed. 1, p. 33. Williams and Wilkins Co., Baltimore, 1969.
7. Rosenbaum, C. P.: The Meaning of Madness, Ed. 1, p. 3. Science House, New York, 1970.
8. Rosenbaum, C. P.: The Meaning of Madness, Ed. 1, p. 17. Science House, New York, 1970.
9. Klein, D. F., and Davis, J. M.: Diagnosis and Drug Treatment of Psychiatric Disorders, Ed. 1, p. 139. Williams and Wilkins Co., Baltimore, 1969.
10. Hollister, L. E.: Drug therapy—mental disorders—antipsychotic and antimanic drugs. N. Engl. J. Med., 286: 984, 1972.
11. Klein, D. F., and Davis, J. M.: Diagnosis and Drug Treatment of Psychiatric Disorders, Ed. 1, p. 139. Williams and Wilkins Co., Baltimore, 1969.
12. Goodman, L. S., and Gilman, A.: The Pharmacological Basis of Therapeutics, Ed. 4, p. 155, MacMillan Co., New York, 1970.
13. Kastrup, E. K.: Facts and Comparisons, Ed. 1, p. 261. Facts and Comparisons, Inc., St. Louis, 1973.
14. Ban, T.: Psychopharmacology, Ed. 1, p. 256. Williams and Wilkins Co., Baltimore, 1969.
15. Ayd, F. J.: Haloperidol: fifteen years of clinical experience. Dis. Nerv. Syst., 33: 459, 1972.
16. Crane, G. E.: Cardiac toxicity and psychotropic drugs. Dis. Nerv. Syst. 31: 534, 1970.
17. Anon.: Haloperidol. Med. Lett. Drugs Ther., 9:70, 1967.
18. Hollister, L. E.: Psychiatric and neurological disorders. In Clinical Pharmacology, Ed. 1, Chap. 11, p. 453, edited by K. L. Melmon and H. F. Morrelli. MacMillan Co., New York, 1972.
19. National Institute of Mental Health: Difference in clinical effects of three phenothiazines in acute schizophrenia. Dis. Nerv. Syst., 28: 369, 1967.
20. Cole, J. O.: Phenothiazine treatment in acute schizophrenia. Arch. Gen. Psychiatry, 10: 246, 1964.
21. Prien, R. F., and Cole, J. O.: High dose chlorpromazine therapy in chronic schizophrenia. Arch. Gen. Psychiatry, 18: 482, 1968.
22. Prien, R. F., Levine, J., and Cole, J. O.: Indications for high dose chlorpromazine therapy in chronic schizophrenia. Dis. Nerv. Syst., 31: 739, 1970.
23. Ayd, F. J.: Int. Drug Ther. Newsl., 7: 33, 1972.

24. Hrushka, M.: Therapeutic effects of different modes of chlorpromazine administration. Dis. Nerv. Syst., 27: 522, 1966.

25. Hollister, L. E.: Clinical use of psychotherapeutic drugs—current status. Clin. Pharmacol. Ther., 10: 170, 1969.

26. Hollister, L. E., Curry, S. H. Derr, J. E., and Kanter, S. L.: Studies of delayed-action medication. Clin. Pharmacol. Ther., 11: 49, 1970.

27. Huang, C. L., and Kurland, A. A.: Chlorpromazine blood levels in psychotic patients. Arch. Gen. Psychiatry, 5: 509, 1961.

28. Bartlett, C.: Comparison of thioridazine tablets to chlorpromazine spansules in the maintenance care of chronic schizophrenics. Curr. Ther. Res., 13: 100, 1971.

29. Crane, G. E.: Tardive dyskinesia in patients treated with major neuroleptics—a review of literature. Am. J. Psychiatry (Suppl.), 124: 40, 1968.

30. Schmidt, W. R., and Jarco, L. W.: Persistent dyskinesia following phenothiazine therapy. Arch. Neurol., 14: 369, 1966.

31. Klawans, H. L.: The pharmacology of tardive dyskinesia. Am. J. Psychiatry, 130: 82, 1973.

32. Ayd, F. J.: Int. Drug Ther. Newsl., 8: 1, 1973.

33. Neu, C., DiMascio, A., and Demirgian, E.: Antiparkinson medication in the treatment of extrapyramidal side effects. Curr. Ther. Res., 14: 246, 1972.

34. Anon.: Med. Lett. Drugs Ther., 7: 21, 1965.

35. Klett, C. J., and Caffey, E.: Evaluating the long-term need for antiparkinson drugs by chronic schizophrenics. Arch. Gen. Psychiatry, 26: 374, 1972.

36. Orlov, P., Kasparian, G., DiMascio, A., and Cole, J. O.: Withdrawal of antiparkinson drugs. Arch. Gen. Psychiatry, 25: 410, 1971.

37. DiMascio, A., and Demirgian, E.: Antiparkinson drug overuse. Psychosomatics, 11: 596, 1970.

38. Winer, J. A.: Loss of teeth with antidepressant therapy. Arch. Gen Psychiatry, 16: 239, 1967.

39. Kane, F. J.: Oral monilias following the use of thorazine. Am. J. Psychiatry, 120: 187, 1963.

40. Kutscher, A. H., Zegarelli, E. V., Seguin, L., Montano, W., and Cryan, R.: Oral moniliasis as a complication of chlorpromazine therapy. Cutis, 2: 176, 1966.

41. Prutting, J.: Pilocarpine nitrate and psychostimulants. J.A.M.A., 193: 236, 1965.

42. Warnes, H., Lehmann, H. E., and Ban, T. A.: Adynamic ileus during psychoactive medication. Can. Med. Assoc. J., 96: 1112, 1967.

43. Shader, R. I., Belfer, M. L., and DiMascio, A.: Endocrine effects of psychotrophic drugs—glucose metabolism. Conn. Med., 32: 389, 1968.

44. Schwarz, L., and Munoz, R.: Blood sugar levels in patients treated with chlorpromazine. Am. J. Psychiatry, 125: 253, 1968.

45. Korenyi, C., and Lowenstein, B.: Chlorpromazine-induced diabetes. Dis. Nerv. Syst., 29: 827, 1968.

46. Kojak, G., Barry, M. J., and Gastineau, C. F.: Severe hypoglycemic reaction with haloperidol—report of a case. Am. J. Psychiatry, 126: 573, 1969.

47. Sigell, L. T., and Flessa, H. C.: Drug interactions with anticoagulants. J.A.M.A., 214: 2035, 1970.

48. Weiner, M.: Effect of centrally active drugs on the action of coumarin anticoagulants. Nature, 212: 1599, 1966.

49. Oakley, D. P., and Lautch, H.: Haloperidol and anticoagulant treatment (Corres.). Lancet, 2: 1231, 1963.

chapter 31

AFFECTIVE DISORDERS

Glen Stimmel, Pharm.D.

Affective disorders are behavior disturbances characterized by persistent moods of depression or elation. Classification has, and continues still, to undergo many changes. For the purposes of this chapter, affective disorders will be divided into manic-depressive illness (bipolar) and depressive illness (unipolar) (Table 31.1). The two categories are considered to be primary disorders, occurring in patients who have no previous history of a psychiatric illness, except for possibly previous similar affective episodes. The two categories must be differentiated from affective disorders secondary to pre-existing illnesses, such as schizophrenia, organic brain syndrome, alcoholism and some neuroses.

The use of the unipolar and bipolar categories can best clarify the classification of affective disorders. Bipolar manic-depressive illness, can consist of manic episodes, either recurrent of alternating with depression; or it can consist primarily of depressive episodes but with a past history of manic episodes. Unipolar depressive illness is characterized by recurrent depressive episodes without mania. Depressive episodes of either category can be clinically indistinguishable. Differentiation depends upon the presence or absence of manic episodes in the past. Genetically, the two categories appear to be separate. The incidence of each is also quite different.

TABLE 31.1
Classification of Affective Disorders

Unipolar depressive illness
    Reactive—includes psychotic depressive reaction
       and neurotic depressions
    Endogenous—includes involutional melancholia
Bipolar manic-depressive illness
    Manic phase
    Depressive phase

Unipolar depressive illness is by far the most common. Manic-depressive illness is much less common, accounting for only about 5% of affective disorders.[1]

Perris followed 131 bipolar and 138 unipolar patients for an average of 20 years.[2] His results showed several important differences in the two categories:

1. Bipolar patients suffer significantly more illness periods than do unipolar patients.

2. Bipolar illness begins with depression more often than with mania.

3. In bipolar illness, only 16% of patients showed three, and only 4% showed more that three consecutive depressive episodes before they had a manic episode.

4. In bipolar illness, sex plays a significant role in the age of onset, depending on the polarity of the first episode. If the first episode is mania, males will have their onset at a significantly younger age than females. If the first episode is depression, females will have their onset at a significantly younger age than males.

5. In unipolar patients, males have their onset of depression much later than females.

The two categories of affective disorders will be discussed separately below, followed by the treatment of both categories.

DEPRESSION (UNIPOLAR)

The magnitude of the depressive illness problem can hardly be overestimated. Although schizophrenia accounts for the most hospitalizations, depression is unquestionably the most frequent cause for psychiatric consultation. About 8% of men and 16% of women can expect to have a depressive illness during their lifetime. Although present in younger age groups, depressive illness frequently presents itself in middle or old age.[1]

The classification of depressive illness is one of constant change and controversy. Classification schemes have been based on etiology (endogenous versus exogenous, autonomous versus reactive) or on symptomatology (agitated versus retarded, neurotic versus psychotic). The most simple scheme, which also correlates best with response to treatment, is one based primarily on etiology. Two broad groups of depressive illness can be identified—reactive and endogenous depression. The major etiological factor is the presence or absence, respectively, of precipitating environmental stress. As will be discussed, however, these two groups also correlate well with clinical symptomatology. Opinion is divided regarding the relationship of these two groups. Some believe the difference is only a matter of degree, while others regard the two to be etiologically distinct and not two opposite ends of one spectrum. Regardless, the separation is useful since the efficacy of the various modes of treatment correlates well with the two groups.[3,4]

Reactive Depression. Reactive depression, by definition, arises as a response to environmental stress. Frequent causes include loss of a family member or friend, illness, divorce or acute disappointment. Reactive depression is thought of as an exaggerated grief reaction. It is usually mild or moderate in severity; vegetative symptoms are either absent or mild; delusions or hallucinations are absent; and reality testing remains relatively intact. The clinical picture consists primarily of low mood, such as low self-esteem dejection, and indecisiveness. The one exception to the above generalizations is the diagnostic category of psychotic depressive reaction. It is a psychotic depression which is clearly reactive in etiology.

Endogenous Depression. Endogenous depression arises without identifiable precipitating events. The cause is thought to be due to internal processes. Recent neurochemical studies of the affective disorders have shed much light on possible etiological factors. Endogenous depression is generally severe in degree; vegetative symptoms are typically present and usually severe; delusions and hallucinations are common; and reality testing and the ability to carry on normal activities are markedly disturbed. Involutional melancholia belongs to this group of depressions. The depression of manic-depressive illness is clinically indistinguishable from unipolar endogenous depression.

Biochemical Etiology

The monoamine hypothesis of affective disorders arose from several simple observations of drugs and depression. It was observed that reserpine caused depression in some patients which was not distinguishable clinically from endogenous depression. It was known also that reserpine caused depletion of biogenic amines within the brain. A second observation was that monoamine oxidase inhibitors (MAOI) were effective antidepressants in some depressed patients. It was known that MAOI increase levels of biogenic amines within the brain. From these observations came the hypothesis that drugs with antidepressant activity must increase the amount of biogenic amines at certain receptor sites in the brain, while drugs causing depression must decrease these biogenic amines. This hypothesis was then extended to the affective disorders. Mania might result from excessive amounts of these biogenic amines while depressions might result from a deficiency in biogenic amines.[5] Such a simple biochemical etiological explanation for the affective disorders has withstood more than 15 years of further research. It has been shown that such diverse somatic treatments as electroconvulsive therapy, MAOI, tricyclic antidepressants and lithium all influence in some way the relative amount of biogenic amines within the brain. Positive evidence for this hypothesis has, and continues still, to slowly accumulate, and negative evidence is thus far lacking. As Lipton stated in regard to the monoamine hypothesis, "the house is far from complete but its foundations seem secure."[6]

Diagnosis and Clinical Findings

The diagnosis of depression is often difficult, since depression can be considered a mood, a symptom or a psychiatric syndrome. In depression, the exaggerated sadness, coupled with pessimism, is more than the ordinary low feelings which most people experience at one time or another. The exaggerated sadness and pessimism constitute the symptom of depression, and it becomes a depressive syndrome when accessory symptoms are present.

The distinction should be made between a depressive reaction and a grief reaction. In a grief reaction, the person's thinking focuses on the actual loss, such as the death of a loved one. Despite the sad mood, dejection and sleep disturbances seen in a grief reaction, they are proportional to the loss and relatively short lived. In depression, the person views himself and his situation unrealistically, and thinking is focused inwardly about his own lack of worth and the hopelessness of the situation.

The characteristic symptoms of depressive illness are:[4]

1. A persistent mood of sadness, apathy or loneliness.

2. Conviction of hopelessness and pessimism.

3. Tendency to blame oneself for problems and for the difficulties of others.

4. Motivational manifestations such as the intense desire to escape through running away, hiding or suicide.

5. Vegetative symptoms and physical symptoms such as loss of appetite, weight loss, insomnia, loss of libido, loss of energy, agitation or retardation.

6. Delusions and hallucinations, which are sometimes present in the severely depressed patients.

The presence or absence and degree of severity of these symptoms correlate well with the separation of depressions into reactive or endogenous depressions, as detailed earlier.

There is a high frequency of medical symptoms that may accompany depressive illness or may even dominate the clinical picture. The chief complaint of a depressed patient often is not the dysphoric mood, but rather somatic complaints. Fatigue, anorexia, dyspepsia, constipation and local or generalized aches and pains all may mask an underlying depression. When a complete medical work-up fails to uncover an explanation for such symptoms, depression should be considered. Whenever such symptoms resist usual treatment methods, then depression should be suspected. And whenever multiple symptoms are present that involve many systems, depression should be considered.[3]

Mention should also be made of the other side of the picture—depressions that mask physical illnesses. Once a diagnosis of depression is made, the possibility of physical illness should not be forgotten. Some illnesses whose clinical picture may be predominately one of depression include Parkinson's disease, brain tumors, peptic ulcer, pancreatic carcinoma, cholelithiasis, cardiovascular disease, early rheumatoid arthritis and the sequelae of infections such as viral pneumonia and infectious mononucleosis.[4,7]

Course and Prognosis

The course of depressive illness is generally self-limiting, but recurrent. Studies of the natural history of depressive illness show an average duration of 6 months. Treatment should be directed toward shortening this period and continued on a maintenance basis, depending on past history of depressive episode duration and frequency. Beck has compiled much information on the course and prognosis of depressive illness, some of which follows:[4]

1. Complete recovery from a depressive episode occurs in 70 to 95% of cases; in younger patients, the percentage is nearer 95%.

2. The median duration of depressive episodes is a little over 6 months for inpatients, about 3 months for outpatients.

3. If the initial depressive episode occurs before 30 years of age, the duration tends to be shorter. Acute onset favors shorter duration also.

4. After an initial depressive episode, long term follow-up studies show nearly 80% will have a recurrence at some time in their lives.

5. After the first depressive episode, most patients have a symptom-free interval of more than 3 years before the next episode. The symptom-free interval tends to decrease with each successive episode.

Suicide is a most important prognostic variable. Because of suicide, depression is one of the few psychiatric disorders with a significant mortality rate. In cases of endogenous depression, the more dangerous suicidal reactions are apt to occur during recurrent episodes. Depressive symptoms characterized by hopelessness, urgent anxiety, agitation, dissatisfaction and demands that something be done immediately are highest in suicidal danger. About 15% of persons who attempt suicide repeat, and about 5% eventually succeed. Half these deaths occur within a year of the previous attempt.[8]

MANIC-DEPRESSIVE ILLNESS (BIPOLAR)

Manic-depressive illness is a distinct diagnostic category, although diagnostic criteria vary from country to country and generation to generation. The occurrence of elation and depression in the same patient had long been recognized, but it was Kraepelin in 1896 who viewed these opposing affective states as variations of a single disorder which he designated manic-depressive insanity.[9]

Etiology

Of the major psychiatric disorders, manic-depressive illness has the best evidence for the existence of a biogenetic factor. Siblings of manic-depressive patients have an incidence 25 times higher than the normal population. Monozygous twin studies show that if one twin becomes manic-depressive, there is a 66 to 96% incidence in the other twin, even when raised in different homes.[9,10] Environmental factors certainly have been shown also to contribute to the etiology. Social class seems to be an important factor. Prevalence in a German clinic shows manic-depressive illness to be 3 times as frequent in the highest social class, and 4 times as frequent in the professional classes as in the general population. American psychiatrists during World War II reported manic-depressive illness to be 3 times more frequent in officers as compared to enlisted men.[9]

No correlation has been found to exist between life stresses and the onset of a manic or depressive episode. This is confirmed by clinical studies as well as clinical experience.[11] Patients frequently report acute onset of illness with no precipitating stress. The depression of manic-depressive illness is described by patients as being very different from the depressed feeling resulting from life stresses or losses. The monoamine hypothesis of affective disorders as discussed earlier applies equally to manic-depressive illness as well as some depressive illnesses.

Phases of Manic-depressive Illness

Manic Phase. The manic phase is characterized by elated mood or irritability, flight of ideas, increased psychomotor activity, diminished fatigability, grandiosity, distractability acute onset of symptoms. The patient is socially aggressive, witty, boastful, argumentative and intolerant of criticism. The patient characteristically may spend his money extravagantly, is full of ambitious schemes and starts enterprises that soon fail or are quickly abandoned. He has little insight as a rule, although there is no clouding of consciousness or forgetfulness.

The mania can vary in severity, which is termed hypomania, acute mania and delirious mania. Hypomania is the milder form, which may not be easily distinguishable from peculiar behavior or personality. Acute mania is a more severe degree, in which the behavior is clearly abnormal. Insight is severely limited or absent. Delirious mania is the extreme manic state where the patient is totally unmanageable. Delusions and hallucinations are most frequent in delirious mania.[9]

Depressive Phase. The depressive phase is clinically similar to unipolar endogenous depression. Only a past history of manic episodes can identify the depression as a phase of manic-depressive illness. Just as in the manic phase, there can be a wide range in the severity of the depression.

Course and Prognosis

The most frequent age for the first manic episode is 20 to 25 years and the first depressive episode is from 30 to 35 years of age. Manic and depressive episodes are generally self-limiting, but recurrent. Duration of an episode can vary from several weeks to a year or 2, but generally they last about 6 months. The frequency of episodes tends to increase with increasing age, meaning there are shorter intervals of remission. Drug treatment can both reduce the duration of the episodes and reduce the frequency of episodes. The patient is usually in good mental health in the intervals between episodes. Personality, intellect and cognition remain intact.

The prognosis for a single affective episode, by the natural course of the illness, is very good. Prognosis for the occurrence of future episodes is variable. The earlier the onset, the worse the prognosis. If the episode is manic, recurrence is almost assured. If the first episode is depressive, it may not be followed by a recurrence. The prognosis is least favorable when episodes are very frequent. Mania does not become chronic, whereas depression is much more likely to become chronic. The over-all prognosis of manic-depressive illness, especially when compared to the other major psychiatric disorders, is good. There is no evidence that

recurrent episodes lead to dementia. Although the episodes may increase in frequency with age, the intervals remain as periods of relatively good mental health.[9]

TREATMENT OF AFFECTIVE DISORDERS

While the treatment of schizophrenia is fairly simple and clear-cut using the antipsychotic drugs, the treatment of affective disorders is complex, controversial and confusing. The many varied treatment modalities for affective disorders are listed in Table 31.2. Of all the psychiatric disorders, affective disorders have the best established etiological hypothesis, and the drugs the best explanation of their mechanism of action. Yet the treatment of affective disorders is represented by many varied drug groups, the efficacy of many still remains a matter of controversy, and a significant number of patients are unresponsive to drug therapy.

Antidepressant Drugs

Tricyclic Antidepressants. Table 31.3 lists the indications for tricyclic antidepressants. The true indications for the tricyclic antidepressants constitute only a small percentage of depressive reactions. It has been consistently shown that tricyclics are the clear choice for endogenous depressions, and generally it is agreed that the tricyclics are effective for this

TABLE 31.2
Treatment Modalities for Affective Disorders

Antidepressants
   Tricyclics
   Stimulants
   Monoamine oxidase inhibitors
   Electroconvulsive therapy
   Psychotherapy—individual, group
Antimanic agents
   Lithium
   Phenothiazines

TABLE 31.3
Indications for Tricyclic Antidepressants

Involutional depressions
Depressive phase of manic-depressive illness (bipolar)
Psychotic depressive illness (unipolar)
Adjunctive treatment for depressions in schizophrenia
   and organic brain syndromes

category of depression.[12,14] Mild reactive depressions clearly are not an indication for tricyclic antidepressants. What confuses interpretation of studies is that the several weeks necessary for tricyclics to take full therapeutic effect is sufficient time for spontaneous recovery to occur in mild reactive depressions.[15] Tricyclics have been promoted for treatment of depressions associated with chronic physical illness, but improved depression scores correlate best with lapse of time and anticipation of discharge from the hospital and not with any pharmacological activity of the drug.[16] Treatment of moderate depression, whether classified as reactive or endogenous, depends primarily on the symptoms. If bodily complaints, anxiety and tension are predominant, antianxiety agents can relieve not only these symptoms but also the resultant depression. If agitation is predominant, phenothiazines such as thioridazine may be most useful. The type of moderate depression responding best to tricyclics occurs when anxiety levels are low and agitation is minimal, which describes a retarded depression.[13,17] However, the tricyclics are used frequently for indications that are contrary to those advocated by the medical literature.

Retarded endogenous depressions account for less than 20% of hospitalized, depressed patients and certainly fewer on an outpatient basis.[18] The widespread use of tricyclic antidepressants indicates they are being used for depressions of many types. The prevalent attitude seems to be that although there is no indication for tricyclics in the more common reactive depressions, many patients seem to respond. Use of tricyclics is considered to be worth a trial, even though the controlled studies in the literature provide little supporting evidence.

Efficacy

Studies of efficacy of tricyclic antidepressants show little and often no difference from placebo. In many studies showing therapeutic superiority of tricyclics over placebo, the difference is small. Additionally, more than 1/3 of patients do not show even moderate improvement on the tricyclic antidepressants.[13,19,20] This kind of evidence clearly illustrates the necessity of utilizing nondrug therapy for many depressive patients, particularly psychotherapy.

The notion that there is a drug to cure everything is most notably a misconception when applied to the treatment of depression. Often drug therapy should be considered only as adjunctive treatment and often not utilized at all.

One explanation offered for the poor showing of tricyclics when compared to placebo is that the sample population is too heterogenous. As mentioned earlier, tricyclics are clearly effective in endogenous depressions, which comprise only a minority of depressions. Thus, studies are diluted by inclusion of other types of depressions that are unresponsive to tricyclics, causing the results to be poor.[18] Such an explanation is certainly a valid one and should serve to re-emphasize the fact that tricyclics do have limited indications.

Dosage

Although effective dosage is an unsettled question, most controlled studies allow a statement of the range of effective dosage for the tricyclic antidepressants. Effective dosage for imipramine and amitriptyline consistently fall into the range of 150 to 300 mg daily. Generally, efficacy correlates best with severity of the depression and the patients receiving the higher doses.[15,19] The stated effective dosage range may be suprising to the community practitioner who is accustomed to seeing much smaller doses being prescribed. From this author's experience, the more common daily dosage being prescribed in the community is in the range of 30 to 100 mg. There are several situations that may justify such a low dosage. These include the initiation period of therapy, the maintenance dose reached after tapering from the higher doses, the use of a tricyclic with a phenothiazine and those patients who are more sensitive to the effects of the drugs. Unfortunately, those four situations can not account for the widespread use of minimal doses. The real answer seems to be that the depressive symptoms are being treated without the underlying cause being identified, resulting in tricyclics being used to treat family and social problems rather than depressive illness. The reasons for such misuse are several, but the primary responsibility necessarily rests with the pharmaceutical industry. The principal source of drug information to prescribers has been advertising through medical journals and manufacturer's representatives. These modalities of information are misleading; they confuse the true indications for the drugs as presented earlier and promote and encourage the use of tricyclics for unproven indications.[21]

Assuming adequate dosage is given, there exists a lag period of up to several weeks before therapeutic effect is achieved. Some of the depressive symptoms, such as insomnia, may respond within several days, but reversal of the depressive syndrome usually begins after several weeks. The claim that the desmethyl derivatives, desipramine and nortriptyline, have a quicker therapeutic onset as yet is unproven. The few studies showing such a nonsignificant trend are equalled by studies showing the opposite.[19] A proper therapeutic trial for the tricyclic antidepressants must consist of at least 4 weeks at a therapeutic dosage. Although some studies report that early signs of response forecast a good therapeutic outcome, use of the drug at therapeutic levels for at least 4 weeks is necessary to allow a judgment that the tricyclic will be a therapeutic failure.

Since the lag time of response is clinically undesirable and troublesome, methods to shorten it have been actively sought. The most interesting finding so far is the use of liothyronine (T_3) with the tricyclic. It had been observed a decade ago that tricyclics were more toxic in hyperthyroid states or when combined with thyroid supplements.[22] Since thyroid seemed to potentiate the effect of the tricyclic drugs, recent research has focused on the use of thyroid hormone hopefully to shorten the lag time of response. Generally, studies have shown that a 14-day course of T_3, 25mg daily, is effective in enhancing the therapeutic effectiveness of tricyclic antidepressants, that the lag time of response is sometimes shortened and that a high proportion of tricyclic drug failures can be converted to therapeutic successes.[23,24] The T_3 usually can be discontinued after 14 days. Most studies show that women respond far better than men to this combined treatment. Side effects due to the T_3 are negligible, and there is little or no effect on peripheral measures of thyroid state. Interestingly, one study included three bipolar patients on the combined therapy, two of whom experienced manic symptoms during recovery.[23]

Duration of Therapy

The duration of tricyclic therapy is based best upon the past history of the individual patient's affective disorder. As mentioned earlier, the natural course of a depressive episode lasts about 6 months. Drug therapy should be directed toward shortening that time and continued for the length of the patient's natural length of depressive episodes. If the depressive episode is the patient's first and he has responded quickly, then treatment can be tapered and discontinued several weeks after remission. If, however, depressive episodes have occurred at closely spaced intervals and have been slow to respond, then prolonged maintenance therapy would be indicated.[13]

Side Effects

The side effects from the tricyclic drugs are generally like the phenothiazines except that extrapyramidal symptoms are rare. Instead, a persistent fine rapid tremor of the hands may occur. This tremor is not responsive to antiparkinson medication.[19] Anticholinergic effects occur with even greater frequency than seen with phenothiazines since tricyclics have more potent anticholinergic activity.[25] Sedation is a frequent effect of amitriptyline, less so with imipramine. The demethylated derivatives are the least sedating of the tricyclics. Orthostatic hypotension is commonly observed with therapeutic doses, and patients should be so warned. The cardiovascular effects of tricyclics are a particular problem, and their use in pre-existing cardiovascular disease should be cautious. The tricyclics in therapeutic doses cause EKG changes in about 20% of patients without any history of cardiovascular disease. Deaths from coronary occlusion, ventricular fibrillation and arrest have been reported, as well as cases of severe arrhythmias. In patients with pre-existing cardiovascular disease, precipitation of congestive heart failure and myocardial infarction have been reported during tricyclic therapy.[19,26]

Withdrawal effects do occur when tricyclics are abruptly discontinued, especially when doses have exceeded 150 mg daily of imipramine or equivalent for several months or more. The effects are usually nonspecific complaints, such as malaise, nausea, vomiting, abdominal cramping, insomnia and irritability.

Overdosage with tricyclic antidepressants constitutes a serious medical situation because of cardiotoxicity. Varying degrees of atrioventricular (AV) block are frequently seen, and ventricular fibrillation and arrest are a frequent cause of death. Ingestion of 1 to 2 g (30 50-mg tablets) of imipramine or amitriptyline constitutes a serious attempt and can be fatal.[2 7]

Interactions

There are two drug interactions with the tricyclic antidepressants that are well documented and highly significant. The first is the combined use of MAOI and tricyclics, which must be absolutely avoided. Severe reactions have occurred, including convulsions, excitation, and death. This interaction is totally predictable, since both drugs increase the amount of norepinephrine available at the adrenergic neuron synapse by different mechanisms. Use of these two drugs, if necessary in the same patient, should be separated by a drug-free interval of at least several weeks.

The other significant interaction is use of guanethidine with tricyclics. The tricyclic blocks the uptake of guanethidine into the neuron, thus blocking its antihypertensive effect. Other antihypertensives, such as methyldopa or hydralazine, may be substituted and used with a tricyclic.

Generally, a hypertensive patient should be carefully evaluated and monitored when using a tricyclic antidepressant. One reason is that many of the antihypertensives can cause depression, reserpine being most notable. The depression being treated may in fact be drug-induced. A second reason for careful monitoring is that the patient may be started on guanethidine by his medical doctor, with the result as explained above. A third reason is that, of the several patients who have experienced a severe hypotensive episode from psychotropic drugs, in this author's experience, all had essential hypertension.

Electroconvulsive Therapy

Electroconvulsive therapy (ECT) is the treatment of choice for severely depressed patients, especially those who are acutely suicidal. The efficacy of ECT is usually superior to antidepressant drugs, and the response is fast. A course of ECT for depression would consist of three treatments per week for a total of six to ten treatments. ECT is most effective in endogenous depressions, either agitated or retarded, the depressed phase of manic-depressive illness and involutional melancholia. It is not particularly effective in reactive depressions, schizoaffective disorders or the manic phase of manic-depressive illness. Although response is fast and efficacy high, relapse is usually certain.[18,19,28] Thus the treatment of choice would be to use ECT when a rapid response is desired, while concurrently initiating tricyclic therapy. The ECT will hold the patient until the tricyclic has had time to take full therapeutic effect.

Monoamine Oxidase Inhibitors

The use of MAOI for treating depression today is severely limited by their toxicity and the superiority of tricyclic drugs in terms of efficacy. The place of MAOI in the treatment of depression is one of being last choice agents when all other treatments have failed. There are patients who are unresponsive to the tricyclics who will respond to MAOI. Their use should be restricted to hospitalized patients.[18,19]

Stimulants

The use of stimulants, such as dextroamphetamine or methylphenidate, has a very small indication in the treatment of depression. At most, stimulants have a very limited value in the short term treatment of mild reactive depressions. They should be used in low doses, such as 5 to 10 mg daily of dextroamphetamine, and used for no more than 4 to 6 weeks. Stimulants have no place in the treatment of moderate or severe depressions, and habituation and overuse can easily complicate successful treatment in any patient.[18,19]

Psychotherapy

The importance of other treatment measures for depression besides drugs can not be overemphasized. Although endogenous depressions do respond well to antidepressant drugs, the addition of some type of psychotherapy can greatly enhance therapeutic response. In the group of reactive depressions, the psychotherapeutic approach to treatment is preferable. Drug therapy at most should be adjunctive. The causes of many reactive depressions involve family and social problems, which no drug can treat or change.

Antimanic Drugs

Lithium. Lithium is a simple alkali metal, the third element in the periodic table. Trace amounts are found throughout nature—in fresh and sea water, minerals and plant and animal tissues. Medical uses of lithium in the past include lithium urate as a treatment for gout, lithium bromide as a sedative and anticonvulsant, and lithium chloride as a salt substitute. Lithium proved to be of no value in the first two and led to toxicity and death in the third. Thus lithium had a poor introduction and history at least in American medicine. The value of lithium as a psychoactive agent was first described in 1949 by an Australian psychiatrist, John F. J. Cade.[29] His reports of lithium's usefulness in psychotic excitement stimulated further trials of lithium in other countries, these results confirmed Cade's original findings. It took until 1965, however, until lithium was first introduced to American psychiatry. Much research quickly followed, and lithium was released for use by the FDA in April, 1970.

Indications. The primary indication for lithium is for the control of manic episodes. No other use is formally sanctioned by the FDA. The value of prophylactic lithium for prevention of manic relapse is now becoming well documented, and preliminary data suggest a lower incidence of depressive relapses as well. Lithium has been tried clinically for a variety of other disorders, including hyperkinesis, reactive depression, schizoaffective disorders and severe premenstrual tension. The results in hyperkinesis and reactive depression are generally poor. The trials in schizoaffective disorders have yielded conflicting results. Generally, it seems that lithium can be effective in treating the affective component of the disorder, but that the psychotic disturbance is unaffected. Much of the conflicting data can be attributed to the variation in diagnostic criteria for mania

versus schizoaffective disorder.[30] It is suggested that lithium can be a useful tool in clarifying an understructure of schizophrenic symptomatology in patients who initially exhibit an affective psychosis.[31] Small doses of lithium during the 10 days preceding menses has been reported useful in treating severe premenstrual tension. The severity of the cases should be emphasized, since the tension in each case was of psychotic or near psychotic proportion and unresponsive to conventional therapies. Results in such cases are outstandingly good, although no controlled studies are yet available. Such use of lithium must be considered to be investigational.[31,32]

Efficacy. Many well controlled studies of lithium in treating manic episodes have been published which clearly demonstrate the efficacy of lithium.[33,35] The results show that 70 to 80% of patients have a good chance of recovery with lithium; that age or sex are not factors in clinical response to lithium; that all types of manic disorder including chronic, recurrent and hypomania respond equally well; and that lithium can often be effective when other treatments such as phenothiazines or ECT are ineffective. By the middle of 1967, 42 papers were published on the use of lithium in mania, representing 1,000 cases, and only 1 paper reported negative results.[36]

When discussing the efficacy of lithium, comparison must be made with the other treatment methods available. Before lithium, phenothiazine drugs were the preferred treatment for manic episodes. Chlorpromazine was the drug of choice because of its sedative effect, while other less sedating phenothiazines were useful for hypomania or prophylactic control. Controlled studies comparing chlorpromazine and lithium in mania generally show their efficacy to be equal but with several important differences. The doses of chlorpromazine necessary for control of a manic episode are higher than those necessary for any other psychiatric disorder. Typically, 2 or 3 g daily are needed. Sedation at that dosage is prominent. Lithium, however, lacks the sedative effect while still being effective in controlling the acute manic episode.[37] An interim report of a double blind study of lithium and chlorpromazine provides several important differences in the two treatments.[38] In manic patients, total remission occurred in 78% of patients on lithium and in 36% on chlorpromazine. Both agents produced a reduction in overactivity, but in optimal doses, chlorpromazine tended to produce sluggishness and drowsiness. Lithium normalized affect and ideation while the chlorpromazine effect was less consistent and slower in onset. Lithium usually takes effect within 4 to 10 days, while chlorpromazine becomes therapeutically effective after 2 to 3 weeks. Chlorpromazine's suppressant effects, however, are evident within a day.

The current evidence seems to establish lithium not just as another acceptable treatment for manic episodes but as an agent superior to other treatment methods. Lithium seems to be the treatment of choice for manic episodes, and in cases of early control problems, moderate amounts of chlorpromazine should be added until lithium takes effect.

While the efficacy of lithium in treating manic episodes has been well established and recognized, its utility prophylactically has raised much controversy. Early evidence for the prophylactic efficacy was based on longitudinal studies which compared the incidence of relapse before lithium therapy with the incidence during lithium therapy. Such studies were severely criticized on methodological grounds. More recent controlled studies have generously supported the findings of the earlier trials, but there still exists an attitude of skepticism regarding prophylactic lithium. The FDA still approves lithium only for the treatment of acute manic episodes. Recent evidence overwhelmingly seems to support the prophylactic value of lithium in preventing recurrence of manic episodes. A VA-NIMH Collaborative Study Group reported that nearly half the patients on prophylactic lithium completed 2 years of treatment without relapse compared to only 10% in the placebo group. Five other double blind prophylactic studies with placbo are cited; they all reported lithium to be significantly more effective than placebo.[39]

The efficacy of lithium in preventing recurrences of depressive episodes in manic-depressive illness has been reported in several studies, although this effect generally has been statistically insignificant. Better studies of this effect are needed. The value of lithium in treatment of depressive episodes in progress is even less certain. Several studies have hinted at such an idea and trend, but the need for controlled studies is clear.[40,41]

Principles of Clinical Use. In contrast to other psychotropic drugs, lithium is a simple element whose blood level can easily be measured and which correlates well with therapeutic and toxic effects. Absorption of lithium carbonate is virtually complete, with less than 1% excreted in the feces. Absorption is independent of the salt form used; the carbohydrate was selected only because of its better stability and smaller molecular weight. Peak serum levels are reached in 2 to 4 hr, with complete absorption in 6 to 8 hr. The complete and rapid absorption gives rise to a practical problem of side effects that correlate with peak blood levels. Trautner et al. demonstrated that nausea, vomiting, vertigo and muscular weakness were present when blood levels went above 1.3 to 1.5 mEq per liter. The syndrome was described as a cross between seasickness and a hangover. These effects disappeared abruptly when the blood level dropped from its peak.[42] For this reason, daily doses of lithium are generally divided even though the drug can be dosed once daily if tolerated. Serum half-life of lithium is about 24 hr, and approaches 30 to 36 hours in elderly patients.

Lithium is not bound to plasma proteins or metabolized but is freely filtered through the glomerular membrane. About 20% is excreted in the urine, while 80% is reabsorbed in the kidney tubules. Reabsorption almost exclusively takes place in the proximal tubules. Lithium clearance is unaffected by large doses of thiazides, furosemide, ethacrynic acid or mercurial diuretics.[43] Sodium intake is an important variable during lithium therapy since there seems to be a common mechanism for reabsorption of sodium and lithium. When sodium intake is low, more lithium is reabsorbed and blood levels rise. The significance of this effect only becomes important when large fluctuations in sodium intake or loss occur, such as crash diets, fasting or excessive sweating. Daily variations in dietary sodium are insignificant and do not require monitoring.[42]

Dosage. For control of manic episodes, the serum level should be from 0.8 to 1.5 mEq per liter, although some patients may require up to 2.0 mEq per liter. A daily dose to achieve such a level would range from 900 to 1,800 mg. The serum level is the variable that is monitored not the daily dose. For maintenance treatment or prophylaxis, serum levels should be maintained at 0.5 to 1.0 mEq per liter, which requires about 600 to 1,500 mg daily. Obviously, dosage must be individualized as needed to achieve the serum level desired.[40] The difference in serum levels necessary between acute mania and maintenance is partially due to the fact that manic phase patients tolerate dosage levels up to 2 to 3 times greater than those tolerated by normal patients.[40]

Serum levels should be done every 2 to 4 days during initiation of treatment, then at least monthly once the dosage and serum level has stabilized. Blood samples for serum lithium level determination must be drawn 8 to 12 hr after the last lithium dose.

Lithium efficacy depends upon its continuous presence in the body at some minimal level. Discontinuing lithium can lead to a recurrence within 3 days. If lithium blood levels are allowed to decline gradually, it has been shown that manic symptoms re-emerge with gradually increasing intensity.[35]

Side Effects and Toxicity. Common side effects related to peak blood levels of lithium have been described earlier, and they should be considered to be harmless rather than the warning signs of impending toxicity. Toxic signs correlate well with the serum lithium level and are presented in Table 31.4.

Several side effects seemingly unrelated to dosage but more often observed as late occurring, are goiter and a diabetes insipidus-like syndrome. Reports of lithium-induced goiter began appearing within the past 5 years and, more recently, cases of hypothyroidism while taking lithium. The goiter reported usually shows a diffuse nontender thyroid enlargement with the patient remaining clinically euthyroid. The goiter usually disappears when lithium is discontinued or thyroid replacement added. Fieve and Platman, however, searched for thyroid abnormalities in manic-depressive patients who never received lithium, and they found the same high incidence as studies show with lithium.[44] What has been found most recently is that lithium decreases the amount of thyroxine secreted by the thyroid gland.[45] In most patients, the decrease is small enough that the body can easily compensate. In patients with latent hypothyroidism or other thyroid abnormalities, this effect of lithium may be enough to cause clinical goiter or even hypothyroidism.

Several cases have now been reported describing a lithium-induced diabetes insipidus-syndrome. Thirst, high urine output and low urine specific gravity are characteristic. Unlike diabetes insipidus, these symptoms can not be counteracted by vasopressin, and infusion of hypertonic saline shows a paradoxical increased diuresis. The explanation has been offered that the kidney tubules become relatively insensitive to vasopressin. No permanent damage to renal function has been seen yet.[46,47] Practitioners of a generation ago should not be surprised at this effect, recalling when lithium salts were used as diuretics.

Overdosage with lithium is an extremely serious medical situation, although there are many signs that can signal lithium intoxication. The effects of late lithium intoxication involve the nervous system primarily. Impairment of consciousness and deep coma are characteristic. Treatment is directed toward hastening the elimination of lithium from the body and preventing the complications of impaired consciousness and coma. Supportive measures similar to those used in the treatment of barbiturate overdosage are necessary, for there are many similarities in the two drugs' complications. Several reported deaths due to lithium were suspected to have resulted from pulmonary complications. The preferred treatment for hastening lithium elimination is to use forced diuresis with urea and alkalinize the

TABLE 31.4
Lithium Side Effects

Mild	Nausea, vomiting
	Abdominal pain, diarrhea
	Muscle weakness
	Fine tremor of hands
Moderate	Coarse tremor
	Ataxia
	Muscle hyperirritability—fasciculation, twitching
	Confusion
	Slurred speech
Severe	Choreo-athetotic movements
	Clonic movement of limbs
	Seizures
	Stupor
	Impaired consciousness
	Coma
	Death

urine. The value of hemodialysis in severe intoxication is not certain, but it may be useful for short periods, especially when the lithium blood level rebounds owing to tissue redistribution.[43,48,49]

CONCLUSION

Affective disorders constitute an area that has clinical relevance for every health practitioner, for these disorders are encountered throughout the practice of medicine and are manifest in a variety of ways. Depressions can be both a cause of illness and a consequence of illness. It is important for all health practitioners to become familiar with the clinical manifestations of affective disorders as well as the various modes of treatment. A knowledgeable and sympathetic pharmacist can help facilitate a successful treatment program by working closely with the prescriber and patient.

REFERENCES

1. Coppen, A.: Depression: a clinical portrait. In Depression, Ed. 1, Chap. 2, p. 11, edited by D. Hill and L. E. Hollister. Medcom Learning System, Medcom, Inc., New York, 1970.
2. Perris, C.: The course of depressive psychoses. Acta Psychiatr. Scand., 44: 238, 1968.
3. Storrow, H. A.: The diagnosis of depression. In Depression in Medical Practice, Ed. 1, Chap. 2, p. 21, edited by A. J. Enelow. Merck and Co., Inc., West Point, Pa., 1970.
4. Beck, A. T.: Depression: Clinical, Experimental and Theoretical Aspects, Ed. 1, p. 10. Harper and Row, New York, 1967.
5. Schildkraut, J. J.: Neuropsychopharmacology and the Affective Disorders, Ed. 1. Little, Brown and Co., Boston, 1970.
6. Lipton, M. A.: Affective disorders: progress, but some unresolved questions remain. Am. J. Psychiatry, 127: 357, 1970.
7. Rossman, P. L.: Organic diseases resembling functional disorders. Hosp. Med., 5: 72, 1969.
8. Litman, R. E.: Evaluation and management of the suicidal patient. In Depression in Medical Practice, Ed. 1, Chap. 7, p. 139, edited by A. J. Enelow. Merck and Co., Inc., West Point, Pa., 1970.
9. Kolb, L. C.: Noyes' Modern Clinical Psychiatry, Ed. 7, p. 326. W. B. Saunders Co., Philadelphia, 1968.
10. Price, J. S.: Genetics of the affective illnesses. Hosp. Med., 2: 1172, 1968.
11. Hudgens, R. W., Morrison, J. R., and Barchha, R. G.: Life events and onset of primary affective disorders. Arch. Gen. Psychiatry, 16: 134, 1967.
12. Hollister, L. E., Overall, J. E., Shelton, J., Penn-

ington, V., Kimbell, I., and Johnson, M.: Drug therapy in depression. Arch. Gen. Psychiatry, 17: 486, 1967.
13. Hollister, L. E.: Drug therapy. N. Engl. J. Med., 286: 1195, 1972.
14. Kiloh, L. G., and Garside, R. F.: The independence of neurotic and endogenous depression. Br. J. Psychiatry, 109: 451, 1963.
15. Cole, J. O.: Therapeutic efficacy of antidepressant drugs: a review. J.A.M.A., 190: 448, 1964.
16. Fryer, D. G., and Timberlake, W. H.: A trial of imipramine in depressed patients with chronic physical disease. J. Chronic Dis., 16: 173, 1967.
17. Rickels, K., Raab, E., DeSilverio, R., and Etemad, B.: Drug treatment in depression: antidepressants or tranquilizers? J.A.M.A., 201: 675, 1967.
18. Hollister, L. E.: Psychiatric and neurological disorders. In Clinical Pharmacology, Ed. 1, Chap. 11, p. 453, edited by K. L. Melmon and H. F. Morelli. The MacMillan Co., New York, 1972.
19. Klein, D. F., and Davis, J. M.: Diagnosis and Drug Treatment of Psychiatric Disorders, Ed. 1, p. 187. Williams and Wilkins Co., Baltimore, 1969.
20. Malitz, S., and Kanzler, M.: Are antidepressants better than placebo? Am. J. Psychiatry, 127: 1605, 1971.
21. Lennard, H. L., Epstein, L. J., Bernstein, A., and Ransom, D. C.: Mystification and Drug Misuse: Hazards in Using Psychoactive Drugs, p. 19. Harper and Row, New York, 1971.
22. Prange, A. J., Jr.: Paroxysmal uaricular tachycardia apparently resulting from combined thyroid imipramine treatment. Am. J. Psychiatry, 119: 994, 1963.
23. Coppen, A., Whybrow, P. C., Noguera, R., Maggs, R., and Prange, A. J.: The comparative antidepressant value of 1-tryptophan and imipramine with and without attempted potentiation of triiodothyronine. Arch. Gen. Psychiatry, 26: 234, 1972.
24. Wheatley, D.: Potentiation of amitriptyline by thyroid hormone. Arch. Gen. Psychiatry, 26: 229, 1972.
25. Vaillant, G. E.: Clinical significance of anticholinergic effects of imipramine-type drugs. Am. J. Psychiatry, 125: 1600, 1969.
26. Crane, G. E.: Cardiac toxicity and psychotropic drugs. Dis. Nerv. Syst., 31: 534, 1970.
27. Davis, J. M.: Overdosage of psychotropic drugs. Ann. Psychiatry, 3: 6, 1973.
28. Impastato, D.: The convulsive therapies in depression. In Depression, Ed. 1, Chap. 6, p. 59, edited by D. Hill and L. E. Hollister. Medcom Learning System, Medcom, Inc., New York, 1970.
29. Cade, J. F. J.: Lithium salts in the treatment of psychotic excitement. Med. J. Aust., 36: 349, 1949.
30. National Institute of Mental Health: Lithium in the treatment of mood disorders. Public Health Service Publication No. 2143, p. 65.

U.S. Government Printing Office, Washington, D.C., 1970.

31. Dinsmore, P. R., and Ryback, R.: Lithium in schizo-affective disorders. Dis. Nerv. Syst., 33: 771, 1972.

32. Sletten, I. W., and Gershon, S.: The premenstrual syndrome. Compr. Psychiatry, 7: 197, 1966.

33. Schou, M., Juel-Neilsen, N., Stromgren, E., and Voldby, H.: The treatment of manic psychoses by the administration of lithium salts. J. Neurol. Neurosurg. Psychiatry, 17: 250, 1954.

34. Wharton, R. N., and Fieve, R. R.: The use of lithium in the affective psychoses. Am. J. Psychiatry, 123: 706, 1966.

35. Bunney, W. E., Jr., Goodwin, F. K., Davis, J. M., and Fawcett, J. A.: A behavioral-biochemical study of lithium treatment. Am. J. Psychiatry, 125: 499, 1968.

36. Schou, M.: Lithium in psychiatric therapy and prophylaxis. J. Psychiatr. Res., 6: 67, 1968.

37. Prien, R. F., Caffey, E. M., and Klett, C. J.: Comparison of lithium and chlorpromazine in the treatment of mania. Arch. Gen. Psychiatry, 26: 146, 1972.

38. Johnson, G., Gershon, S., and Hekimian, L. J.: Controlled evaluation of lithium and chlorpromazine in the treatment of manic states: an interim report. Compr. Psychiatry, 9: 563, 1968.

39. Prien, R. F., Caffey, E. M., and Klett, C. J.: Prophylactic efficacy of lithium carbonate in manic-depressive illness. Arch. Gen. Psychiatry, 28: 337, 1973.

40. Gershon, S.: Use of lithium salts in psychiatric disorders. Dis. Nerv. Syst., 29: 51, 1968.

41. Goodwin, F. K., Murphy, D. L., and Bunney, W. E.: Lithium carbonate treatment in depression and mania. A longitudinal double-blind study. Arch. Gen. Psychiatry, 21: 486, 1969.

42. Trautner, E. M., Morris, R., Noack, C. H., and Gershon, S.: The excretion and retention of ingested lithium and its effects on the ionic balance of man. Med. J. Aust., 42: 280, 1955.

43. Thomsen, K.: Renal lithium elimination in man and active treatment of lithium poisoning. Acta Psychiatr. Scand., Suppl., 207: 83, 1969.

44. Fieve, R. R., and Platman, S. R.: Follow-up studies of lithium and thyroid function in manic-depressive illness. Am. J. Psychiatry, 125: 149, 1969.

45. National Institute of Mental Health: Lithium in the treatment of mood disorders. Public Health Service Publication No. 2143, p. 83. U.S. Government Printing Office, Washington, D.C., 1970.

46. Lee, R. V., Jampol, L. M., and Brown, W. V.: Nephrogenic diabetes insipidus and lithium intoxication—complications of lithium carbonate therapy. N. Engl. J. Med., 284: 93, 1971.

47. Ramsey, T. A., Mendels, J., Stokes, J. W., and Fitzgerald, R. G.: Lithium carbonate and kidney function. J.A.M.A., 219: 1446, 1972.

48. Schou, M., Amdisen, A., and Trap-Jensen, J.: Lithium poisoning. Am. J. Psychiatry, 125: 520, 1968.

49. Amdisen, A., and Skjoldborg, H.: Hemodialysis for lithium poisoning. Lancet, 2: 213, 1969.

chapter 32

MYASTHENIA GRAVIS

Rex S. Lott, B. Pharm.

Myasthenia gravis is a chronic disease of neuromuscular function which characteristically results in weakness and ease of fatigue of the skeletal muscles. This weakness most commonly affects the oculomotor, oropharyngeal and facial muscles. It accounts for the more common presenting signs and symptoms: diplopia, ptosis, dysarthria, dysphagia and the characteristic "myasthenic smile or snarl." In these patients, muscle strength is usually greatest after periods of rest but gradually decreases with continued activity. There are also characteristic variations in the severity of the weakness over longer time periods—there are remissions and exacerbations.

The over-all incidence of myasthenia gravis is estimated at approximately one case in 15,000 to 20,000, but an equal number of mild cases probably go undiagnosed.[1] In adult patients, women develop the disease approximately 2 to 3 times as often as do men, but in children there seems to be an equal distribution between sexes. The incidence of myasthenia gravis is highest among women between 20 and 30 years of age and among men after the age of 40.[2]

The disease occurs in members of the same family more frequently than one would predict on the basis of its normal incidence, but no available evidence indicates that myasthenia is genetically transmitted. Also, it has been suggested that familial occurrence of the disease may result from common exposure to some unidentified etiological agent.[3]

A condition known as neonatal myasthenia

occurs in approximately 15% of the children born to mothers with mysasthenia gravis. The affected infant may lack the ability to nurse properly, and he sometimes displays an abnormally low level of spontaneous movement. Neonatal myasthenia rarely lasts longer than a few weeks and, except in a few cases where there is respiratory involvement, the only treatment necessary is nasogastric feeding to insure proper nutrition. Neonatal myasthenia usually disappears without recurrence, although some children do develop myasthenia gravis later in life.[4]

Congenital myasthenia can occur in children whose parents do not have myasthenia gravis.[4] Although it may be recognized at birth owing to early development of ocular symptoms, it is usually not diagnosed until after the child becomes older and certain motor functions become noticeably abnormal.

MOTOR END PLATE PHYSIOLOGY

In order to appreciate both the effects of myasthenia gravis and the relationships between clinical observations and some theories concerning the disease's etiology, one should be familiar with the normal function of the neuromuscular system. Skeletal or striated muscles are innervated by somatic motor neurons. The point at which one of these motor neurons comes in contact with muscular tissue is called the neuromuscular or myoneural junction (Fig. 32.1). At this junction the nerve fiber expands into an "end foot" which fits into a thickened convoluted depression in the muscle cell membrane known as the motor end plate. A small gap between the end foot and the motor end plate corresponds anatomically to the synaptic cleft of the nervous system.

There is an electrical potential across the resting muscle cell membrane which is due to a higher intracellular concentration of potassium ions and a higher extracellular sodium ion concentration. These concentration gradients result in polarization of the cell; the interior is negative with respect to the exterior.

When a motor neuron action potential reaches the myoneural junction, the electrical impulse causes release of discrete packets or quanta of acetylcholine (ACh) from the terminal end of the nerve fiber. If sufficient quanta of ACh are released and travel across the gap between nerve and muscle tissue, a shift of sodium and potassium ions across the cell membrane causes depolarization of the motor end plate. This deplorization spreads throughout the muscle tissue and initiates contraction. As soon as ACh is released and causes depolarization, it is rapidly broken down into choline and acetic acid and inactivated by the enzyme acetylcholinesterase (AChE) which is concentrated at the myoneural junction. This action of AChE prevents continuous stimulation of muscle contractions by previously released ACh.

When the action of ACh is terminated, the muscle cells are rapidly repolarized through reestablishment of the ionic concentration gradients. The muscle is then ready to be stimulated by another nerve action potential.

The actions of ACh at the neuromuscular junction should be distinguished from those at peripheral autonomic effector cells and smooth muscle. The latter actions are blocked by anticholinergic agents such as atropine and are termed muscarinic or parasympathetic actions, *e.g.,* increased salivation, increased gastrointestinal motility with cramping and diarrhea and perspiration. The neuromuscular or nicotinic effects of ACh are antagonized by neuromuscular blocking agents such as curare (*d*-tubocurarine), gallamine and succinylcholine,

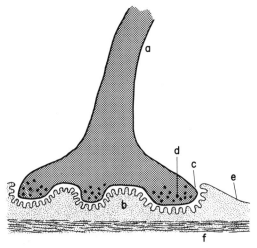

FIG. 32.1. a, Motor neuron (axon); b, motor end plate; c, motor neuron end foot; d, quanta of acetylcholine; e, muscle cell membrane; f, contractile muscle tissue.

but they are not affected by anticholinergic agents.

ETIOLOGY AND PATHOPHYSIOLOGY

Although myasthenia gravis was described over 300 years ago by Thomas Willis, it has been studied intensively only during the last 50 years. Neither the nature of the primary lesion nor any one single etiology has been proven, and they are still the subjects of several different theories. One of the first etiological theories was undoubtedly based on the observation that the symptoms of myasthenia closely resemble those produced by the competitive neuromuscular blocking agent, curare; and that both myasthenia gravis and curare intoxication are relieved by anticholinesterase drugs which inhibit AChE and make more ACh available for stimulation of motor end plates. However, the presence of a circulating substance with curare-like actions has never been demonstrated in patients with myasthenia.[4]

Examination of the myoneural junction, muscle tissue and motor neurons has led to several other theories concerning myasthenia's etiology. A number of these are depicted in Figure 32.2. Among these are:

1. A decreased size of the quanta or a decrease in the amount of ACh produced by motor neurons has been suggested on the basis

of miniature end plate potentials (MEPPs) of subnormal amplitude in patients with myasthenia. When microelectrodes are placed at the myoneural junction of normal patients, infrequent tiny electrical pulses (MEPPs) are recorded. These are thought to be due to spontaneous release of individual quanta of ACh in the absence of a nerve action potential.[2]

2. Electron microscopic studies of myasthenic muscle have revealed nerve terminals of subnormal area and an apparent misplacement of motor neuron end feet in relationship to motor end plates. These microscopic examinations have also revealed areas of muscle tissue in which nerve terminals are completely absent.[5]

3. And, there is some experimental evidence which seems to indicate a decreased sensitivity to ACh in the motor end plate. This same study also showed that the disease most probably does not result from an increased activity of AChE.[6]

Myasthenia may be caused by an autoimmune process. It has long been recognized that myasthenia frequently occurs in patients with systemic lupus erythematosus, another disease believed to result from formation of autoantibodies.[2] The thymus, an endocrine gland located in the chest, is often abnormal in myasthenic patients. It is known to be of major importance to immunological functions in humans. Thymoma, a frequently benign, noninvasive tumor of the thymus, is seen in 10% of the cases of myasthenia; or, more commonly, large numbers of antibody-producing cells are found in the gland. These antibody-producing cells, lymphocytes, also are observed in collections of lymphorrhages around blood vessels in muscles affected by myasthenia.[2, 6]

Antibodies specific for the striations of skeletal muscle have been found in serum samples from myasthenic patients. These antibodies are present in only 30% of all patients with the disease, but they are found in 85% of those with both myasthenia and thymoma.[14] The significance of these antibodies is controversial. Most physiological evidence indicates that an alteration in transmission at the myoneural junction is responsible for myasthenia, but these antibodies are not directed toward this area. However, it has recently been shown that these antibodies are also specific for thymic myoid cells, which are histologically and antigenically very similar to muscle cells.[4, 7]

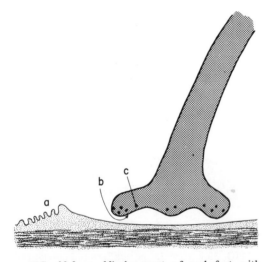

FIG. 32.2. a, Misplacement of end feet with respect to motor end plate; b, decreased area of neuron ending; c, subnormal quantal size for acetylcholine and decreased numbers of quanta.

These antibodies may cause autoimmune thymitis resulting in hyperscretion of thymin, a thymic hormone which has been shown to cause myasthenic symptoms in experimental animals.[6, 7] The presence of thymin in maternal blood could account for the appearance of neonatal myasthenia.

Drug-induced Myasthenia Gravis

There have been a few cases in which administration of certain drugs has been associated with development of clinical myasthenia. These drugs include: methoxyflurane,[8] trimethadione,[9] and busulfan.[10] However, these cases may have been due to activation of subclinical myasthenia rather than initiation of the disease state *de novo*. It is also possible that these drugs initiated an autoimmune response which caused myasthenia in the same manner that certain drugs are thought to cause systemic lupus erythematosus and other autoimmune phenomena.

Neuromuscular blockade produced by curare and related drugs is probably one of the few examples of "drug-induced" myasthenia gravis, but this effect is due to pharmacological actions and not to production of the actual disease. These actions are easily terminated in most cases by withdrawal of the drug and/or by administration of anticholinesterase agents. (It should be noted that, while the actions of the competitive neuromuscular blocking drugs, *d*-tubocurarine and gallamine, are reversed by anticholinesterases such as neostigmine, the actions of the depolarizing blockers, decamethonium and succinylcholine, are not affected by these enzyme inhibitors.) Certain antibiotics such as the polymyxins and the aminoglycosides (streptomycin, kanamycin, neomycin and gentamicin) also possess the ability to block neuromuscular transmission probably by an effect on the mobilization of ACh into quanta in motor neurons.[11] Postsurgical use of these antibiotics in patients who have received neuromuscular blocking agents has resulted in a number of cases of prolonged respiratory paralysis. This has occurred even with their use in prophylactic washes for the thoracic or peritoneal cavities.[12] Again, this appears to be a pharmacological action and does not represent a truly drug-induced disease.

In addition, other drugs are known to aggravate the weakness of myasthenia. These include: ether,[13] quinine and quinidine[14,15] and procainamide.[16] If possible, such agents should be avoided in the myasthenic's therapeutic regimen. Myasthenic patients are also particularly sensitive to the respiratory depressant effects of sedative hypnotics and opiates. These drugs should be administered cautiously and in reduced dosages to these people.

CLINICAL FINDINGS

The clinical manifestations of myasthenia gravis are all due to muscular weakness. In general, this weakness is worsened by fatigue and continued use of the affected muscle group, and it is characteristically relieved by periods of rest and the administration of anticholinesterases.

The clinical course of the disease may vary considerably among individual patients. In some cases, the disease appears gradually, progresses to a certain point and remains stable for many years. However, a fulminant case of myasthenia may progress from simple ocular involvement to respiratory paralysis and death within 6 months.[17] For many patients, fluctuation rather than stability is the rule. Swings between periods of severe relapse and symptomatic remission may occur unpredictably and rapidly.

Most patients initially present symptoms of ocular and facial muscle involvement. Progression of the disease usually follows the order: ocular→facial and orpharyngeal→proximal muscles of the extremities such as the shoulder and pelvic muscle groups→respiratory musculature. If either progression of the disease to other muscle groups or spontaneous remission is to occur, they will usually do so within 2 to 5 years of the onset of symptoms.[18, 19]

Ocular Weakness

Diplopia and ptosis are two quite characteristic findings in myasthenic patients. The ocular muscles seem to be the group most easily affected by the disease, and generally it is in these muscles that it first manifests its presence. Ptosis is demonstrated easily in myasthenics by requiring the patient to maintain an upward gaze. The eyelids gradually droop and cover the iris as strength is lost in the levator muscles. The disease's symptoms remain limited to the ocular muscles in approximately 1/3 of the patients.[19]

Facial and Oropharyngeal Symptoms

Progression of myasthenia into these muscles causes other commonly described symptoms of the disease: dysphagia, dysarthria and weakness of the jaw muscles with continued chewing or speaking. Fatigue of the muscles of the palate causes the myasthenic's voice to have a flat, nasal quality and also results in nasal regurgitation. The "myasthenic snarl" is seen when the patient attempts to smile. The retractor muscles at the corners of the mouth are more severely affected by the disease, allowing the patient only to lift the upper lip and expose the teeth.

Symptoms of Involvement of the Extremities

Weakness in peripheral skeletal muscles is usually a sign of advanced myasthenia gravis, but it can occur without previous ocular or facial involvement in up to 15% of the cases.[19] The patient will complain of difficulty in climbing stairs, lifting objects and rising from a supine position. Further progression of the disease into the more distal limb muscles causes a loss of strength in the hands, fingers and feet. The severely affected patient has difficulty walking and may be completely incapacitated.

Respiratory Muscle Involvement

Compromised respiratory function due to the effects of myasthenia gravis on the diaphragm and intercostal muscles is a poor prognostic sign. It often indicates severe progression of the disease and a high risk of complications or mortality. Weakness of these muscles seldom occurs without prior involvement of the ocular, facial or proximal limb muscles.[2]

Patients with myasthenia commonly do not suffer from muscular atrophy or degeneration except in a few severe cases of long duration. In addition, the tendon reflexes are almost never decreased in these patients. The presence of hyporeflexia and muscle wasting is usually indicative of a process other than myasthenia gravis.[2]

Associated Diseases

As mentioned above, myasthenia frequently occurs with autoimmune diseases such as systemic lupus erythematosus. Also it is commonly preceded or accompanied by thyroid disease—usually thyrotoxicosis. Some clinicians feel that this is actually a separate disease, "thyrotoxic myopathy," since correction of the thyroid disorder often produces dramatic improvement of the muscular strength.[20] However, patients with thyrotoxic myopathy are very often further benefited by anticholinesterase medication.[2] This condition may provide further evidence for the autoimmune nature of myasthenia, since at least one form of thyrotoxicosis, Graves' disease, also is thought to result from an autoimmune process.[7]

Myasthenic syndrome or Eaton-Lambert syndrome, which occurs in some patients with bronchial carcinoma, is similar to myasthenia gravis in many respects. However, this syndrome differs from true myasthenia in several ways: the muscular weakness is not as markedly relieved by anticholinesterase therapy; there may be atrophy of the affected muscles; there is reduction or loss of tendon reflexes; and the limb muscles are often affected first.[4,21]

DIAGNOSIS

Myasthenia often is diagnosed solely on the basis of symptomatology and the total clinical picture presented by the patient. When necessary, confirmation of the diagnosis or differentiation of true myasthenia gravis from similar diseases or conditions—myasthenic syndrome, neurasthenia and weakness associated with mental depression—is accomplished easily with edrophonium chloride, a rapidly acting anticholinesterase with a brief duration of effect. When edrophonium is administered to myasthenic patients, it causes a brief but dramatic increase in muscle strength.

The edrophonium chloride test is best performed when the pre- and postinjection performance of a single muscle group such as the hand or arm muscles can be measured carefully. Also it is desirable to employ a placebo injection to compensate for effects due to patient enthusiasm. After a baseline measurement of muscle strength is obtained, the same muscle group is evaluated 30 sec after rapid intravenous administration of 2, 6 and a total dose of 10 mg of edrophonium. A positive response is usually quite evident: the patient's oculomotor function improves; muscle strength returns to the extremities; and his voice may regain a more normal tone.[22] The muscarinic side effects of edrophonium are also short-lived and cause only minor discomfort to the patient.

Owing to edrophonium's brief duration of action, intramuscular administration of 1.5 mg neostigmine, a longer acting agent, is preferred by some clinicians for evaluation of limb muscle strength. Neostigmine's duration of action results in the occurrence of more severe muscarinic symptoms than are seen with edrophonium. Atropine may be employed prophylactically with this test at a dosage of 0.5 to 1.0 mg. The anticholinergic can serve a dual purpose in that it also may be used as a placebo control for baseline evaluation.[2]

Provocative tests with curare-like agents were used at one time. A positive response consisted of dramatic worsening of myasthenic symptoms because of increased sensitivity to these drugs. Such tests are dangerous and should be avoided. The increased muscle weakness produced by neuromuscular blockade may cause respiratory paralysis.

Electromyograms are also useful in establishing a diagnosis of myasthenia. These tests involve electrical stimulation of a motor neuron and measurement of the electrical or mechanical responses evoked in affected muscles. Most commonly, the ulnar nerve is stimulated at a frequency of 25 impulses per sec. In normal persons, the evoked electrical responses will all be of approximately equal amplitude; however, in a myasthenic individual, a phenomenon known as decrement occurs.[2] The amplitude of the muscular responses, although approximately normal at first, becomes progressively smaller, and response may completely cease. The administration of edrophonium during such a test will restore the amplitude of evoked responses to nearly normal levels.[23, 24]

Other tests which may be useful in diagnosing myasthenia gravis or assessing the progression of the disease include: measurement of the palpebral fissures, timing of the patient's ability to sustain an upward gaze, timing the ability to bite a tongue depressor without fatigue, measurement of the speaking time required for the voice to develop a nasal tone and counting the number of times one leg can be crossed over the other before fatigue occurs.[19] These tests are rough guides, however, and they can only reinforce an impression of the patient's clinical status obtained by more objective methods.

COMPLICATIONS

Myasthenic and cholinergic crisis are the major complications of myasthenia gravis. Respiratory paralysis due to weakness of the intercostal muscles and the diaphragm is the major symptom in both types of crisis, but it occurs for different reasons.

Myasthenic Crisis

This form of crisis is due to an acute exacerbation of the disease state. It may result from rapid, unrecognized progression of myasthenia with involvement of the respiratory musculature, failure of anticholinesterase medications to control the disease or improper administration of anticholinesterase medications. Upper respiratory infections and general physical fatigue are common precipitating factors.

Cholinergic Crisis

Overmedication with anticholinesterase drugs may result in cholinergic paralysis owing to sustained depolarization of motor end plates by large amounts of unmetabolized ACh. This type of paralysis is often preceded by uncoordinated twitching (fasciculation) of affected skeletal muscles. Paralysis due to cholinergic crisis may also result if a patient has become relatively resistant to the therapeutic effects of anticholinesterase drugs. Administration of increasing amounts of these drugs may cause cholinergic crisis rather than control of muscle weakness.[19] A patient in cholinergic crisis also may show characteristic symptoms of increased parasympathetic activity in addition to the generalized muscular weakness and respiratory paralysis seen in myasthenic crisis.

Although it would appear that differentiation of these crisis states would be quite easy, this is not always the case. Parasympathetic symptoms are not always apparent in cholinergic crisis. Clinically, attempts at differentiation are time-consuming and unnecessary, since initial treatment of both forms is the same.[19]

The patient in crisis is on the verge of total respiratory arrest. He should be placed under intensive care; all anticholinesterase medications should be discontinued; a tracheotomy should be performed; a cuffed endotracheal tube should be inserted to prevent aspiration of saliva and other liquids; and the patient should be attached to a positive pressure breathing apparatus. If, as is often the case, respiratory infection is a contributing factor, appropriate, vigorous antibiotic therapy should be instituted. As mentioned above, caution is required with the use of aminoglycoside or polymixin antibiotics in myasthenic patients since these drugs may produce neuromuscular blockade. The trachea, mouth and throat should be frequently cleared by suction, using a sterile catheter each time to reduce the risk of infection.[19] Administration of atropine as a "drying agent" to patients in crisis is not advocated by most clinicians since it may mask some symptoms of cholinergic crisis or produce plugging of the respiratory tree by tenacious mucus.

After the patient is out of immediate danger, edrophonium chloride may be administered in doses of 1 to 2 mg to evaluate the nature of the crisis. If there is a positive response to edrophonium indicating myasthenic crisis, then parenteral anticholinesterase therapy may be maintained until the patient can be stabilized with an oral agent. If the patient is in cholinergic crisis, his symptoms should improve 12 to 24 hr after withdrawal of anticholinesterase medication.

TREATMENT

Although treatment of myasthenia gravis is primarily pharmacological, general principles of management of myasthenia are particularly important to the outpatient's control of his disease. These patients should avoid any form of vigorous physical activity or any situation which might lead to fatigue. Avoiding emotional stress is equally important as this also tends to increase weakness. Since respiratory infections and other contagious diseases may be extremely dangerous to the myasthenic, he should be cautioned to avoid contracting "colds" and influenza at all costs. Numerous "gimmicks" or tricks can be used as aids in symptomatic management, *e.g.,* taping the eyelids with plastic tape to relieve ptosis and alternating an eyepatch from side to side to reduce diplopia. Although these tricks may be awkward, they are used with some success by a few patients.

Anticholinesterase Drugs

The long term pharmacological management of myasthenia gravis usually depends upon oral therapy with one of three anticholinesterase drugs: neostigmine, pyridostigmine and ambenonium (Table 32.1). While advantages are claimed for each of these drugs on the basis of specificity of effect and greater ability to control muscular weakness, the only clinically significant difference seen is usually in duration of effect.

Neostigmine is available in both oral and parenteral forms. Although parenteral neostigmine is normally used only for diagnostic testing, it may be used therapeutically in patients who are unable to swallow oral medications. Patients treated with neostigmine are usually started at a dose of 15 mg (1 tablet) every 3 to 5 hr. Neostigmine's short duration of action often necessitates too frequent dosing with too many tablets and results in low patient compliance. Thus, it is used only occasionally for maintenance therapy.

Pyridostigmine is the anticholinesterase most commonly used in myasthenia. Its duration of action allows more convenient dosing intervals, and it is available in several dosage forms. Treatment is begun at a dose of 60 mg (1 tablet or 1 teaspoonful of syrup) every 4 hr. As with the other anticholinesterases, the patient is titrated until he achieves optimal control with a minimum of side effects. The use of prolonged action pyridostigmine can be of value in patients who need the effects of anticholinesterase drugs during sleep. It should not be used to initiate therapy; titration of patients with this type of preparation is difficult and unreliable.

Although ambenonium has a longer duration of action than neostigmine or pyridostigmine, it is sometimes less effective in producing symptomatic control, and it tends to cause more undesirable effects.[25] For these reasons, it seldom is used except as an alternative drug when optimal relief is not obtained from the other available drugs.

Dosage adjustments for these drugs are usually based on the patient's clinical status and subjective evaluation of his response to therapy. However, this practice may be dangerous; cholinergic crisis may result from inadvertent overdosage during futile attempts at the total relief of symptoms. Edrophonium testing may be of use in evaluating the adequacy of anticholinesterase therapy. Patients showing dramatic responses to the test drug just prior to their next scheduled dose of neostigmine or pyri-

TABLE 32.1
Anticholinesterase Drugs Used in the Treatment of Myasthenia Gravis

Drug	Available Preparations	Initial Dose *mg*	Duration of Action *hr*
neostigmine (Prostigmin)	0.5 mg/ml. 0.1 mg/ml. 15 mg/tablet	1.0-1.5 I M 15	2-3 2-3
pyridostigmine (Mestinon)	60 mg/tablet 60 mg/5 ml 180 mg/tablet (timespan)	60 orally 60 orally (see text)	4-6 8-12
ambenonium (Mytelase)	10 mg/tablet 25 mg/tablet	10-25 orally	5-7

dostigmine often will respond favorably to an increased dose of their maintenance drug. If edrophonium causes increased parasympathetic side effects and unchanged or decreased muscle strength, the patient is being overdosed and he may be on the verge of cholinergic crisis. Optimal response to anticholinesterase therapy is indicated by no change in muscle strength and minimal parasympathetic effects after administration of edrophonium. The dosage should always be increased gradually, *e.g.*, in increments of 60 mg of pyridostigmine daily, to avoid cholinergic crisis. It should be remembered that complete restoration of muscle strength occurs very rarely, and that, at best, only 50 % of the patients will exhibit excellent response to anticholinesterase therapy.[19] Even adjustments of dosage based on response to edrophonium may be misleading since the dose of anticholinesterase required for maximal benefit may vary considerably even over short periods of time. Several independently variable factors including stress, febrile illness and emotions play a significant role in determining drug requirements and may necessitate temporary increases in dosage. An additional complicating factor is the differential sensitivity of muscle groups in the same patient to anticholinesterase therapy. For example, some patients find that they must accept a certain level of ocular weakness to avoid cholinergic paralysis of the limb or respiratory muscles.[18]

Adjuvant Drug Therapy

Atropine, at a dose of 0.1 mg 3 to 4 times daily, usually controls muscarinic side effects of anticholinesterase therapy (Table 32.2). Although this seems desirable, these effects of atropine also may eliminate some early symptoms of cholinergic crisis. For this reason, some physicians avoid using anticholinergics except on an infrequent basis. Avoidance of atropine-like drugs may be especially important in "brit-

TABLE 32.2
Adjunctive Drugs for Myasthenia Gravis

Drug	Dose	Effect
Atropine	0.1 mg 3-4 X daily	Relieves muscarinic side effects of anti-AChE agents
Ephedrine	25 mg 2-3 X daily	Not known
Potassium chloride	10-15 mEq. 2-3 X daily	May act to facilitate muscle contraction CAUTION: excess *or* deficiency produce increased weakness
Calcium gluconate	1 g 3-4 X daily	Essential for muscle contraction CAUTION: excess *or* deficiency produce increased weakness
Spironolactone (Aldactone)	25 mg 4 X daily	Increases potassium levels CAUTION: hyperkalemia
Triamterene (Dyrenium)	100-200 mg daily	Same as spironolactone

tle" patients who are subject to wide variations in control.

Patients who have achieved optimal benefit from anticholinesterase drugs, as evidenced by negative edrophonium chloride tests or failure to show objective improvement with further increases in dosage, may improve further upon addition of ephedrine, potassium chloride or calcium salts to their therapeutic regimens. The mechanisms by which these drugs act are not well understood.

Calcium ions are known to play a major role in neuromuscular transmission and muscular contraction, and potassium is essential for proper function of nerve and muscle cells; but it is essential to realize that both deficiency and excess of these electrolytes can result in muscular paralysis. Caution is required with their use as adjunctive therapy, and serum levels should be determined frequently.

Spironolactone and triamterene have also been used with some success in myasthenia. Their usefulness probably stems from their potassium-retaining properties; however, potassium supplements are far less expensive and cause fewer unnecessary pharmacological effects, *e.g.,* diuresis.[25, 26]

Thymectomy

Although surgical removal of the thymus has been performed in myasthenics for over 30 years, the cumulated results of large series of thymectomies have recently become available. Prior to this time the operation was performed empirically in patients with thymoma, or it was reserved for patients with severe myasthenia not relieved by anticholinesterases. An analysis of the results in large series of thymectomies indicates that 70 to 80% result in definite improvement or complete remission of the disease, and, interestingly, it appears that patients with thymoma may benefit less from surgery. On a statistical basis, patients with long standing severe disease appear to develop irreversible neuromuscular disability and may not show improvement after thymectomy.[7]

Some clinicians now advocate routine thymectomy early in the course of myasthenia. This recommendation seems reasonable in light of two factors: there are known relationships between the thymus and myasthenia; and many severely affected patients who are unable to withstand the stress of chest surgery may be deprived of the benefits of this form of therapy.

An alternative to thymectomy in severely ill patients or those with thymic malignancy limited to spread within the thoracic-cavity is thymic irradiation. This may result in remission of symptoms within a few weeks. Unfortunately, remission is only temporary in some cases.[4, 27]

Corticosteroid and ACTH Therapy

The use of adrenocorticotropic hormone and glucocorticoids is aimed at correcting any immunological abnormalities underlying myasthenia gravis. These agents suppress the body's immune response by inhibiting the functions of antibody-producing lymphocytes. However, if one accepts the theory that myasthenia results from an autoimmune thymic inflammation, then it also becomes necessary to consider the anti-inflammatory actions of these drugs. Although ACTH therapy was first used in myasthenia, it has been replaced by individual glucocorticoids, prednisone in most cases. At present, steroid therapy is usually reserved for patients in whom anticholinesterase drugs and thymectomy have failed to provide adequate control or remission of symptoms.[28-30]

Therapy with prednisone is usually started at a dosage of 50 mg daily. It is preferable to administer the total day's dose in the early morning. During the initial period, the patient should be maintained on anticholinesterase drugs since exacerbation of symptoms often occurs during the first few days of steroid treatment. Admitting the patient to an intensive care unit may be advisable as severe complications can occur. After initial worsening of their symptoms, most patients improve dramatically and their anticholinesterase requirements may be drastically reduced or entirely eliminated.

As soon as possible, an attempt should be made to convert the patient from 50 mg of prednisone each morning to 100 mg *every other morning*. This dosage regimen greatly reduces the undesirable effects of prednisone such as Cushingoid symptoms and suppression of the patient's adrenocortical function but remains therapeutically effective in most instances. The dose of steroid may be gradually reduced to a minimal effective level which can be supplemented by anticholinesterase therapy. Additional anticholinesterase supplementation occasionally is necessary during the days the patient does not receive prednisone.[31, 32]

CONCLUSION

Although there is no cure for myasthenia gravis, the mortality rate for the disease is surprisingly low—approximately 15%. This is a considerable decrease below death rates observed 4 decades ago. Reduction in mortality is a result of more efficient methods of treatment, better general management and more effective crisis therapy. The mortality rate from crisis and respiratory paralysis, the most commonly fatal complications, has been reduced from 50% to 10% as a result of the ready availability of intensive care facilities. The myasthenic patient today more commonly dies from intercurrent or unrelated disease processes than from myasthenia itself.[2,18]

Significant improvement in at least some aspects of the disease can be expected in virtually every patient with myasthenia gravis, and with proper management and supportive care, most of these people can live reasonably full and normal lives.

REFERENCES

1. Flacke, W. Treatment of myasthenia gravis. N. Engl. J. Med., 288: 27, 1973.
2. Beeson, P. B., and McDermot, W. (editors): Cecil-Loeb Textbook of Internal Medicine, Ed. 13, p. 350. W. B. Saunders Co., Philadelphia, 1971.
3. Herrmann, C. J., Jr.: The familial occurrence of myasthenia gravis. Ann. N.Y. Acad. Sci., 183: 334, 1971.
4. Herrmann, C. J., Jr.: Myasthenia gravis and the myasthenic syndrome. Calif. Med., 113: 27, 1970.
5. Bergman, R. A., and Johns, R. J.: Ultrastructural alterations in muscle from patients with myasthenia gravis and Eaton-Lambert syndrome. Ann. N.Y. Acad. Sci., 183: 88, 1971.
6. Goldstein, G., and Manganaro, A.: Thymin: a thymic polypeptide causing the neuromuscular block of myasthenia gravis. Ann. N.Y. Acad. Sci., 183: 230, 1971.
7. Goldstein, G.: Myasthenia gravis and the thymus. Annu. Rev. Med., 22: 119, 1971.
8. Elder, B. F., Beal, H., DeWald, W., and Cobb, S.: Exacerbation of subclinical myasthenia by occupational exposure to an anesthetic. Anesth. Analg., 50: 383, 1971.
9. Booker, H. E., Chun, R. W. M., and Sanguino, M.:

Myasthenia gravis syndrome associated with trimethadione. J.A.M.A., 212: 2262, 1970.
10. Djaldetti, M., Pinkhas, J., DeVries, A., Kott, E., Joshua, H., and Dollberg, L.: Myasthenia gravis in a patient with chronic myeloid leukemia treated by busulfan. Blood, 32: 336, 1968.
11. Wright, E. A., and McQuillen, M. P.: Antibiotic-induced neuromuscular blockade. Ann. N.Y. Acad. Sci., 183: 358, 1971.
12. Davia, J. E., Siemsen, A. W., and Anderson, R. W.: Uremia, deafness, and paralysis due to irrigating antibiotic solutions. Arch. Intern. Med., 125: 135, 1970.
13. Goodman, L. S., and Gilman, A. (editors): The Pharmacological Basis of Therapeutics, Ed. 4, p. 80. The Macmillan Co., Toronto, 1970.
14. Goodman, L. S., and Gilman, A. (editors): The Pharmacological Basis of Therapeutics, Ed. 4, pp. 464, 1121. The Macmillan Co., Toronto, 1970.
15. Way, W. L., Katzung, B. G., and Larson, C. P.: Recurarization with quinidine. J.A.M.A., 200: 153, 1967.
16. Drachman, D. A., and Skom, H.: Procainamide: a hazard in myasthenia gravis. Arch. Neurol., 13: 316, 1965.
17. Osserman, K. E., Kornfeld, P., Cohen, E., Genkins, G., Mendelow, H., Goldberg, H., Windsley, H., and Kaplan, L. I.: Studies in myasthenia gravis. Review of two hundred eighty-two cases at the Mount Sinai Hospital, New York City. Arch. Intern. Med., 102: 72, 1958.
18. Brain, W. R., and Walton, J. N.: Brain's Diseases of the Nervous System, Ed. 7, p. 863. Oxford University Press, New York, 1969.
19. Gilroy, J., and Meyer, J. S.: Medical Neurology, Ed. 1, p. 682. The Macmillan Co., Toronto, 1969.
20. Gilroy, J., and Meyer, J. S.: Medical Neurology, Ed. 1, p. 672. The Macmillan Co., Toronto, 1969.
21. Wintrobe, M. M., Thorn, G. W., Adams, R. D., Bennett, I. L., and Petersdorf, R. D. (editors): Harrison's Principles of Internal Medicine, Ed. 6, Sect. 11, Chap. 377, p. 1913. McGraw-Hill Book Co., N.Y., 1970.
22. Osserman, K. E., and Genkins, G.: Critical reappraisal of edrophonium (tensilon) chloride tests in myasthenia gravis and significance of clinical classification. Ann. N.Y. Acad. Sci., 135: 312, 1966.
23. Ozdemir, C., and Young, R. R.: Electrical testing in myasthenia gravis. Ann. N.Y. Acad. Sci., 183: 287, 1971.
24. Foldes, F. F., and Glaser, G. H.: Diagnostic tests in myasthenia gravis: an overview. Ann. N.Y. Acad. Sci., 183: 275, 1971.
25. Herrmann, C. J., Jr.: Myasthenia gravis. In Current Therapy, Ed. 24, p. 676, edited by H. F. Conn. W. B. Saunders Co., Philadelphia, 1972.
26. Walton, J. N.: Essentials of Neurology, Ed. 3, p. 365. J. B. Lippincott Co., Philadelphia, 1971.

27. Schulz, M. D., and Schwab, R. S.: Results of thymic (medrastinal) irradiation in patients with myasthenia gravis. Ann. N.Y. Acad. Sci., 183: 303, 1971.
28. Anon: Management of myasthenia gravis. Lancet, (editorial) 1: 780, 1972.
29. Genkins, G., Kornfeld, P., and Osserman, K. E.: The use of ACTH and corticosteroids in myasthenia gravis. Ann. N.Y. Acad. Sci., 183: 369, 1971.
30. Engel, W. K., and Warmolts, J. R.: Myasthenia gravis: a new hypothisis of the pathogenesis and a new form of treatment. Ann. N.Y. Acad. Sci., 183: 72, 1971.
31. Jenkins, R. B.: Treatment of myasthenia gravis with prednisone. Lancet, 1: 765, 1972.
32. Warmolts, J. R., and Engel, W. K.: Benefit from alternate-day prednisone in myasthenia gravis. N. Engl. J. Med., 286: 17, 1972.

chapter 33

HEADACHE

Robert A. Miller, Pharm.D.

The headache, of all the common symptomatic ailments seen by the physician, constitutes the major complaint in more than 50% of patients seen in office practice.[1] Treating headaches is primarily symptomatic, but selecting the appropriate drug depends upon the physician being able to classify properly the patient's head pain. Headaches may be classified simply as: vascular; associated with severe psychiatric disease; associated with intracranial or extracranial structural disease; or due to systemic disease.[2] A more detailed classification has been prepared by the American Association for the Study of Headache and may be found in a modified form in Table 33.1. As pharmacists, we are called upon constantly to suggest over-the-counter drugs for the relief of the simple, short duration headache which usually is relieved by salicylates or similar drugs and defies classification. The term "Excedrin headache" is as good as any way to describe it.

When a patient complains of a headache, a number of possibilities exist. The complaint may be a social excuse, a symptom of a pri-marily psychiatric illness such as depression or the first symptom of many life-threatening diseases such as a malignant cerebral neoplasm or malignant hypertension. On the other hand, headaches can be a syndrome in their own right, as with tension, cluster or migraine headaches.

The headache can be primarily muscular, vascular or neurological in nature, but usually more than one of these tissues is involved in varying degrees. Changes in these tissues of the magnitude necessary to trigger headache can be induced by increased stress, strain, anxiety, frustration, repressed hostility, guilt and other unresolved emotional conflicts.

Headache also can occur independently of any tissue changes. This is possible by means of the psychiatric mechanism of hysteria, in which the headache is a symbolic expression of some otherwise unexpressed emotional feeling or conflict. This is due mainly to the patient's lack of expressing or venting his repressed emotions. The quiet individual who "never gets angry" and "is always in control" may express his anger or frustration through recurring bouts of

TABLE 33.1
Classification of Headaches

I. Traction and inflammation
   A. Mass lesions (tumors, edema, hematoma, etc.)
   B. Diseases of the eye, ear, nose, throat, teeth
   C. Cranial neuralgia
   D. Allergy
   E. Infection
   F. Arteritis, phlebitis

II. Muscle contraction
   A. Cervical osteoarthritis
   B. Chronic myositis
   C. Tension (anxiety)
   D. Depressive

III. Vascular headache
   A. Migraine
      1. Classical
      2. Nonclassical
   B. Cluster
   C. Facial—unilateral episodic facial pain
   D. Ophthalmoplegic—attacks associated with paresis of the extraocular muscles
   E. Hemiplegic—rare condition in which headaches are associated with hemiplegia
   F. Hypertensive
   G. Toxic

headache. This is worth remembering when faced with a patient who fails to get complete relief from any of the common drugs available. This patient is a candidate for discovering the reality of his life, *e.g.,* his job, family, goals and life style rather than the "two aspirin every four hours."

It is well to realize that, in spite of the many conditions (physical, emotional, psychosomatic, psychogenic, pyrexial, metabolic, endocrine, and chemical changes in the head or other parts of the body) that can lead to headaches, there are only a few physical changes in the tissue in and about the head which can cause pain. These include changes in or pressure upon the skeletal muscles; certain arterial or venous channels; and several pain-sensitive cervical and cranial nerves or their branches.[3]

PAIN-SENSITIVE STRUCTURES AND MECHANISM OF HEADACHE

A brief discussion of those structures which may be involved in the production of a headache will be helpful in understanding the pathophysiology of this condition. The following cranial structures are sensitive to mechanical stimulation: skin, subcutaneous tissue, muscles, arteries and the membrane covering the skull; delicate structures of the eye, ear and nasal cavity; intracranial venous sinuses and their tributary veins; parts of the dura (the outer and toughest of the three membranes covering the brain and spinal cord) at the base of the brain and the arteries within this and the next inner level of membrane, the parachnoid; the trigeminal (V), glossopharyngeal (IX), vagus (X) and the first three cervical nerves. Interestingly, pain is practically the only sensation produced by stimulation of the structures mentioned above. Also it should be noted that the nerves just mentioned constitute the pathways whereby sensory stimuli, whatever their source, are conveyed to the central nervous system.

By analysis of several types of headaches, Wolf and his colleagues[5] have demonstrated that most "spontaneous" cranial pains can be traced to the operation of one or more of the following mechanisms:

1. Distention, traction and dilation of the intracranial or extracranial arteries.

2. Traction or displacement of large intra-cranial veins or the membranous envelope in which they live.

3. Compression, traction or inflammation of sensory, cranial and spinal nerves.

4. Voluntary or involuntary spasm and possibly inflammation of cranial and cervical muscles.

In an infection or blockage of the nasal sinuses, the accompanying headache is manifested by pain in the forehead. The mechanism involves changes in pressure and irritation of the pain-sensitive sinus walls. Usually this is associated with tenderness of the surrounding skin. The pain may have two remarkable properties. First, when throbbing, it may be terminated by compressing the carotid artery on the same side. Second, the pain tends to recur and subside at the same hours, *i.e.,* on awakening, with a gradual disappearance while in an upright posture only to come on again in the late morning hours. These time relations are believed to correspond to the possible mechanism of action. The morning pain is ascribed to the sinuses filling at night, and its relief on arising, from emptying after the patient stands up. Stooping intensifies the pain by pressure change, as does blowing the nose sometimes. Vasoconstrictor drugs (inhalants, sprays and drops) which reduce swelling and congestion tend to relieve the pain.

Headache of ocular origin, located as a rule in the orbit, forehead or temple, is believed to be the result of ocular muscle imbalance. There is some experimental evidence to show that the main faults are farsightedness (hypermetropia) and astigmatism, which result in sustained contraction of the extraocular as well as frontal, temporal and occipital muscles. Correction of the refractive error eliminates the headache. Another mechanism involved is the increased intraocular pressure seen in acute glaucoma, which produces a steady aching pain in the region of the eye.[4]

The headache of meningeal irritation (infection or hemorrhage) has been linked by some investigators to increased intracranial pressure. This has been supported by the observation that withdrawal of cerebral spinal fluid may lead to relief of pain. However, most workers agree that dilation and congestion or inflamed meningeal vessels must also be a factor. It also seems reasonable that much of the pain is due to chemical irritation of nerve endings in the meninges. The mechanism of the pain, therefore, is probably identical with that occurring in acute inflammatory conditions elsewhere.

The mechanism of the throbbing or steady headache which accompanies febrile illnesses (acute tonsillitis, typhoid fever and malaria) is probably vascular. It is similar to a histamine headache in being relieved on one side by carotid artery compression and on both sides by jugular vein compression or the subarachnoid injection of saline.

The mechanism responsible for tension headaches is contraction of the cranial and cervical muscles. The contraction itself is quite painful; however, another factor exists. The contraction reduces the blood flow to the involved muscles and the ischemia which results produces additional pain.

PRINCIPLE VARIETIES OF HEADACHE

Traction and Inflammatory Headaches

Included in this group are the headaches caused by brain tumor; diseases of the eye, ear, nose, throat and teeth; infection; arteritis; phlebitis and cranial neuralgia. Diamond and Baltes[6] reported that these categories account for only about 2% of the headaches seen in their clinic. Headache is the primary symptom of cerebral tumor. The pain tends to be deep-seated, aching or bursting and may or may not be throbbing. Attacks may last from a few minutes to an hour or more and may occur once or many times during the day. The pain can be provoked by activity and the frequent change in the position of the head. As might be suspected, bedrest reduces the frequency of attacks. In the latter stages of the illness, unexpected and sometimes violent attacks of vomiting may occur. As the tumor grows, the pain becomes more frequent, severe and sometimes nearly continuous terminally. Of course, there are exceptions—some headaches being mild and tolerable, others as agonizing as that of bacterial meningitis and subarachnoid hemorrhage. An interesting note is that when the headache is unilateral, *i.e.,* it occurs on one side of the head; it is on the same side of the head as the tumor 90% of the time.[4]

The pain of ocular, nasal and paranasal headache varies in intensity from mild to the fulminating pain of glaucoma. This pain is felt in and around the eyes. (Note: while eye strain may produce headache, it is not a common cause of chronic headache.) Nasal and sinus headache is dull, deep and aching. The pain usually occurs in the frontal and maxillary regions. Sinus headache pain is seldom as severe as that of migraine. It is most severe in the morning and diminishes later in the day.

Pyrexial and Toxic Headache

The headache pain produced by fever, sepsis and toxic agents may be pulsating or dull, deep and aching. It is made worse by coughing and body movement. The headache is controlled when the primary disease is cured.

Headaches Due to Muscle Contraction

The two most common types of muscle contraction headaches are those caused by tension (anxiety) and depression.

The tension headache is usually bilateral, and the patient will frequently describe other sensations than pain. These include fullness, tightness and pressure (as if the head is in a vise, or has a rubber band wound tightly around it). The onset of this type of headache is more gradual than that of a migraine and often adds to a pressure ache, which can last for weeks or months. It should be noted that this is the only type of headache which can be continuous day and night for long periods of time. The tension headache is frontal in 90% of the patients.[7] While a typical profile of a migraine headache sufferer is periodic and lifelong, with a tendency to lessen as he becomes older, tension headache occurs more often in the middle years. It is during this period of life that most patients undergo difficult and stressful times, and the chance of suffering from anxiety and depression greatly increases during this time of life. Many premenstrual headaches are of this type, and there is an increased incidence of this type at menopause.[8]

For patients suffering headaches caused by depression, the back of the head is the most frequently affected location. These headaches tend to occur regularly, are usually worse on Sundays, holidays and the first day of vacation. A common complaint is that of early and frequent awakening during the night.[6] The headache is usually described as worse in the morning than in the evening. In the clinic of Diamond and Baltes,[6] 70 to 75% of patients complaining of headache were diagnosed as suffering from a depressive reaction. Here, the headache may have been the outward manifestation of turmoil and confusion.

Traumatic Headache

The headache which is the result of trauma (*i.e.,* scalp lacerations and contusions with increased intracranial pressure) may last from a few days to 1 to 2 weeks. Following this initial period, severe, chronic, continuous or intermittent headaches may appear as the cardinal symptom of two post-traumatic syndromes.[3]

The first is chronic subdural hematoma. The usual symptoms are headache and dizziness, which fluctuate in severity, followed by drowsiness, stupor, coma and partial paralysis. The injury itself may have been minor and forgotten by both the patient and family. The headache is deep-seated, steady and unilateral or generalized. The typical attack profile of the headache and other symptoms is one of increasing frequency and severity of symptoms over many weeks or months. Diagnosis is established by arteriography.

The second syndrome is that of post-traumatic nervous instability. In this case, headache is a primary symptom of a complex syndrome consisting of giddiness, fatigability, insomnia, nervousness, trembling, irritability, inability to concentrate and tearfulness. The pain varies from day to day and its location varies from patient to patient.

The symptoms are apt to be made worse by exercise, changes of posture, exposure to the sun or bright light, noise, confusion and ingestion of alcohol. The patient may look and act like a person in an agitated depression. In fact, many neurologists believe such a state to be a post-traumatic neurosis or depression. A final point of interest is that the severity and duration of the headache have little or nothing to do with the magnitude of the injury; some of the worst cases have had minor injuries without loss of consciousness, and major injuries may produce no headache symptoms at all.

Hypertensive Headache

Hypertension is, of course, frequent in the general population and is difficult to prove as a cause of recurrent headaches. No doubt severe hypertension with diastolic blood pressure of over 110 mg Hg are associated regularly with headache; and it has been shown that when the pressure is reduced, the headache is relieved. However, it is the moderate hypertensive patient who, when subject to numerous and severe headaches, gives concern. When this happens, there is usually a secondary anxiety or tension state or a common migraine syndrome which is exacerbated by the hypertension. The intensity and severity of this type of headache are not related directly to the level of blood pressure.[9] It is often present upon arising and usually improves once the patient is up and around. Nausea and vomiting may occur and frequently there is a feeling of vertigo and a full or congested feeling in the head.

Vascular Headache

Vascular headaches can be classified as migraine, either classic or common; cluster headache (histamine cephalgia, Horton's syndrome); and migraine equivalents.

Migraine can be defined as a paroxysmal headache which lasts for hours, sometimes days, interspersed with periods of complete freedom. Attacks almost always affect either the gastrointestinal tract (anorexia, nausea, vomiting, constipation or, rarely, diarrhea) or the visual system (teichopsial or photophobia). The pain is not always unilateral and often is felt in the middle of the head as a deep seated ache. At some time during the attack the pain becomes throbbing in nature and may be accompanied by coughing, sneezing or head movement. At this time the patient's face is usually pale.[10]

As stated above, migraine can be classified as classic or common. In classic migraine the prodromes (a warning symptom indicating the onset of a disease) are usually well defined and consistent. Scotoma and other neurological symptoms precede the headache, which actually begins as these symptoms diminish. The headache usually takes almost 1 hr to reach its peak and lasts 4 to 6 hr. Nausea and vomiting usually, although not always, follow the onset of the pain. The scotoma and other neurological symptoms usually occur on the side opposite to that which the headache occurs. As the attack repeats itself, the site of the headache alternates from one side of the head to the other.

The other type of migraine, namely common or nonclassic, differs significantly in its profile. The prodromes are vague and variable. They usually involve the autonomic nervous system and may precede the headache by hours or even days. The total duration of the pain is 12 to 24 to 48 hr, followed by nausea, vomiting, polyuria, diarrhea, chills and exhaustion. The headache is most often unilateral and is associated with nasal congestion or rhinorrhea of the affected side. These symptoms can be confused easily with those produced by a typical sinus headache attack. The physician, therefore, must exercise his judgment in identifying these symptoms as an integral part of the migraine attack.

The third type of vascular headache, the cluster headache, often begins with a short (5 min) period of burning discomfort in or around the temple or eye. This is followed by increasing severe pain of a steady or throbbing nature. The attacks seem to come with clock-like regularity especially during sleep or after relaxation and naps. The duration varies from a few minutes to a few hours, although 30 to 90 minutes is most common. Pain is associated with tearing, myosis, nasal congestion and/or rhinorrhea and sweating. Pain may be experienced in the neck and its appearance and disappearance may be sudden. Cluster headaches may go into a remission stage for months or even years.[10]

The final class to be examined is the migraine equivalents. These attacks may consist of abdominal pain associated with nausea, vomiting and diarrhea, pain localized in the chest, pelvis, or extremities, fever, tachycardia, vertigo and edema.

The incidence of migraine in the general population ranges between 5 and 10%. There is no conclusive evidence that migraine and intelligence are linked. It does appear, however, that social levels increase the chance of a patient visiting the physician and seeking help for the control of head pain. Thus, when a study is performed on a patient population suffering from migraine, the chance of including the well educated, intelligent middle to upper class patient is increased significantly.[12] Also, contrary to popular notion, migraine is not worsened during the menopause.

The question of inheritance of migraine is not clear yet. However, heredity has been emphasized by all observers as an important etiological factor. About 60% of the patients report a history of migraine in their families.[12]

It has been found over the years that certain factors can precipitate a migraine attack.[9] The recognition of these precipitating factors by the patient can play an important role in reducing the number and severity of attacks. (A list of these factors may be found in Table 33.2.) Another problem facing the physician treating a patient for migraine headaches is the recognition of certain aggravating factors.[13] When the patient's attacks become worse and the usual remedies fail to achieve their intended results, the recognition and exclusion of these aggravating factors are definitely indicated. These factors may be found in Table 33.3.

TABLE 33.2
Precipitating Factors

1. Physical factors
   a. Heat
   b. Cold
   c. Noise
   d. Flashes of bright light
   e. Watching TV
   f. Intense odors

2. Dietary factors
   a. Dairy products (cheese)
   b. Chocolate
   c. Fruits (citrus)
   d. Fatty fried foods
   e. Vegetables (onion)
   f. Tea
   g. Coffee
   h. Meat (pork)
   i. Seafood
   j. Missing meals
   k. Alcohol
   l. Low fasting blood glucose

3. Sleeping too long

4. Hormones
   a. Estrogen
   b. Progesterone

5. Local head pain
   a. From upper cervical region
   b. Ocular causes
   c. Dental causes

TABLE 33.3
Aggravating Factors

1. Hypertension
2. Anxiety
3. Depression
4. Cervical spondylosis
5. Menopause
6. Pregnancy—rarely it becomes worse

ETIOLOGY AND PATHOGENESIS OF MIGRANE

Migraine attacks have been attributed wholly or in part to genetics, intelligence, social class, endocrine disorders, various psychological mechanisms and other possible causes. However, the biochemical changes occurring in patients with migraine have proven to be the most revealing and productive in discovering the actual cause of this disease. Studies by Wolf[5] appeared to indicate that the pain of migraine headache is due to a combination of arterial dilation and the effect of agents having the capacity to reduce pain thresholds, accumulating locally in the walls of the arteries and surrounding tissues. The underlying pathophysiology which accounts for the migraine syndrome is still unknown. However, there are certain factors which appear to be present in the majority of cases. It is quite clear that no single process or mechanism is responsible in all cases of migraine.

The vasomotor theory of the production of migraine has been recognized for a long time. More than 100 years ago, DuBois-Reymond[14] ascribed the symptoms to tonic (continuous) spasm of the muscular walls of the vessels. Today, most investigators feel that changes in the cerebral and meningeal circulation are basic causes of the prodroma, course, symptoms, signs and sequela of the disease. Three distinct phases have been identified.[16]

The first phase is vasoconstriction of certain cranial arteries which in turn produces central visual and other preheadache signs prior to the onset of the actual head pain. These signs may include flashes of light, blind spots, intolerance to light, speech difficulty, dizziness or weakness. This prodromal period of the attack is followed by the second phase which is dilation and distension of the cranial arteries; these are primarily branches of the external carotid artery. In this phase, one side of the head begins to throb. As the throbbing increases, the pain can become excruciating. The persistent vasodilation of the arteries results in a thickening of their walls and often in edema of the surrounding tissues. This is the third phase—edema. Now the headache becomes dull and steady as the soft, collapsible arteries become rigid. Nausea, vomiting, excessive sweating, dryness of the mouth and chills may be seen in this phase. Following such prolonged pain and distension of the cranial arteries, contraction of the skeletal muscles of the head and neck may occur. These become painful, thus adding another component to the migraine headache which may outlast the original vascular pain.

Wolf and his associates added to this concept of vasoconstriction and vasodilation by isolating a humoral factor which appeared to be significant in the development of the migraine attack.[14] This factor, called neurokinin, was shown to be related directly to the intensity of the headache. Neurokinin, which is a biologically active polypeptide and closely related if not identical to bradykinin, causes vasodilation and increases the permeability of the capillaries. At the same time the pain threshold is lowered, and the vulnerability of the tissues to injury is increased. Whether neurokinin escapes coincidently during the phase of vasodilation or initiates this phase is not known.

Sicuteri[16] and his colleagues put forth the hypothesis that the observed vasospasm was induced by the release of catecholamines such as norepinephrine, epinephrine and serotonin in patients whose blood vessels were peculiarly sensitive. These substances are known to be powerful vasoconstrictors. It was observed that some patients excreted increased amounts of the terminal metabolites 5-hydroxyindoleacetic acid (5-HIAA) and 3-methoxy-4-hydroxy mandelic acid (VMA) during their migraine attacks. These metabolites are derived from serotonin (5-HIAA) and norepinephrine and epinephrine (VMA). In addition, it was observed that reserpine, which reduces the level of serotonin in the platelets, brain and other tissues, may provoke migraine; the injection of serotonin gives partial or complete relief of the headache; and a number of serotonin antagonists (see section on treatment) have been employed successfully in the prevention of migraine attacks. There is much work being carried on presently to unravel the mystery surrounding the scope, mechanism of action and clinical manifestatiQns of the kinins. The chances seem good that, when this is accomplished, our knowledge of the specific mechanisms responsible for the migraine headache will be advanced significantly.

TREATMENT OF HEADACHES

The most important steps in treating a headache are the discovery and removal of the underlying disease or functional disturbance that is producing the pain. For the common everyday headache caused by fatigue, stuffy atmosphere or too much alcohol and tobacco, the answer simply is to avoid the offending activity or agent. This becomes more difficult when the headache is caused by your mother-in-law, children, spouse, boss or the stock market. As all pharmacists (and physicians, for that matter) are aware, the next step is to suggest two aspirin every 4 hr. This drug will work adequately in most cases. The vast number of both prescription and over-the-counter analgesics available to treat a headache is only outdone by the number of television commercials and journal advertisements helping the layman and professional alike to decide on the "best" treatment. After the patient is buffered, fizzed, extra strengthed and had "the ingredient that most doctors prescribe," both he and you probably will come to the same conclusion on the treatment of the common headache: two aspirin every 4 hr.

There are however, situations that do warrant other simple analgestic treatment. The patient who cannot tolerate plain aspirin because of ulcer, bleeding tendencies, allergies and the like should be treated with acetaminophen. The literature is replete with papers on the major advantages and disadvantages of the various O-T-C preparations. The reader is also directed to the *Handbook of Non-Prescription Drugs*[17] for a comprehensive look at this class of drugs. A general outline of drugs used to treat headache will be found in Table 33.4. This table, which is modified from Diamond and Baltes,[6] is included as a handy reference guide rather than a definitive collection of wonder drugs. It should be used accordingly.

Now let us look again at the major types of headaches mentioned previously and examine briefly how they are treated. It is not this author's intention to go into the pharmacology, biopharmaceutics or pharmaceutical chemistry of all possible analgesics, psychoactive drugs, depressant drugs, etc., which can and are used every day to treat headaches. The reader is directed to the appropriate textbooks for discussion of this nature. Instead, the purpose here is to give an overview on the type of drugs used and the rationale (where possible) for their selection.

Traction and Inflammatory Headaches. Treatment in this group is directed at exposing the primary disease. Once this is accomplished, surgical correction, antibiotic therapy and other specific treatment for the organic cause will usually relieve the headache. Nasal and sinus headache may be relieved by decongestant agents (nasal sprays are preferred) and the creation of drainage. The pharmacist should educate the patient in the proper use of nasal spray (*i.e.*, spray once into each nostril, wait 5 min and spray again).

Pyrexial and Toxic Headache. These headaches disappear upon removal of the offending agent or the treatment of the primary underlying disease. Symptomatic relief is achieved by antipyretics and analgesics.

Muscle Contraction Headache. Tension headaches respond well to common analgesics such as the salicylates and to any of the common sedative or minor tranquilizers (see Table 33.4). The most effective in this group seems to be diazepam because of its muscle relaxant and sedative properties.[6] Actually, relatively few patients are seen with tension headaches due to anxiety, probably because these patients respond well to common analgesics like aspirin. Depressive headaches respond to antidepressant drugs. The tricyclic agents appear to be the most effective. There is no conclusive evidence to date to indicate that the demethylated congeners of the tricyclics are more effective or produce a more rapid rate of relief. There is little significant difference between all of these agents except that protriptyline should not be used at bedtime because of its stimulant effects. Depressive headaches usually do not respond well to the common analgesics.[6]

Traumatic Headache. The pain of chronic subdural hematoma and post-traumatic nervous instability must be handled with great care. Again, the primary thrust of treatment is directed at exposing and curing the underlying

TABLE 33.4
Headache Therapy Chart[a]

Class	Type	Treatment	Route	Drug	Dosage
Vascular	Migraine Classic Nonclassic	Prophylactic	Oral	Ergotamine tartrate	1 mg 4 times daily
				Ergotamine, phenobarbital and belladonna	1 tablet 4 times a day 1 sustained action tablet twice a day twice a day
				Methysergide maleate	2 mg 3 times daily
				MAO inhibitors Phenelzine sulfate Isocarboxazid	15 mg 3 times daily 10 mg 3 times daily (reduce to maintenance dose in 1 month)
		Abortive	Oral	Ergotamine tartrate	1 mg immediately; repeat every ½ hr, if necessary, to a maximum of 6 mg/day
				Ergotamine, caffeine, belladonna Ergotamine and caffeine	
			Sublingual	Ergotamine	2 mg immediately, under the tongue; repeat in 2 hr if necessary
			Inhalation	Ergotamine	1 dose immediately; repeat every 5 min to a maximum of 6/day, if necessary
			Intra-muscular	Ergotamine tartrate	0.5–1 mg immediately and no more than 3 mg/week
				Dihydroergotamine	1 mg at hourly intervals; up to 3 mg/day, if necessary

TABLE 34.4—*Continued*
Headache Therapy Chart[a]

Class	Type	Treatment	Route	Drug	Dosage
			Rectal	Ergotamine and caffeine	Insert 1 suppository in rectum immediately; repeat in 1 hr, if necessary
				Ergotamine, caffeine, belladonna	
	Cluster	Prophylactic	Oral	Methysergide maleate	2 mg 3 times daily
				Triamcinolone	4 mg 4 times daily
				Methylprednisolone	16 mg every other day
				Cyproheptadine	4 mg 4 times daily; maximum of 2 tablets at bedtime
				Ergotamine preparations	Same dosage as for migraine
			Intra-venous	Histamine	3 mg histamine diphosphate in 250 ml of saline; drip at a rate sufficient to produce a flush but not a headache; 21 treatments, 1 or 2 daily
		Abortive		Ergotamine preparations	Same dosage as for migraine
Muscle contraction	Tension and anxiety	Prophylactic	Oral	Diazepam	2–10 mg 4 times daily
				Chlordiazepoxide	5–25 mg 4 times daily
				Hydroxyzine pamoate	25–100 mg 4 times daily
				Meprobamate	300–400 mg 4 times daily
				Major tranquilizers only rarely used	
		Abortive	Oral	Analgesics: aspirin, codeine, propoxyphene and combinations with caffeine and phenacetin	2 tablets every 4 hr

	Intra-muscular	Diazepam	5–10 mg immediately
		Hydroxyzine hydro-chloride	25–100 mg immediately
Depression	Prophylactic	Oral	Amitriptyline hydro-chloride	5–50 mg 4 times daily
		Protriptyline hydro-chloride	5–10 mg 3 times daily
		Imipramine	25–50 mg 3 times daily
		Desipramine hydro-chloride	25–50 mg 3 times daily
		Nortriptyline	25 mg 4 times daily
		MAO inhibitors	Same dosage as for migraine
	Abortive	Oral	Analgesics as above are usually ineffective but may give partial relief	
Depression with agitation	Prophylactic	Oral	Add minor or major tranquilizers to antidepressant medications above; the combinations below are useful:	
		Perphenazine and amitriptyline	Usual dosage: 1 tablet 3 times daily; 2 tablets at bedtime; 2–10, 2–25, 4–10 and 4–25

aReprinted with permission from Ref. 8.

condition. Most, if not all, of the effort will be directed toward this goal, rather than relieving the head pain *per se*. Treatment might include sedation, maintenance of fluid and acid-base balance, corticosteroids, hypertonic solutions to reduce the intracranial pressure (of cerebral edema), vigorous use of antibiotics, mechanical respiratory support and definitive surgery.

Hypertensive Headache. This headache responds to agents which lower blood pressure and relieve muscle tension. For a discussion on antihypertensive drug therapy, the reader is directed to Chapter 15. For the relief of pain from the muscle tension component, besides those measures already mentioned, relaxation and freedom from emotional stress are of primary importance. Heat to the involved muscles by means of hot towels, a heating pad or a warm bath will help relieve the discomfort. Gentle massage of the muscles also will usually be of benefit. Specific drug therapy might combine an analgesic, such as aspirin, to raise the pain threshold and a sedative, such as phenobarbital, to relieve the nervous tension which triggers the headache. Many times just the use of the mild analgesic in conjunction with a few moments of complete quiet and relaxation is all that is required to obtain relief.

Migraine Headache. As with other types of headache, the most important factor in treating a patient with migraine is to treat the whole person, rather than a specific symptom. Most controlled studies have shown that the results of the prophylactic treatment of migraine with drugs are very similar and only a few of these agents are more effective than a placebo. An improvement rate of about 60% commonly results from any therapeutic trial in migraine.[9] The treatment of migraine is 2-fold. First is the treatment of the acute attack and second is the prevention of further attacks.

In treating the acute attack of migrane, the most common drugs used are the ergot derivatives and their varied formulations. A few contain only ergotamine tartrate, while many contain a combination of ergotamine with caffeine, or antispasmodics, antiemetics and sedatives. Almost all routes of administration (oral, rectal, parenteral, sublingual and inhalation) are included in these various preparations. Ergotamine's beneficial effect most likely is related to its vasoconstrictive action in the smooth muscle of the cranial blood vessels. The ratio-

nale for adding caffeine to ergotamine is based on the observation that it acts synergistically with the ergot alkaloids and, therefore, the total dosage of ergotamine may be reduced. Agents such as antispasmodics and antiemetics may decrease the possible side effects of ergotamine and help to control the nausea and vomiting. There is some current work being done in England with an effervescent ergotamine preparation which appears to work more rapidly than the solid dosage form.[19] This is based on the fact that there is some evidence that absorption of solid dosage forms is impaired in patients under attack.

The importance of administering the medication, regardless of which preparation is used, at the first sign of an attack and in adequate doses can not be overemphasized. One reason for seeing differences in therapeutic results from various studies using the same drug and dosage form is the difference in the initial and total dose employed. Table 33.4 gives guidelines to these doses. The pharmacist must take the time to explain both the mechanics of how to administer the medication and the rationale for the selection of that particular dosage form to the patient. This is especially true of meter-dose inhalation devices such as Medihaler-Ergotamine. When the patient feels an attack starting, the anxiety and fear which accompany the first signs may tend to obliterate hastily given instructions on the proper use of the drugs.

Habituation to ergotamine can result in the possibility of a rebound reaction of constriction, dilation and headache, as the patient takes the drug ritually. Friedman reported that a number of patients who took 2 to 3 mg of ergotamine tartrate daily for 3 to 30 years complained of daily headaches and required an increased dose for continued relief.[20] The Princess Margaret Migraine Clinic in London recommends that no patient take more than 10 to 12 mg of the drug per week.[19] According to Dr. Marcia Wilkinson of the Clinic, the symptoms of overdose are those of a continuing migraine headache so that patients may think their attack is still going on, so they take more ergotamine. The symptoms from withdrawal of ergotamine are increasing frequency of headaches (which may continue for several days or weeks), loss of feeling of well-being, fatigue and depression. Many of these patients suffer from an underlying depression, and this should be dealt with first since the headache may prove to be secondary to the depression.

If migraine headaches occur only occasionally, abortive therapy is the best approach. If, however, the headaches occur with enough frequency and severity to interfere with the patient's daily routine, prophylactic therapy should be attempted. The drug of choice is ergotamine tartrate, administered 4 times daily in divided doses. In many cases this type of therapy not only will reduce the number and severity of attacks, but may even eliminate them.

Methysergide maleate is a very potent antiserotonin agent. It is currently the most widely used drug for prophylactic treatment. It will suppress migraine completely or in part in approximately 60% of patients.[21] However, 20 to 40% of patients experience such adverse side effects as abdominal discomfort, muscle cramps, and in some instances swelling, depression, numbness and tingling of the extremities. Of this group, about 10% are unable to tolerate the drugs because of symptoms of peripheral vasoconstriction. The drug has also been implicated in the production of retroperitoneal fibrosis as well as fibrotic changes in the heart. Because of this risk, it should be discontinued for 6 to 8 weeks after every 6 months of use. Although it must be used cautiously, methysergide is the most effective preparation available in the United States for the prevention of migraine.

Cyproheptadine, an antihistamine with mild to moderate antiserotonin activity, is also used as a prophylactic agent. No fibrosis has been reported after the use of this drug, but the patient may experience dry mouth, pronounced drowsiness and increased appetite stimulation. Some controlled studies have shown that cyproheptadine is not significantly different from other agents which are available.

Another agent similar in its action is pizotyline (BC 105), a tricyclic derivative, similar to cyproheptadine which has recently undergone clinical trials for the prophylaxis of migraine.[22] The reports on this drug are conflicting and the studies short term. It would appear that the drug is more effective than a placebo and less effective than methysergide.

Anthony and Lance[22] reported a 2-year study with phenelzine sulfate, a MAO inhibitor.

It was shown that the drug reduced the severity and frequency of attacks to less than half the original number. In the last few years, however, MAO inhibitors have seldom been used because of their potential for dangerous drug interactions, toxicities and the extremely variable response to them.

Corticosteroids have also been used in the treatment of cluster headaches, but the results have been ambiguous when they are the only agent used.

One of the most promising of the prophylactic drugs is clonidine.[24,26] This drug appears to work by reducing the sensitivity of the blood vessels to circulating amines. The drug seems to be even safe in patients with cardiovascular disease.

Propranolol hydrochloride, a beta-adrenergic blocker, has been used successfully in patients with migraine who are unable to tolerate other drugs.

Other types of treatment which have met with limited success include the use of oxygen (breathing 100% oxygen for 5 min to terminate an attack), carotid artery freezing and acupuncture.

PROGNOSIS

The general prognosis for patients suffering from headache is usually good. Once the underlying cause for the headache has been discovered, numerous methods of effective treatment are available. A final impression worth noting is that some patients may never get relief from their headaches, regardless of the diagnostic efforts of the physician and the pharmacological efforts of the numerous drugs which abound. There seems to be strong, but generally undocumented, evidence that a primary reason for this is that the headache, regardless of type, is an expression of frustration. The frustration may be based upon guilt, a never ending attempt at peer acceptance, lack of love or the fact that the patient cannot develop a proper relationship with the people around him or adjust to his environment. If this is a cause of the pain, then the prognosis is not optimistic.

REFERENCES

1. Friedman, A. P., and Merritt, H. H.: Headache: Diagnosis and Treatment. F. A. Davis Co.,

Philadelphia, 1959.

2. Rose, J. A.: Managing headaches. Postgrad. Med., 12: 69, 1969.

3. Blumenthal, L., and Fuchs, M.: Diagnostic Criteria: Vascular Headaches, Vol. 6, p. 5 Lederle Labs., Pearl River, N.Y., 1964.

4. Griffith, J. F., and Adams, R. D. (editors): Harrison's Principles of Internal Medicine, p. 52. McGraw-Hill Book Co., New York, 1970.

5. Wolf, H. G.: Headache and Other Pain. Oxford University Press, Fair Lawn, N.J., 1947.

6. Diamond, S., and Baltes, B.: Management of headache by the family physician. Am. Fam. Physician, 5: 68, 1972.

7. Diamond, S., and Baltes, B.: Chemotherapy of severe headache. Drug Ther., 5: 72, 1972.

8. Blau, J. N.: Migraine-research. Br. Med. J., 2: 751, 1971.

9. Nelson, R.: Cluster migraine—an unrecognized common entity. Can. Med. Assoc. J., 103: 1026, 1970.

10. Waters, W. E.: Migraine: intelligence, social class, and familial prevalence. Br. Med. J., 2: 77, 1971.

11. Selby, G., and Lance, J.: Observations of 500 cases of migraine and allied vascular headache. J. Neurol. Neurosurg. Psychiatry, 23: 23, 1968.

12. Carroll, J. D.: Migraine—general management. Br. Med. J., 2: 756, 1971.

13. Chapman, L. F., Ramos, A. O., Goodell, H., Silverman, G., and Wolf, H. G.: A humoral agent implicated in vascular headache of the migraine type. Arch. Neurol., 3: 223, 1960.

14. Dubois-Reymond, E.: Zur kenntness der hemikrania. Arch. F. Anat. Physiol. U. Wissensch. Med., p. 461, 1860.

15. Anon: Headache. Sandoz-Wander, Inc., p. 21, 1970.

16. Sicuteri, F.: Vasoneuroreactive substances and their implication in vascular pain. In Research and Clinical Studies in Headache: An International Review. The Williams and Wilkins Co., Baltimore, 1967.

17. Anon: Handbook of Non-Prescription Drugs. American Pharmaceutical Association, Washington, D.C., 1973.

18. Wilkinson, M.: Medical news. J.A.M.A., 222: 1400, 1972.

19. Friedman, A.: Migraine headaches. J.A.M.A., 225: 567, 1973.

20. Curran, D. A., and Lance, J. W.: Clinical trial of methysergide and other preparations in the management of migraine. J. Neurol. Neurosurg. Psychiatry, 27: 463, 1964.

21. Lance, J. W., Anthony, M., and Somerville, B.: Br. Med. J., 2: 227, 1970.

22. Anthony, M., and Lance, J.: Monoamine oxidase inhibition in the treatment of migraine. Arch. Neurol., 21: 263, 1969.

23. Wilkinson, M.: Proceedings of the International Migraine-Headache Symposium, Florence, Italy, 117, 1970.

24. Sjaastad, O., and Sjaastad, E.: The histaminuria in vascular headache. Acta Neurol. Scand., 46: 331, 1970.

25. Shafar, J., Tullett, E. R., and Knowlson, P. A.: Evaluation of clonidine in prophylaxis of migraine. Lancet, 1: 403, 1972.

26. Anon: Freeze-thaw procedure proven effective against chronic headache J.A.M.A., 213: 385, 1970.

section 10

Diseases of the eye

chapter 34

GLAUCOMA

Theodore G. Tong, Pharm. D.
Robert J. Ignoffo, Pharm. D.

Glaucoma is an ocular disease characterized by an abnormally elevated intraocular pressure. Degeneration of the optic nerve and retina, which may result in irreversible visual impairment, is the pathological consequence of the disorder. It is estimated that 2,000,000 people in the United States are afflicted with glaucoma and 10 to 20% of the blindness in this country can be attributed to the disease. Although glaucoma can occur at any age, the incidence is markedly increased in persons over the age of 40. Nearly 2% of the population in this age group is afflicted with glaucoma and fewer than ½ of those involved are even aware of its presence. Permanent visual impairment occurs frequently as a result of failure to implement prompt and appropriate therapeutic measures. Glaucoma often goes unnoticed until it is too late to treat because most forms of the disease are insidious at their onset and asymptomatic during most of their clinical course. Optic nerve and retinal damage from rising intraocular pressure often is not detected until later stages of the disease.

Glaucoma can be classified conveniently into primary, secondary and congenital types. The cause of the elevation of intraocular tension which brings about the condition of primary glaucoma can be further divided into simple open angle or wide angle and angle closure or narrow angle forms. Open angle glaucoma is the most commonly occurring form and accounts for about 90% of the cases diagnosed. Less than 5% of the glaucomas are of the angle closure or narrow angle type.

Primary open angle glaucoma occurs with greater frequency in middle-aged than in young people. A significant percentage of people in their 60's and 70's are afflicted with open angle glaucoma, and it is common in people who are in their 80's. The familial relationship of glaucoma has been well established; whether the hereditary pattern is one consistent with a dominant or recessive autosomal trait remains equivocal. Particular attention to factors which contribute to greater risk of developing this disease should be paid for any patient with a familial history of glaucoma. Although there are more males with primary open angle glaucoma, sex predilection for the disease is not clinically significant. Primary open angle glaucoma is a relatively more common disorder in Caucasians and Blacks than American Indians and Asians. Although many patients may present with unilateral involvement initially, it can be anticipated that the other eye will be involved within 5 years. Myopia has been suggested to be a high risk factor in predisposition to glaucoma. Although it is more common to find open angle glaucoma in patients with myopia, especially in the younger age group, the evidence of association between the two factors remains equivocal.

ETIOLOGY

Glaucoma can occur as a secondary manifestation of systemic disorders, trauma or drugs.[1] Elevation of intraocular tension induced by pupillary block and angle occlusion is a frequent complication of lens dislocation, advanced cataractous changes of the lens or exfoliation of the lens capsule. Uveitis and melanomas of the uveal tract, hemorrhaging into the anterior and posterior chambers, corneal or limbal laceration of the iris, impaired wound healing following cataract surgery and contusions or penetrating injuries to the eye are frequent causes. Intraocular pressure elevation is often a consequence of rubeosis iritis in advanced diabetes mellitus. Secondary glaucoma is most often unilateral, affecting one eye, and it is temporary until the underlying disorder has been corrected.

Primary congenital or infantile glaucoma is a rare disorder in which intraocular pressure is elevated as a result of developmental abnormalities of structures in the eye. Inadequate drainage of the aqueous humor is the primary defect. This form of glaucoma may occur in association with congenital abnormalities and anomalies such as homocystinuria and Marfan's syndrome. Congenital glaucoma can occur at birth and most often is detected soon thereafter. Sensitivity to light, excessive tearing and spasms of the eyelids in an infant should arouse suspicion for the presence of this disorder. Gonioscopic findings of chamber angle abnormalities accompanied by an elevated intraocular tension and atrophy of the iris or glaucomatous cupping of the optic disk are diagnostically important. Early detection and control of the condition are most important for an optimistic prognosis.

PATHOGENESIS

The onset of primary open angle glaucoma is insidious.[2] Patients are often oblivious of any symptoms until their vision is markedly impaired. Frequently, the disease will have progressed gradually to the point where it is minimally, if at all, alterable by therapy.

The genesis of primary open angle glaucoma is the malfunction of the trabecular meshwork interfering with the outflow of aqueous humor from the anterior chamber to the drainage channel of the eye. Normally aqueous humor is secreted by the ciliary processes into the posterior chamber. It is circulated from there through the pupil into the anterior chamber. The aqueous humor then leaves the eye by way of the trabecular meshwork and the canal of Schlemm reaching the episcleral and conjunctival vessels. Impairment of this drainage system causes the rise in intraocular tension experienced in open angle glaucoma. The elevation in intraocular pressure is usually not dramatic; the pressure usually ranges between 25 and 35 mm Hg, compared to the normal of 10 to 20 mm Hg.

The increase in intraocular pressure leads to characteristic deterioration of the optic disk

and defect in the visual field. The optic and retinal nerve fibers also are affected adversely. Detachment of the corneal epithelium and formation of bullae produce corneal edema as the trabecular spaces become obliterated. In chronic primary open angle glaucoma, scotomas (blind areas) appear often in the visual field. These abnormalities are not noticed readily since the visual loss in most cases does not affect the acuity of perception until rather late. All field losses are irreversible.

An acute angle closure attack occurs as a consequence of a rapid and sudden rise in intraocular pressure. Apposition of the peripheral iris against the corneal and trabecular meshwork obstructs the outflow of aqueous humor; the aqueous fluids can not reach the filtering channels but are confined within the posterior chamber. As these fluids accumulate, the intraocular tension rises.

Relaxation of the ciliary zonule and constriction of the ciliary fibers can induce angle closure by pupillary blockade. As the iris root is folded against the trabecular epithelium during pupillary dilation, the filtration processes become isolated from the anterior chamber. Pupillary dilation is a common factor associated with angle closure attacks. Dim lights or darkness, emotion, shock and drugs can precipitate an attack, especially where the anterior chamber angle is already chronically narrowed. For a number of drug-induced angle closure glaucoma cases, the mechanism of induction is unknown. Other factors also may cause narrowing of the anterior chamber. A large lens in a small eye decreases the convexity of the iris with shallowing of the anterior chamber. In an eye with a shallow chamber, the iris may be displaced anteriorly by the surface of the enlarged lens. The lens continues to grow throughout life, progressively shallowing and narrowing the angle.

DIAGNOSIS AND CLINICAL FINDINGS

During the early stages of primary open angle glaucoma, the intraocular tension may be elevated only slightly. However, the onset of elevated intraocular pressure appears very abruptly in many cases where young adults are involved.[1, 2] Intraocular tensions of 40 to 70 mm Hg may be found with minimal or no impairment of the optic disk or visual field. Transient blurring and colored halos are experienced during these episodes of abrupt elevations of intraocular tension. It is important on these occasions for the clinician to identify the type of glaucoma being experienced since similar symptoms can be associated with acute angle closure glaucoma. A choice of treatment can not be made until the form of glaucoma is clearly determined. An intraocular tension of 22 to 24 mm Hg or more should arouse suspicion of possible glaucoma. Repeated tonometric studies should be done before diagnosis of glaucoma is made definite. The diurnal variations of intraocular pressure must be considered with the tension highest when the patient arises in the morning and lowest during late evening. The magnitude of diurnal variations of intraocular tension is greater than normal in primary open angle glaucoma, and it is not unusual for some patients to experience a peak in intraocular tension at other times of the day.

Primary angle closure glaucoma occurs much less frequently than the open angle type. An acute attack of angle closure glaucoma is an emergency situation and must be treated vigorously at its onset. An uncontrolled attack can lead to permanent visual impairment and blindness in 2 to 3 days. Symptoms experienced at onset are severe ocular congestion, pain, the appearance of colored halos around lights and diminished visual acuity. The intraocular tension during an acute attack may rise from 40 to over 100 mm Hg.

The onset and course of angle closure glaucoma are variable but on most occasions are intermittent and acute. The condition, however, can be subacute. In such a case, there is an asymptomatic but rapid rise in intraocular tension to a level below those usually experienced during acute attacks. Chronic angle closure glaucoma is gradual and symptomatic until advanced stages of the disease are reached.

Measurement of intraocular pressure by tonometry, however, can not be relied upon as the sole means of detecting whether an individual is predisposed to angle closure glaucoma since the intraocular tension may be normal. Shortly after recovery from an attack, the tension in the affected eye temporarily may become normal or even lower than in the unaffected eye. Prior to any attempt at dilating the pupil, gonioscopic examination of the depth of the anterior chambers' angle should be performed.

Angle closure glaucoma almost always involves both eyes. The unaffected eye probably will be subject to attack within a year. Females and late middle-aged people are the group most commonly afflicted with angle closure glaucoma.

Pathological complications of angle closure glaucoma include formation of cataracts, peripheral anterior synechias, further atrophy of optic nerve and retina and absolute glaucoma. The development of cataracts can increase the existing pupillary blockade and degree of angle closure. Following repeated or prolonged attacks, anterior synechias are formed between the iris and corneal surface in the trabecular epithelium. The outflow of aqueous humor is further obstructed. The more congestion and edema of the iris and ciliary processes, the greater the tendency to form these adhesions. Table 34.1 summarizes the clinical findings and symptoms of primary glaucoma. Table 34.2 summarizes the diagnostic studies for glaucoma.

DRUGS CONTRAINDICATED IN GLAUCOMA

Specific classes of drugs such as anticholinergics, adrenergics and corticosteroids have been implicated in inducing glaucoma. Any drugs with atropine-like side effects can produce pupillary dilation and paralysis of accommodation for near vision. Concern for this iatrogenic complication has prompted Food and Drug Administration requirements for warnings on the systemic use of anticholinergics in the presence of glaucoma.

It appears that the absolute contraindication for the use of sympathomimetics and anticholinergics in patients with glaucoma is an empirical evaluation. One must distinguish between open angle and angle closure glaucoma in arriving at a therapeutic decision because drug effects are different in the two cases. Drugs that dilate the pupil, for instance, may precipitate an acute attack of angle closure glaucoma but will produce no harmful effect in open angle cases. Dilation of the pupil may cause the peripheral iris to bulge forward, blocking the trabecular meshwork, preventing the aqueous humor from reaching the outflow channels and bringing about an increase in intraocular pres-

TABLE 34.1

Clinical Findings and Symptoms of Primary Glaucomas

Disease	Onset	Early Findings and Symptoms	Late Findings and Symptoms
Open angle glaucoma	Insidious	Asymptomatic slight rise in intraocular pressure decrease rate of aqueous humor outflow; optic disk changes	Gradual loss of peripheral vision (over months to years); persistent elevation of intraocular pressure; optic nerve degeneration; retinal nerve atrophy; edema of the cornea; cataracts; trabecular meshwork degeneration
Angle closure glaucoma	Sudden	Blurred vision; severe ocular pain and congestion; conjunctival redness; cloudy cornea; moderately dilated pupil; poor pupil response to light; intraocular pressure markedly elevated; nausea and vomiting	Complete blindness in 2-5 days

sure. Since excessive resistance to outflow in open angle glaucoma is caused primarily by changes within the trabecular epithelium outflow channels, dilation of the pupil will not exacerbate the intraocular pressure. Remarkably few medications, other than those used locally to treat glaucoma, will alter intraocular pressure significantly.[3] Systemic medications usually produce intraocular pressure alterations for only brief durations. Factors implicated in potential drug induction of angle closure glaucoma are summarized in Table 34.3.

Anticholinergics

In patients with normal eyes, topically instilled anticholinergics[4] such as atropine, scopolamine and cyclopentolate produce no significant elevations in intraocular pressure. However, in patients over 30 years of age who have abnormally shallow anterior chambers, there is a significant risk of precipitating acute attacks of angle closure glaucoma. The incidence has been estimated to be nearly 1 in 4,000.[5] Atropine and scopolamine have profound effect on the eye because of their longer duration of action than other agents with anticholinergic effects, *i.e.*, phenothiazines, tricyclic antidepressants and antihistamines. These locally instilled agents cause mydriasis and cycloplegia which may persist for as long as 2 weeks. In some open angle patients, they can produce a slight rise of intraocular tension (less than 6 mm Hg) when instilled into the eyes.[6] Other mydriatics, however, do not appear to have this effect. Conventional doses of atropine systemically administered for preanesthesia have little ocular effect; in contrast, equivalent therapeutic doses of scopolamine can cause definite pupillary dilation.[7-9] Belladonna, of which atropine is the main component, has been reported to exacerbate preglaucomatous eyes, although this is rare.[10] Nevertheless, it is prudent to exercise caution in administering drugs which cause pupillary dilation in patients predisposed to glaucoma.

Propantheline, a commonly used anticholinergic, has been shown to produce no significant elevation in intraocular tension in either normal or angle closure patients.[11] Anticholinergics, in fact, can deepen the anterior chamber by inhibiting the contraction of the ciliary body and produce cycloplegia which widens rather than narrows the anterior chamber angle making angle closure less likely to occur.[3] Anticholinergic drugs such as anisotropine, dicyclomine or methixene have little effect on the pupil and therefore, rarely induce either open

TABLE 34.2
Diagnostic Studies for Glaucoma

	Procedure
Tonometry	Measures intraocular tension; routinely used for mass screening studies; diurnal variations of intraocular tension in open angle glaucoma should be considered; repeated readings should be done before definite diagnosis; between acute attacks of angle closure glaucoma, the intraocular tension may be normal
Gonioscopy	Differentiates the type of glaucoma; gonioscopic appearance of narrowed anterior chamber angle is usually diagnostic of angle closure glaucoma
Tonography	May reveal impaired facility of aqueous humor outflow; early open angle glaucoma can be detected by this technique; tonometer is applied to the eye and the resultant reduction in the intraocular tension is measured as an indicator of outflow facility
Water-drinking test	Rise in intraocular tension after rapid ingestion of a quart of water is significant indication of glaucoma; positive result occurs in 30% of open angle glaucoma cases; negative result does not rule out glaucoma
	Tonography and water-drinking test will reveal open angle glaucoma with 90% reliability
Ophthalmoscopy	Glaucomatous excavation or cupping of the optic disk is found in chronic primary open angle and congenital glaucomas; glaucomatous changes of optic disk and/or occlusion of the central retinal vein in absence of elevated intraocular tension should arouse suspicion of glaucoma in early stage
Visual field examination	Isolated areas of impaired vision surrounded by normal areas in a visual field is indicative of open angle glaucoma; visual field changes are irreversible and parallel optic disk changes
Corticosteroid instillation	Striking differences in ocular tension (between primary open angle glaucoma patients and normal subjects) are produced by topic-

TABLE 34.2—*Continued*
Diagnostic Studies for Glaucoma

	Procedure
	ally instilled corticosteroids; steroid provocative test is used to evaluate genetic predisposition to glaucoma; response of primary angle closure glaucoma to corticosteroid instillation is much more similar to normal subjects
Dark room test	Intraocular tension is assessed in patient before and after being placed in a dark room; in chronic angle closure glaucoma, a considerable rise in the intraocular tension is observed after being in the dark

TABLE 34.3
Factors Implicated in Potential Drug Induction of Angle Closure Glaucoma

1. Age—usually over thirty
2. History—familial, genetic basis
3. Race—usually Caucasian
4. Sex—usually female
5. Anterior chamber angle—shallow and narrow
6. Vision—hyperopia, hypermetropia
7. Convexity of the iris—flattened
8. Dose and duration of the offending drug used
9. Duration of effect on the eye—longer duration
10. Route of administration—topical more than systemic

angle or angle closure glaucoma.[11-15] No recent reports of exacerbations of glaucoma with diazepam or amitriptyline have appeared in the literature, although the manufacturers of these drugs contraindicate their use in patients with the disorder.[16] Very high doses of phenothiazines given for schizophrenia have reportedly been observed to produce slight elevations of intraocular pressure.[16] Treatment with miotics easily overcame the effect. Prolonged use of anticholinergics can exacerbate open angle glaucoma to some extent, but studies have shown that oral atropine at a dose of 0.6 mg every 4 hr for 1 week produced only slight elevations of intraocular tension.[17, 18]

In summary, withholding systemic anticholinergics for fear of inducing open angle glaucoma probably is not justified. This is true especially with regard to the use of parenteral atropine or scopolamine given preoperatively prior to general anesthesia. Sensitivity of the eye to systemic drugs is relatively low.[3, 11] Although these agents can induce angle closure in rare instances, the concomitant use of parasympathomimetic miotics will overcome any of the intraocular pressure effects. However, ocularly instilled potent anticholinergics, such as atropine, scopolamine, cyclopentolate and homatropine should not be used in patients diagnosed or predisposed to having angle closure glaucoma.[19]

Sympathomimetics

Adrenergic agents commonly found in appetite suppressants, bronchodilators, central nervous stimulants and vasoconstrictors produce slight pupillary dilations. No adverse effects on open angle glaucoma have been experienced while the incidence of deleterious effects on angle closure glaucoma has been extremely small after systemic administration.[20] Adrenergic agents such as epinephrine and phenylephrine have been used ocularly to treat open angle glaucoma. It is important to note, however, that these agents will elevate the intraocular pressure by narrowing the anterior chamber angle when instilled into eyes of angle closure patients.[21, 22]

General anesthetics producing parasympathetic and sympathetic imbalance may cause pupillary block. Topical pilocarpine 1% may be instilled into the eye an hour prior to inducing anesthesia to prevent this complication.[3, 16]

Steroids

Corticosteroids instilled locally in the eye will induce elevations of intraocular tension.[16, 23-29] The degree of rise in pressure appears to be associated with the anti-inflammatory potency of the agents involved. The rise in ocular tension is most marked with dexamethasone and betamethasone. Equivalent doses of ophthalmic prednisolone and triamcinolone used 4 times daily gave similar elevations of intraocular pressure to betamethasone instilled only once daily. Duration of corticosteroid treatment and the age of the patient

influence the degree of ocular hypertension that is experienced. In some instances, topical epinephrine or systemic carbonic anhydrase inhibitors can maintain the ocular tension within normal limits. On other occasions, it may be necessary to reduce the frequency of administration or substitute a less potent steroid. Withdrawal of the drug may even be necessary to return ocular tension to normal levels. In some cases, irreversible eye damage is caused as ocular tension persists for 1 to 2 months or even longer. In addition, cupping of the optic disk and defects of visual field may develop a few months after topical administration of corticosteroids is begun. Patients on chronic topical steroid therapy should, therefore, have tonometric examinations performed every 2 months.

Steroids administered systemically can make pre-existing open angle glaucoma more difficult to control, but their effect on intraocular pressure is much smaller than topically applied steroids. Ocular hypertension may occur during prolonged systemic therapy, usually over a period of 1 year or more, in patients with such conditions as rheumatoid arthritis or disseminated lupus erythematosis. This complication, however, should not deter one from using systemic corticosteroids in situations where they are appropriate.

Cardiovascular drugs

There is no convincing evidence that vasodilators significantly can aggravate glaucoma despite the fact that subconjunctival injection of strong vasodilators such as isoxsuprine and tolazoline can induce transient elevations in intraocular pressure, particularly in chronic open angle glaucoma.[5] Nitrates, nitrites, aminophylline, nylidirin and cyclandelate can be used safely in glaucoma.[5, 40] Antihypertensives will decrease intraocular blood flow which can lead to loss of small visual fields in the patient with a high intraocular pressure. Therefore, it is probably best to decrease blood pressure gradually in angle closure patients. If it is necessary to decrease blood pressure rapidly, one should either increase the patient's miotic medication or simultaneously lower the intraocular tension rapidly with an agent such as acetazolamide.

Miscellaneous agents

Amphetamines, tricyclic antidepressants, monoamine oxidase inhibitors, indomethacin and cocaine[41] produce slight degrees of mydriasis, but the likelihood of inducing angle closure with these drugs is very low.[42] Strong miotics such as pilocarpine 4 to 8% and the indirect acting nonreversible cholinesterase inhibitors may lead to pupillary block and inhibition of aqueous humor outflow and increase vascular congestion of the peripheral part of the iris so that the swollen iris becomes opposed to the cornea.[3, 7, 43, 44]

Polarizing neuromuscular blocking agents such as succinylcholine used as adjuvants to general anesthesia can cause a marked rise in intraocular pressure if the patient is not adequately anesthetized.[45] They should not be used in glaucomatous patients. A nondepolarizing neuromuscular blocking agent such as gallamine is effective in preventing the rise in intraocular pressure.[16]

An acute transient myopia has occurred following vaginal absorption of AVC cream which contains sulfanilamide, complicated by retinal edema, shallowing anterior chambers and acute angle closure.[46] Similar reactions have occurred involving carbonic anhydrase inhibitors,[47-49] tetracycline,[50] prochlorperazine and promethazine.[51] A few of these may be responsible for ocular hypertension but, more commonly, they act to increase retinal fluid production. These reactions can be classified as idiosyncratic phenomena.

Patients who have received alpha-chymotrypsin while undergoing cataract extraction characteristically show an increase in intraocular tension 2 to 5 days after surgery for a week or more.[52, 53] Deep anterior chambers and open angles are seen, differentiating alpha-chymotrypsin from pupillary block-induced glaucoma. The ocular hypertension induced appears to be a dose-related and self-limiting event.[54] Table 34.4 lists those drugs which can induce glaucoma.

It is important to consider the following factors when appraising a problem of drug-induced glaucoma. Topically administered drugs will induce glaucoma more frequently than those given systemically; acute angle closure glaucoma should be regarded as an emergency; and any agent which might precipitate an attack must be used cautiously. A diagnosed case of angle closure glaucoma should be a contraindication to the use of such drugs. Conditions under which any drugs are contraindicated should be made specific. Seldom, if ever, in a package insert or other form of information available to the pharmacist does a recommendation against the use of a particular agent in glaucoma indicate which type of glaucoma is meant.

THERAPY

The goal of treatment in glaucoma is the immediate and sustained reduction of intraocular pressure to prevent deterioration of the optic nerve and loss of visual function. Drugs used in the treatment of glaucoma may be divided conveniently into those that increase the elimination of aqueous humor or decrease its formation. Parasympathomimetic miotic agents act by removing the obstruction to the outflow channels thereby facilitating the elimination of aqueous humor.[55] Sympathomimetic mydriatic agents lower elevated intraocular pressure by decreasing the rate of aqueous humor formation.[55] Secretion and inflow of aqueous humor are most effectively decreased by the carbonic anhydrase inhibitors.[56] Hyperosmotic agents reduce intraocular pressure by increasing the osmolarity of the plasma relative to the aqueous and vitreous humors.[57] Ocularly instilled parasympathomimetic miotics, sympathomimetic mydriatics and orally administered carbonic anhydrase inhibitors find their greatest clinical application in primary open angle glaucoma. The management of acute angle closure glaucoma and congenital glaucoma is essentially surgical. Medical treatment is limited to preparing the patient for surgery. Treatment of secondary glaucoma should be directed at correcting the underlying cause as well as the elevation of intraocular pressure. Table 34.5 summarizes the basis of medical treatment of glaucoma.

Miotics

Miotics are cholinergic agents which facilitate the outflow of aqueous humor from the

TABLE 34.4
Ability of Drugs to Induce Glaucoma

Drug	Route	Open angle	Angle closure
Anticholinergics			
Atropine			
Scopolamine	Topical	Rarely	Frequently
Belladonna			
Propantheline	Systemic	Rarely	Rarely
Adrenergics			
Phenylephrine 10%[a]	Topical	Never	Occasionally
Epinephrine	Systemic	Never	Rarely
Miotics			
Pilocarpine 4-8%			
Echothiophate	Topical	Never	Occasionally
Isoflurophate			
Carbonic anhydrase inhibitors	Systemic	Never	Rarely
Acetazolamide			
Alpha-chymotrypsin[b]	Topical	Rarely	Occasionally
Antihypertensives[c]	Systemic	Never	Never
Prochlorperazine[b]	Systemic	Never	Never
Promethazine[b] (high doses)	Systemic	Never	Rarely
Corticosteroids (at equipotent doses)			
Betamethasone	Topical	Frequently	Never
Dexamethasone			
Hydrocortisone			
Prednisolone	Topical	Occasionally	Never
Triamcinolone			
Dexamethasone			
Hydrocortisone	Systemic	Occasionally	Never
Prednisolone			

[a]Phenylephrine 10% can induce acute angle closure which is refractory to medical management. Pretreatment with miotics and carbonic anhydrase inhibitors does not prevent this occurence.

[b]These agents have produced idiosyncratic increases in intraocular pressure on rare occasions.

[c]Antihypertensives can provoke the loss of visual fields if the blood pressure is decreased too rapidly, but in general they lower intraocular pressure transiently and this may even benefit glaucoma patients.

anterior chamber of the eye (Table 34.6). This is accomplished primarily by their action on the musculature of the iris and the ciliary body. The exact mechanism of improved fluid drainage remains poorly understood. The contraction of the ciliary musculature appears to be a primary mechanism by which the intraocular tension is reduced. It is widely held that the

TABLE 34.5
Basis of Medical Treatment for Glaucoma

A. Increase elimination of aqueous humor via drainage system
   Drugs: Parasympathomimetics
   Sympathomimetics
B. Decrease formation of aqueous humor by the ciliary processes
   Drugs: Sympathomimetics
   Carbonic anhydrase inhibitors
C. Reduction of volume of aqueous humor in anterior chamber
   Drugs: Hyperosmotics

trabecular meshwork and veins peripheral to the canal of Schlemm also become dilated, thereby facilitating the outflow of aqueous humor. This action is independent of the pupillary constriction or miosis produced by the cholinergic miotic since outflow has been demonstrated to be unaffected in its absence. Miotics can directly lower intraocular tension by stimulating the postjunctional effector cells innervated by the cholinergic fibers. Structurally, these agents are similar to acetylcholine, the endogenous mediator of nerve impulses which produces miosis and facilitates the outflow of aqueous fluid through the canal of Schlemm. Cholinergic miotics are therapeutically beneficial for treatment of open angle glaucoma and preoperative preparation for surgery in narrow angle. Their disadvantage is their short duration of action requiring frequent administration.

Acetylcholine is not used in glaucoma therapy because of its poor corneal penetration upon ocular instillation and rapid inactivation by cholinesterase. Pilocarpine is the drug most commonly used for initial and maintenance therapy of chronic primary open angle glaucoma.[58,59] Pilocarpine penetrates the cornea after ocular instillation with miosis and fall in intraocular tension reaching their maximal levels in 30 to 40 min.[55,60,61] It is employed in solution strengths varying from ½ to 10% (although there appears to be little if any therapeutic advantages in the use of concentrations above 4%). The duration of intraocular pressure lowering is 4 to 8 hr. The usual frequency of instillation is 2 to 3 times daily, but it may be given as often as every 2 hr.

Carbachol is a synthetic derivative of choline with a direct action like that of pilocarpine on parasympathetic receptors. It is more resistant to inactivation by cholinesterase and, therefore, is considered to be more effective than pilocarpine in comparable strengths for intraocular tension control. The solution is available in strengths of 0.75 to 3.0%. In the treatment of open angle glaucoma 1 drop is instilled usually 2 or 3 times daily. Response has been shown to vary with the dose, and weaker strength solutions may require more frequent administration than usually suggested.[62] In circumstances where pilocarpine and other miotics can not be used owing either to allergy or to intolerable side effects, carbachol may be a suitable alternative. However, if the glaucoma is uncontrollable with pilocarpine, it is doubtful that carbachol would yield much, if any, therapeutic improvement.

Diurnal fluctuations of intraocular tension have been shown to be diminished more effectively by carbachol than by pilocarpine. The major disadvantage of carbachol is its poor corneal penetration. In addition, it must be prepared in a vehicle such as methylcellulose to insure prolonged contact with the cornea or with a wetting agent such as benzalkonium chloride in an effort to enhance corneal permeability. In the treatment of nonedematous glaucoma, an ointment of carbachol applied locally twice daily causes blurring of vision, a disadvantage of any ophthalmic ointment.

Methacholine bromide pharmacologically is very similar to acetylcholine with the exception of being very resistant to cholinesterase. However, poor corneal penetration and instability in solution make it an unsuitable miotic for clinical use in glaucoma.

The anticholinesterase miotics act by inhibiting the cholinesterase enzyme, thereby permitting the accumulation of acetylcholine and prolonging the parasympathetic activity on the effector end organs of the eye.

Intraocular pressure is reduced by facilitating aqueous outflow. Cholinesterase inhibitors used in the management of glaucoma, such as physostigmine and neostigmine, are relatively short acting. Organophosphate compounds, such as demecarium, echothiophate and isoflurophate, have long durations of action. The essential pharmacological difference between these compounds is the relative reversibility or permanency of their parasympathomimetic activity. Although the direct and indirect acting

TABLE 34.6
Miotic Drugs Used in the Management of Glaucoma

Drug	Dosage[a]	Comment
Parasympathomimetic		
Pilocarpine hydrochloride	0.5% to 10%, instilled	Most commonly used;
Pilocarpine nitrate	1 or 2 drops in	onset of intraocular
	affected eye from every	pressure lowering effect
	6-8 hr to as often	rapid with 4-8 hr
	as every 4 hr	duration
Carbachol	0.75%-3% instilled 1	Response varies with dose;
	or 2 drops in affected	may require frequent ad-
	eye every 8-12 hr	ministration for weaker
	to as often as every 4	solutions than usually
	hr	suggested; a suitable
		alternative when other
		miotics cannot be used
		due to allergy or side
		effects; poor corneal
		penetration; contraindi-
		cated in presence of corneal
		injury
Short acting anticholinesterases	0.25%-1.0% instilled	Onset of intraocular
Physostigmine salicylate	1 or 2 drops in	pressure lowering effect
Physostigmine sulfate	affected eye every 6-	similar to pilocarpine;
	12 hr; 0.25%	considered to be stronger
	ointment applied at	miotic than pilocarpine;
	bedtime	aqueous solutions unstable;
		decomposition on exposure
		to light
Neostigmine bromide	3%-5% instilled 1 or	More stable and less
	2 drops in affected	irritating than
	eye every 4-6 hr	physostigmine; less
		effective due to poor
		corneal permeability
Long acting anticholinesterases	0.06%-0.25% instilled	Potent, long acting;
Echothiophate iodide	1 drop in affected eye	maximum effects in 10-
	no more frequently than	20 hr and may persist
	every 12 hr	for several days; unstable
		in solution; should be used
		when shorter acting miotics
		are inadequate; contraindi-
		cated prior to filtering surger;
		not used prior to cataract
		extraction
Demecarium bromide	0.125%-0.25% instilled 1	Potent, long acting;
	or 2 drops in affected	should be used only when
	eye every 12 hr to once	shorter acting miotics
	or twice weekly	do not give desired result;
		duration of miosis is
		prolonged
Isoflurophate	0.025%-0.1% instilled	Potent; long acting;
	1 or 2 drops in	should be used when shorter
	affected eye every 12-	acting miotics are
	24 hr or longer	inadequate; unstable;
		ointment supposedly most
		stable and less irritating;
		blurring of vision common
		complaint with ointment

[a]For open angle glaucoma.

parasympathomimetic miotics pharmacologically act on different sites of action, their clinical effects on lowering elevated intraocular pressure in glaucoma are quite similar.[60, 63]

Anticholinesterase miotics are therapeutically beneficial for the treatment of primary open angle glaucoma; they are not advised for the treatment of angle closure glaucoma or congenital glaucoma. Since these agents act indirectly by inhibiting cholinesterase activity prolonging the effects of endogenous acetylcholine, parasympathetic activity of the fibers to the pupil must be functional. They are not effective if given after retrobulbar injections of anesthesia such as during cataract extraction since liberation of acetylcholine is impaired.

Physostigmine lowers intraocular tension by facilitating the outflow of aqueous humor. It has a longer duration of action and is considered to be a stronger miotic than pilocarpine. Physostigmine can be given in strengths of 0.25 to 1.0% every 4 to 6 hr. The onset of reduction in intraocular pressure usually occurs within 10 to 30 min, reaching its maximal effect within 1 to 2 hr and lasting 4 hr or more after instillation. The miotic effects, however, may persist much longer. Aqueous solutions of physostigmine are unstable. Decomposition occurs with pH changes and upon exposure to light. This is detected by the presence of progressive darkening of the solution. Decomposition products of physostigmine solutions are quite irritating and therapeutically ineffective. Physostigmine ointment perhaps should be reserved for bedtime use since the intense miosis produced soon after application would be less discomforting for the patient while asleep. The prolonged duration of increased aqueous humor outflow facilitation is ideal and convenient since the patient need not be interrupted from his sleep to administer miotics.

Neostigmine is more stable but less effective than physostigmine because of poorer corneal permeability. It is less irritating and has fewer unpleasant side effects than physostigmine. Ocular instillation of 3 to 5% aqueous solutions of neostigmine can be given every 4 to 6 hr alone or on an alternating schedule with pilocarpine. Demecarium is chemically similar to neostigmine with comparable miotic and intraocular tension-lowering activity to that of echothiophate and isoflurophate. In contrast to the organophosphates, the inhibition of cholinesterase activity by demecarium 0.06 to 0.25% instilled every 12 to 48 hr will give beneficial effects on intraocular tension lasting from 12 hr to several days. In open angle glaucoma, maximal reduction of intraocular pressure with demecarium is seen in 24 to 36 hr. The rapidity of the onset and duration of miosis is related directly to the concentrations used. Tolerance and refractoriness to demecarium occur earlier than reported for echothiophate and isoflurophate.

Echothiophate is a slow onset but long acting cholinesterase inhibitor.[64, 65] Aqueous solutions of 0.06 to 0.25% instilled 1 drop every 12 to 24 hr for open angle glaucoma can produce miosis within 10 to 15 min, although maximal effect on lowering intraocular tension is not seen until 10 to 20 hr later and may persist as long as 96 hr. Instillation of 0.25% solution more often than twice daily does not appear to enhance the effectiveness on the reduction of intraocular tension.[66]

The advantage of echothiophate is its long duration of action requiring fewer instillations and better control of the intraocular tension on a diurnal basis. The intense miosis can produce a pupillary block and resultant shallowing of the anterior chamber of the eye. Therefore, in the presence of subacute narrow angle or angle closure glaucoma, echothiophate should not be used. Aqueous solutions of echothiophate are unstable and must be prepared just prior to dispensing. Storage under refrigeration for no more than 6 months should be recommended to the patient.

Isoflurophate possesses more potent and longer duration of action than physostigmine. A drop of 0.01 to 0.1% concentration once or twice daily produces effects on intraocular tension similar to those of echothiophate in open angle glaucoma. Miosis is maximally experienced within 15 to 20 min. Intraocular tension is maximally reduced within 24 hr after instillation. Instillation of 0.1% solution more than twice daily yields very minimal additional therapeutic benefit.

A direct and short acting miotic such as pilocarpine can produce local conjunctival irritation as a result of frequent instillations. Allergic sensitivity or refractoriness to pilocarpine has developed after prolonged use. Frequent instillation of the short acting miotics can exacerbate .chronic allergic conjunctivitis or blepharitis.

Discontinuation of the offending agent most often will eliminate the symptoms, and other miotics can be tried. Miotics may stimulate progressive deterioration of the visual field defect associated with glaucoma. Poor vision in dim light and blurring of vision from pupillary constriction and accommodative myopia are particularly troublesome for some patients. It is likely that the elderly patient already has diminished visual acuity and, therefore, should be made aware of the drug's effect. This problem can be further complicated in those aged patients who have cataracts in addition to impairment of visual function.

Miotics can produce annoying side effects such as transient headaches, ocular and periorbital pain, twitching of the eyelids, ciliary congestion and spasms.

The indirect long acting anticholinesterase miotics produce the most severe symptoms including discomfort associated with bright lights and close-up work. The affected eye is extremely sensitive to efforts in accommodating to light, and it is extremely myopic. These symptoms are particularly intense in younger patients who have active accommodation and are myopic to begin with. Patients should be reassured that these difficulties will usually diminish within a week or so. Severe fibrinous iritis can be induced by miotics and is most likely to occur with the long and indirect acting cholinesterase inhibitors. After intense and prolonged administration of the stronger miotics, pupillary cyst production is likely to occur.[67] This is seen more commonly in children, but the reason is not known.

Anticholinesterase miotics also may produce vitreous hemorrhaging, contact dermatitis and allergic conjunctivitis. Retinal detachment and cataracts have been associated with use of anticholinesterase miotics; however, their role is probably as a contributing factor secondary to underlying retinal pathology.

Glaucoma secondary to ocular inflammation may be exacerbated by these agents as a result of further vascular disruption. Lens opacities have been reported in patients treated with anticholinesterase miotics.[68-74] The incidence of cataractogenic lens changes appears related to the drug, the concentration the patient is

receiving and the duration of treatment. Cataract formation does not appear to be associated directly with glaucomatous eyes; patients not receiving treatment with anticholinesterase miotics are less likely to develop lens opacity. The lens changes may be partly reversible when the drug is discontinued. Progressive worsening of the cataract may occur, however, necessitating surgical extraction.

Systemic absorption of antiglaucoma drugs following ocular instillation has an undesirable stimulating effect.[75-78] This is seen more commonly after administration of the indirect and longer acting anticholinesterase agents. Gastrointestinal (GI) disturbances, i.e., nausea, diarrhea, abdominal pain, muscle spasm and weakness, sweating, lacrimation, salivation, hypotension, bradycardia, bronchial constriction and respiratory failure are systemic effects that have been experienced.[76, 79] Most systemic effects rapidly reverse after discontinuation of the drug. In severe cholinergic toxicity, atropine sulfate 2 mg or pralidoxime chloride 25 mg per kg intravenously or subcutaneously can be given without affecting the control of the glaucoma. Caution with the use of any potent long acting miotic agent should be exercised when a patient has bronchial asthma, parkinsonism, peptic ulcer of other GI disease or cardiac disease since anticholinesterase systemic effects can exacerbate their clinical course. There is evidence that echothiophate can traverse the placental barrier; therefore, its use should be dictated by considerations for the potential risks and benefits during pregnancy.[80]

When known sensitivities to these agents exist, they should not be used. Considerable inhibition of plasma cholinesterases can be produced by prolonged topical anticholinesterase therapy.[81,82] A patient who is receiving these agents must be monitored closely for prolongation of apnea when given succinylcholine chloride during surgery.[83,84]

Patients who may be exposed to insecticides containing organophosphates should be made aware of the potential problems and risks associated with prolonged topical anticholinesterase therapy: there is an additive and cumulative inhibitory effect on the cholinesterase enzyme potentiating parasympathetic nervous system effects.[78] Systemically administered cholinergic agents such as ambenonium, neostigmine and pyridostigmine used in disorders such as myasthenia gravis can potentiate the action of the anticholinesterase miotics.

The long acting, irreversible anticholinesterase miotics should be reserved for use in chronic primary noncongestive glaucomas and secondary glaucomas when the shorter acting miotics have not been successful in reducing intraocular tension. Undesirable side effects from these agents also can be minimized by instillation of their lowest effective concentrations at reasonable intervals.

Sympathomimetics

Reduction of intraocular tension in open angle glaucoma may be accomplished successfully by ocular instillation of sympathomimetic mydriatics. The mechanism of their action is not understood fully, but the main effects appear to be decreasing the rate of aqueous humor secretion and increasing its outflow.

Epinephrine, 1 to 2% solution instilled every 8 to 24 hr can reduce intraocular tension in open angle glaucoma. The rate of aqueous secretion initially is decreased probably through or by means of adrenergic stimulation at receptor sites in the ciliary epithelium. Improved facility of outflow is not immediate but may be seen after several months of epinephrine therapy. The probable mechanism suggested is beta-adrenergic response to epinephrine at the trabecular meshwork. The pressure lowering by epinephrine from 3 to 15 mm Hg is not great; maximal effect occurs in 6 to 8 hr. The duration of action varies from several hours to days. Patient response appears to be highly variable from individual to individual. Epinephrine is seldom used alone for open angle glaucoma but usually with miotics.[85, 86] Epinephrine does not disturb accommodation and is especially beneficial in overcoming the disabling miosis induced by the parasympathomimetics. When used in combination, it should be given 5 to 10 min after the miotic has been instilled. Comparative effects of epinephrine bitartrate 2% and epinephrine borate 1% have been studied and no statistical differences in ability to reduce intraocular tension in glaucomatous eyes can be found between individual preparations.[86] The commercial borate salt is buffered to enhance corneal penetration and is perhaps better tolerated than the others.[87]

Phenylephrine has not proven to be any more effective than epinephrine in lowering intraocular tension. A 10% solution of phenylephrine is less effective in lowering intraocular tension than a 2% solution of epinephrine. Phenylephrine is used primarily in assisting with ophthalmoscopic examination as it is without disturbing cycloplegic effects.[88] Guanethidine interferes with sympathetic transmission by interrupting normal release or synthesis of norepinephrine at sympathetic nerve endings.[89-91] Its major clinical use is as an antihypertensive agent. When 2, 5 and 10% solutions are instilled ocularly, the reduction in intraocular tension is relatively minor. The onset of effects occurs within an hour, and duration varies widely from 3 to 24 hr. Its action has been considered comparable to a 1% solution of pilocarpine. Propranolol is a beta-adrenergic blocker used in the management of angina and cardiac arrhythmias. It has been demonstrated that 20 mg given orally is able to reduce intraocular tension in open angle glaucoma quite effectively. However, in many cases, the dose had to be increased with time to maintain effective reduction of intraocular tension. The fall in systemic blood pressure and the potential for cardiac difficulties attendant with the use of propranolol make it very unlikely that widespread use is warranted.

Isoproterenol in 5% solutions produces effects comparable to those of epinephrine with maximal reduction of intraocular tension in 6 hours persisting for 12 to 60 hr. The widespread use of isoproterenol for ocular instillation is militated against by the common occurrence of systemic side effects such as tachycardia and palpitation.[92]

Appreciable local and systemic side effects are experienced by patients who use ocular sympathomimetics for long periods of time.[93, 94] Local side effects include melanin deposits on the conjunctiva and cornea, hyperemia and corneal edema and allergic blepharoconjunctivitis.[95-98] Headache, periorbital pain and lacrimation with intermittent visual blurring and distortion are common complaints. Although the incidence is relatively low, cardiac irregularities and elevations of blood pressure after ocular administration of epinephrine have been reported.[99] Side effects, both local and systemic, are relieved promptly after the epinephrine is discontinued. Close supervision and caution should be exercised for patients who are receiving anesthetics in preparation for surgery since the reported incidence of systemic side effects of the ocular sympathomimetics is higher in such cases. Sympathomimetics are contraindicated in angle closure glaucoma prior to peripheral iridectomy. Gonioscopic examinations must be advised before the ocular instillation of sympathomimetic mydriatics in order to rule out the existence of asymptomatic or subacute angle closure glaucoma. After the iridectomy is performed, ocular epinephrine can be useful, especially if aqueous humor outflow is impaired. It should not be used, however, if intraocular pressures can be managed adequately by miotics alone.

Carbonic Anhydrase Inhibitors

The lowering of intraocular tension can be achieved by systemic administration of carbonic anhydrase inhibitors (Table 34.7).[56, 100] These agents are of particular value where control of glaucoma is unobtainable with parasympathomimetic miotics. Carbonic anhydrase is a widely distributed enzyme in the body that catalyzes the reversible reaction of water and carbon dioxide to form carbonic acid and, subsequently, the bicarbonate ion.[101] In the eye, large concentrations of carbonic anhydrase are found in the ciliary process and retina. The mechanism of action of the carbonic anhydrase inhibitor on the intraocular tension is not understood clearly.[102] Acetazolamide has been found to increase the outflow of aqueous fluid in some glaucoma patients, while a decrease in outflow also has been reported to occur in normal eyes and in eyes with very early glaucoma. The lowering of the intraocular volume is not dependent upon its diuretic effect and can not be explained simply as a depletion of the bicarbonate ion content. It is probable that the

TABLE 34.7
Carbonic Anhydrase Inhibitors Used in the Management of Glaucoma

Drug	Dosage	Comment
Acetazolamide	125 mg to 1.0 g daily	Used in short term therapy for primary and secondary glaucoma especially if refractory or uncontrollable by miotics; used with miotics and hyperosmotics in emergency treatment of primary angle closure glaucoma; fair success with long term use in open angle glaucoma; failures frequently due to side effects; carbonic anhydrase inhibitor of choice in management of glaucoma
Methazolamide	100-130 mg daily	50 mg is equivalent to 250 mg of acetazolamide; little significant difference from acetazolamide with exception of side effects and slower onset of action; drowsiness, fatigue and malaise with minimal GI disturbance are common; main indication for chronic glaucoma insufficiently controlled by miotics or acetazolamide
Dichlorphenamide	100-300 mg daily	Metabolic acidosis occurs less frequently with dichlorphenamide than other carbonic anhydrase inhibitors; patient intolerant or refractory to acetazolamide (may not be to dichlorphenamide); anorexia, nausea, paresthesias, dizziness or ataxia and tremor should alert one to the possibility of toxicity
Ethoxozolamide	60-600 mg daily	125 mg is equivalent to 250 mg of acetazolamide; therapeutic effects achieved essentially the same with acetazolamides; side effects are similar; patients intolerant to acetazolamide may not be to ethoxozolamide

buffer system necessary for maintaining secretory functions in the ciliary epithelium is impaired or inhibited thus reducing aqueous formation. Only slight, if any, changes in intraocular tension are experienced in normal tensive eyes when carbonic anhydrase inhibitors are administered. There is no effect on the intraocular pressure when carbonic anhydrase inhibitors are instilled locally. These drugs are concomitantly employed with cholinergic miotics and hyperosmotic agents for the emergency treatment of primary angle closure glaucoma. The prompt and vigorous reduction of intraocular tension to normal levels prior to peripheral iridectomy is necessary for a better postoperative prognosis.

A single dose of oral or intravenous acetazolamide can maintain reduced intraocular tension for 4 to 6 hr. The maximal effect is seen in about 2 hr after oral administration. Following intravenous administration, the maximal effect is attained within 20 min. The rarely seen hypersecretion glaucoma can respond to treatment with carbonic anhydrase inhibitors alone. In chronic primary glaucoma where control has been difficult to obtain with miotics or during acute exacerbations, addition of a carbonic anhydrase inhibitor to cholinergic and sympathomimetic agents may produce satisfactory ocular tension control. Carbonic anhydrase inhibitors are useful in the short term management of glaucomas secondary to trauma or uveitis and in the preoperative management of congenital glaucoma. Their use in chronic angle closure glaucoma should be discouraged since symptoms of progressive angle narrowing can be obscured easily. The prognosis for a successful iridectomy may be compromised by the severity of involvement when surgical intervention is the remaining alternative.

Long term use of carbonic anhydrase inhibitors is frequently unsuccessful owing to their side effects. Patients differ in their ability to tolerate the various carbonic anhydrase inhibitors; however, the side effects produced are similar with variations in severity and intensity. The GI effects are a common cause of discomfort for the patient and often become so severe that their use is discontinued. Nausea, vomiting, intestinal colic, diarrhea and anorexia and paresthesis of the face and extremities are common side effects experienced. Transient myopia is an unusual and rare occurrence. Long term treatment with a carbonic anhydrase inhibitor does not appear to deplete intracellular potassium, although, when treatment with the agent is begun, there may be marked depletion of electrolytes, including potassium.[103] Careful monitoring of serum potassium levels and clinical manifestation of cellular potassium depletion should be undertaken.[104] However, the routine supplementation of potassium for glaucoma patients receiving carbonic anhydrase inhibitors is not encouraged and is of doubtful value in the absence of depletion.

Acetazolamide reportedly can produce a significant hyperglycemia in prediabetics and diabetics receiving oral hypoglycemic agents. Hyperuricemia has occurred following treatment with carbonic anhydrase inhibitors. Prolonged use of these drug inhibitors can lead to production of urinary and renal colic secondary to formation of calcium calculi.[105,106] Alkalinization of the urine by acetazolamide results in an enhanced renal tubular reabsorption of drugs such as quinidine, amphetamine and the tricyclic antidepressants which may magnify their desired and undesired effects. Alkalinization of the urine also can decrease significantly the acid-dependent and antibacterial activity of methenamine. Exfoliative dermatitis secondary to these agents is similar to those dermatological reactions encountered with the sulfonamides. Rare occurrences of idiosyncratic reactions such as cholestatic jaundice, drug fever, blood dyscrasias including thrombocytopenia, agranulocytosis and aplastic anemia have been reported. Carbonic anhydrase inhibitors should not be recommended for patients with hemorrhagic glaucoma, hepatic or renal or adrenocorticol hypofunction or a history of prior sensitivity to the drugs.

Hyperosmotic Agents

Hyperosmotic agents lower the intraocular pressure by creating an osmotic gradient between the plasma and the aqueous humor from the anterior chamber of the eye (Table 34.8).[107,108] Given systemically, these agents induce withdrawal of fluids from the anterior chamber of the eye to the plasma. Hyperosmotic agents are most useful in the preoperative management of primary acute angle closure glaucoma. The degree of intraocular pressure

TABLE 34.8

Hyperosmotic Agents Used in the Management of Glaucoma

Drug	Dosage	Comment
Mannitol	1.5-2 g/kg of body weight	Given intravenously; require larger volumes than other hyperosmotics; rapid diuresis produced; not metabolized; can be used in the diabetic; less irritating and free of tissue necrosis when solution extravasates; not contraindicated in patients with renal disease; monitor for cellular dehydration, hypokalemia, cardiac irregularities, urinary output and chest pain; more effective for glaucoma with inflammation than urea or glycerin; avoid excessive hydration or therapeutic effect diminishes
Urea	0.5-2.0 g/kg of body weight	Given intravenously over 30 min; unstable, sloughing, phlebitis, acute psychosis, severe headaches, nausea, vomiting, hemolysis and "rebound diuresis"; contraindicated in nephrotic patients; caution in hepatic impairment; use freshly made solutions only; maximal effect in 1 hr
Ascorbic acid	0.4-1.0 g/kg of body weight	Given intravenously or orally; gastric distress and diarrhea follow oral administration; seldom used since more effective agents are available
Glycerol	0.7-1.5 g/kg of body weight	Given orally; nausea, vomiting and hyperglycemia can occur; caution in diabetic patients; as effective as intravenous hyperosmotic agents; less diuresis produced
Isosorbid	1-2 g/kg of body weight	Investigational; given orally; can be given to diabetic; effects on intraocular tension comparable to intravenous hyperosmotics; diarrhea, nausea and vomiting less frequently experienced
Ethyl alcohol	0.8-1.5 g/kg of body weight	Given orally; pressure reduction slower than other hyperosmotics; can produce nausea, vomiting, central nervous systems effects and potential drug-drug interactions; rarely used since more effective agents are available[a]

[a]Reprinted with premission from Ref. 131.

lowering depends upon the tension elevation and the osmotic gradient induced. The greatest effect of rapid changes in plasma osmolarity is on the eye with very profound pressure elevations. The hyperosmotics used most commonly are mannitol, urea and glycerol.[109]

Mannitol can effectively reduce acutely elevated intraocular pressures if given slowly by the intravenous route to adults in a 20% solution and a 10% solution to children.[110-116] The ocular hypotensive effect is produced in 30 to 60 min and lasts from 4 to 6 hr. The degree of effectiveness of the hyperosmotic agents depends upon rate of administration and amount absorbed. Some are metabolized and others are excreted unchanged. Mannitol is not metabolized; therefore it is a suitable preparation for the diabetic who requires rapid reduction of intraocular tension. Mannitol is preferred in the management of secondary glaucomas accompanied by hyperemia or uveitis since it penetrates the eye less readily, which is particularly advantageous where inflammatory processes are active. Agents which enter the eye rapidly produce a less osmotic gradient and shorter duration of action than those which do so slowly or not at all. Inflammation greatly increases the ocular permeability of agents such as urea; therefore, it is less desirable under those circumstances. There is relatively less local tissue irritation, thrombophlebitis and necrosis occurring with mannitol than urea when either is given intravenously. Renal disease does not contraindicate the use of mannitol.

Excessive thirst is a common sensation experienced by patients following infusion of hyperosmotic agents. However, these patients should not be given fluids during the period of osmotic dehydration. Secondary rises in intraocular tension will occur following administration of fluids, diminishing the therapeutic effects of the hyperosmotics. Headache is also a common occurrence but can be minimized simply by bed rest. Monitoring for symptoms of cellular dehydration, hypokalemia and cardiac irregularities secondary to mannitol therapy should be carried out. Since mannitol is not absorbed orally, it is not effective when given by that route. On rare occasions, disorientation and severe agitation may be observed. Pulmonary edema and congestive heart failure may be precipitated in the elderly, especially with mannitol infusions. Potassium deficiency is a complication which can accompany diuresis following hyperosmotic infusion; cautious monitoring of cardiac patients or patients with hepatic or renal disorders should be routinely maintained.

Urea given by the intravenous route as a 30% solution will reduce elevated intraocular tension within 30 to 40 min.[117-119] Miotics and carbonic anhydrase inhibitors are used concomitantly with urea in the management of acute glaucoma prior to surgery. Nausea, vomiting, confusion, disorientation and anxiety are seen. Severe headache is a common complaint, and it can begin soon after initiation and last for the duration of the intravenous infusion. The patient's head should not be elevated during this time.

Although urea produces less cellular dehydration because of its ease of penetrability into the cell, a "rebound phenomenon" can occur as the plasma level of the hyperosmotic agent drops below that of the vitreous fluid. As the urea is cleared from the circulation rapidly with diuresis, the osmolality of the blood will decline. The hyperosmotic vitreous in turn induces the entrance of fluid into the eye resulting in an increased intraocular tension or pressure "rebound" effect.

Ascorbic acid has been shown to reduce successfully intraocular tension in glaucoma patients.[120,121] It has been claimed that in cases of refractoriness to acetazolamide and miotics, ascorbic acid given intravenously was able to lower the ocular hypertension. A 20% solution of sodium ascorbate at a pH of 7.2 to 7.4 can produce normal ocular tensions in 60 to 90 min.

Oral hyperosmotic agents will effectively reduce elevated intraocular tension and are useful where the rapid action-infused preparations are not required. Glycerol is a convenient hyperosmotic agent when given as a 50 or 75% solution. The ocular penetration of glycerol is poor; therefore, a substantial osmotic gradient can be produced between the plasma and aqueous humor. Intraocular tension reduction is considered as effective as hyperosmotic agents given by intravenous infusion. Intraocular pressures normally return to pretreatment levels within 5 to 6 hr. Hyperglycemia and glycosuria can occur following glycerol and should be used with particular caution in labile diabetics. There have been reports of acute diabetic acidosis, ketosis being experienced following treatment with glycerol.[122] Nausea, diarrhea and headache are also common complaints following oral glycerol.[113,114,123-126]

The reduction of intraocular pressure with isosorbide is comparable to that of intravenous mannitol or urea or oral glycerol. Given as a 50% solution orally, its absorption is rapid and primarily unchanged upon excretion in the urine. Effective reduction in intraocular pressure occurs within 30 min following ingestion and remains for 1 to 2 or more hr depending on dosage. Side effects include transient headaches and diarrhea. Other GI disturbances such as nausea are usually less of a problem with isosorbide than glycerol.[127-130]

MEDICAL MANAGEMENT

Conservative medical management can control successfully the majority of cases of chronic open angle glaucoma. Consideration for the stage or severity of the disease as evidenced by the condition of the optic disk and quality of the visual field should be the major influence in the choice of treatment implemented. Mild elevations of intraocular tension (less than 30 mm Hg) in the presence of a normal optic disk and visual field are not an absolute indication for therapy. The patients with this condition should have routine, periodic follow-ups in order to detect any optic disk changes which may occur since such changes can be detected long before permanent visual field impairment will be experienced. There is no absolute level of intraocular tension that must be maintained in order to be assured of therapeutic success. The intraocular tension should be maintained at the level where further deterioration of the optic disk and impairment of visual field are prevented. If the disk on gonioscopic examination is normal, intraocular tension in the high 20's is not as clinically significant as one with concurrent disk involvement or abnormal visual field. The former situation may warrant only close periodic following, while in the latter, appropriate medical treatment should deserve immediate consideration. If there is the slightest indication of disk pathology, the intraocular tension should be preferably maintained at 20 mm Hg or even lower by medical management. In cases of considerable disk degeneration and visual field loss, vigorous treatment should be undertaken to attain a level of 15 mm Hg or lower.

In situations where advanced cupping of the optic disk and visual loss are not apparent in the presence of high intraocular tension (greater than 30 mm Hg), medical therapy should be considered a priority. The aim of therapy is to lower the intraocular tension adequately to interrupt the course of the disease. One always should keep in mind problems common to antiglaucoma therapy before proceeding to reduce intraocular tension with drugs. The expense and inconvenience of the medication used should be considered as well as whether the side effects and toxicities secondary to the drugs constitute greater risk to the patient than even the level of intraocular tension measured.

For primary open angle glaucoma, a miotic agent should be given at its lowest effective concentration and at intervals no more frequent than necessary to maintain a satisfactory level of intraocular tension. Generally, pilocarpine 1% or its equivalent is tried first. The intraocular tension should be measured prior to beginning therapy. The effects of therapy on the intraocular pressure can be determined within a week or so. If the reduction of intraocular tension is not satisfactory, the concentration of the miotic agent should be increased, keeping in mind, however, that there is little advantage in using concentrations of pilocarpine solutions greater than 4% or its equivalent.

Refractoriness, following prolonged use of cholinergic miotics, often occurs. Rather than increasing the frequency of instillation or strength used, the selection of an alternative agent should be considered. Responsiveness to the cholinergic miotics often is restored following their replacement for a brief period of time by an anticholinesterase miotic. Various combinations of glaucoma medications often are given together with the intention of potentiating their therapeutic effects. Not all combinations, however, produce an additive pharmacological response. Enhancement of intraocular tension-lowering effect following concomitant instillation of pilocarpine with physostigmine or isoflurophate has not been unequivocally demonstrated.[55]

Epinephrine or phenylephrine may be added to miotic therapy provided that gonioscopic examination has failed to demonstrate excessive narrowing of the anterior chamber angle if intraocular tension control is inadequate.[130] There is evidence suggesting that greater activity is produced when pilocarpine and epinephrine are applied separately rather than in combination.[132,133] Combinations of anticholinesterase miotics can reduce rather than potentiate the effectiveness of each other. Prior instillation of physostigmine or demecarium will reduce the activity of subsequently instilled echothiophate or isoflurophate by a competitive inhibition of the acetylcholinesterase. Pretreatment with either echothiophate or isoflurophate will enhance only slightly the activity of physostigmine or demecarium. However, the action of physostigmine and demecarium is additive rather than competitive regardless of their order of instillation. Differences in the duration of action and type of cholinesterase-inhibiting activity inherent with each miotic given in combination contribute to these predictable responses. Concomitant instillation of miotics, particularly those that act indirectly, offer very few advantages and should not be encouraged in attempts to treat difficult to control open angle glaucoma. Addition of an agent from another class of antiglaucoma drugs is preferred to substitution or addition of an agent from the same group. Deterioration of the glaucomatous condition should always be ruled out. The pharmacist should inquire into the medication's storage condition, expiration date and method of administration when a patient experiences diminished effects from the eye drops. The patient's physician should then be made aware of the situation and consulted on whether increasing the frequency of instillation or strength of the patient's medication or substituting with another agent would be appropriate.

Surgical management of open angle glaucoma should be reserved for situations in which maximal efforts utilizing miotics, sympathomimetics and carbonic anhydrase inhibitors have been unsuccessful in maintaining an acceptable level of intraocular tension and preventing exacerbation of the disease. An acute angle closure glaucoma attack must receive prompt and intensive attention in order to avoid irreparable damage to the eye. Pilocarpine 1 to 4% or an equivalent cholinergic miotic is instilled into the affected eye at frequent intervals until the intraocular tension is reduced to levels at which surgery can be performed. Cholinesterase-inhibiting miotics should be avoided. Concurrent administration of intravenous or oral carbonic anhydrase inhibitors or hyperosmotic agents to an acutely dilated pupil not responsive to the miotic agent may be required. Control of an attack should be established within 1 to 2 hr following the initiation of this intensive treatment. Experience has suggested that the incidence of subsequent involvement in the unaffected eye is significantly reduced when pilocarpine is given as a prophylactic measure.[1][3][4] Instillation of pilocarpine at normal intervals into the unaffected eye following an episode of acute angle closure glaucoma is considered appropriate. Treatment of secondary glaucomas should be directed at the underlying and contributory factors. Medical treatment of congenital glaucoma may lower intraocular tension levels, but this disorder can be corrected successfully only by surgery.

CONCLUSION

The successful outcome of treatment in glaucoma is greatly dependent upon the patient's proper use of his medications. Pharmacists frequently encounter patients who fail to adhere to instructions regarding the use of their medications. It is not unreasonable to suspect that an asymptomatic patient who does not understand why he must continue to use expensive and inconvenient to administer eyedrops will be less inclined to use them according to prescribed instructions. The blurring of vision and occasional discomfort associated with the use of these medications further enhance the likelihood of noncompliance. As a consequence, visual function is often irreversibly impaired and therapeutic intervention no longer influences the clinical course of the disease. It is vital that the glaucoma patient be given an understanding of the nature of his disorder and appropriate expectations of the therapeutic measures being employed against it. A pharmacist can make significant contributions to reducing the incidences of therapeutic failures by virtue of his accessibility to the glaucoma patient. Conscientious monitoring of patient adherence to a prescribed therapeutic regimen, increasing the patient's awareness of the nature of glaucoma and participating with the patient's physician in evaluating the effectiveness of therapy should be responsibilities of a pharmacist. Success at this formidable task can be achieved only if the pharmacist understands the nature of the disease and is aware of the capabilities and limitations of available therapeutic approaches.

REFERENCES

1. Duke-Elder, S., and Jay, B.: Simple glaucoma. In Systems of Ophthalmology: Diseases of the Lens and Vitreous Glaucoma and Hypotony, Vol 11, p. 392. C.V. Mosby Co., St. Louis, 1969.
2. Vaughan, D., Asbury, T., and Book, R.: Glaucoma. In General Ophthalmology, Ed. 6, p. 193. Lange Medical Publications, Los Altos, Calif., 1971.
3. Spaeth, G. L.: General medications, glaucoma and disturbances of intraocular pressure. Med. Clin. North Am., 53: 1109, 1969.
4. Kitazawa, Y.: Primary angle-closure glaucoma. Arch. Ophthalmol., 84: 724, 1970.
5. Grant, W. M.: Ocular complications of drugs—glaucoma. J.A.M.A., 2071: 2089, 1969.
6. Harris, L. S.: Cycloplegic-induced intraocular pressure elevations. Arch Ophthalmol., 79: 242, 1968.
7. Leopold, I. H., and Comroe, J. H., Jr.: Effect of

intramuscular administration of morphine, atropine, scopolamine and neostigmine on the human eye. Arch. Ophthalmol., 40: 285, 1948.

8. Mehra, K. S., Chandra, P., and Khare, B. B.: Ocular manifestations of parenteral administration of scopolamine (hyoscine). Br. J. Ophthalmol., 49: 557, 1965.

9. Schwartz, H., De Roetth, A., and Papper, E. M.: Preanesthetic use of atropine and scopolamine in patients with glaucoma. J.A.M.A., 165: 144, 1957.

10. Ullman, E. V., and Mossman, F. D.: Glaucoma and orally administered belladonna. Am. J. Ophthalmol., 33: 757, 1950.

11. Hiatt, R. L., Fuller, I. B., Smith, L., Swartz, J., and Risser, C.: Systemically administered anticholinergic drugs and intraocular pressure. Arch. Ophthalmol., 84: 735, 1970.

12. Cholst, M., Goodstein, S., Berenes, C., and Cinotti, A.: Glaucoma in medical practice. J.A.M.A., 166: 1276, 1958.

13. Lowe, R. F.: Amitriptyline and glaucoma. Med. J. Aust., 2: 509, 1966.

14. Marcotta, D.: Use of a new antispasmodic in glaucomatous patients. Rocky Mt. Med. J., 63: 66, 1966.

15. Gorin, G.: Angle-closure glaucoma induced by miotics. Am. J. Ophthalmol., 62: 1063, 1966.

16. Bryant, J. A.: Effects of systemic drugs on intraocular pressure. Hosp. Form. Mgmt., 4: 15, 1969.

17. Lazenby, G. W., Reed, J. W., and Grant, W. M.: Short-term tests of anticholinergic medication in open-angle glaucoma. Arch. Ophthalmol, 80: 443, 1968.

18. Lazenby, G. W., Reed, J. W., and Grant, W. M.: Anticholinergic medications in open-angle glaucoma. Arch. Ophthalmol., 84: 719, 1970.

19. Roberts, W.: Rapid progression of cupping in glaucoma. Am. J. Ophthalmol, 66: 520, 1968.

20. Grant, W. M.: Systemic drugs and adverse influence on ocular pressure. In Symposium on Ocular Therapy, Vol. 3, Ed. 1, p. 57, edited by I. H. Leopold. C. V. Mosby Co., St. Louis, 1968.

21. Ballin, N,, Becker, B., and Goldman, M. L.: Systemic effects of epinephrine applied topically to the eye. Invest. Ophthalmol, 5: 125, 1966.

22. Becker, B., Cage, T., Kolker, A. E., and Gay, A. J.: The effect of phenylephrine hydrochloride on the miotic-treated eye. Am. J. Ophthalmol, 48: 313, 1959.

23. Armaly, M. F.: Inheritance of dexamethasone hypertension and glaucoma. Arch. Ophthalmol, 77: 747, 1967.

24. Armaly, M. F.: Effect of corticosteroids on intraocular pressure and fluid dynamics. I. The effect of dexamethasone in the normal eye. Arch. Ophthalmol, 70: 482, 1963.

25. Armaly, M. F.: Effect of corticosteroids on intraocular pressure and fluid dynamics. II. The effect of dexamethasone in the glaucomatous eye. Arch. Ophthalmol, 70: 492, 1963.

26. Becker, B., and Mills, D. W.: Corticosteroids and intraocular pressure. Arch. Ophthalmol, 70: 500, 1963.

27. Becker, B., and Mills, D. M.: Intraocular pressure after topical corticosteroids. J.A.M.A., 185: 884, 1963.

28. Becker, B., and Hahn, K. A.: Topical corticosteroids and heredity in primary open-angle glaucoma. Am. J. Ophthalmol, 57: 543, 1964.

29. Becker, B., and Chevrette, L.: Topical corticosteroid testing in glaucoma siblings. Arch. Ophthalmol, 76: 484, 1966.

30. Bernstein, H. N., and Schwartz, B.: Effects of long-term systemic steroids on ocular pressure and tonographic values. Arch. Ophthalmol, 68: 742, 1962.

31. Bernstein, H. N., Mills, D. W., and Becker, B.: Steroid-induced elevation of intraocular pressure. Arch. Ophthalmol, 70: 15, 1963.

32. Burde, R. M., and Becker, B.: Steroid-induced glaucoma and cataracts in contact lens wearers. J.A.M.A., 213: 2075, 1970.

33. Diotallevi, M., and Bocci, M.: Effect of systemically administered corticosteroids on intraocular pressure and fluid dynamics. Acta Ophthalmol, 43: 524, 1965.

34. Goldmann, H.: Cortisone glaucoma. Arch. Ophthalmol, 68: 621, 1962.

35. Kolker, A. E., Becker, B., and Mills, D. W.: Topical corticosteroids in secondary glaucoma. Arch. Ophthalmol, 72: 772, 1964.

36. Nicholas, J. P.: Topical corticosteroids and aqueous humor dynamics. Arch. Ophthalmol, 72: 189, 1964.

37. Romano, J.: Anterior chamber depth in medically-treated open-angle glaucoma. Br. J. Ophthalmol, 52: 361, 1968.

38. Smith, C. L.: Corticosteroid glaucoma—a summary and review of the literature. Am. J. Med. Sci., 252: 239, 1966.

39. Spiers, F.: A case of irreversible steroid-induced rise in intraocular pressure. Acta Ophthalmol, 13: 419, 1965.

40. Whiteworth, C. G., and Grant, W. M.: Use of nitrate and nitrate vasodilators by glaucomatous patients. Arch. Ophthalmol, 71: 492, 1964.

41. Peczon, J. D., and Grant, W. M.: Sedatives, stimulants, and intraocular pressure in glaucoma. Arch Ophthalmol, 72: 188, 1964.

42. Willetts, G. S.: Ocular side-effects of drugs. Br. J. Ophthalmol, 53: 252, 1969.

43. Drance, S. M.: The effects of phospholine iodide on the lens and anterior chamber depth. The Symposium on Ocular Therapy, Vol. 4, Ed. 1, p. 25, edited by I. H. Leopold. C. V. Mosby Co., St. Louis, 2969.

44. Zeckman, T. H., and Syndacker, D.: Increase intraocular pressure produced by di-isopro-

pyl fluorophosphate (DEP). Am. J. Ophthalmol, 36: 1709, 1953.

45. Lincoff, H. A., Ellis, E. H., De Voe, G. A., DeBeer, E. J., Impastato, D. J. Berg, S., Orkin, L., and Magda, H.: The effect of succinylcholine on intraocular pressure. Am. J. Ophthalmol, 40: 501, 1955.

46. Maddalena, M. A.: Transient myopia associated with acute glaucoma and retinal edema following vaginal administration of sulfanilamide. Arch. Ophthalmol, 80: 186, 1968.

47. Beasley, F. J.: Transient myopia and retinal edema during ethoxzalamide (Cardrase) therapy. Arch. Ophthalmol, 68: 490, 1962.

48. Galin, M. A., Baras, I., and Zweifach, P.: Diamox-induced myopia. Am. J. Ophthalmol, 54: 237, 1962.

49. Halpren, A., and Kulvin, M. M.: Transient myopia: during treatment with carbonic anhydrase inhibitors. Am. J. Ophthalmol, 48: 534, 1959.

50. Edwards, T. S.: Transient myopia due to tetracycline. J.A.M.A., 186: 69, 1963.

51. Bard, L. A.: Transient myopia associated with promethazine therapy. Am. J. Ophthalmol, 58: 682, 1964.

52. Jocson, V. L.: Tonograph and gonioscopy—before and after cataract extraction with alpha chymotrypsin. Am. J. Ophthalmol, 60: 318, 1965.

53. Scheie, H. G., Edwards, D. L., and Yanoff, M. C.: Clinical and experimental observations using alpha chymotrypsin. Am. J. Ophthalmol, 59: 469, 1965.

54. Havener, W. F.: Alpha-chymotrypsin. In Ocular Pharmacology, Vol. 1, Ed. 2, p. 32, edited by W. F. Havner. C. V. Mosby Co., St. Louis, 1970.

55. Ellis, P. P.: Carbonic anhydrase inhibitors: pharmacologic effects and problems of long-term therapy. In Symposium on Ocular Therapy, Vol. 4, Ed. 1, p. 32, edited by I.H. Leopold. C.V. Mosby Co., St. Louis, 1969.

56. Ellis, P. P.: Carbonic anhydrase inhibitors: pharmacologic effects and problems of long-term therapy. In Symposium on Ocular Therapy, Vol. 4, Ed. 1, p. 32, edited by I.H. Leopold. C.V. Mosby Co., St. Louis, 1969.

57. Peczon, J. D., and Grant, W. M.: Diuretic drugs in glaucoma. Am. J. Ophthalmol, 65: 680, 1968.

58. Atchoo, P. D., and Vogel, H. P.: Phospholine iodide (0.03%) in the therapy of glaucoma. Am. J. Ophthalmol, 62: 1044, 1966.

59. Klayman, J., and Taffet, S.: Low-concentration phospholine iodide therapy in open-angle glaucoma. Am. J. Ophthalmol, 55: 1233, 1963.

60. Drance, S. M.: Comparison of action of cholinergic and anticholinesterase agents in glaucoma. Invest. Ophthalmol, 5: 130, 1966.

61. Fenton, R. H., and Schwartz, B.: The effect of two percent pilocarpine on the normal and glaucomatous eye. I. The time response of pressure. Invest. Ophthalmol, 2: 289, 1963.

62. Flindall, R. J., and Drance, S. M.: Dose response of intraocular pressures of single installations of carbaminoylocholine chloride. Can. J. Ophthalmol, 1: 292, 1966.

63. Leopold, I. H.: Ocular cholinesterase and cholinesterase inhibitors: the Friedenwald memorial lecture. Am. J. Ophthalmol, 51: 885, 1961.

64. Kellerman, L., and King, A. D.: Echothiophate iodide in glaucoma. Am. J. Ophthalmol, 62: 278, 1966.

65. Wahl, J. W., and Tyner, G. A.: Echothiophate iodide. Am. J. Ophthalmol, 60: 419, 1965.

66. Harris, L. S.: Dose response analysis of echothiophate iodide. Arch. Ophthalmol, 86: 502, 1971.

67. Chin, N. B., Gold, A. A., and Breinin, G. M.: Iris cysts and miotics. Arch. Ophthalmol, 71: 611, 1964.

68. Axelsson, U., and Holmberg, A.: The frequency of cataract after miotic therapy. Acta Ophthalmol, 44: 421, 1966.

69. De Roetth, A., Jr.: Lens opacities in glaucoma patients on phospholine iodide therapy. Am. J. Ophthalmol, 62: 619, 1966.

70. Drance, S. M.: The effects of phospholine iodide on the lens and anterior chamber depth. In Symposium on Ocular Therapy, Vol. 4, Ed. 1, p. 25, edited by I. H. Leopold. C. V. Mosby Co., St. Louis, 1969.

71. Harrison, R.: Bilateral lens opacities associated with use of di-isopropylflurophosphate eye drops. Am. J. Ophthalmol, 50: 153, 1960.

72. Levene, R. Z.: Echothiophate iodide and lens changes. In Symposium on Ocular Therapy, Vol. 4, Ed. 1, p. 45, edited by I.H. Leopold. C.V. Mosby Co., St. Louis, 1969.

73. Scheie, H., and Day, R. M.: Simulated progression of visual field defects of glaucoma. Arch. Ophthalmol, 50: 418, 1953.

74. Shaffer, R. N., and Hetherington, J.: Anticholinesterase and cataracts. Am. J. Ophthalmol, 62: 613, 1966.

75. Ellis, P. P.: Systemic effects of locally applied anticholinesterase agents. Invest. Ophthalmol, 5: 146, 1966.

76. Humphreys, J. A., and Holmes, J. H.: Systemic effects of echothiophate iodide in treatment of glaucoma. Arch. Ophthalmol, 69: 737, 1963.

77. Leopold, I. H.: Cholinesterases and the effects and side effects of drugs affecting cholinergic systemic. Am. J. Ophthalmol, 62: 771, 1966.

78. Quinby, G. E.: Further therapeutic experiences with pralidoximes in organic phosphorus poisoning. J.A.M.A., 187: 202, 1964.

79. Hiscox, P. E. A., and McCulloch, C.: Cardiac arrest occurring in a patient on echothiophate iodide therapy. Am. J. Ophthalmol, 60: 425, 1965.

80. Birks, D. A., Prior, V. J., and Silk, E.: Echothiophate iodide treatment of glau-

coma in pregnancy. Arch. Ophthalmol, 79: 283, 1968.

81. De Roetth, A., Jr., Wong, A., Wolf-Dietrich, D., Rosenberg, P., and Wilensky, J. S.: Blood cholinesterase activity of glaucoma patients treated with phospholine iodide. Am. J. Ophthalmol, 62: 834, 1966.

82. Eilderton, T. E., Farmati, O., and Zsigmond, E. K.: Reduction in plasma cholinesterase levels after prolonged administration of echothiophate iodide eyedrops. Can. Anaesth. Soc. J., 15: 291, 1968.

83. Gesztes, T.: Prolonged apnea after suxamethonium injection associated with eyedrops containing an anticholinesterase agent. Br. J. Anesth., 38: 408, 1966.

84. Pantuck, E. J.: Echothiophate iodide eyedrops and prolonged response suxamethonium. Br. J. Anaesth., 38: 406, 1966.

85. Becker, B. Petitt, T. H., and Gay, A. J.: Topical epinephrine therapy in open-angle glaucoma. Arch. Ophthalmol, 66: 219, 1961.

86. Briswick, V. G., and Drance, S. M.: Epinephrine salts and intraocular pressure. Arch. Ophthalmol, 75: 768, 1966.

87. Vaughan, G., Shaffer, R., and Riegelman, S.: A new stabilized form of epinephrine for treatment of open-angle glaucoma. Arch. Ophthalmol, 66: 232, 1961.

88. Becker, B., Gage, T., Kolker, A. E., and Gay, A. J.: The effect of phenylephrine hydrochloride on the miotic-treated eye. Am. J. Ophthalmol, 48: 313, 1959.

89. Bonomi, L., and DiComite, P.: Effect of guanethidine and other sympatholytic drugs. Am. J. Ophthalmol, 61: 544, 1965.

90. Bonomi, L., and DiComite, P.: Outflow facility after guanethidine sulfate. Arch. Ophthalmol, 78: 337, 1967.

91. Sneddon, J. M., and Turner, P.: The interactions of local guanethidine and sympathomimetic amines in the human eye. Arch. Ophthalmol, 81: 622, 1969.

92. Ross, R. A., and Drance, S. M.: Effects of topically applied isoproterenol on aqueous dynamics in man. Arch. Ophthalmol, 83: 39, 1970.

93. Aronson, S. B., and Yamamoto, E. A.: Ocular hypersensitivity to epinephrine. Invest. Ophthalmol, 5: 75, 1966.

94. Ballin, N., Becker, B., and Goldman, M. L.: Systemic effects of epinephrine applied topically to the eye. Invest. Ophthalmol, 5: 125, 1966.

95. Corwin, M. E., and Spencer, W. H.: Conjunctival melanin depositions—side effects of topical epinephrine therapy. Arch. Ophthalmol, 69: 317, 1963.

96. Donaldson, D, D.: Epinephrine pigmentation of the cornea. Arch. Ophthalmol, 78: 74, 1966.

97. Mooney, D.: Pigmentation after long-term topical usage of adrenaline compounds. Br. J. Ophthalmol, 54: 823, 1970.

98. Reinecke, R. E., and Kuwabara, T.: Corneal deposits secondary to topical epinephrine. Arch. Ophthalmol, 70: 170, 1963.

99. Lansche, R. K.: Reaction to epinephrine and phenylephrine. Am. J. Ophthalmol, 61: 95, 1966.

100. Gallin, M. A., and Harris, L. S.: Acetazolamide and outflow facility. Arch. Ophthalmol, 76: 493, 1966.

101. Maren, T. H.: Carbonic anhydrase: chemistry, physiology and inhibition. Physiol. Rev., 47: 595, 1967.

102. Thomas, R. P., and Riley, M. W.: Acetazolamide and ocular tension: notes concerning the mechanism of action. Am. J. Ophthalmol, 60: 241, 1965.

103. Draeger, J., Gtuttner, R., and Theilmann, W.: Avoidance of side-reactions and loss of drug efficacy during long-term administration of carbonic anhydrase inhibitors by concomitant supplement electrolyte administration. Br. J. Ophthalmol, 47: 457, 1963.

104. Spaeth, G. L.: Potassium, acetazolamide, and intraocular pressure. Arch. Ophthalmol, 78: 578, 1967.

105. Parfitt, A. M.: Acetazolamide and sodium bicarbonate induced nephrocalcinosis and nephrolithiasis. Arch. Intern. Med., 124: 736, 1969.

106. Peyes, M. B.: Acetazolamide and renal stone formation. Lancet, 1: 837, 1970.

107. Becker, B., Kolker, A. E., and Krupin, T.: Hyperosmotic agents. In Symposium on Ocular Therapy, Vol. 3, Ed. 1, p. 42, edited by I. H. Leopold. C. V. Mosby Co., St. Louis, 1968.

108. Galin, M. A., Davidson, R., and Schachter, N.: Ophthalmological use of osmotic therapy. Am. J. Ophthalmol, 62: 629, 1966.

109. Kronfeld, P. C.: The efficacy of combinations of ocular hypotensive drugs. Arch. Ophthalmol, 78: 140, 1967.

110. Adams, R. E., Kirschner, R. J., and Leopold, I. H.: Ocular hypotensive effect of intravenously administered mannitol. Arch. Ophthalmol, 69: 55, 1963.

111. Smith, E. W., and Drance, S. M.: Reduction of human intraocular pressure with intravenous mannitol. Arch. Ophthalmol, 68: 734, 1962.

112. Spaeth, E. W., Spaeth, E. B., Spaeth, P. G., and Lucier, A. C.: Anaphylactic reaction to mannitol. Arch. Ophthalmol, 78: 583, 1967.

113. Thomas, R. P.: Glycerin. Arch. Ophthalmol, 625, 1963.

114. Virno, M., Cantore, P., Bietti, C., and Bucci, M. G.: Oral glycerol in ophthalmology—a valuable new method for the reduction of intraocular pressure. Am. J. Ophthalmol, 55: 1133, 1963.

115. Weiss, D. I., Shaffer, R. N., and Wise, B. L.: Mannitol infusion to reduce intraocular pressure. Arch. Ophthalmol, 68: 341, 1962.

116. Weiss, D. I., Shaffer, R. N., and Harrington, D. D.: Treatment of malignant glaucoma with intravenous mannitol infusion. Arch. Ophthalmol., 69: 154, 1963.

117. Davis, M., Duehr, P., and Javid, M.: The clinical use of urea for reduction of intraocular pressure. Arch. Ophthalmol., 65: 526, 1961.

118. Galin, M. A., Aizawa, F., and McLean, J. M.: Urea as an osmotic ocular hypotensive agent in glaucoma. Arch. Ophthalmol., 62: 347, 1959.

119. Hill, K., Whitney, J., and Trotter, R.: Intravenous hypertonic urea in the management of acute angle-closure glaucoma. Arch. Ophthalmol., 65: 497, 1961.

120. Linner, E.: Intraocular pressure regulation and ascorbic acid. Acta Soc. Med. Uspal., 69: 225, 1966.

121. Suzuki, Y.,: Studies on the effect of ascorbic acid on the intraocular pressure of rabbits. Acta Ophthalmol., 75: 201, 1966.

122. D'Alena, P., and Ferguson, W.: Adverse effects after glycerol orally and mannitol parenterally. Arch. Ophthalmol., 75: 201, 1966.

123. Casey, T. A.: Oral glycerol in glaucoma. Br. Med. J., 2: 851, 1963.

124. Consul, B. N., and Kulshrestha, O. P.: Oral glycerol in glaucoma. Am. J. Ophthalmol., 60: 900, 1965.

125. Drance, S. M.: Effect of oral glycerol on intraocular pressure in normal and glaucomatous eyes. Arch. Ophthalmol., 72: 491, 1964.

126. McCurdy, D. K., Schneider, B., and Scheic, H. G.: Oral glycerol: the mechanism of intraocular hypotension. Am. J. Ophthalmol., 61: 1244, 1966.

127. Barry, K. G., Khoury, A. H., and Brooks, M. H.: Mannitol and isosorbide. Arch. Ophthalmol., 81: 695, 1969.

128. Becker, B., Kolker, A. E., and Krupin, T.: Isosorbide: an oral hyperosmotic agent. Arch. Ophthalmol., 78: 147, 1967.

129. Krupin, T., Kolker, A. E., and Becker, B.: A comparison of isosorbide and glycerol for cataract surgery. Am. J. Ophthalmol., 69: 373, 1970.

130. Becker, B., and Morton, R. W.: Topical epinephrine in glaucoma suspects. Am. J. Ophthalmol., 62: 272, 1966.

131. Peczon, J. D., and Grant, W. M.: Glaucoms, alcohol, and intraocular pressure. Arch. Ophthalmol., 73: 495, 1965.

132. Becker, B.: Round table discussion from fifteenth annual session of the New Orleans Academy of Ophthalmology. In Symposium on Glaucoma. Transaction of the New Orleans Academy of Ophthalmology, Vol. 1, Ed. 1, p. 239, edited by M.F. Armaly. C.V. Mosby Co., St. Louis, 1967.

133. Swan, K. C.: Problems in the use of combinations of drugs in ophthalmology. In Ocular Therapy-Complications and Management, Vol. 2, Ed. 1, p. 29, edited by I. H. Leopold. C. V. Mosby Co., St. Louis, 1967.

134. Winter, F. G.: The second eye in acute primary shallow-chamber angle glaucoma. Am. J. Ophthalmol., 40: 557, 1955.

Skin diseases

chapter 35

ACNE VULGARIS

C. A. Bond, Pharm. D.

Acne is a self-limiting disease primarily affecting adolescents. Ninety percent of all teenagers are affected to varying degrees of severity. The lesions will usually clear during the early twenties but occasionally may persist for many years into adulthood. The primary lesion involves an inflammation of the pilosebaceous follicles resulting in a variety of lesions. Among these are comedones, cysts, papules, pustules and nodules. Acne is almost exclusively limited to the seborrheic or oily areas of the skin. These areas include the face, ears, neck, upper back and occasionally the upper arms. The disease is not life-threatening by any means but can lead to a great deal of emotional distress. Unfortunately, acne affects adolescents at a period when they are undergoing tremendous growing stress and, as a consequence, the disease can have profound social and psychological effects on these patients which may permanently affect their personality.

ETIOLOGY

The exact cause of acne is not well understood. Hereditary and environmental factors play a role in determining susceptibility; and it is well documented that androgens seem to trigger the onset of the disease at adolescence.[1,2] In males, androgen levels are higher than in females and, as one might expect, males have a slightly higher incidence of the disease and generally have a more severe form. The exact source of the female androgenic substance is unknown. Current theories suggest this female androgenic substance may be evolved by ovarian tissue or possibly the adrenal glands.[3,4] Also, it is believed by some that progesterone may be metabolically converted in the body to an androgenic substance. Androgens increase sebaceous gland activity and thus increase sebum production. This increased sebum production has been shown experimentally, and this is one of the reasons acne occurs most often during puberty.

The highest incidence of acne occurs between the ages of 14 and 20, but the disease can be found from the neonatal period all the way up to the 7th or 8th decades of life. When acne is found during periods of life where it normally does not occur or when there is a sudden appearance of symptoms, endocrine abnormalities or the possibility of drug-induced acne must be considered. When acne is drug-induced, the lesions are identical to common acne lesions except there usually is an absence of comedones. Also, pre-existing acne may be made worse by certain drugs. Drugs that have been reported to induce acneform eruptions may be found in Table 35.1.[5]

PATHOGENESIS

The basic lesion of acne, as previously mentioned, is an inflammation of the pilosebaceous follicles of the skin. Only certain areas of the body are affected due to the fact that, whereas with most hair follicles, the size of the sebaceous gland is roughly proportional to the size of the hair,[2] in the areas of the body where acne occurs large sebaceous glands are present with small or rudimentary hairs. This combination is much more favorable for the development of acne, which explains why acne occurs on the face but only rarely on the scalp.

At puberty, under the influence of androgens, the sebaceous glands increase in size and activity. As part of the response to the androgens, the follicular walls hypertrophy. When this increase in keratinization or hypertrophy of the follicular walls occurs, the flow of sebum to the outside skin becomes mechanically

TABLE 35.1
Drugs Reported to Induce Acneform Eruptions[a]

ACTH	Iodides
Androgens	Quinine
Bromides	Scopolamine
Chloral hydrate	Thiouracil
Cod liver oil	Thiourea
Diphenylhydantoin	Trimethadione
Disulfiram	Vitamin B_{12}
INH	

[a]Reprinted with permission from Ref. 5.

blocked.[2,6] The pilosebaceous follicle starts to dilate and becomes filled with entrapped sebum and cellular debris. At this point the lesion is known as a comedo or blackhead. The follicular orifice of the blackhead usually remains partially open and allows varying amounts of sebum to reach the outside skin, but it can close off completely.

When the comedo forms, bacteria that are present normally on the skin and in the follicular canal are especially favored in this nutrient-rich environment of plugged pilosebaceous gland. Organisms most often found in the pilosebaceous follicle are the acid-producing bacteria *Corynebacterium acnes, Staphylococcus albus* and the fungi *Pityrosporon ovale.*[2,7] Of these, *Corynebacterium acne* and, to a lesser extent, the other bacteria produce lipolytic enzymes.[8] These enzymes are capable of converting the sebum, which is composed normally of esterified long chain fatty acids, into short chain free fatty acids. It has been shown that free fatty acids, especially those of carbon chains between 8 and 14, have the ability to provoke a nonspecific type of inflammatory response. Thus, while these bacteria do not take an active role in producing acne, they act as mediators or catalysts in the inflammatory response.

As the free fatty acid content of the entrapped sebum builds up, an inflammatory reaction occurs with its characteristic leukocytic infiltrates. As this process continues, bacterial by-products and dead leukocytes cause the walls of the sebaceous gland and follicular canal to become thinner and more brittle. Trauma to this area can cause the pilosebaceous follicle to rupture, spilling its contents into the surrounding dermis. If this occurs, the follicular contents produce a foreign body reaction and a cyst

generally will form. At this point, the hair follicle is usually destroyed and will not regenerate.[2] Sometimes these cysts will rupture again and again, forming larger and larger cysts. When a large number of cysts occur in any given area, they can form interconnecting channels.[4] This type of acne is known as *acne conglobata* and is a very severe form of the disease often leading to scarring. Systemic therapeutic agents should be used with this type of acne to lessen the chance of scarring.

DIAGNOSIS

The diagnosis of acne is a relatively easy one to make. Since 90% of the adult population has had the disease during their adolescence, the lay public is quite familiar with the signs and symptoms. Only when acne occurs very suddenly or in age periods where it is not generally seen should the clinician suspect underlying endocrine dysfunctions or drug-induced types of acne.

Acne does not lead to any major physical complications. Its most severe effect on most patients is the psychic trauma induced by the disease. Unfortunately, the disease occurs during a period of unusual emotional, physical and social upheaval, and it tends to complicate already pre-existing problems. It is not uncommon to see a patient's personality dramatically affected by the disease. Therefore, often it is beneficial to give these patients good counseling regarding their disease and have a sympathetic attitude when explaining the proper therapy. The physical complications of acne are limited to the scarring that sometimes remains after the acne has cleared. Although not actually a complication of acne, seborrhea or dandruff often accompanies this disease. This can be explained by the fact that both diseases are related to increased sebum production and thus often occur together.

TOPICAL THERAPY

The goal of acne therapy is to interrupt the degeneration of the pilosebaceous follicles so that cysts do not form and scarring will not occur. Treatment is directed toward keeping the skin clean and to the peeling of skin so that the follicular orifices are kept open and draining properly. The role of soaps or other cleans-

TABLE 35.2
Agents Commonly Used to Treat Acne[3,4,6,9,10,15,16]

Abrasives
1. Polyethylene granules
2. Aluminum oxide

Mild to moderate keratolytics

Concentrations most often employed
1. Sulfur   3-12%
2. Resorsinol   2-20%
3. Salicylic acid   1/2-3%

Potent keratolytic or peeling agents

Concentrations most often employed
1. Benzoyl peroxide   5-10%
2. Vleminckx solution (sulfurated lime)   Diluted 10-20 times
3. Vitamin A acid   0.1% solution
4. Veleminckx powder   2 tbs. in 500 cc hot water
5. Carbon dioxide slush and acetone   Not applicable

Drying agents

Concentrations most often employed
1. Alcohol   10-70%
2. Acetone   Varying concentrations
3. Phenol   0.5-2%

Systemic agents

Dosage
1. Hydrochlorthiazide (or equivalent)   25-100 mg/day
2. Prednisone (or equivalent)   20-30 mg with gradual withdrawal over
                                                   1 month
3. Interlesional steroids, Triamcinolone   1 mg or less is generally all that is
   (or equivalent)   required
4. Tetracycline   250 mg qid decreasing to the minimal
                                                   effective dose over 3-4 weeks
                                                   (this usually is 250 mg/day)
5. Erythromycin   Dosing similar to tetracycline
6. Lincomycin   500 mg qid decreasing to the minimal
                                                   effective does over 3-4 weeks
                                                   (this usually is 500 mg/day)
7. Estrogens
   a. Ethynylestradiol   0.1 mg/day
   b. Mestranol   0.1 mg/day
   c. Equivalent estrogenic substance

ing agents has been somewhat overplayed.[4] As one can see from the discussion on the pathology of the disease, acne lesions occur beneath the skin and soaps, regardless of their ingredients, only affect the surface of the skin. Since sebum and bacteria on the skin do not play an active role in the pathogenesis of acne, any soap's usefulness lies in its ability to remove sebum from the skin and thus help promote a state of dryness.

For mild to moderate cases of acne, topical therapy is generally all that is required to control the symptoms. There are two classes of compounds that are used in proprietary acne preparations, the mild keratolytic agents and the potent keratolytic or peeling agents.[4,9,10] The mild keratolytic agents are the most often used preparations. These agents have both keratolytic and keratoplastic properties depending on the concentration of each individual agent.

In the treatment of acne, it is important to maximize the keratolytic effects and minimize the keratoplastic properties. The most often used keratolytic is sulfur. It is used in concentrations of 3 to 12% and has keratoplastic properties at the 3% level which rapidly moves into the keratolytic range as the concentration is increased. Another often used agent is salicylic acid which is used in concentrations of 1/2 to 3%. Salicylic acid has keratoplastic properties below 2% and keratolytic effects above 2% concentration. Resorcinol also is used in many proprietary preparations and generally is used in concentrations of 2 to 20%. It is not uncommon to find several keratolytic agents used in combination in the same product. When this is the case, the concentration of each keratolytic agent can be lowered while still maintaining an adequate keratolytic effect.[6]

The second class of compounds used in the topical treatment of acne are the potent keratolytic or peeling agents. These agents are designed to remove the skin from around the comedones and skin covering superficial acne pustules. This helps to keep sebaceous follicles patent and draining properly.[6,9] Benzyol peroxide is one of the more popular nonprescription peeling agents. It is converted to hydrogen peroxide on the skin and acts as an oxidizing agent to promote peeling. Retinoic acid, one of the newer peeling agents, has proved to be very effective in promoting peeling despite its high irritant properties.[11] Hot Vleminckx compresses and carbon dioxide slush are peeling agents which should be used only under the close supervision of a physician owing to their low therapeutic indices.[4,6,10]

Hot Vleminckx compresses utilize a cloth compress soaked in a hot, sulfurated lime solution, which is then applied to the skin for varying lengths of time. Carbon dioxide slush treatment uses pulverized carbon dioxide in a cloth bag that is soaked in acetone and applied to the skin. Both of these treatments can produce severe irritation if allowed to stay in contact with the skin too long. Ultraviolet light treatments are sometimes used to produce mild peeling. The light treatments act by producing a mild burn which then causes peeling. There are also several types of mechanical peeling agents available. These agents contain an abrasive compound, usually a fine sand or small plastic balls and are used to produce peeling and also

to help keep the skin clean. When using any of the peeling agents, there should be a mild or tolerable level of irritation produced. There is considerable variance from patient to patient in the amount of peeling agent tolerated. In the case of retinoic acid, some patients can tolerate three or four applications per day while other patients may not be able to use the agent at all because of the severe irritation produced. Therefore, it is often necessary to individualize treatment regimens when using these agents.

SYSTEMIC THERAPY

The use of systemic agents in the management of acne should be reserved for the more severe forms of the disease. Antibiotics are the most often used systemic agents and are used for their suppressive effects on the bacteria responsible for producing the lipolytic enzymes in the sebum. Tetracycline is the most often used antibiotic, but lincomycin and erythromycin appear to be equally effective although they are more expensive.[6] When initiating antibiotic therapy, a normal dosing regimen should be employed. In the case of tetracycline, this is usually 250 mg 4 times a day.[6,12] After several weeks of therapy, the dosage should be tapered gradually until the minimal effective dose is found. With tetracycline, this usually is only 250 mg per day. The bacteria responsible for producing the free fatty acids are uniformly sensitive to these antibiotics and thus sensitivity tests are not employed. The epithelium lining the pilosebaceous follicle is considered to be an effective barrier against the penetration of these antibiotics. It is thought that these antibiotics gain entry into the sebum by sequestering in cells surrounding the sebaceous follicle and then being shed into the sebum. Such a sequestering process would explain why such low doses of antibiotics are effective and also explain the lag time observed between administration of the various drugs and their therapeutic effects.

X-ray therapy and estrogens sometimes are employed for their suppressive effects on the production of sebum. X-ray therapy is quite effective because it reduces the size of the sebaceous glands. However, due to the dangers involved with repeated X-ray treatments, this therapeutic modality is used only infrequently and usually in cases that are refractory to other types of therapy. Estrogen therapy sometimes is employed in women and, if adequate doses are used, is usually very effective. Oral contraceptive agents are the most often used agents for this purpose and have been shown to decrease sebum production as much as 40% in some patients. Sedatives also may be of benefit in anxious patients.[6,13] Anxiety increases sebum production and in these patients sedatives often prove to be beneficial.[14]

Diuretics seem to produce improvement in some patients, especially those women who have premenstrual flares of their acne. If diuretics are to be used for this purpose, they should be given 5 to 7 days prior to menses and continued during the menstrual period.[4] When acne is very severe, systemic corticosteroids may be employed. The rationale for using these drugs is to interrupt the inflammatory reaction and thus hopefully reduce the chance of scarring. Unfortunately, once steroid therapy is started, it often has to be continued to maintain its beneficial effect.[4,10] The side effects of these drugs must be weighed against the potential therapeutic benefits. For this reason, corticosteroids usually are reserved for very severe cases of acne or when other therapeutic modalities have failed.

SURGERY

Surgical procedures very often are employed by the dermatologist. These include the sterile rupturing of the comedones, pustules and cysts to allow proper drainage. Usually scarring will not result from these surgical procedures unless the lesion is very deep and requires extensive cutting. Dermabrasion is a surgical procedure employed to remove acne scars. This procedure involves the freezing of the skin and then abrading it with a high speed rotating wire brush. After dermabrasion, the patient should be instructed to avoid excessive sunlight for 6 to 8 weeks to reduce the chances of hyperpigmentation of the area.

DIET

The role of diet as a means of acne therapy has been exaggerated, and opinions on the usefulness of diet vary greatly from practitioner to practitioner. There is no evidence to support the value of eliminating various dietary items in helping the course of disease.[3,4,6,10] Some patients, though, insist they have flareups of their disease from certain foods. In these cases, despite no evidence to support the role of diet in acne, the patient should be cautioned to avoid those foods he thinks worsen his condition.

PROGNOSIS

The prognosis of acne vulgaris is very favorable. In most cases, the disease will undergo spontaneous remission. The only major sequela to acne is scarring. With proper treatment early in the course of the disease, the scarring often can be minimized. When treating acne, it is extremely important to discuss fully the disease and the proper treatment with the patient; it is the patient himself who must determine whether or not he will adhere to his therapeutic regimen and thus make his acne better or worse.

CONCLUSION

While there is no specific cure for acne, many of the physical symptoms can be made more tolerable by the use of various topical and systemic medicinals. The average case of acne certainly can not be considered a threat to the physical well-being of the emerging adolescent, but the disease can cause severe emotional problems for the patient. Thus, the most severe problems of acne may penetrate deeper than the acne lesions of the skin. An appreciation of the impact that acne can have on the psyche of the adolescent is paramount in establishing a successful therapeutic regimen.

REFERENCES

1. Cunlis, W. J., and Shuster, S.: Pathogenesis of acne. Lancet, 1: 685, 1969.
2. Freinkel, R. K.: Pathogenesis of acne vulgaris. N. Engl. J. Med., 280: 1161, 1969.
3. Andrews, C. C.: Acne vulgaris. Med. Clin. North Am., 49: 737, 1965.
4. Fitzpatrick, T. B.: Dermatology in General Medicine, Ed. 1, p. 353. McGraw Hill Book Co., New York 1971.
5. Hitch, J. M.: Acneform eruptions induced by drugs and chemicals. J.A.M.A., 200: 879, 1967.
6. Frank, S. B.: Acne Vulgaris, Ed. 1. Charles C Thomas Co., Springfield, Ill., 1971.
7. Scehadeh, N. H., and Kligman, A. M.: The bacteriology of acne. Arch. Dermatol, 88: 829, 1963.

8. Reisner, R. M., Silver, S., Puhvel, M., and Sternberg, T. H.: Lipolytic activity of corvnebacterium acne. J. Invest. Dermatol, 51: 190, 1968.

9. American Society of Hospital Pharmacists: American Hospital Formulary. Washington, D. C., 1972.

10. Domonkas, A. N.: Andrews' Diseases of the Skin, Ed. 6, p. 254. W.B. Saunders Co., Philadelphia, 1971.

11. Kligman, E. M., Fulton, J. E., and Plewig, G.: Topical vitamin A acid in acne vulgaris. Arch. Dermatol, 99: 469, 1969.

12. Ashurst, P. J.: Tetracycline in acne vulgaris. The Practitioner, 200: 539, 1968.

13. Strauss, J. S.: Effect of cyclic progestin estrogen therapy on sebum and acne in women. J.A.M.A., 190:815, 1964.

14. Kraus, S. J.: Stress, acne and skin surface free fatty acids. Psychosom. Med., 32: 503, 1970.

15. Freinkel, R. K., Strauss, J., Yip, S., and Pochi, P.: Effect of tetracycline on the composition of sebum in acne vulgaris. N. Engl. J. Med., 273: 850, 1965.

16. Reisner, R. M.: Systemic agents in the management of acne. Calif. Med. 106: 28, 1967.

chapter 36

PSORIASIS

C. A. Bond, Pharm. D.

Psoriasis as a disease state has been mentioned in literature for thousands of years, although often it has been confused with other disease states, such as leprosy and syphilis. The first well documented description of the disease was made early during the 19th Century in England, but most knowledge and development of effective treatments have been limited to the last 20 years.[1] The disease is estimated to occur in 2 to 3% of the population of the United States when mild as well as severe cases are counted.[2,3] Psoriasis does not affect all populations equally. It is seen only rarely in North and South American Indians and Eskimos. The disease is also rare in American Negroes probably owing to the fact that this racial group has ancestral origins in West Africa where the disease is extremely rare.[4] There is no difference in incidence with regard to sex except women generally will observe symptoms of the disease earlier in life than males.[2]

ETIOLOGY AND PATHOGENESIS

The exact cause of psoriasis is not known. While hereditary factors play a role in determining susceptibility, environmental factors also seem to influence the occurrence of the disease. Although the cause is unknown, a great deal of work has been done in regard to the pathogenesis of the disease.[5] The basic lesion of psoriasis is due to a loss in control of the normal growth-regulating mechanisms in the epidermis.[6] The normal turnover time for a cell to proceed from the generative layer of the skin to the point where it sloughs off is 27 days. In the psoriatic, the turnover time is decreased to 3 or 4 days. With the shortened transit time, the cells do not mature and keratinization fails to reach completion.[4,7,8] The epidermis is thickened owing to the increase in mitotic activity of the generative layer. Along with the increased cell turnover, there is also a corresponding increase in nucleoprotein synthesis as well as an increase in certain enzymes responsible for growth. Vascular changes are noted as the blood vessels become dilated and tortuous. The blood vessels extend further up into the skin than normal, thus allowing bleeding when the lesions are subjected to trauma. Inflammation with leukocyte infiltrates into the skin also is seen to varying degrees and is a secondary process to the underlying psoriatic lesion.

DIAGNOSIS

Psoriasis is classified as one of the papulosquamous dermatoses.[4] The common denominator among these types of dermatoses is a scaling papule. With psoriasis this papule is erythematous and is topped by a silvery scale which is loosely adherent. When this scale is removed, several bleeding sites are noted (called Auspitz signs). These signs, while not entirely diagnostic of psoriasis, are strongly suggestive of this disease. The primary lesions may coalesce to form plaques which can lead to significant cosmetic disfigurements. Common areas for these large plaques are on the extremities and the trunk. The individual lesions are usually symmetrical and can occur on any part of the body, although some areas are more prone to developing lesions than others. The most common sites of involvement are the knees and elbows. Often the scalp is affected and lesions here are often confined to this area. Mucuous membrane involvement can occur, but it is rare. Nail involvement, while not absolutely characteristic of psoriasis, often provides considerable assistance in establishing the diagnosis. The nails may have a brownish yellow discoloration, uplifting of the front of the nailbed, and a cracking of the edge of the nails. There is usually a characteristic pitting of the nails associated with psoriasis.

The clinical course of psoriasis is extremely variable. The mean age of onset of the disease is 27 years, but generally the earlier the appearance of the disease, the more severe it is.[2] The disease is characterized by remissions and exacerbations. People who have been known to be in remission for years may suddenly have explosive exacerbations for unknown reasons. Likewise, people with only minor degrees of psoriasis may continue to have only slight involvement for decades then suddenly may develop severe psoriasis. Among the many things thought to have caused psoriasis to become worse are injury or trauma to the skin (known as "Koebner's" response), cold weather and psychic upsets. Hot weather, sunlight and, sometimes, pregnancy are factors which have been associated with causing psoriasis to get better.[2] Remissions, although hard to calculate, have been shown to occur in approximately 40% of males and 60% of females sometime during the course of the disease.[2]

COMPLICATIONS

Approximately 25% of patients afflicted with psoriasis have arthritis.[9] While mimicking rheumatoid arthritis, this condition is actually a separate clinical entity. Females usually have a higher incidence of arthritis than males, and usually rheumatoid factor tests are negative in this type of arthritis. Another severe complication that can arise with psoriasis is an exfoliative dermatitis. This can be a life-threatening situation, as the patient is severely ill, and often the situation is complicated owing to large amounts of fluid loss. Severe secondary bacterial infections also may occur with an exfoliative dermatitis. It is thought that withdrawal of systemic corticosteroid therapy, use of synthetic antimalarial drugs, a too harsh topical therapy, and some systemic infections may precipitate a psoriatic exfoliative dermatitis. Occasionally, increases in serum uric acid levels and steatorrhea may be present along with psoriasis, but this is rare. Diabetes mellitus and increase in serum lipids and cholesterol have been reported to occur in psoriasis, but well controlled studies indicate that these states occur no more frequently than in the normal population.[4,7]

TREATMENT

A variety of treatments is available to combat psoriasis. The two most popular methods of topical treatment of psoriasis are the Goeckerman and the Ingram techniques. The Goeckerman regimen employs the use of coal tar or its derivatives and the use of ultraviolet light. A coal tar ointment is applied several times a day and removed after 24 hr followed by exposure to ultraviolet light. In addition, a coal tar bath is given at least once a day. With successive daily treatments, the exposure to ultraviolet light is increased. This particular regimen has resulted in a significant number of remissions usually lasting from 6 to 18 months.[4,11] The Ingram regimen differs in that an anthralin paste is applied to each psoriatic plaque instead of the coal tar ointment, and a stockinette dressing is applied over the lesions.[4,11] This regimen is very effective but requires close supervision. Hospitalization is required for both of these methods of treatment. Many variants of each of these two regimens may be used, such as the addition of corticosteroids or systemic therapy. When steroid creams and ointments are used, there is usually a prompt response noted. When the scalp is involved, a steroid is suspended in a propylene glycol vehicle and then applied. The corticosteroids, in addition to having anti-inflammatory actions, also depress mitotic activity, which is very beneficial to psoriatics. To facilitate penetration of steroids into the skin, an occlusive dressing is often applied; this is usually Saran wrap or a space suit and is left on from 12 to 24 hr at a time.[1,4] Intralesional steroid injections are sometimes employed, especially where only small lesions exist. With use of intralesional steroids, there is often atrophy of the subcutaneous tissue which can lead to a depression in the skin that may take months to resolve. While steroids are initially quite effective, the lesions usually return within a short time and other therapy must be started.

Tars

There are many different tar-containing products available in oil or several water-soluble bases.[3,12] Next to corticosteroids, these agents are most often used. Tar-containing products have mild anti-inflammatory and mild anti-pruritic effects as well as keratoplastic and keratolytic properties. These agents increase the skin's sensitivity to ultraviolet light which decreases mitotic activity, thus benefiting psoriasis. While this mechanism has been proposed to totally explain the beneficial effects seen with tars, it has never been proven, despite intensive study. The antipsoriatic effects seen with coal tar probably are not totally due to this mechanism, and other mechanisms have yet to be elucidated. While most psoriatics are benefited from tars and ultraviolet light, some psoriatics are made worse by sunlight and tars are definitely contraindicated in these patients.

Anthralin[3,4,11]

Anthralin, incorporated in Lassar's paste and paraffin, is extremely effective in the treatment of psoriasis.[3,4,11] Salicylic acid usually is added to the mixture. The paste is applied only to the psoriatic plaques, as it is very irritating to unaffected skin. The problem with treatments with anthralin is that it is messy and sometimes very irritating. While anthralin treatment is very effective in producing remission, the relapse rate approaches 100% in patients treated with this agent.

Ammoniated Mercury

This agent is sometimes used for its keratolytic activity and its effect on reducing mitotic activity. Generally, ammoniated mercury ointments have been less effective than coal tar.[4,12] If topical ammoniated mercury-containing products are used, one must be aware of systemic mercury toxicity, as mercury can be absorbed through the skin. For this reason, this agent should not be used in children under 5 years old, pregnant women and patients with a history of kidney disorders.

Methotrexate

Most of the drugs used in systemic therapy are used for their suppressive activity on rapidly proliferating skin. Methotrexate is the most often used systemic antipsoriatic agent. The side effects of the agent are similar to other antimetabolites, i.e., blood dyscrasias, gastrointestinal tract ulceration and hepatotoxicity. There are several dosing schedules available with methotrexate. Among these are 12.5 mg daily for 12 days, stop 1 week, then repeat; 3.75 to 5 mg per day for 12 days, stop for 1 week and repeat; and 25 to 37.5 mg once a week, divided in 3 or 4 doses given 8 to 12 hr apart. The use of this drug by the I.V. or I.M. route is not recommended, as it is more toxic by these routes, and it is not any more effective than the oral route.[7,13] The most often used dosing schedule is the 25 to 37.5 mg P.O. dose once a week, but this is only a guideline, as the smallest effective dose should be used. Since methotrexate is primarily excreted via the kidney, adequate renal function is vital to reduce the chances of toxicity.

Methotrexate is normally 50% bound to plasma proteins, and this bound form can be displaced from its binding sites by a number of drugs, thus potentiating the toxic effects of the drug.[3] Among these are: PAS, the sulfonamides, the sulfonylureas and aspirin. Methotrexate is contraindicated in patients with a history of liver disease, peptic ulcer disease, renal disorders and in patients who are pregnant.[12] Since liver toxicity can occur with methotrexate, it is prudent to follow liver function tests and take liver biopsies at regular intervals. It is extremely important to obtain regular blood counts to determine the suppressive effect of the drug on bone marrow and blood elements. Treatment is generally successful with this agent with about 70% of the patients gaining remissions.[2,3] Psoriasis treated with methotrexate generally clears or improves fairly rapidly which may be followed by prolonged periods of remission or marked suppression of the lesions. However, methotrexate is not a cure for the disease. It only suppresses it, and the beneficial effects with this treatment must be weighed against the life-threatening side effects of the drug.

Miscellaneous Agents

Various other agents are used topically. Keratolytics such as salicylic acid are used to remove scales. Nitrogen mustards occasionally are used topically, although effective in treating psoriasis, these compounds lead to a very high degree of sensitization and thus can not be used by most patients. Topical therapy is the mainstay in the treatment of psoriasis. Systemic therapy usually is employed only in severe cases of psoriasis where topical therapy has proved inadequate in controlling the disease.

A few other agents sometimes are used systemically in the treatment of psoriasis. These are usually other antimetabolites, such as aza-uridine.[3] Systemic arsenic still is used occasionally, even though in order to be effective in psoriasis, doses large enough to cause arsenical toxicity must be employed. Systemic corticosteroids, while very effective in treating psoriasis, are generally not used owing to the fact that with most psoriatics, after systemic corticosteroids are tapered or stopped, there generally is a severe rebound of the disease.[4] The side effects of systemic corticosteroids also greatly limit their long term use.

PROGNOSIS

Since psoriasis follows such an unpredictable course, it is most difficult to make any statement regarding the prognosis. The disease is characterized by spontaneous remissions as well as severe exacerbations. In most cases, all a patient can do is "learn to live with it" and carry on his life as normally as possible.

CONCLUSION

Although the medical literature contains reports proclaiming the discovery of the cause of psoriasis, the actual origin of the disease is still obscure. Treatment to date largely has been aimed at suppression of the disease, rather than producing a cure. In the future, drugs must be developed to maximize their effects on tissue that is abnormally proliferating without interfering with normal tissue growth. At present, toxicity greatly limits many of the drugs that would be very effective in treating psoriasis; and when antimetabolite therapy is employed, the patient must be closely monitored. Although remissions do occur for long periods, exacerbations are common. Thus, treatment is directed toward suppression of the disease to the point where the psoriatic can live comfortably and interact reasonably well with his environment.

REFERENCES

1. Farber, E., and McClintock, R., Jr.: A current review of psoriasis. Calif. Med., 108: 440, 1968.
2. Farber, E., Bright, R. D., and Nall, M. L.: Psoriasis—a questionnaire survey of 2,144 patients. Arch. Dermatol., 98: 248, 1968.
3. Farber, E.: International Symposium on Psoriasis, Stanford University, 1971. Ed. 1. Stanford University Press, Stanford, Calif., 1971.
4. Fitzpatrick, T. B.: Dermatology in General Medicine, Ed. 1, p. 353. McGraw-Hill Book Co., New York, 1971.
5. Shuster, S.: Research into psoriasis, the last decade, Br. J. Med., 3: 236, 1971.
6. Sidi, E., Zagula-Mally, Z., and Hincky, M.: Psoriasis. Charles C Thomas, Co., Springfield, Ill., 1968.
7. Farber, E.: Studies on the nature and management of psoriasis. Calif. Med., 114: 1, 1971.
8. Van Scott, E. J., and Ekel, T. M.: Kinetics of hyperplasia in psoriasis. Arch. Dermatol., 88: 373, 1963.
9. Reed, W. B., Becker, S. W., Rohde, R., and Heiskell, C. L.: Psoriasis and arthritis. Arch. Dermatol., 83: 541, 1961.
10. Perry, H., Soderstrom, C., and Schulze, R.: The Goeckerman treatment of psoriasis. Arch. Dermatol., 78: 176, 1968.
11. Comaish, S.: Ingram method of treating psoriasis. Arch. Dermatol., 92: 56, 1965.
12. Anon.: American Hospital Formulary. American Society of Hospital Pharmacists, Washington, D.C., 1972.

chapter 37

DRUG ERUPTIONS

C. A. Bond, Pharm. D.

Drug eruptions present one of the most difficult diagnostic problems that a clinician might encounter. Statistics regarding the incidence of drug eruptions in the community are almost nonexistent, but it has been shown that between 1 and 5% of hospitalized patients will experience a drug-induced skin eruption. Clinically recognizable adverse drug reactions are seen more often in the skin than in any other organ or organ system.[1,2] The statement often has been made that any drug can produce any type of eruption; however, drug eruptions are rarely described accurately,[2-5] and in most cases, adverse reactions involving the skin are described only as a "rash." Accurate statistics on the type and incidence of drug eruptions have been kept only recently and, thus, statistical inference with regard to drug eruptions is difficult, except in those cases where large numbers of specific reactions have been reported.

Another problem in accurately documenting most drug eruptions is the lack of test procedures available. Generally, all one can do to prove a drug hypersensitivity is to withdraw therapy, wait for the lesions to clear and rechallenge the patient with the suspected agent. This type of challenge-testing procedure obviously is not always practical. Drug eruptions also have a remarkable ability to mimic other types of dermatitis, but usually can be differentiated by the fact that they generally occur quite suddenly and are usually symmetrical and widespread.

Many mechanisms have been offered to explain drug eruptions, but true allergy probably accounts for a majority of cases.[4,6,7] However, allergic mechanisms rarely are demonstrable; in most cases drugs act as haptens and not as complete antigens. In addition, the drug itself may not be the causative agent, and the eruption may be due to a metabolite or an impurity in the formulation. Allergic skin responses generally are classified in two ways. The first is an immediate reaction in which urticarial, angioneurotic edema or anaphylaxis may occur—serum antibodies often are demonstrable and desensitization is possible. The second type of response, and the one to which most drug eruptions belong, is the delayed or tuberculin-like reaction. With this type of eruption, serum antibodies can not usually be demonstrated and variable responses with regard to desensitization are observed.[1,2,6,8-10]

Drug eruptions usually are limited to the skin. In rare instances, other organs may be involved. The time interval between the first dose of the drug and the appearance of the rash is determined by the state of sensitivity. Most drug eruptions appear early after drug therapy is begun, but in some cases, eruptions may appear months after a drug is discontinued. A good history is paramount when a drug eruption is suspected. In some cases, pre-existing lesions can be made worse by the use of certain drugs. It has been shown that patients with acne are more susceptible to acneform eruptions caused by iodides, bromides, androgens and other steroids; persons with purpuric and hemorrhagic conditions may be more susceptible to purpuric lesions caused by barbiturates, arsenicals, gold salts, sulfornamides and salicylates. Patients who are susceptible to the development of urticarial eruptions are more likely to experience such reactons from salicylates, iodides and bromides. It should be pointed out that large doses or prolonged therapy may be necessary to elicit an eruption but, once it appears, small doses of the offending agent at a much later date may cause a recurrence. Certain drugs, especially penicillin, are more likely to cause drug eruptions than others.[11,12] Other drugs that are implicated most often in causing drug eruptions may be found in Table 37.1. It has been suggested that if the same agent is used both systemically and topically, there appears to be an increased chance of a drug eruption occurring.[1-3,6]

EXANTHEMATIC ERUPTIONS

Exanthematic eruptions are subdivided into two groups: scarlatiniform and morbilliform. Most drug eruptions fall within these two groups. Scarlatiniform eruptions are erythematous and usually involve extensive areas.[6,8] They. are differentiated from scarlet fever by the lack of other diagnostic signs and laboratory studies. Morbilliform eruptions usually begin as discrete, reddish brown macules which may coalesce to form a diffuse rash. Likewise, morbilliform eruptions are differentiated from measles by the lack of other diagnostic signs and lab studies.[6,13] In either type of exanthematic eruption, pruritus may or may not be present. Drugs reported to have caused these types of reactions are found in Table 37.2.

URTICARIA

Urticarial eruptions usually appear as sharply circumscribed, edematous and erythematous plaques with an abrupt onset. In most cases, the lesions disappear within a few hours and are associated with intense itching, stinging or prickling sensation. Urticarial eruptions are commonly called hives and are frequently associated with certain drugs, foods, psychic upsets and serum sickness. Rarely, parasites or neoplasms may precipitate hives,[14-16] Angioneurotic edema, a variation of urticaria, can be explained best as a more severe form where giant hives predominate. Drugs associated with the development of urticarial and angioneurotic edema reactions may be found in Table 37.3.

ERYTHEMA MULTIFORME ERUPTIONS

As the name implies, erythema multiforme eruptions take on a variety of morphological

TABLE 37.1
Drugs Most Often Causing Drug Eruptions

Arsenicals
Barbiturates
Bromides
Gold salts
Hydantoins
Iodides
Mercurials
Quinine
Salicylates
Streptomycin
Sulfonamides
Thiouracils

TABLE 37.2
Exanthematic Eruptions

Allopurinol
Antipyrine
Arsenic
Atropine
Bismuth
Chloral hydrate
Codeine
Digitalis
Diphenylhydantoin
Gold salts
Griseofulvin
INH
Insulin
Meprobamate
Mercury compounds
Morphine
Novobiocin
PAS
Penicillin
Phenothiazines
Phenylbutazone
Quinidine
Quinine
Salicylates
Sulfonamides
Tetracycline
Thiazides
Thiouracil

forms. The lesions are discrete and sharply circumscribed and usually are arranged symmetrically. They appear as acute, polymorphous, bright or dark red macules, papules, vesicles or bulla; however, only one type lesion usually predominates in a given patient. Erythema multiforme is more common in children and young adults. Sometimes malaise and a low grade fever and, occasionally, itching or burning may be seen with this type of eruption. Etiological factors associated with erythema multiforme include drugs, infections, deep x-ray therapy, foods and sometimes neoplasms. Sulfonamides are the drugs most often implicated in erythema multiforme eruptions.[1,8,11] Other drugs implicated in causing this eruption may be found in Table 37.4.

STEVENS-JOHNSON SYNDROME

The Stevens-Johnson syndrome is probably the most common type of severe drug eruption.[17] It is classified as a serious variant of

TABLE 37.3
Urticaria Eruptions

ACTH	Liver extracts
Adrenalin (possibly from	
chlorbutanol)	Meperidine
Allopurinol	Meprobamate
Aminopyrine	Mercury compounds
Antitoxins	Morphine
Arsenic	Nalidixic acid
ASA	Nitrofurantoin
Barbiturates	Novobiocin
Bismuth	Penicillin
Bromides	Penicillinase
BSP	Phenacetin
Chlordiazepoxide	Phenolpthalein
Chloral hydrate	Phenothiazines
Chloramphenicol	Phenylbutazone
Chlorpropamide	Pilocarpine
Codeine	Pituitary extracts
Dextran	Procaine
Digitalis	Propoxyphene
Ephedrine	Pyribenzamide
Erythromycin	Quinine
Fluorides	Saccharin
Gold salts	Sulfonamides
Griseofulvin	Tetanus toxoid
Heparin	Thiamine
Hydantoins	Tragacanth
Insulin	Tuberculin skin test
Iodides	Warfarin
INH	Vaccines

bullous erythema multiforme. In addition to what has already been described previously, the Stevens-Johnson syndrome usually involves the mucous membranes and includes constitutional symptoms of fever and malaise. The skin can become hemorrhagic and pneumonia and joint pains may occur. Serious ocular involvement is common and can culminate in partial or complete blindness. Besides drugs, this syndrome has been associated with infections, pregnancy, foods, deep x-ray therapy and neoplasms. Mortality is estimated to be in the range of 5 to 18%[17,18] The duration of the syndrome is usually 4 to 6 weeks and the long acting sulfonamides most often are implicated in the development of the syndrome. Other drugs associated with causing the Stevens—Johnson syndrome may be found in Table 37.5.

ERYTHEMA NODOSUM ERUPTIONS

Drug-induced erythema nodosum is quite rare. It appears as red, tender nodules usually located around the shins, but they can occur elsewhere. Occasionally, there may be mild constitutional symptoms, but there is usually no mucous membrane involvement. Etiological factors associated with the development of erythema nodosum are drugs, rheumatic fever, leprosy, certain bacterial infections and systemic fungal infections. Usually the lesions slowly heal several weeks after the offending agent is removed.[1,6] Drugs that have been reported to cause this type of eruption may be found in Table 37.6.

FIXED DRUG ERUPTIONS

This eruption, unlike the others mentioned, is caused exclusively by drugs. The lesions are

TABLE 37.4
Erythema Multiforme Eruptions

Acetazolamide
Diphenylhydantoin
Furosemide
Gold salts
Griseofulvin
Iodides
Mechlorethamine
PAS
Penicillin
Phenolphthalein
Phenothiazines
Phenylbutazone
Propranolol
Salicylates
Smallpox vaccine
Sulfonamides
Thiazides
Tolbutamide

TABLE 37.5
Stevens-Johnson Syndrome

Antipyrine
ASA
Chloramphenicol
Chlorpropamide
Diphenylhydantoin
Hydralazine
Measles vaccine
Penicillin
Phenobarbital
Phensuximide
Phenylbutazone
Smallpox vaccine
Sulfonamides
Tetracycline
Trimethadione

erythematous, sharply bordered and have a tendency to be darker than the surrounding, unaffected skin. They also may be eczematous, urticarial, vesicular, bullous or nodular. Because these lesions have a marked propensity to recur at the same location, the word "fixed" is applied.[1,19] Although the eruptions heal after withdrawal of the causative drug, there usually is a marked hyperpigmentation of the area which may take months to resolve. The mechanism by which fixed drug eruptions occur has not been elucidated but is believed to be allergic in nature.[2,20] It can be described figuratively as islands of hypersensitivity, one area of the skin having the ability to evoke an allergic response and other areas lacking this ability. Drugs that have been reported to cause this type of eruption may be found in Table 37.7.

TABLE 37.6
Erythema Nodosum Eruptions

Aspirin
Bromides
Codeine
Iodides
Oral contraceptive agents
Penicillin
Streptomycin
Sulfonamides
Tuberculin skin test

TABLE 37.7
Fixed Drug Eruptions

Acetaminophen	Hydralazine
Acetanilid	Licorice
Aminopyrine	Mandelic acid
Amphetamine	Meprobamate
Antimonial compounds	Mercury compounds
Barbiturates	Morphine
Belladonna alkaloids	PAS
Bromides	Pentaerythritol tetranitrate
BSP	Phenacetin
Chloral hydrate	Phenolphthalein
Chlordiazepoxide	Phenothiazines
Chloramphenicol	Phenylbutazone
Codeine	Quinacrine
Diethylstilbestrol	Quinine
Digitalis	Reserpine
Diphenylhydantoin	Saccharin
Disulfiram	Salicylates
Ephedrine	Sulfonamides
Ergot	Tetracyclines
Ethchlorvynol	Vermouth
Gold salts	

PURPURA

Purpuric lesions are characterized as hemorrhages into the skin. They are purplish, sharply bordered and have a tendency to become brownish as they get older. These lesions may or may not be associated with thrombocytopenia. Etiological factors other than drugs that are associated with purpura are: vitamin C deficiency, snake bites and infections. The mechanism by which these lesions are produced is not known, but they have a tendency to recur with re-exposure to the causative agent. Sometimes purpura may develop from other types of eruptions, such as erythema multiforme. It is worth noting that a clot retraction test is available to document quinidine-induced purpura. Although not commonly associated with drugs, purpuric lesions have been observed following therapy with the drugs listed in Table 37.8.

ACNEFORM ERUPTIONS

Acneform eruptions appear very much like common acne.[21] They are differentiated from

TABLE 37.8
Purpuric Eruptions

Antitoxins
Aspirin
Bromides
Carbromal
Chloral hydrate
Chloroform
Chlorpromazine
DDT
Diethylstilbestrol
Ephedrine
Ergot
Fluoxymestrone
Gold salts
Griseofulvin
INH
Insulin
Iodides
Meprobamate
Phenylbutazone
Quinidine
Quinine
Sulfonamides
Tetracycline
Thiazides
Thiouracils
Warfarin

acne by their sudden occurrence, the absence of comedones in affected areas and the fact that they can occur on any part of the body. Eruptions can also occur during any period of a patient's life and, thus, acne that appears in age brackets where it does not appear normally may be suspected of being caused by drugs.[21,22] Someone who already has acne may have the existing lesion made worse. Table 37.9 lists the drugs that have been reported to cause this type of lesion.

PHOTOSENSITIVE-PHOTOALLERGIC-PHOTOTOXIC ERUPTIONS

These eruptions require the presence of both drug and light source to occur. Photosensitive eruptions are divided into two subtypes based on different mechanisms of action. The first type is called photoallergic and requires the presence of light to alter the drug so that it becomes an antigen or acts as a hapten.[23,24] Photoallergic eruptions require previous contact with the offending drug, are not dose-related, exhibit cross sensitivity with chemically related compounds, and may appear as a variety of lesions including urticaria, bulla and sunburn. These lesions are usually secondary to the use of topical agents. The second type of photosensitive eruption is known as phototoxic reaction in which the light source alters the drug to a toxic form, resulting in tissue damage independent of allergic response. This eruption may occur on first exposure to a drug, is dose-related, usually has no cross sensitivity and almost always appears as an exaggerated sunburn. In some instances, a drug may produce both photoallergic and phototoxic reactions.[25] Drugs that have been reported to cause photosensitive eruptions may be found in Table 37.10[25,26]

LICHEN PLANUS-LIKE ERUPTIONS

These lesions appear as flat-topped papules which have a distinct sheen. Pruritus is usually quite pronounced and any part of the body may be affected, including mucous membranes. The lesions are sometimes confused with fixed eruptions but can easily be differentiated histologically. Drugs reported to cause lichen planus eruptions may be found in Table 37.11.

TABLE 37.9
Acneform Eruptions

ACTH
Androgens
Anovulatory agents
    (although pre-existing acne may
    improve with anovulatory agents)
Bromides
Chloral hydrate
Cod liver oil
Diphenylhydantoin
Disulfiram
INH
Iodides
Quinine
Scopolamine
Thiouracil
Thiourea
Trimethadione
Vitamin B_{12}

TABLE 37.10
Photosensitive-Photoallergic-Phototoxic Eruptions

Antimalarials
Barbiturates
Chlorpromazine
Gold salts
Griseofulvin
Nalidixic acid
Norethynodrel
Mestranol
Phenothiazines
Psoralens
Quinethazone
Quinine
Smallpox vaccine
Sulfonamides
Sulfonylureas
Tetracycline
Thiazides

TABLE 37.11
Lichen Planus-like Eruptions

Chloral hydrate
Chlordiazepoxide
Chloroquine
Diphenylhydantoin
Gold salts
Meprobamate
PAS
PTU
Quinacrine
Quinidine
Thiazides

TOXIC EPIDERMAL NECROLYSIS

This type of eruption was first described by Lyell in 1956 and may be preceded by a prodrome characterized by malaise, lethargy, fever and occasionally throat or mucous membrane soreness.[27] Epidermal changes follow and consist of erythema and massive bulla formation which easily rupture and peel. The skin appears as if scalded. Hairy parts of the body are usually not affected, but mucous membrane involvement is common. Approximately 30% of the patients with toxic epidermal necrolysis succumb, often within 8 days after bulla appear.[17] The usual cause of death is infection complicated by massive fluid and electrolyte loss. Even though the skin takes on a very grave appearance, healing occurs within 2 weeks in about 70% of patients, usually with no scarring.[6,8] In addition to drugs, certain bacterial infections and foods are believed to cause this type of eruption. Most cases of toxic epidermal necrolysis in children are due to infection; *Staphylococcus aureus* has been implicated. Drugs thought to cause toxic epidermal necrolysis are listed in Table 37.12.

EXFOLIATIVE DERMATITIS

Exfoliative dermatitis, as the name would imply, is characterized by large areas of skin becoming scaly and erythematous and then sloughing off. Hair and nails sometimes are lost.

In most patients, a generalized systemic toxicity also accompanies the eruption. Secondary bacterial infection may occur and most fatalities are due to infection. Exfoliative dermatitis also may follow other drug eruptions; thus, a less severe eruption may culminate with an exfoliative dermatitis.[1,17] This type of eruption may take weeks or months to resolve, even after withdrawal of the offending agent. Drugs implicated in causing this type of eruption may be found in Table 37.13[6,8,28,29]

BULLOUS ERUPTIONS

Bullous lesions may occur in combination with other drug eruptions, such as erythema multiforme or toxic epidermal necrolysis, or by themselves. The lesions may be round or irregular in shape and contain a clear, serous fluid. The fluid-filled sacs may be either tense or flaccid and can occur in mucous membranes as well as the skin. Table 37.14 lists the drugs that have been reported to cause these eruptions.

TABLE 37.12
Toxic Epidermal Necrolysis

Acetazolamide
Aminopyrine
Barbiturates
Brompheniramine
Dapsone
Diphtheria innoculations
Diphenylhydantoin
Gold salts
Nitrofurantoin
Penicillin
Phenolphthalein
Phenylbutazone
Polio vaccine
Sulfonamides
Tetanus antitoxin
Tetracycline
Tolbutamide

TABLE 37.13
Exfoliative Dermatitis

Actinomycin D
Allopurinol
Antimony compounds
Arsenic
Barbiturates
Boric acid (internally)
Chlorpropamide
Codeine
Diethylstilbestrol
Diphenylhydantoin
Gold salts
Iodides
Mercury compounds
Mesantoin
Methantheline
Methylphenidate
PAS
Penicillin
Phenacemide
Phenolphthalein
Quinacrine
Quinidine
Streptomycin
Sulfonamides
Tetracycline
Vitamin A

TABLE 37.14
Bullous Eruptions

Acetazolamide
Aminopyrine
Arsenicals
Atropine
Barbiturates
Bismuth
Bromides
Chloral hydrate
Digitalis
Diphenylhydantoin
Ergot
Gold salts
Licorice
Mercury compounds
Mesatoin
Penicillin
Phenolphthalein
Promethazine
Quinine
Streptomycin
Sulfonamides

MISCELLANEOUS DRUG ERUPTIONS

Pigmentary changes usually are not allergic in nature but are classified as idiosyncratic reactions. Examples of drugs that cause pigmentary disorders are: ACTH, bismuth, corticosteroids, mesantoin, phenolphthalein, phenothiazines, quinacrine and silver compounds.[8,30] Drug-induced tumor-like lesions involving the skin are extremely rare; a few cases have been reported with iodides, bromides and arsenic compounds. Eczematous lesions are seen more often with contact sensitizers than with internally administered compounds. However, drugs that can produce this type of reaction after internal ingestion are chloramphenicol, meprobamate, penicillin and tetracyclines. Although alopecia is not a true drug eruption, hair may occasionally be lost when such reactions occur. Eruptions which may lead to alopecia are exfoliative dermatitis and erythema multiforme. Hair loss may be attributed to a toxic action of a drug, such as an antimetabolite, or to an interference with the normal growth phases of hair, as is the case with warfarin.[29,31,32]

TREATMENT

Diagnosis is very important in determining adequate therapy. For the more severe erup-tions, early diagnosis and prompt treatment may modify the severity and eventual course of the eruption. The treatment of drug eruptions is mostly supportive. After withdrawal of the causative compound, most drug eruptions resolve in a matter of days. For less severe cases, topical therapy may be all that is needed. This usually includes a topical corticosteroid cream and/or antipruritic lotion or cream. Supportive care includes decreasing the frequency of bathing, using nonabrasive soaps or cleansing agents, eliminating harsh or abrasive clothing and avoiding high temperatures and humidity. The use of a wet dressing may be used to help soothe inflamed skin. For more severe eruptions, systemic steroids should be used to control symptoms. Antihistamines also may be beneficial. In lesions where large amounts of fluid are lost, parenteral replacement is mandatory. Although patients with severe drug eruptions are more prone to infection, the prophylactic use of antibiotics is not warranted, as they should be used only when an infection occurs.

REFERENCES

1. Baer, R. L., and Harris, H.: Types of cutaneous reactions to drugs. J.A.M.A., 192: 189, 1965.
2. Coleman, W. P.: Unusual cutaneous manifestations of drug hypersensitivity. Med. Clin. North Am., 51: 4, 1969.
3. Kirshbaum, B. A., Beerman, H., and Stahl, E. B.: Drug eruptions: a review of some of the recent literature. Am. J. Med. Sci., 240: 512, 1960.
4. Kopf, A., and Andrade, R.: Year Book of Dermatology, p. 146. Year Book Medical Publishers, Chicago, 1969.
5. Sternberg, T. H., and Biermiau, S. M.: Unique syndromes involving the skin induced by drugs, food additives and environmental contaminants. Arch. Dermatol., 88: 779, 1963.
6. Fitzpatrick, T. B.: Dermatology in General Medicine, Ed. 1, p. 1281. McGraw-Hill Book Co., New York, 1971.
7. Baer, R. L., and Witten V. H.: Drug eruptions: a review of selected aspects of an age old, but always timely and fascinating subject. In Year Book of Dermatology, p. 9, 1961.
8. Domonkos, A. N.: Andrews Diseases of the Skin, Ed. 6, p. 109. W. B. Saunders Co., Philadelphia, 1971.
9. Newbold, P. C.: Drug eruptions. Calif. Med., 113: No. 1, 23, 1970.
10. Rostenberg, A.: Mechanism of cutaneous drug reactions. J.A.M.A., 154: 211, 1954.
11. Torok, H.: Dermatitis medicamentosa: a ten-year

study. Dermatol. Int., p. 57, April–December, 1969.

12. Burrows, D., Shanks, R. G., and Stevenson, C. J.: Adverse reactions in a dermatology ward. Br. J. Dermatol., 81: 391, 1969.

13. Dickey, R. F., and Hartman, D. L.: Photogermatitis induced by drugs, Part II. Skin, p. 198, July, 1964.

14. Tatro, D. S.: Drug induced cutaneous eruptions. Alta Bates Newsletter Vol. II, No. 7, July, 1970.

15. Tatro, D. S.: Drug induced cutaneous eruptions. Alta Bates Newsletter Vol. II, No. 9, September, 1970.

16. Tatro, D. S.: Drug induced cutaneous eruptions. Alta Bates Newsletter Vol. II, No. 10, October, 1970.

17. Rostenberg, A., and Fagelson, H. J.: Life threatening drug eruptions. J.A.M.A., 194: 660, 1965.

18. Bianchine, J., Macaraeg, P., Lasagna, L., Azarnoff, D., Brunk, S., Huidberg, E., and Owen, J.: Drugs as etiologic factors in Stevens-Johnson syndrome. Am. J. Med., 44: 390, 1968.

19. Derbes, V. J.: The fixed eruption. J.A.M.A., 190: 765, 1964.

20. Savin, J. A.: Current causes of fixed drug eruption. Br. J. Dermatol., 83: 546, 1970.

21. Weary, P. E., Russell, C. M., Butler, H. K., and Hsu, Y. T.: Acneform eruptions resulting from antibiotic administration. Arch. Dermatol., 100: 179, 1969.

22. Hitch, J. M.: Acneform eruptions induced by drugs and chemicals. J.A.M.A., 200: 879, 1967.

23. Pillsbury, D. M., and Baro, W. A.: The increasing problem of photosensitivity. Med. Clin. North Am., 50: 1295, 1965.

24. Sams, W. M.: Photosensitizing therapeutic agents. J.A.M.A., 174: 2043, 1960.

25. Dickey, R. F., and Hartman, D. L.: Photodermatitis induced by drugs. Skin, 3: 169, 1964.

26. Baer, R., and Harber, L.: Photosensitivity induced by drugs. J.A.M.A., 192: 189, 1965.

27. Bailey, G., Rosenbaum, J. M., and Anderson, B.: Toxic epidermal necrolysis. J.A.M.A., 191: 979, 1965.

28. Meyler, L., and Herxheimer, A.: Side Effects of Drugs, Vol. 2, p. 320. The Williams and Wilkins Co., Baltimore, 1968.

29. Shelley, W. B.: Consultations in Dermatology, Ed. 1. W. B. Saunders Co., Philadelphia, 1972.

30. Santanouf, J.: Pigmentation due to phenothiazines in high and prolonged dosages. J.A.M.A., 191: 263, 1965.

31. Crounse, R., and Van Scott, E.: Changes in scalp hair roots as a measure of toxicity from cancer chemotherapeutic drugs. J. Invest. Dermatol., 35: 83, 1960.

32. Simister, J. M.: Alopecia and cytotoxic drugs. Br. Med. J.: 2: 1138, 1966.

section 12

Neoplastic diseases

chapter **38**

THE ACUTE LEUKEMIAS

Douglas G. Christian, B.S.
William A. Cornelis, B.S.
Clarence L. Fortner, M.S.

The leukemias are a group of related malignant diseases characterized by quantitative and morphological alterations in the peripheral blood white cells and in the precursors of the affected white cell series in the bone marrow and by secondary anemia, granulocytopenia and thrombocytopenia due to leukemic cell infiltration of the bone marrow and crowding out of normal myeloid elements. Untreated, the patient ultimately succumbs to progression of the disease, infection and/or hemorrhage. The approximate incidence of leukemia is 6.5 cases per 100,000 population;[1] approximately 40% of the total incidence are acute varieties of leukemia. Leukemias will be responsible for an estimated 15,000 deaths this year with 2,000 of its victims children under 15 years of age.

There is generally an acute and a chronic form of leukemia for each main type of white cell, and the varying histories and clinical courses of these diseases allow that each may have a different pathogenesis. Although theories of the etiology of leukemias and scattered case reports describe infective (viral) agents, genetic factors and chemical (or environmental) inducers, the fact remains that no etiology other than high dose radiation exposure has been proved for any of the human leukemias. Any one of the above agents could, however, alter genetic structure, and predisposition to the disease by this means is feasible.

Acute and chronic forms of leukemia are defined by expected length of survival after diagnosis, which is closely related to the morphology of the predominating white cell. Immature cells in the peripheral blood exhibit less than optimal normal activity for their type, and leukemic cells, by virtue of structural and biological errors in development, are even less effective. It is not surprising therefore, that prognosis of the various types of leukemias depends on the stage of white cell maturation at which the malignancy has centered. In general, the less mature the predominating cell type, the worse the prognosis. Acute leukemias are detected by a high percentage of very immature forms of the white cell series involved in the peripheral blood and bone marrow. The prognosis for untreated acute leukemias is a lifespan of 2 to 3 months or less. Chronic leukemias, in contrast, would be expected to permit a lifespan of 2 to 5 years untreated, and the predominating white cell would be a more mature form.

CLASSIFICATION OF LEUKEMIAS

Besides general division of leukemias into "acute" and "chronic" categories, it is necessary to subclassify the disease in terms of white blood cell morphology, as each type responds differently to treatment. Acute lymphocytic leukemia, for instance, responds to therapy with a much greater degree of success than acute myelocytic leukemia.

There are five series of white blood cells and each follows a similar pathway of maturation, deriving from a "blast" cell (itself arising from a fixed tissue reticulum cell) and progressing through histologically defined stages to the mature form which is then released into the blood stream (Fig. 38.1). The normal percentage distribution of the white cell types in peripheral blood is described in Table 38.1.

In circumstances of physiological stress, it is not uncommon for the less mature leukocyte forms to appear in the peripheral blood. The

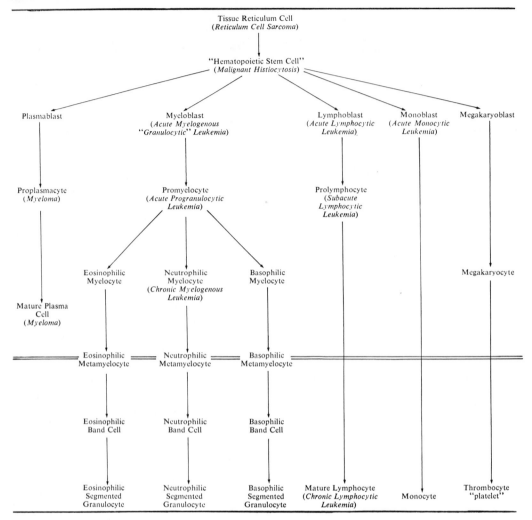

FIG. 38.1. White blood cell series maturation sequence (The names of malignant proliferative diseases which can be associated with each cell type are indicated in parentheses and italics.)

very primitive blastic stage of white cell, however, should not be present in the peripheral blood, and its appearance introduces clinical suspicion of leukemia. The diagnostic process necessarily includes complete history, physical examination, peripheral blood studies and bone marrow sampling to differentiate leukemias from other possible causes of peripheral leukocytosis and occurrence of atypical white blood cells. Some of these causes include toxic bone marrow stimulation by chemicals (e.g., lead), aplastic anemics, certain viral diseases including infectious mononucleosis, tissue destruction and the normal granulocytic response to infection. At diagnosis, the actual white cell count

may be within normal limits, depressed or elevated. If secondary anemia is present, it may be of the normocytic, normochromic type or macrocytic, normochromic type.

Acute lymphocytic leukemia (ALL), as shown in Figure 38.1, is defined by proliferation within the lymphocytic series. This disease, especially in children aged 2 to 19 years, has begun to yield to therapeutic advances. Several drugs, in specified dosage ranges and treatment regimens to be discussed, can be expected to prolong the life of 20% of childhood ALL patients for 5 or more years.

Acute myelocytic leukemia (AML) involves the precursors of the granulocytes, or poly-

TABLE 38.1
The Normal Differential White Blood Cell Count[a]

	%
Total neutrophils	50-70
Segmented neutrophils (polys)	50-70
Band cells	3-5
Metamyelocytes	0-1
Lymphocytes	20-40
Monocytes	0-7
Eosinophils	0-5
Basophils	0-1
Blasts (of any type)	0-0

[a]Total white cell count is in the range of 5,000 to 10,000 mm³, with considerable normal variation. Of this number, the above percentage distribution of cell types is normal in the peripheral blood.

morphonuclear leukocytes. Relative to discussion, therapeutic considerations and prognosis, AML is often grouped with acute monocytic leukemia (AMOL) and acute myelomonocytic leukemia (AMML). The three entities together are referred to as acute nonlymphocytic leukemia (ANLL). ANLL has responded much less dramatically to therapeutic attempts than has ALL, with median survival for all treated ANLL patients about 6 months. Patients who do not respond to therapy survive an average of 2.5 months, and those who respond to treatment may expect an average 12-month survival.

CLINICAL COURSE OF ACUTE LEUKEMIAS

The presenting symptomatology of patients with acute leukemia varies greatly but usually can be referred to the underlying disorders of the disease. Displacement of normal elements from the bone marrow by neoplastic cells leads to anemia, thrombocytopenia and granulocytopenia. Symptoms referrable to these conditions would include the possibilities listed in Table 38.2. Fever and weight loss can be ascribed to increased metabolic activity of the bone marrow tissue. Many signs of organ infiltration are absent in the acute forms of leukemia, but lymphadenopathy and splenomegaly are not uncommon.

These clinical findings are vague at best, and diagnosis always must be based as mentioned on complete evaluations, including bone marrow studies. Because the patient can often relate these symptoms to more benign disorders he has previously experienced, tentative diagnosis of leukemia often is made upon blood studies drawn for less specific purposes.

Whichever cell type is prevalent, there are many factors which will influence the clinical course of a patient with an acute leukemia. At diagnosis, these factors include the age and general condition of the patient (presence or absence of other underlying conditions such as diabetes, cardiovascular disease or impaired renal or hepatic function) and the interval from onset of symptoms to diagnosis and treatment. Occurrence of septicemia while the patient's immune response is compromised and toxicity of the vigorous treatment regimen will greatly affect the progress of treatment. The greatest factor in successful therapy, however, is achievement of the state of "complete remission" (CR), wherein all symptoms of the disease including peripheral blood and bone

TABLE 38.2
Clinical Symptoms from Leukemic Replacement of Normal Bone Marrow Elements

Anemia	Thrombocytopenia	Granulocytopenia
Fatigue	Conjunctival and fundal	Infection
Pallor	hemorrhages	(fever and/or chills)
Shortness of	Gingival hemorrhages	"Flu" symptoms; frequent
breath	Gastrointestinal bleeding	or prolonged colds
Headache	(emesis or melena)	
Tachycardia	Renal hemorrhages	
	(blood in urine)	
	Petechiae; ecchymosis	
	Purpura	
	Subarachnoid hemorrhages	

marrow appearance are normalized.[2] The treatment leading to remission status from clinical disease is termed "induction." Although undetectable by current methods, leukemic stem cells undoubtedly linger even when the patient is in complete remission. Treatment which is given during remission in an attempt to destroy newly activating leukemic cells is termed "maintenance." "Reinduction" courses will be necessary to treat each successive relapse, or return of active disease, which is recognized by return of symptoms and of "blasts" in the bone marrow. Complete remission status infers functional as well as morphological normalization, and the patient in remission no longer is subject to abnormal hemorrhagic risk or the greatly lowered resistance to infection. It is established that increased survival for a remitting patient is very comparable to the total time spent in complete remission.[2] Thus, therapy of acute leukemia has been aimed at achievement and maintenance of remission(s) and supportive therapy during granulocytopenic and thrombocytopenic phases before remission can be induced.

One reason that acute nonlymphocytic leukemias have responded less to therapeutic efforts than the acute lymphocytic variety may be that inducing remission in ANLL requires a more lengthy and profound marrow aplasia before new, normalized myeloid elements reappear. Therefore, morbidity due to infection and bleeding during the induction period is higher in ANLL than ALL. The granulocytopenia seen in ALL is only secondary to marrow crowding and competition for nutrients by the abnormal lymphoid elements.[3] Chemotherapy directed against lymphocytic precursors allows relatively rapid recovery of the granulocytic (myelocytic) precursors remaining after treatment. In ANLL, the malignant myeloid precursors are the target of chemotherapy, so suppression of that series of white blood cells is more profound. Survival during this compromised period may reflect, again, on the age and general condition of the patient as lymphoblastic malignancy occurs largely in a very young (i.e., more immunologically resilient) patient population. This does not account adequately for the large disparity between achievement of successful first complete remission inductions in acute lymphocytic leukemia (currently 90 to 95% in some series of children)[4] and in acute nonlymphocytic leukemia (favorable reports list complete remission rates of 50 to 65%).[4] Chemotherapy seems to exhibit less activity against ANLL than ALL. In both diseases, duration of each succeeding remission tends to be progressively shorter, though exceptions are noted. Present figures for median survival among childhood ALL patients achieving at least one complete remission averages 36 months.[4] Among adult ALL patients, survival averages 18 months. Comparable data for ANLL patients in a series from the Baltimore Cancer Research Center list median survival at 11.5 months.[5]

Leukemic cell infiltration of many organs and tissues of the body (bowel, liver, spleen, lymph nodes, kidneys, bone marrow and subcutaneous lesions) presents little morbidity in acute varieties of leukemia, if the leukemic cell line is responsive to therapy. Central nervous system (CNS) involvement, however, is a serious and not uncommon development. Ultimately but not acutely life-threatening is the fact that the CNS can be a reservoir for leukemic cells (not reached by therapeutic agents which can not cross the blood-brain barrier) and may give rise to systemic relapse. Another CNS leukemic involvement of concern is development of meningeal leukemia. This CNS leukemic proliferation can occur independently of bone marrow condition and indeed may arise and progress while the patient is in bone marrow and peripheral blood remission. This complication has become more prevalent in all varieties of leukemia as their respective survival times have lengthened. Meningeal leukemia can be treated with varying degrees of success by intrathecal administration of methotrexate or cytosine arabinoside and/or external irradiation of the spinal column and brain. Neurological manifestations of CNS leukemia may be minimal or flagrant, but symptoms of increased intracranial pressure and cranial nerve palsies are reason for concern. Leukemic cells which have infiltrated or proliferated in the CNS can be identified by lumbar puncture and cerebrospinal fluid (CSF) sampling, followed by Cytocentrifuging and examining a preparation of the resultant material. CSF samples as well as bone marrow and peripheral blood samples become important in monitoring progression of the disease as well as success of treatment, especially in the later stages. Leukemic cell infiltration of intra-cerebral alveolar structures (rather than the meninges and subarachnoid space) may occur, especially when peripheral white cell counts exceed 200,000 cells per mm^3. Intracerebral intravascular plugging with increased local pressure on vessel walls is a critical situation predisposing one to intracranial hemorrhage, and it must be treated vigorously. At present, effective means of lowering the very high peripheral white cell levels are available in the form of hydroxyurea.

AVAILABLE MODALITIES OF TREATMENT

In all malignant conditions, therapy may utilize one or more of the following agents: surgery, ionizing irradiation, immunotherapy or chemotherapy.

In leukemias, surgical excision of the tumor tissue is impossible, which relegates this modality to a minor supportive role.

Irradiation also has a supportive role in antileukemic therapy, particularly in reducing the size of an infiltrative leukemic mass. This is useful when functional impairment of some organ or vessel has occurred, or when pain is the result of marrow hyperactivity (i.e., sternal tenderness) or leukemic infiltration in an area such as a joint. Irradiation also is used to decrease numbers of proliferating leukemic cells when they occur in the CNS.

Immunotherapy has received some attention in recent years with the demonstration of specific tumor antigenic sites in two cancerous states, Burkitt's lymphoma and choriocarcinoma. BCG vaccine is being investigated clinically as a means of rallying the body's total immune response (after a patient has achieved remission). Specific active immunotherapeutic response may be feasible if a viral agent is proven as the etiology of the disorder, or if specific "foreign tissue" antigenic sites are described for other tumors and responsive antibody stimulation can be developed.

To date, successful treatment of the acute leukemias has rested almost entirely on chemotherapy. Briefly, the history of antileukemic chemotherapy began with demonstration of the lympholytic properties of adrenocortical steroids in 1947 and extrapolation of this activity of prednisone and prednisolone to acute leukemia in 1949. Development of antineoplastic

drugs has been steady since that time. Attrition has left us with fewer than 10 drugs presently in common use against acute leukemias. Many of the basic pharmacological and pharmacokinetic/pharmacodynamic characteristics of these are still being investigated, while clinical use of the agents has produced therapeutic advances. We have mentioned that science has not yet elucidated the external agent or biological errors which cause leukemias. Because of this, many theories, proposals and models of antileukemic chemotherapy were developed in an empiric manner. Progress to date represents refined extrapolation of the original principles, plus a tremendous effort to demonstrate in well controlled clinical trials the added benefit or toxicity of each proposed improvement, whether in drug moiety or schedule of drug administration.

CONCEPTS RELATIVE TO CHEMOTHERAPY

Understanding antineoplastic chemotherapy requires exposure to the concepts of cytotoxicity in general, as modified by the principle of selective toxicity when antineoplastic agents are used in a tumor-bearing human. In addition, supportive therapy is important in all malignant conditions but has even greater significance for the course and prognosis of a patient with acute leukemia.

Modern growth-kinetic studies have disproved the concept of the leukemic cell population as a runaway prolific body. Analogous to growth of a bacterial colony, as the leukemic cell population expands and nutrient supplies dwindle, rate of growth seems to "plateau." Henderson has thus described leukemic cell populations as "self-renewal systems which, though they march to a different drummer, depend upon external stimuli and internal mechanisms similar to other living tissue."[6]

It is worthwhile to review the cell cycle as it is depicted by Figure 38.2. This description applies to both normal and malignant cells. The portion of the cycle labeled "D" represents cellular division (mitosis). "G_1" (which is also referred to as "Go" in chemotherapy literature) is a resting phase, until recently considered to be relatively quiescent. The "S" phase is that of active deoxyribonucleic acid (DNA) synthesis, which is followed by "G_2," another resting phase. The S, G_2 and D phases are relatively

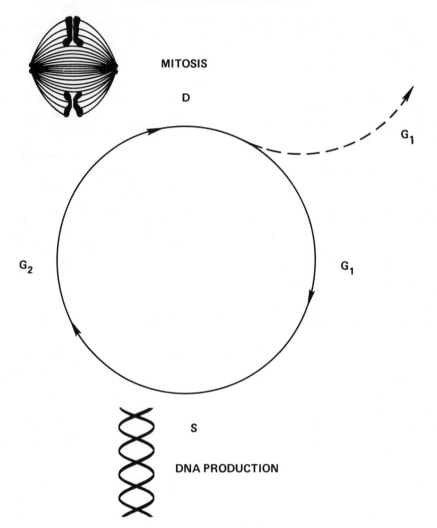

FIG. 38.2. The mitotic cell cycle.

fixed periods of time for a given cell population, and if rate of division (length of the average cell cycle) varies, it is usually the G_1 phase which accommodates. When cells stop proliferating and come to rest, they do so in the G_1 phase, and when proliferative activity is high, the G_1 may become very short. Certain aspects of ribonucleic acid (RNA) production are known to occur during the G_1 phase, but it is not known how a cell receives the biological message to proceed to DNA synthesis.[7]

In a malignant body of cells, the immediately premitotic event of spindle formation and the cell division, as well as the S-phase of DNA replication necessary for reproduction of the cell line, have been the specific targets of antineoplastic chemotherapy. Drugs which act at these or some other defined phase of cell life are called cycle-specific. Drugs are also in effective use, however, for which no phase specificity has been demonstrated and these are designated cycle-nonspecific. The classification is relative rather than absolute.

Antileukemic chemotherapeutic approaches must take advantage of very subtle differences in rate of growth and cellular metabolism between the leukemic cell population and the patient's normal tissues. Both irradiation and chemotherapeutic drugs are basically toxic or injurious to all cells, and selectivity of response depends on the vulnerability of malignant versus normal cells.

Cycle-specific drugs tend to be more effective in rapidly proliferating tissues, where their incorporation into disruptive cytotoxic events will kill maximal tumor cells with minimal effect on normal cells. Predictably, toxic manifestations of most antineoplastic drugs are borne by normal tissues (i.e., the bone marrow, gastrointestinal mucosa, skin and hair follicles) in which the rate of cell division approaches or exceeds that of the malignant tissue under treatment. In antileukemic chemotherapy, toxicity to certain elements of the bone marrow is the object of treatment, but the need for careful titration of dosage is obvious.

Recalling the mechanism of drug activity above, remission induction involves lysis of the many immature leukocytes present in the peripheral circulation and bone marrow. Maintenance phases are designed to suppress only those newly proliferating leukemic stem cells (in an otherwise normal hematological state) before they cause relapse to clinical disease. Though exceptions exist cell cycle-specific drugs are generally used in induction while cell cycle-nonspecific drugs are most effective in maintenance.

The timing of sequential doses of chemotherapeutic agents to catch larger numbers of neoplastic cells in their susceptible phase is of clinical importance. Like normal tissues, leukemic cell lines do not exhibit synchronized division. That is, at a given moment, different cells within the leukemic cell population are in different phases of their individual cycle. As such, only a percentage will be vulnerable to the effects of a cycle-specific drug while that drug is present in an active form in the body.

The experience to date has shown that combinations of agents which produce qualitatively different toxicities can produce additive and perhaps synergistic increases in remission induction rate and remission duration. The administration of combinations of antineoplastic drugs in some cancers has two cytotoxic objectives. The first is to combine drugs which act at different points of the cell cycle and thus expose a larger percentage of the cancerous cells to the drug when they are in a susceptible state. The second (analogous in many respects to theories of antimicrobial therapy) is to expose susceptible cancer cells to toxic effects

by as many mechanisms as possible to suppress selective emergence of cell strains which are resistant to further therapy. With the addition of each drug in a proposed combination regimen, the following considerations must be made. Is the tumor type uniformly and reliably susceptible to one drug, or does resistance to repeated therapy occur? Does the proposed combination produce additive toxicity to particular normal tissues, or are the combined expected toxicities spread to different organs of the body? Is an effective dose of one drug (or all drugs) in the combination influenced by concomitant or subsequent administration of the other drugs? Is the effective dosage schedule of one drug (or all drugs) in the combination altered by administration of the other drugs? As can be seen, complexity of the variables involved in combination antineoplastic chemotherapy dictates that this approach be undertaken by physicians with the background and sufficient laboratory and supportive facilities to monitor results of drug administration.

ANTILEUKEMIC DRUGS IN USE

The two drugs of choice when used singly in acute lymphocytic leukemia are prednisone (Pred) and vincristine sulfate (VCR). The average successful complete remission (CR) rates with either approach is 50%. Other agents can produce the following CR rates when used in ALL: L-asparaginase (L-ASP, investigational), 45%; daunorubicin (daunomycin, DMN, investigational), 40%; 6-mercaptopurine (6-MP), 36%; and methotrexate (MTX), 31 to 100% (the last on a schedule of intermittent massive infusion). MTX administered daily, cyclophosphamide (CTX), and cytarabine (arabinosyl cytosine = ARA–C) are less effective but do demonstrate some activity when used alone against ALL.[8]

Several two-, three- and four-drug combinations are in current use against acute lymphocytic leukemia. PRED and VCR together produce CR rates near 88%. It can be seen that this figure is better than for either agent used alone, but it is not equal to or greater than the additive CR rates of the two drugs used alone. Other two-drug combinations and their respective expected CR rates are as follows: Pred and 6-MP, 78%; Pred and DMN, 65% and Pred and CTX, 52%. Many others have been tried which do not exhibit better CR rates than the constituent drugs when used alone. A three-drug combination of Pred, VCR and DMN has produced CR rates above 95%, and in a specific dose schedule by Mathe and coworkers (Lancet 2:380, 1967) a CR rate of 100% was reported. This combination is not in widespread use because daunorubicin is still investigational, and because that drug has a very narrow therapeutic margin. The doses and schedule for administration of the four-drug combination known as "POMP" (Pred, Oncovin or VCR, MTX, and Purinethol or 6-MP) in common use across the nation and produces CR rates approaching 95%.[8]

In acute nonlymphocytic leukemia, the results are less gratifying though progress has been made. Pred, so effective as a single agent against ALL, produces CRs in only 15% of AML cases. DMN, however, will produce CR rates of up to 50%. ARA-C produces CR rates varying from 20 to 45% (or higher) depending on dose, schedule of administration and the age of the patient. Expected CRs with other agents when used alone in AML are: VCR, 36% (one study, patients mostly children); 6-MP, 11%; and MTX, 10%. CTX and L-ASP are active but less effective.[8]

Compared to success of single drug chemotherapy against AML, some of the combination regimens are decided improvements. Most two-drug combinations have not demonstrated greater efficacy than the individual agents used alone. Exceptions are ARA-C and 6-thioguanine, which gave 65% CRs in adults under 65 years of age, and ARA-C with CTX yielding 40% CRs.[8] Studies continue concerning the combination of Pred, MTX, 6-MP and VCR in varying doses and schedules of administration. DMN has been substituted for VCR in the above regimen. With proper supportive care, CRs have been achieved in up to 50% of patients.

Remission maintenance therapy of acute leukemias can and often must use different drugs in different administration schedules than the successful induction program.

Pharmacological mechanisms, commonly encountered toxicities and the clinical applications of current antileukemic drugs are listed briefly in Table 38.3. Further information can be obtained from pharmacology and therapeutics textbooks.

One exception to those drugs which act by some interference with cell division is that of L-asparaginase which will be discussed briefly because of its historic interest. Development of this agent followed the discovery that some leukemic cells did not have the capacity to synthesize their own requirements of the amino acid, L-asparagine. These cells utilized circulating asparagine produced by other cells. It was postulated that sensitive leukemic cells could be starved out if endogenous asparagine were eliminated, and it was shown that the enzyme asparaginase from bacteria (especially *Escherichia coli*) inhibits replication of susceptible leukemic cells *in vitro* and *in vivo*. This is an apparent effect of catalyzing hydrolysis of L-asparagine in the blood and extracellular fluid. Asparaginase thus exploits a difference in metabolic requirements between leukemic and normal cells. Theoretically, L-ASP should be the most specific cytotoxic drug available to date and less toxic to normal tissues, especially those of the hematopoietic system. Because of this potential for relative marrow-sparing specificity, it was investigated in combination chemotherapy with myelotoxic drugs.

Unfortunately, the specificity of the drug does not appear as great as postulated. Evidence has accumulated to suggest that some leukemic cells can produce sufficient asparagine for survival and that normal tissue may, in contrast, be damaged. Hepatic toxicity is of particular concern at present. Allergic responses have also been frequent. The drug has proven more effective in ALL than AML and those CRs induced by L-ASP have been of relatively short duration. Although the experience to date with L-ASP has been disappointing, the approach is promising and future developments along similar lines may evolve clinically effective agents.

SUPPORTIVE THERAPY

As has been stressed, terminal pathology of the acute leukemias has been associated in many cases with two morbid states, infection and hemorrhage. Hyperuricemia and resultant urate nephropathy were formerly a third complication which now may be largely circumvented.

As recently as 1959, hemorrhages were responsible for nearly 67% of deaths from acute leukemias.[9] Many of these were generalized hemorrhages, although the greatest percentage

TABLE 38.3

Drugs in Current Use Against Acute Leukemias

Drug Name	Pharmacological Category	Cycle-Specificity	Mechanism of Action	Outstanding Toxicities And Side Effects	Application in Acute Leukemias
L-Asparaginase (investigational)	Enzyme	Unknown	Depletion of endogenous extracellular asparagine	Multiple defects in protein synthesis; clotting abnormalities, hypoalbuminemia; hepatic and pancreatic toxicities; allergic response	ALL remission induction; intrathecal use in CNS leukemic infiltration
Cyclophosphamide	Polyfunctional alkylating agent	?Nonspecific	Requires *in vivo* activation; believed to act by cross-linking macromolecules including DNA	Nausea and vomiting; myelosuppression; chemically-induced sterile hemorrhagic cystitis; alopecia	ALL remission induction
Cytarabine (Arabinosyl cytosine; cytosine arabinoside)	Pyrimidine analog	Specific	Interferes with conversion of cytidylic to deoxycytidylic acid; inhibits DNA synthesis	Nausea and vomiting; myelosuppression; hepatic dysfunction; esophagitis	AML and ALL remission induction and maintenance; intrathecal use in CNS leukemic infiltration
Daunorubicin (Daunomycin; rubidomycin) (investigational)	Antibiotic	Unknown	Inhibition of RNA and DNA synthesis	Nausea and vomiting; myelosuppression; cardiotoxicity	AML and ALL remission induction only
6-Mercaptopurine	Purine analog	Specific	Inhibition of purine synthesis; inhibition of DNA synthesis	Nausea and vomiting; myelosuppression; hepatic dysfunction; stomatitis; diarrhea	ALL remission induction and maintenance
Methotrexate	Folic acid antagonist	Specific	Inhibits activity of enzyme dehydrofolate reductase; interferes with synthesis of tetra hydrofolic acid, a coenzyme necessary in metabolic transformations in the production of DNA	Myelosuppression; oral and gastrointestinal ulceration; hepatic dysfunction; alopecia; dermatitis	AML and ALL remission induction and maintenance; intrathecal use in CNS leukemic infiltration
Prednisone, Prednisolone	Adrenocortical steroids	?Nonspecific	Direct lysis of lymphoid tissue; ? inhibition of DNA synthesis	Psychoses; acute hypertension, peptic ulcer, fluid retention, immunosuppression, etc.; osteoporosis	ALL remission induction
6-Thioguanine	Purine analog	Specific	Inhibition of purine systhesis; inhibition of DNA synthesis	Nausea and vomiting; myelosuppression; hepatic dysfunction; stomatitis; diarrhea	ALL remission induction and maintenance
Vincristine SO4	Vinca alkaloid	Specific	Disruption of mitotic spindle formation; inhibition of RNA and DNA synthesis	Peripheral neuropathies; paralytic ileus; alopecia	ALL remission induction

were pulmonary hemorrhages associated with pneumonias. Other difficulties included bleeding into the subarachnoid space and into the GI tract. Complex coagulation problems exist in these patients, but the greatest cause of secondary hemmorrhage is an insufficient quantity of platelets due to leukemic crowding of platelet precursors (megakaryocytes) or myelosuppression by chemotherapy.

Freshly collected platelets obtained from whole blood or plasmapheresis techniques are able to maintain effective levels of circulating platelets when given by transfusion. Since this procedure became available in 1961, the percentage of hermorrhagic deaths in acute leukemias has dropped from 66.8% to 37.2%, as discussed by Hersh et al.[9] The category most greatly affected has been that of generalized (systemic) hemorrhage. Half-life of transfused platelets is approximately 24 to 48 hr in the thrombocytopenic recipient. Repeated infusions, thus, are necessary as dictated by circulating platelet levels until the patient's marrow regains the ability to sustain platelet counts above a hemostatic level. This requires adequate blood-banking facilities with relatively great platelet sources.

Infections in the granulocytopenic patient continue to be a serious problem. The number of leukemic deaths precipitated by infection has remained at 70%. Since deaths due to hemorrhage have been reduced in proportion to the total over the past few years, it is reasonable that figures for infections may have been inflated in spite of the numerous advances in antibacterial chemotherapy during the same period. Owing to effective suppression of some species, the pattern of infective organisms involved has been altered quite drastically. With the use of penicillinase-resistant antibiotics, incidence of fatal staphylococcal infection has dropped from 23.5 to 3.1% of those deaths due to infection.[9] Decrease in prevalence of this organism has been supplanted in turn by *Pseudomonas aeruginosa, E. coli* and *Klebsiella* sp. In an attempt to reduce morbidity due to these three species of bacteria, the Baltimore Cancer Research Center currently employs a "triple antibiotic" regimen consisting of intravenous carbenicillin disodium, gentamicin sulfate and cephalothin sodium. Because progression of a septicemia or pneumonia is so rapid in the immunologically compromised patient, our protocol states that the above drugs shall be started at the first sign of systemic infection in granulocytopenic patients. Cultures of suspected sites of origin plus blood, urine, stool, nose, gingiva and axilla are taken at the time the antibiotics are begun. Once the cultures from a patient become available, drugs can be altered to suit the sensitivities as determined by disc and tube-dilution methods.

With relative success of this and similar antibacterial regimens,[10] *Enterobacter* sp., *Klebsiella* sp., group D streptococcus and *Candida* sp. (monilia) appear on the upswing. Treatment of infections in the acute leukemic patient promises to continue as a therapeutic challenge.

Effective prophylaxis against infection would provide more reasonable therapeutics than treating infections when they occur. Current investigation along this line is evaluating reverse isolation (isolating the patient from contact with bacteria from exogenous sources) in programs at several institutions with the aim of protecting the patient from nosocomial micro-organisms as well as protecting him prophylactically from opportunistic invasion by his own normal flora. The latter frequently occurs with GI lesions, including hemorrhoids, as the portal of entry.

In very stringent approaches, "life island" and laminar air flow (LAF) rooms place the patient in a virtually sterile environment. Supplies are sterilized before being passed to patients confined in these units, uncooked foods are avoided and contamination from all sources (including drug products) must be considered. In addition, topical flora of the patient's body is suppressed by rigid hygienic efforts and flora of the GI tract is suppressed by administration of oral, nonabsorbable antibiotics (nystatin, gentamicin and vancomycin). BCRC is conducting a controlled study utilizing LAF rooms in conjunction with the oral nonabsorbable antibiotics. The group of patients treated on this program will be compared with those having the same disease (ANLL) maintained in the usual hospital environment, with and without the oral antibiotics.

Another rational prophylactic measure and means of supportive treatment against infection in granulocytopenic patients would seem to be the transfusion of granulocytes from donors. This approach has not been investigated on a controlled basis because, until recently, the procedure presented several technical problems.

Elaborate selective centrifuging techniques have been unsuccessful in yielding great enough numbers of granulocytes to transfuse effectively. Red cells and platelets can be obtained in pure fractions for transfusion because their specific gravities and other physical characteristics allow successful filtration, sedimentation and centrifugation procedures. Leukocytes are relatively few in number in the prospective donor (red cells: platelets: leukocytes = 500:20:1) and are intermediate in size and specific gravity. Thus, collected leukocytes generally have been contaminated with the other two formed elements. A new plastic wool filtering device (Leukopak, Baxter Laboratories) is currently under investigation and, hopefully, will yield much higher numbers of viable cells.

It should be emphasized that efficacy of LAF protection, the oral nonabsorbable antibiotic regimen and granulocyte transfusion has not been determined though controlled studies, which are now in progress for this purpose. There well may be major toxic reactions to orally administered gentamicin, vancomycin and nystatin (i.e., acquisition and infection with *Pseudomonas* sp. after discontinuing these drugs) or the Leukopak (i.e., shaking chills and liver function abnormalities in the donor after return of blood). As with all experimental trials, these and other reactions as yet undetected may eventually lead to abandonment of the described procedures.

Anemia, as a result of leukemic crowding of red cell precursors in the marrow, chemotherapeutically induced aplasia or hemorrhage can be treated by transfusion of packed red cells or whole blood.

Hyperuricemia and resultant obstructive urate nephropathy can result from the increased nucleoprotein production of large numbers of neoplastic cells. The problem is compounded when chemotherapy produces lysis of large numbers of tumor cells and release of their contents. Degradation of the purine by-products of these nucleoproteins to the final metabolite, uric acid, is mediated by the enzyme, xanthine oxidase. Administration of the xanthine oxidase inhibitor, allopurinol, interferes with the process at this point, leaving purine degradation products in the form of xanthines, which are more soluble metabolic

precursors of uric acid. Prevention of hyperuricemia, a nearly inevitable consequence of the leukemia and its treatment, is much more satisfactory than treating urate nephropathy once it occurs. Additional measures utilized in prevention and treatment of hyperuricemia, with differing degrees of success, include adequate hydration of the patient and alkalinization of the urine with sodium bicarbonate or acetazolamide to favor solubility of uric acid. Routine use of allopurinol, recognizing its possible untoward effects, can circumvent the problem in most cases.[11]

CLINICAL MONITORING OF CHEMOTHERAPY

Having noted the clinical course of acute leukemias, the concepts relative to antineoplastic chemotherapy and supportive therapy, it is obvious that this patient population requires intensive surveillance efforts by all health professionals concerned with their care. The drug therapy each patient receives is the specific end result of diagnostic procedures, clinical evaluations and efforts to minimize toxicities, side effects and complicating secondary problems. The pharmacist, utilizing support of current medication profiles and accurate dispensing records (including intravenous drugs and fluids), is in an excellent position to review all aspects of the patient's status.

Surveillance efforts relative to chemotherapy are directed at the emergence of toxic effects, side reactions and drug interactions of clinical significance and adherence to rational utilization of antineoplastic drugs. "Rational utilization" is a relative term in this instance, since the optimal doses, dosage schedules and the complete indications for most of the antineoplastic drugs are not fully known yet. Effective doses for any of these agents in a given disease state in fact may be much different from the dosage range expressed in the product literature. Balanced against this is the fact that the drugs are not completely selective for neoplastic cells and exhibit a narrow therapeutic margin. The effectiveness of many antineoplastic agents is measured by appearance of their toxic effects, and the doses prescribed are often titrated against "tolerable" levels of adverse effects, especially against hematopoietic tissues. With respect to drug interactions, this delicate balance assumes special significance. If the biological availability of antineoplastic agents is enhanced, or their metabolism or excretion inhibited, the danger of increased toxicity should be readily apparent. To date, few reported drug interactions involving cancer chemotherapeutic agents have been well documented.[12] A working understanding of the pharmacology of the drugs involved and the mechanisms which are plausible for a suspected potential interaction is invaluable to the pharmacist, who should expect to do some reasonable extrapolation from those principles. The pharmacist who is interested in monitoring effects of these drugs in patients will have to be familiar also with laboratory indices, especially those concerning bone marrow function, peripheral blood counts and coagulation parameters. Additionally, hepatic and renal function can be reviewed. With respect to renal function in leukemic patients it should be remembered that as systemic infection occurs, several antibiotics (including all those of the aminoglycoside class) might be needed and can, themselves, produce acute tubular necrosis. When decreased renal function is noted, doses of gentamicin sulfate may be adjusted on the basis of serum creatinine values. Evaluation of the clinical situation might suggest similar alterations for other drugs the patient is taking which normally are excreted in active forms in the urine. Electrolytes and acid-base balance can be monitored as indicated.

In addition to their leukemia, these patients present a normal cross-section of other medical problems, including hypertension, diabetes, congestive heart failure, etc. Treatment for these conditions must continue, but the patient should be observed carefully for adverse response in the face of chemotherapy. Steroids used to lyse neoplastic lymphoid tissue, for example, may aggravate or precipitate a diabetic condition. Drugs used for treating underlying problems will have their contraindications and toxicities, and adequate monitoring can avoid additive complications of these and the antineoplastic drugs.

CONCLUSION

The acute leukemias are malignancies of the white blood cell-forming tissue of bone marrow. Chemotherapy, administered in sequential or concomitant doses of combinations of toxic drugs, may prolong the useful life of the victim if complete, though temporary, remission of the disease is achieved. Side effects of the treatment regimen and complications of the disease are severe, and success in achieving remission status is variable. Nearly 95% of children with ALL and approximately 50 to 60% of adults with ANLL will achieve CR, extending their useful life up to 5 years and 1 year or more, respectively. Thus, significant progress has been noted and hopeful avenues of research have been opened to investigation. More selective cytotoxic agents, improved techniques to limit infection as a complication of treatment and approaches utilizing specific active immunotherapy will be goals of future development.

It is anticipated that, for several years to come, effective induction therapy of acute nonlymphocytic leukemias will, of necessity, be restricted to specialized treatment centers where supportive facilities can adequately serve the needs of the patient. Well evaluated therapeutic regimens and more completely elucidated appreciation for possible complications allow the successful chemotherapy of acute lymphocytic leukemia in children in conventional medical facilities.

Through multifaceted surveillance efforts, assurance of an accurate and well documented drug delivery system and constant involvement in the clinical area with patients, physicians and nurses, the pharmacist can serve a vital function in the direct care of those patients being treated for acute leukemias.

REFERENCES

1. Serpick, A.: Acute versus chronic leukemia: differential features and treatment. Hosp. Med., 6: 7, 1970.
2. Henderson, E.: Treatment of acute leukemia. Semin. Hematol, 6: 297, 1969.
3. Serpick, A.: Acute versus chronic leukemia: differential features and treatment. Hosp. Med., 6: 15, 1970.
4. Bernard, J., Jacquillat, C., and Weil, M.: Treatment of the acute leukemias. Semin. Hematol, 9: 185, 1972.
5. Wiernick, P. H., and Serpick, A. A.: Factors affecting remission and survival in adult acute nonlymphocytic leukemia (ANLL). Medicine, 49: 506, 1970.
6. Henderson, E.: Treatment of acute leukemia. Semin. Hematol, 6: 273, 1969.
7. Cline, M. J.: Cancer chemotherapy, In Major Problems in Internal Medicine, Vol. 1, p. 4,

edited by L.H. Smith. W.B. Saunders Co., Philadelphia, 1971.

8. Goldin, A., Sandberg, J., Henderson, E., Newman, J., Frei, E., and Holland, J.: The chemotherapy of human and adult acute leukemia. Cancer Chemother. Rep., 55: 310, 1971.

9. Hersh, E. M., Bodey, G. P., Niles, B. A., and Freireich, E. J.: Causes of death in acute leukemia. J.A.M.A., 193: 99, 1965.

10. Schimpff, S., Satterlee, W., Young, V. M., and Serpick, A. A.: Empiric therapy with carbenicillin and gentamicin for febrile patients with cancer and granulocytopenia. N. Engl. J. Med., 284: 1061, 1971.

11. Modell, W. (editor): Drugs of Choice, 1972–1973 Edition, p. 561. C.V. Mosby Co., St. Louis, 1972.

12. Hansten, P. D.: Drug Interactions, Ed. 1, p. 143. Lea and Febiger, Philadelphia, 1971.

chapter 39

HODGKIN'S DISEASE

William A. Cornelis, B.S.
Douglas G. Christian, B.S.
Clarence L. Fortner, M.S.

The malignant lymphomas and lymphatic (lymphocytic) leukemias are lymphoreticular malignancies. The malignant lymphomas are derived from reticuloendothelial tissue (histiocytic lymphoma) or from lymphatic tissue (lymphocytic lymphoma).[1] The lymphatic leukemias are derived from lymphatic tissue within the bone marrow and, at times, may resemble the lymphocytic lymphomas. The lymphatic leukemias affect the bone marrow with resulting peripheral blood abnormalities associated with leukemic infiltration of the spleen, liver, lymph nodes and other tissue. In contrast, the malignant lymphomas may originate either as extensive involvement of tissue or as localized involvement of one or more lymph nodes in a single anatomic region or a solitary extranodal site.[2]

The differences between the malignant lymphomas are found in microscopic examination of diseased tissue where characteristic cellular composition will distinguish them. Hodgkin's disease is a malignant lymphoma and, like all other malignant lymphomas, it is termed a lymphoreticular disorder.

Hodgkin's disease was first described in 1832 by the British physician, Thomas Hodgkin, in his paper "On some morbid appearances of the absorbent glands and spleen" after he had made some initial anatomical investigations of patients who had this disease of the lymphoreticular system. Another British physician, Sir Samuel Wilks, independently had described several cases of the same disease and had reassessed Hodgkin's paper; several years later, Wilks named the disease after Hodgkin in another paper. The later work of two pathologists, Carl Sternberg (1898) and Dorothy Reed (1902), led to the subsequent naming of the Sternberg-Reed cell, the cell which is considered the actual malignant cell of Hodgkin's disease.

For many years there existed a great deal of controversy concerning whether Hodgkin's disease was a true neoplastic disease or an infectious disease of micro-organismal etiology. The proponents of the microbial etiology of the disease argued that the afflicted nodes resembled granulomatous changes found in the lymph nodes of patients with tuberculosis, brucellosis and a variety of systemic fungal infections. In addition, some of the symptoms of Hodgkin's disease such as lymphadenopathy, fever and night sweats were also impressive clinical features which suggested an infectious process. Various workers even cultured brucella organisms, diphtheroids, *Histoplasma capsulatum, Cryptococcus neoformans* and avian strains of mycobacteria from the lymph nodes of patients with Hodgkin's disease, though later studies and follow-up work found these microorganisms to be contaminants in the tissue culture. Studies investigating possible viral etiology have been performed with inconclusive results. The histopathology of a lymph node invaded with Hodgkin's disease reveals that the number of Sternberg-Reed cells is remarkably sparse when compared to the great number of neoplastic cells in other malignancies. In the past, this finding cast further doubt on the neoplastic nature of Hodgkin's disease.

The support for the neoplastic basis of Hodgkin's disease comes from the metastatic nature of Hodgkin's disease (characteristic of all untreated malignancies) with eventual disease infiltration into organs. Also, the typical infectious disease spreads via horizontal transmission from one person to the next, but to date, this has never been proven conclusively for Hodgkin's disease. Currently, studies are being conducted in certain geographical areas where the incidence of Hodgkin's disease among the resident population has been unusually high.[3] These studies attempt to suggest an infectious etiology of Hodgkin's disease, but concrete evidence to support the implications of these studies is still lacking. Hodgkin's disease presently is considered a malignant neoplastic process and associated therapy is conceived along the same lines as therapy for other malignant diseases.

PATHOLOGY

Lymph nodes are discrete nodules of lymphatic tissue anatomically located along lymphatic vessels. Lymphatic tissue is not uniquely found in lymph nodes, for lymphatic aggregates also are found in intestinal submucosa, bone marrow, bronchi, spleen and thymus. As distinct structures, the lymph nodes have a fibrous capsule from which connective tissue forms a framework by radiating throughout the node. The capsule is perforated by afferent lymphatic vessels which lead to a peripheral sinus. Branches of the sinus extend throughout the node and finally terminate at the hilus where efferent lymphatic vessels emerge. The lymphatic vessels within the node are lined with reticuloendothelial cells. The lymph nodes have the following three functions: formation of lymphocytes, production of antibodies and filtration of the lymph.[4]

Diagnosis of Hodgkin's disease can be made only by microscopic examination of biopsied tissue from a suspicious lymph node or organ invaded by the disease. The presence of the Sternberg-Reed cell, in the appropriate cellular picture, will confirm the diagnosis. The diagnosis of suspected tissue can, at times, be difficult owing to the relative paucity of Sternberg-Reed cells within diseased tissue. Sternberg-Reed cells are thought to arise from mononuclear reticulum cells which are found as a normal component of lymphatic tissue and ordinarily are associated with the connective tissue network

found within a lymph node. Microscopic examination of a disease node not only reveals Sternberg-Reed cells, but predominant cellular elements also may include normal lymphocytes, histiocytes, occasional eosinophils, plasma cells, polymorphonuclear leukocytes, a hyperplasia of reticulum cells and varying degrees of collagen deposits.[5] As Hodgkin's disease progresses, the normal nodal architecture is destroyed and concurrent disease infiltration of the node capsule occurs.

The histopathology of lymph nodes invaded by Hodgkin's disease can be classified into four distinct tissue types: lymphocyte-predominant, nodular sclerosis, mixed cellularity and lymphocyte-depleted. The differences between each tissue type are described in Table 39.1. Lymphocyte-predominant offers the best prognosis with nodular sclerosing offering the second best prognosis. Mixed cellularity is considered to have a poor prognosis, and lymphocyte-depleted has the poorest prognosis.[6] It has been shown that as the relative number of Sternberg-Reed cells within diseased nodes increases, the tissue type prognosis becomes poorer.

The establishment of Hodgkin's disease as a neoplastic process brought about questions as to whether the disease was unicentric or multicentric in origin. Some cases suggested a unicentric origin because the disease could be localized to a single lymph node or lymph node chain. Other cases suggested a multicentric origin since they presented with involvement of virtually all lymph nodes. It is now agreed that Hodgkin's disease is probably unicentric in origin and spreads via contiguous lymph node chains and hematogenous routes. The natural course of the disease can be followed rather well, and it has been observed that the disease generally spreads caudad rather than cephalad, suggesting a spread against the normal direction of lymph flow. Characteristically, 60 to 80% of the patients present with complaints of unilateral lymphadenopathy either in the cervical or supraclavicular region. The disease may spread in a retrograde fashion from cervical and supraclavicular regions to adjacent nodes in the ipsilateral axilla. If unchecked, the disease eventually may spread to lymph nodes in the chest or abdomen, including the spleen. This may open a portal for the disease to invade

TABLE 39.1

Histological Subtypes Found in Hodgkin's Disease

---

1. Lymphocyte predominance
   A. Lymphocytic and/or histiocytic diffuse
      Sinusoids of lymph nodes become filled with lymphocytic cells and general normal architecture of the lymph node becomes obscured; this picture does not occur uniformly throughout the node and normal foci may be found; the lymph node capsule is not invaded by lymphocytes in early stages of the disease
   B. Nodular proliferative type
      This form differs little from the diffuse form except for the tendency of the lymphocytic cells to be placed into poorly defined large and closely arranged nodules
2. Nodular sclerosis
      This tissue type is characterized by formation of bands of connective tissue which intercommunicate and separate the cellular and necrotic areas into islands
3. Mixed cellularity
      Presents a picture between lymphocyte predominance and lymphocyte-depleted and is characterized by having a variable number of lymphocytes and the presence of neutrophils, eosinophils and plasma cells
4. Lymphocyte-depleted
   A. Diffuse fibrosis
      Characterized by widespread disorderly fibrosis with depletion of lymphoid cells and eventually of all other cellular elements
   B. Reticular type
      Lesions in this category have no significant characteristics other than a predominance of Sternberg-Reed cells to distinguish them from other diffuse, fibrotic, mixed or even nodular sclerotic lesions

---

such visceral organs as the liver as well as invasion of the bone marrow. There are some cases of Hodgkin's disease where spread of the disease is in a noncontiguous fashion and as the disease progresses, certain contiguous lymph node chains are skipped and remain uninvolved. These cases of noncontiguous dissemination probably reflect hematogenous spread and represent a poor prognosis since the anatomic involvement of the disease can not be predicted. Noncontiguous spread is common with the lymphocyte-depleted and mixed cellularity varieties and may be a major reason for the poorer prognosis of these two histological subtypes.

STAGING

After Hodgkin's disease has been diagnosed and the cell type established, the patient must be staged; that is, the anatomic extent of the disease must be determined. Just as the histopathology was one factor in determining prognosis, so too is staging. Staging is important in order to identify and treat all involved areas, since untreated areas may continue to serve as a source for the dissemination of the disease. There are four agreed upon stages of Hodgkin's disease: I, II, III and IV (Table 39.2). As the disease progresses from stage I to stage IV, the prognosis becomes poorer. The presence of symptoms within the individual stages of Hodgkin's disease reflects a poorer prognosis than if no symptoms were present. The clinical symptoms of Hodgkin's disease are general rather than specific; they are unexplained

TABLE 39.2

Ann Arbor Classification for the Staging of Hodgkin's Disease[a]

Stage I–	Disease involvement of a single contiguous lymph node region (I) or of a single localized extralymphatic organ or site (I_E) on the same side of the diaphragm
Stage II–	Disease involvement of two or more contiguous lymph node regions on the same side of the diaphragm (II) or localized involvement of an extralymphatic organ or site and of one or more lymph node regions on the same side of the diaphragm (II_E); an optional recommendation is that the number of node regions involved be indicated by a subscript (e.g., II_3)
Stage III–	Disease involvement of lymph node regions on both sides of the diaphragm (III) which may also be accompanied by localized involvement of an extralymphatic organ or site (III_E) or by involvement of the spleen (III_S), or both (III_{SE})
Stage IV–	Diffuse or disseminated disease involvement of one or more extralymphatic organs or tissues with or without associated lymph node enlargement; the extralymphatic sites of involvement should be identified by symbols

---

[a]Each stage subdivided into A (asymptomatic) and B (symptomatic). Symptoms are—(a) weight loss greater than 10 per cent of body weight, (b) unexplained fever with temperature above 38°C (100.4°F) and (c) night sweats.

weight loss of more than 10% of the body weight, unexplained fever with temperature above 38°C (100.4°F) and night sweats. A patient may experience additional symptoms such as pruritis or alcohol-induced pain, but they do not correlate with severity of disease and, therefore, are not considered in the staging evaluation.

The anatomic landmark which has key significance in the staging of Hodgkin's disease is the diaphragm, which is the reference point from which the extent or stage of Hodgkin's disease is measured. If the disease is confined to lymph nodes only on one side (above or below) of the diaphragm, the disease is considered to be localized and the prognosis is better than if the disease were more disseminated and present on both sides of the diaphragm.

Clinical staging (CS) involves an intensive compilation of data obtained from the patient's history, physical examination and results of laboratory tests and procedures, the purpose of which is to determine the "clinical" extent of disease short of a diagnostic laparotomy. A detailed patient history is obtained, making note of the presence or absence of unexplained fevers, night sweats and weight loss. Other important historical facts include a familial history of Hodgkin's disease or other neoplastic diseases. A complete and thorough physical examination must be performed, giving particular attention to areas where lymphadenopathy usually occurs, areas of bone tenderness and the size of the liver and spleen.

The laboratory tests and procedures which are conducted are designed to detect any clinical abnormality which may implicate a specific organ or organ system invaded by Hodgkin's disease. The necessary laboratory tests are as follows: a complete hematological work-up consisting of a complete blood count, white blood cell count and differential, platelet count, hemoglobin and/or hematocrit; evaluation of renal function including routine urinalysis, serum creatinine, blood urea nitrogen and creatinine clearance; evaluation of liver function by measuring albumin, bilirubin, lactic dehydrogenase, serum glutamic oxaloacetic transaminase and alkaline phosphatase (elevated alkaline phosphatase also may imply bone disease and require further work-up). Radiological studies which are advised consist of: chest x-ray with posteroanterior and lateral views and

tomograms if the chest x-ray is suspicious; views of the skeletal system to include the thoracic and lumbar vertebra, the pelvis, proximal extremities and other areas of bone pain and tenderness; a bilateral lower extremity lymphangiogram for visualization of deeper lymph nodes in the abdomen which may be diseased; and an intravenous pyelogram, if indicated, for visualization of the renal system and detection of any obstruction or organ displacement. Required evaluation procedures in the presence of suspected organ involvement with Hodgkin's disease include scintiscans of osseous tissue, liver, spleen and bone marrow biopsy by needle or open surgical method. Other laboratory tests and diagnostic procedures are indicated if involvement of Hodgkin's disease is suspected in other organs.[7]

Clinical staging, therefore, serves only as a means of estimating disease extent or identifying organs or organ systems in which disease is suspected, but does not serve to diagnose Hodgkin's disease within organs. Positive diagnosis can be made only by tissue biopsy and subsequent identification of Sternberg-Reed cells within lymphatic or nonlymphatic tissue.

Pathological staging (PS) serves as a scheme to diagnose Hodgkin's disease in various tissues which have been implicated by the clinical staging procedure. Pathological staging involves biopsying and examining microscopically lymphatic tissue, organs and other tissue clinically evidenced as being diseased. Exploratory laparotomy is the surgical procedure employed. During laparotomy, various biopsies of abdominal lymph nodes, bone and liver may be undertaken.

Adequate tissue biopsies are important since tissue diagnosis of Hodgkin's disease depends on the presence of the sparse Sternberg-Reed cells, and tissue which is clinically evidenced as diseased will not always show pathological evidence of disease.

The abdominal lymph nodes which should be biopsied include: an upper periaortic node; a splenic hilar node (located on the fissure of the gastric surface of the spleen where vessels and nerves enter); an iliac node (located on the expansive superior portion of the pelvis); a porta hepatis node (located on the transverse fissure of the visceral surface of the liver where portal vein and hepatic artery enter and hepatic ducts leave); and a mesenteric node. It is important that a porta hepatis node and a mesenteric node be biopsied because lymph nodes in these two regions can not be clinically evidenced as diseased (they are not visualized in a lower extremity lymphangiogram), and later radiation therapy normally does not include these anatomic areas within radiation fields or "ports." If Hodgkin's disease is present in these areas, the radiation ports may have to be extended to include them or chemotherapy used instead, if appropriate ports can not be designed.

Tissue sampling of the liver should include two needle biopsies (one in each lobe of the liver) and a wedge biopsy where a 2-cm cube of hepatic tissue is excised. Bone marrow biopsy, if indicated, is performed on the iliac crest region of the pelvis by obtaining a core of osseous tissue via a needly biopsy or an open surgical biopsy where an actual piece of bone is removed.

In addition to the various biopsies, a splenectomy also is performed during the laparotomy procedure. There are three reasons for removal of the spleen: disease involvement of the spleen may be impossible to determine grossly and may be found only if the spleen is carefully sectioned; the spleen overlies the left kidney and is adjacent to the left lung; if radiation therapy to the spleen were necessary, this would increase the risk of radiation-induced nephritis and/or pneumonitis; and the spleen is involved with normal destruction of formed blood elements, and patients receiving radiation therapy and/or chemotherapy will have falling blood counts because of bone marrow toxicities; this will be exacerbated if blood elements are sequestered and destroyed by the spleen.

The findings from pathological staging procedures are subscripted by symbols indicating the tissue sampled. The results of histopathological examination are indicated by + when positive for Hodgkin's disease and by - when negative. The recommended abbreviations used in the pathological staging procedure are as follows:

N+ or N- for lymph node positive or negative for disease by biopsy.

H+ or H- for liver positive or negative by liver biopsy.

S+ or S- for spleen positive or negative following splenectomy.

L+ or L- for lung positive or negative by biopsy.

M+ or M- for bone marrow positive or negative by biopsy or smear.

P+ or P- for pleura positive or negative by biopsy or cytological examination.

O+ or O- for osseous tissue positive or negative by biopsy.

D+ or D- for dermal tissue positive or negative by biopsy.

Examples of staging classification utilizing results of CS and PS procedures are given in Table 39.3.

The data collected over the past several years have revealed some interesting statistics regarding the correlation of the clinical stage of Hodgkin's disease with histological tissue type. Review of the literature has shown that patients presenting with the lymphocyte-predominant variety have a strong association with clinical stages I and II while the lymphocyte-depleted variety is seen mainly in patients presenting

TABLE 39.3
Staging Classification Examples

CS IA PS I$_{S- H- N- M-}$	Implies clinical stage I without symptoms and pathological stage I without disease involvement of the spleen, liver, additional lymph nodes and bone marrow
CS IIA$_3$ PS III$_{S+ N+ H- M-}$	Implies clinical stage II without symptoms and three lymph node regions involved; pathological stage III with spleen and additional lymph nodes positive for disease; liver and bone marrow negative for disease
CS IIIB PS IV$_{H+ M- S-}$	Implies clinical stage III with symptoms; pathological stage IV with liver positive for disease; bone marrow and spleen negative for disease
CS IVB$_{L H}$ PS IV$_{H+ M-}$	Implies clinical stage IV with symptoms and clinical evidence for lung and liver disease; pathological stage IV with liver positive for disease and bone marrow negative for disease; lung involvement was only documented clinically, but not pathologically

with clinical stages III and IV. The mixed cellularity variety occurs in all clinical stages of the disease without any strong correlations. The nodular sclerosis variety is seen primarily in patients presenting with clinical stage II disease and is the one histological subtype which presents with a distinctive anatomic pattern of distribution, namely, a predilection to involve the lower cervical lymph nodes and mediastinum.[8] The lymphocyte-predominant, lymphocyte-depleted and mixed cellularity varieties exhibit a variable propensity for anatomic involvement when compared within the same clinical stage. Contrasting the other three histological subtypes, nodular sclerosis occurs primarily in females within all age groups. As previously mentioned, lymphocyte predominance has the best prognosis with nodular sclerosis having the second best prognosis; however, studies have shown that the prognostic advantage of nodular sclerosis diminishes as the disease advances to stages III and IV in contrast to lymphocyte predominance which retains its prognostic favorability as the disease progresses to these later stages. The poorer prognosis for lymphocyte-depleted and mixed cellularity remains constant in all stages of the disease.

CLINICAL COURSE AND COMPLICATIONS

Hodgkin's disease usually manifests itself initially with patients noting lymphadenopathy and often the Hodgkin's disease symptoms of fever, night sweats and weight loss. Patients presenting with these symptoms frequently will undergo a short course of antibiotic therapy since some infectious process frequently will be suspected by the attending physician. Since the symptoms will not subside with antibiotic therapy, patients may be hospitalized and further work-up will reveal Hodgkin's disease as the underlying problem. Routine chest X-rays may show an enlarged mediastinum with some displacement or obstruction of the trachea and/or esophagus due to an impinging mass. The patient may be symptomatic and may complain of dysphagia or coughing.

The lymphadenopathy of Hodgkin's disease is usually a painless enlargement of peripheral lymph nodes (cervical, axillary and inguinal) presenting with or without additional symptoms. Rapid enlargement of the lymph nodes,

however, may cause them to become tender. In the early stages of the disease, the affected lymph nodes are discrete and easily palpable, but as the disease progresses, these nodes become matted.[9] If the lymphadenopathy is present initially above the diaphragm, the disease, if unchecked, can be expected to spread to areas below the diaphragm by dissemination via contiguous lymphatics. Disease presentation below the diaphragm, if checked, in most cases will remain below the diaphragm since dissemination to areas above the diaphragm would suggest a cephalad spread which is not generally characteristic of Hodgkin's disease.

The classic symptoms of Hodgkin's disease include fever, night sweats, and weight loss. It has been postulated that the fever may be a consequence of some immune response to the disease and may be brought about by pyrogens released from lysed granulocytes involved in the immune mechanism. Whatever the cause, the fever is fluctuating in nature and frequently responds to salicylates or acetaminophen. In refractory cases, indomethacin has been found effective in reducing the fever of patients who do not respond to the usual antipyretics.[10] The etiology of the weight loss and night sweats remains unclear, but it is noted that the night sweats can, at times, be so profuse as to warrant the changing of bed clothes several times during the night. There is one unique symptom experienced by a minority of the patients, and this is alcohol-induced pain. This phenomenon is characterized by severe pain localized in anatomic areas of active disease after the patient has ingested alcohol; the pain eventually subsides as the alcohol is metabolized.[11] The alcohol intolerance syndrome has remained an enigma, for no etiology has been found.

Stage IV Hodgkin's disease is characterized by invasion of the disease into various organs or organ systems culminating in a variety of complications and clinical problems. A frequent physical and radiographic finding of stage IV patients is invasion of the disease into the pleura. This causes the pleural tissue to leak fluid into the pleural cavity and results in accumulation of fluid known as a pleural effusion. The patient complains of difficult or labored breathing (dyspnea), and he has severe dyspnea upon exertion. Treatment involves repeated removal of this pleural fluid (thoracentesis). If the fluid continues to accumulate, this may necessitate the intrapleural instillation of sclerosing agents such as quinacrine.

Invasion of osseous tissue may cause local destruction of bone (osteolytic lesions) or may cause local osseous reactions characterized by the formation of new bone tissue (osteoblastic lesions). This bone destruction and local attempts at repair will alter the clinical chemistry of the patient by causing an elevation of serum alkaline phosphatase. Bone involvement will lead to severe bone pain in the patient, and palliative relief can be obtained by local radiation.

Hepatic involvement is not uncommon in stage IV Hodgkin's disease and may manifest itself by showing an elevation of serum hepatic enzymes, elevated bilirubin and suspicious liver scans. A notable observation found in staging procedures is that hepatic presence of Hodgkin's disease almost always is found with attendant disease in the spleen, but the converse is not true.[12,13]

Some disease involvement may occur in the gastrointestinal (GI) tract and renal system, but it is rare; symptoms can be related to organ displacement or obstruction. Neurological complications occur in 12% of the cases and consist mainly of spinal cord compression, peripheral nerve palsies and cranial nerve palsies.[14]

One notable finding that has been reported is that some Hodgkin's disease patients may be free of their disease for several years only to present again with a diagnosis of leukemia.[15] This observation has stirred some debate. It is uncertain whether the leukemia is a normal manifestation of the disease, now being noted owing to longer survival rates of Hodgkin's disease patients, or if the leukemia is indeed induced by prior radiation or drug therapy. It is known that high dose radiation can induce leukemia, but to accuse radiation therapy as the sole cause of subsequent leukemia is still conjectural.

Infectious complications have a high incidence in Hodgkin's disease patients, especially in the later stages of their disease. These patients have a great tendency toward infections because, as a manifestation of their disease, they are immunologically deficient. This deficiency is not clearly understood, but it has been noted that some of these patients are unable to react to various intradermal antigens such as mumps and chemical agents such as dinitrochlorobenzene (DNCB); patients unable to react to dermal antigens are termed anergic. A patient with Hodgkin's disease even may have active tuberculosis but may be unreactive to a tuberculin skin test. This finding shows that there exists some cellular immunological deficiency, since a delayed immunological reaction (characteristic of dermal antigens) is mediated by cells, unlike an immediate immunological response which is mediated by antibodies. Normal antibody formation is found in Hodgkin's disease except in the terminal state. Also important to note is that this delayed immunological reactivity may be present in early stages of the disease but may disappear as the disease progresses.

Tuberculosis was the major infection attending patients with Hodgkin's disease but is to a lesser degree now because of improved chemotherapy of tuberculosis. Bacteria still remain the most common cause of infection, but recently viruses such as herpes zoster, herpes simplex and cytomegalovirus (CMV) have been recognized to cause infection in these patients. Systemic fungal infections such as actinomycosis, nocardiosis, histoplasmosis, cryptococcosis, candidiasis and aspergillosis and the protozoal infection toxoplasmosis also have an unusually high incidence of infecting Hodgkin's disease patients.

THERAPY

The treatment of Hodgkin's disease centers mainly around radiation therapy and/or chemotherapy. Surgery, although useful in the management of some other malignancies, does not play a role directly in the treatment of Hodgkin's disease and is employed primarily in staging and diagnostic procedures. Therapy of Hodgkin's disease is aimed at eliminating all clinical signs and symptoms of the disease. If all symptomatic and objective parameters for monitoring the disease resolve (approach normal), the disease is considered inactive, and the patient is said to be in "remission." If symptoms or abnormal objective parameters recur, the disease is considered again present, and the patient is said to be in "relapse." Effective therapy of Hodgkin's disease is a highly controversial topic and several research centers around the country are evaluating radiation therapy, chemotherapy and various combinations of both in the treatment of the different stages of Hodgkin's disease.

Stage I and II disease is very amenable to radical radiation therapy (radical implying high doses of radiation with curative intent) because in these stages the disease is present in a few well defined focal areas, not disseminated, and it can be effectively treated with radiation of involved and adjacent lymph nodes. Some investigators, however, are subjecting stage I and II patients initially to radiation therapy followed by chemotherapy and have found these patients to have a lesser incidence of relapse than those patients treated with radiation alone.[16]

Stage IV disease is not well suited for radiation therapy since sites of the disease in this stage may be so numerous and diffuse that localized radiation can not be carried out effectively. Parenchymal organs can not tolerate curative doses of radiation, and the presence of Hodgkin's disease in these areas precludes the use of radical radiation. Stage IV disease is, therefore, treated primarily with systemic chemotherapy which has access to all sites of disease. "Spot" radiation is also used in stage IV disease for palliative treatment to anatomic areas of disease involvement not responding to chemotherapy and causing pain, tenderness or obstruction.

The therapy of Stage III patients is not well defined and is debatable among clinicians. Accepted therapy has been to treat all stage III patients with radical radiation therapy. However, recent findings reported by some researchers have shown that patients with stage IIIA disease will do well (in terms of lesser incidence of relapse) when treated with radiation therapy while patients with stage IIIB disease will do poorly. From these findings, it has been suggested that stage IIIA disease should be treated like stage I or II disease utilizing radiation therapy alone or radiation therapy followed by chemotherapy, and that stage IIIB disease should be treated like stage IV disease using only chemotherapy with palliative doses of radiation therapy.[17]

RADIATION THERAPY

The use of radiation has been employed in treating Hodgkin's disease since the early 1900's when it was shown that the disease responded to small doses of x-irradiation, although a response of only temporary benefit. These early attempts were rather crude since the radiation did not penetrate to the tumor but delivered its maximal effect on the skin. The 1950's brought about advances in equipment (use of Co^{60} and linear accelerators for clinical use) so that megavoltage radiation could be given, increasing the penetration and dose rate of radiation with skin-sparing effect. These devices allow the practical use of large fields exposing entire lymph node regions to radiation in the range of 3,500 to 4,000 rads ("rad" stands for radiation absorbed dose and equals 100 ergs per g tissue). Radiation therapy essentially has the same effect on cellular biochemistry as do the alkylating agents employed in chemotherapy. Deoxyribonucleic acid (DNA) replication is prevented by interfering with cross links necessary for the double helix integrity of the DNA molecule. Rapidly proliferating tissue, characteristic of malignancies, is especially radiosensitive owing to constant DNA production necessary for cell division. The epithelial lining of the GI tract also is rapidly dividing tissue, and frequently encountered side effects with radiation therapy are radiation-induced pharyngitis, esophagitis and gastroenteritis. The rapid production of cells in the bone marrow also makes this site very susceptible to radiation-induced bone marrow suppression. It is, therefore, important that vital, uninvolved organs and viscera be shielded during radiation therapy to minimize radiation-induced toxicities.

Radiation techniques in treating Hodgkin's disease also are debatable and differ in various treatment centers. In stage I and II disease, tumorcidal doses of radiation are given to diseased nodes over a period of 4 to 6 weeks and radiation also is administered prophylactically to areas uninvolved with disease.[17] The controversy centers on which uninvolved areas should be irradiated. Extended field radiation therapy involves irradiating all localized areas of disease and uninvolved adjacent areas. Some centers will irradiate all lymph nodes, contiguous or not, above the diaphragm in the presence of stage I or II disease above the diaphragm; this technique is known as radiation to the upper mantle. Stage I and II disease below the diaphragm will receive radiation to all abdominal and inguinal nodes. This technique is known as an inverted "Y," owing to the anatomic pattern formed by the lymph nodes below the diaphragm. Total nodal radiation therapy involves irradiating diseased nodes and prophylactic irradiation of all other nodes in the body. As an example, if stage I or II disease were localized in the cervical area, total nodal irradiation would involve treating all lymph node regions above the diaphragm (cervical, supra- and infraclavicular, axillary and mediastinal) and lymph node regions below the diaphragm (periaortic, retroperitoneal, inguinal and splenic regions) with tumorcidal doses. Clinical trials have shown that stage I and II disease has a lesser incidence of relapse when treated with total nodal radiation therapy compared to localized and extended field radiation therapy.[17] Clinical trials have also shown that patients with stage IIIA disease should be treated with at least total nodal radiation therapy.[17]

CHEMOTHERAPY

Malignant growths are characterized by rapidly proliferating tissues which synthesize and assimilate DNA quickly for cell division and growth. Chemotherapy is not selective against malignant growths because cytotoxic effects also are exerted against normal tissue whose rates of proliferation parallel that of the malignancy: bone marrow elements, GI epithelial cells and cells of hair follicles.

The use of chemotherapy in the treatment of Hodgkin's disease relies upon using combinations of drugs rather than single drugs. This approach is true for many malignancies. Combination chemotherapy employs drugs with different mechanisms of action which attack rapidly proliferating cells at different stages of cell replication. This allows the use of lower doses of individual drugs. The resulting toxicities are varied owing to the different drugs employed but are lower in magnitude than if high doses of a single agent were used.[18]

Combination chemotherapy also minimizes the emergence of resistant malignant cell lines which are refractory to drug therapy. A number of cellular mechanisms may be involved in drug resistance: altered drug metabolism, cell impermeability to the active compound, elevations of drug inhibitory enzymes and increased activity of cellular repair.[18] Drugs in combination attack the malignant cell at different stages

of the cell cycle making it more difficult for the cell population to acquire multiple drug resistance than if only a single drug were used (this concept is analogous to antibiotic therapy utilizing combinations to prevent emergence of resistant bacterial strains).

The scheduling of combination chemotherapy is important. Drug doses ideally should be administered at a time when malignant cells are actively synthesizing and assimilating DNA components so that maximal cell kill can occur. Chemotherapy should continue at specified time intervals to destroy any newly formed malignant cells and keep the total number of malignant cells at a level where clinical signs of disease are not evident. An example can illustrate this facet of multiple drug therapy.

Assume that a patient with disseminated Hodgkin's disease has 10^{16} malignant cells in his body. If a single drug is 99.9999% effective in killing the malignant cells, then 10^{10} malignant cells still remain after therapy. Increasing the dose of the drug will not significantly increase the percentage of kill (no drug is 100% effective). It will, however, increase the risk of drug toxicity while not further suppressing the emergence of resistant malignant cell strains. A second drug, with a different mode of action, which is say 99.999% effective may then be administered, and the number of malignant cells would drop to 10^5. Theoretically, the therapy could be continued with other drugs until the number of malignant cells remaining is 0, but, in truth, this never happens since toxicities occur before the malignant cell population approaches 0. Drug therapy should continue in intermittent doses to maintain the malignant cell population below some point where the disease is not manifest.

The drug combination which has been very successful in obtaining the induction of remissions in Hodgkin's disease is MOPP (mechlorethamine or Mustargen, vincristine or Oncovin, prednisone and procarbazine).[19] MOPP also has been used as maintenance therapy during the remission state to prolong remission.[19] Alternate choice to MOPP therapy presently being evaluated for remission induction is COP (cyclophosphamide, Oncovin and prednisone).[19] Other drug combinations currently being evaluated include new combinations of established chemotherapeutic agents and newer investigational drugs.

The classes of antineoplastic drugs used in

the treatment of Hodgkin's disease are outlined in Table 39.4. The mechanisms of action of the various antineoplastic agents are as follows:[20]

Alkylating Agents

These drugs attack functional groups on the various purine and pyrimidine bases interfering with necessary cross linking between the two strands of DNA. This prevents DNA replication and transcription of ribonucleic acid (RNA). Alkylating agents are considered radiomimetic since the chromosome damage incurred, when examined microscopically, resembles the damage caused by radiation.

Vinca Alkaloids

Two alkaloids, vincristine (VCR) and vinblastine (VLB), isolated from the periwinkle plant (*Vinca rosea*) have been used in combination chemotherapy of Hodgkin's disease. VLB has been used in remission induction regimens when the disease has become refractory to regimens employing alkylating agents. VCR has a similar spectrum of clinical activity as VLB, but one important distinction between these two drugs is that Hodgkin's disease appears not to have cross resistance between them. VCR has relatively little myelosuppression, its outstanding side effect being neurotoxicity manifested by peripheral paresthesias and numbness, loss of deep tendon reflexes, and constipation due to autonomic nervous neuromuscular toxicity. Because of this last side effect, patients who received VCR therapy should be maintained on stool softeners.

The mechanism of action of the vinca alkaloids is unknown, but they have been observed to cause an arrest of cell division during metaphase; this arrest of cell division is also characteristic of colchicine and its derivatives.

Adrenocorticosteroids

Drugs in this class are employed in very high doses (for prednisone, 40 mg per m^2 of body surface area per day or higher) when used in the treatment of Hodgkin's disease. The mechanism of action of these drugs in Hodgkin's disease therapy is unknown but resides in lympholytic effects and the ability to supress mitosis. Side effects observed are typical of corticosteroid therapy (*e.g.,* fluid retention, electrolyte imbalance and ulcerogenic possibilities).

Methylhydrazine Derivatives

Procarbazine is the sole drug in this new class of antineoplastic agents which has found application in the treatment of Hodgkin's disease. The mechanism of action is not clearly understood, but the drug is believed to undergo auto-oxidation *in vivo* resulting in the formation of hydrogen peroxide. The hydrogen peroxide then presumably interacts with DNA, preventing cross linkage. The drug is also a weak monoamine oxidase inhibitor. Therapeutic incompatabilities with alcohol, similar to disulfiram type reactions, have been observed.

Nitrosoureas

All the drugs in this class are under investigation in treating neoplastic disease. The prototype which has shown activity against Hodgkin's disease is BCNU (1, 3-bis—(β-chloroethyl)—1—nitrosourea). This drug has a mechanism of action similar to the alkylating agents and is under evaluation at some centers as a maintenance drug for Hodgkin's disease while patients are in remission. The most outstanding toxicity which has been observed to date with BCNU is myelosuppression.

PROGNOSIS

Hodgkin's disease once was thought of as a rapidly fatal disease, but statistics compiled from the past several years are not so bleak. Institutions engaged in the research and treatment of Hodgkin's disease consistently are reporting longer survival rates for patients in all stages of their disease. Data have shown that many patients with stage I and II disease can be expected to survive 20 years or longer and approach a point in time where they could be considered "cured" of their disease. The prognosis of stage III and IV disease, although not as good as that of stage I and II, also is steadily improving to the point where survival in some patients can be expected to be 5 years and beyond.[21] Advances in therapy have allowed many patients to remain clinically free of their

TABLE 39.4
Drugs Currently Used in Treatment of Hodgkin's Disease

Pharmacological Class	Drug Name	Mechanism of Action	Side Effects and Outstanding Toxicities
Alkylating agents	Cyclophosphamide	Requires *in vivo* activation by hepatic enzymes; attacks functional groups on purine and pyrimidine bases preventing DNA cross linking necessary for DNA replication and RNA transcription	Nausea and vomiting Alopecia Myelosuppression Drug-induced hemorrhagic cystitis
	Mechlorethamine	Same as for cyclophosphamide, except does not require *in vivo* activation	Nausea and vomiting Pain at injection site Alopecia Myelosuppression
Vinca alkaloids	Vincristine	Unknown exactly; observed to disrupt mitosis by interfering with spindle formation in metaphase	Neurotoxicity causing peripheral neuropathies and constipation Alopecia
	Vinblastine	Same as vincristine	Myelosuppression Neurotoxicity (but less than vincristine)
Adrenocorticosteroids	Prednisone Prednisolone	Unknown exactly; observed to have lympholytic effects and interference with mitosis	Fluid retention Electrolyte imbalance Ulcerogenic Adrenal dysfunction Psychoses
Methylhydrazines	Procarbazine	Unknown exactly; believed to auto-oxidize with formation of hydrogen peroxide which exerts cytotoxic effects	Nausea and vomiting Myelosuppression Central nervous system toxicity Dermatitis
Nitrosoureas (investigational)	1, 3-bis-(β-chloroethyl)-1-nitrosourea (BCNU)	Same as alkylating agents	Nausea and vomiting Pain at injection site Myelosuppression

disease for years and have decreased relapse rates during the first 5 years after initial therapy to 50% for patients with stage I and II disease and 70% for patients with stage III and IV disease. It has been observed also that 90% of patients who do relapse will do so within 3 to 4 years after initial therapy and only infrequently does disease recur after 5 years of freedom from clinical signs of the disease.[22]

Cure for Hodgkin's disease sometimes is discussed in the literature, but this does not imply a state where all microscopic foci of disease are eradicated. Cure, as discussed in literature, relates to a "statistical cure" which states that after a certain period of time—perhaps a decade—there remains a population of patients whose death rate from all causes is similar to that of a normal population of the same age and sex constitution.[22]

CONCLUSION

Hodgkin's disease is a malignant lymphoma which originates in the lymphoreticular system, disseminates via contiguous lymphatics and possibly the blood stream to other lymph nodes, and if unchecked, eventually will invade organ systems and bone marrow. The prognosis and treatment of the disease are related to histopathology of diseased lymph nodes and the anatomic extent of the disease determined by staging procedures. Available therapy relying on radiation therapy and chemotherapy or judicious combinations of both has greatly improved the outlook and length of survival for patients, but 3,400 deaths per year in the United States are still attributed to Hodgkin's disease.

Therapeutic concepts of Hodgkin's disease involve an understanding of the diagnostic and staging procedures and the rationale behind the available modes of treatment. Prospects for the future include new chemotherapeutic agents and combinations of both new and old antineoplastic drugs with minimization of attendant toxicities. Advances in diagnostic procedures promise to locate disease presence more accurately and efficiently. Improvements in radiation therapy and therapeutic plans employing radiation therapy and combination chemotherapy also promise more effective treatment. The future also holds a better understanding and insight into the nature of the Hodgkin's disease itself.

REFERENCES

1. Williams, W. J., Beutler, E., Erslev, A. J., and Rundles, R. W. (editors): Hematology, p. 829. McGraw-Hill Book Co., New York, 1972.
2. Williams, W. J., Beutler, E., Erslev, A. J., and Rundles, R. W. (editors): Hematology, p. 901. McGraw-Hill Book Co., New York, 1972.
3. Vianna, N. J., Greenwald, P., Brady, J., Palan, A. K., Swork, A., Mauro, J., and Davies, J. N. P.: Hodgkin's disease: cases with features of a community outbreak. Ann. Intern. Med., 77: 169, 1972.
4. Anderson, W. A. D.: Pathology, Ed. 6, p. 1325. C. V. Mosby Co., St. Louis, 1971.
5. Anderson, W. A. D.: Pathology, Ed. 6, p. 1325. C. V. Mosby Co., St. Louis, 1971.
6. Lukes, R. J., Butler, J. J., and Hicks, E. B.: Natural history of Hodgkin's disease as related to its pathologic picture. Cancer, 19: 317, 1966.
7. Carbone, P. P., Kaplan, J. S., Musshoff, K., Smithers, D. W., and Tubiana, M.: Report of the committee on Hodgkin's disease staging classification. Cancer Res., 31: 1860, 1971.
8. Berard, C. W., Thomas, L. B., Axtell, L. M., Kruse, M., Newell, and Kagan, R.: The relationship of histopathological subtype to clinical stage of Hodgkin's disease of diagnosis. Cancer Res., 31: 1776, 1971.
9. Beeson, P. B., and McDermott, W. (editors): Cecil-Loeb Textbook of Medicine, Ed. 13, p. 1557. W. B. Saunders Co., Philadelphia, 1971.
10. Goodman, L. S., and Gilman, A. (editors): The Pharmacologic Basis of Therapeutics, Ed. 4, p. 338. The MacMillan Co., New York, 1970.
11. Beeson, P. B., and McDermott, W., (editors): Cecil-Loeb Textbook of Medicine, Ed. 13, p. 1558. W. B. Saunders Co., Philadelphia, 1971.
12. Kadin, M. E., Glatstein, E., and Dorfman, R. F.: Clinicopathologic studies of 117 untreated patients subject to laparotomy for the staging of Hodgkin's disease. Cancer, 27: 1277, 1971.
13. Wiernik, P. H., O'Connell, M. J., Abt, A., Kirschner, R., Murphy, W. L., Sutherland, J., and Sklansky, D. B.: Detection, incidence, and prognostic significance (abstract). In Symposium (with international participation): The Romania, May, 1973.
14. Beeson, P. B., and McDermott, W. (editors): Cecil-Loeb Textbook of Medicine, Ed. 13, p. 1558. W. B. Saunders Co., Philadelphia, 1971.
15. Ezdinli, E. Z., Sokal, J. E., Aungst, C. W., Kim, U., and Sandberg, A. A.: Myeloid leukemia in Hodgkin's disease: chromosomal abnormalities. Ann. Intern. Med., 71: 1097, 1969.
16. Moore, M. R., Bull, J. M., Jones, S. E., Rosenberg,

S. A., and Kaplan, H. S.: Sequential radiotherapy and chemotherapy in the treatment of Hodgkin's disease. Ann. Intern. Med., 77: 1, 1972.

17. Johnson, R. E.: Modern approaches to the radiotherapy of lymphoma. Semin. Hematol., 6: 357, 1969.

18. Cline, M. J.: Cancer chemotherapy In Major Problems in Internal Medicine, Vol. 1, p. 13, edited by L. H. Smith. W. B. Saunders Co., Philadelphia, 1971.

19. Gutterman, J., and Rodriguez, V.: Combination chemotherapy of advanced lymphoma. Milit. Med., 137: 255, 1972.

20. Goodman, L. S., and Gilman, A. (editors): The Pharmacologic Basis of Therapeutics, Ed. 4, p. 1344. The MacMillan Co., New York, 1970.

21. Tubiana, M., Attie, E., Flamant, R., Gerard-Marchant, R., and Hayat, M.: Prognostic factors in 454 cases of Hodgkin's disease. Cancer Res., 31: 1801, 1971.

22. Frei, E., and Gehan, E. A.: Definition of cure for Hodgkin's disease. Cancer Res., 31: 1828, 1971.

chapter 40

CARCINOMA OF THE BREAST

William R. Grove, B.S.
Clarence L. Fortner, M.S.

Breast cancer has become the most common malignancy among women in this country, with an estimated 90,000 new cases to be diagnosed during 1974. During this same year, approximately 33,000 women of all ages will die of this disease. The number of newly diagnosed cases of breast cancer per year has been steadily on the rise since 1935, while the mortality rate per population base has remained essentially constant.[1] This trend suggests that progress is being made slowly in this disease which claims more female victims between the ages of 40 and 44 than any other single disease. The most notable advances in the management of breast cancer have been in the areas of improved methods of diagnosis and increased public awareness. Intensive public education campaigns on the importance of self-examination and early diagnosis are being conducted by the American Cancer Society and the National Cancer Institute, and we should continue to realize their benefits in the years to come. In addition, studies are in progress evaluating new surgical and radiotherapeutic techniques and new chemotherapeutic agents alone and in combinations to improve the rate and duration of responses in breast cancer.

INCIDENCE

The risk of a woman developing breast cancer in the United States is about 1 in 15 during her lifetime.† Several factors have been identified, however, which influence one's chances of ever developing breast cancer. The two risk factors considered most significant are a family history of breast cancer and previous breast cancer in the contralateral breast. There is a genetic component involved in developing breast cancer, thereby imparting a greater risk to relatives, especially daughters and sisters of patients who have breast cancer. In fact, a 2- to 3-fold increased incidence has been demonstrated. More evidence of this is reflected in the fact that daughters of women who have breast cancer develop it 10 to 12 years earlier than their mothers. The second factor accepted as an increased risk factor is a past history of breast cancer. Women who are treated for breast cancer are candidates of developing cancer in the other breast at a rate 7 times the expected incidence.

A definite pattern is evident when age at diagnosis is compared against incidence. Breast cancer occurring under the age of 30 is rare and is nearly unheard of under the age of 15. Over 30, however, the incidence sharply rises with

The authors would like to express their gratitude to Dr. Peter H. Wiernik, Chief, Medical Oncology, Baltimore Cancer Research Center, National Cancer Institue, National Institutes of Health; Dr. Mark Green, Robert DeChristoforo, and Robert L. West for their thoughtful comments in reviewing the manuscript.

†Breast cancer does occur in males but is rare. Many of the principles described in this paper are applicable to male breast cancer. Owing to the magnitude of the problem of female breast cancer, further discussion of male breast cancer is beyond the scope of this paper.

age, levelling off slightly around the age of menopause. .This gives evidence of the influence hormones have in breast cancer.

Recognizing that these hormonal influences exist on breast tissue and the development of breast cancer, studies are in progress investigating what effect, if any, oral contraceptives may have on carcinogenesis. Because long term studies of significant numbers of premenopausal women are not yet available to evaluate adequately this carcinogenic potential, experts caution against the use of oral contraceptives in a particular population defined as high risk candidates. This includes women who have a positive family history of breast cancer, a previous history of cancer of the breast, gross cystic disease, recurrent chronic cystic mastitis or women who have had an abnormal or suspicious mammogram in the past. It should be noted, however, that there is no evidence to date linking an increased incidence of breast cancer to women who have taken oral contraceptives.

Several other variables have been identified which appear to place certain women in a higher risk category, although proof of this is lacking. The longer the total menstrual life is, the greater is the tendency for developing malignant breast disease. Women who reach menarche earlier and menopause later, thereby experiencing more menstrual cycles, are at greater risk. Women whose menstrual life is surgically ended through an oophorectomy years prior to their expected natural menopause develop breast cancer at a much reduced rate. Parity is a variable, as evidenced by the fact that childless women develop breast cancer with a greater incidence than do women who have borne children. A tendency also exists that the longer a women breast feeds her children the lower is her risk of developing breast cancer. The difficulty in evaluating these variables is that many of them are interrelated and do not lend themselves to independent analysis. In any event, a high risk population has been identified as women who have one of the first two following variables, plus one or more of the others: a positive family history of breast cancer, a previous history of malignant breast disease, a short (or nonexistent) history of breast feeding, few (or no) pregnancies and an age of 30 years or over.

ETIOLOGY

Intensive animal research has demonstrated that a virus particle is capable of causing mammary cancer in the mouse and in the monkey. The relationship between this discovery and the etiology of human breast cancer is unknown and is currently under investigation.

Adequate treatment requires knowledge of the pathological process involved in the development of breast cancer, whatever the etiology may be. A gradual process appears to affect breast epithelia diffusely, rather than at a single focus. The etiological agent responsible for the original hyperplastic transformation is unknown, as are the various factors associated with the direction the process takes. Cellular environment, particularly including supply of nutrition and growth factors, undoubtedly plays a role. The surrounding supportive connective tissue also may be affected by the pathological process. This means that microscopically involved breast tissue may exist some distance away from a breast tumor.

DIAGNOSIS

Approximately 95% of all patients with breast cancer first detect some breast abnormality themselves. The symptom most frequently found (75 to 80%) is a mass or lump and is usually found accidentally while bathing or dressing. Occasionally (10%), the presenting sign is a stabbing or aching pain. Other symptoms which are noticed less frequently are signs of nipple retraction (most notable when the arms are raised), spontaneous nipple discharge or areas of skin redness. Breast tissue undergoes cyclic hormonally influenced changes during the menstrual cycle. A breast mass which appears prior to menstruation and disappears afterward most likely is not a malignancy, especially in a young woman, but rather normal breast tissue. For this reason, women who practice breast self-examination should do so at approximately the same phase of their menstrual cycle each month.

One critical factor in the early diagnosis of breast cancer is the interval between the patient's first noticing some breast abnormality, nearly always a lump, and her seeking medical attention. In the period between 1915 and 1942, the average delay in seeking medical advice was 10.7 months. Between 1956 and 1967 it was 4.9 months.[2] A direct correlation of increased delay and increased axillary lymph node metastases is demonstrated in Table 40.1. It is seen that the earlier the diagnosis is made, the greater is the chance of limited disease. The increased public awareness which has resulted in a shorter period of patient delay is in no small way responsible for the general improved prognosis of breast cancer today.

The initial approach to evaluate a possible breast cancer is a careful and complete history and physical examination. Certain characteristics of a mass, such as size, shape, firmness, movability and tenderness can be determined by palpation. Along with the patient's history, these are frequently sufficient to suspect carcinoma which then can be confirmed by biopsy. Further diagnostic procedures may be performed, however, which can provide additional more specific information. It is important to realize that these additional methods work best when they complement each other. They are meant to identify areas of clinical suspicion which should be biopsied to obtain a histological diagnosis. No single method short of biopsy can diagnose unequivocally a breast malignancy.

Mammography is a commonly used procedure which employs the diagnostic role of x-rays to detect areas of increased density in breast tissue. It is much more sensitive than palpation and may detect densities which are, as yet, undetectable by palpation. Expertly done mammography can detect a cancer at least

2 years before it becomes clinically palpable.[3] Both false positive and false negative interpretations, however, do occur in 10 to 20% of mammographic studies. A recent refinement of this technique, called xeroradiography, allows greater resolution and involves less radiation exposure and should improve the results obtained by conventional mammography. For either of these two procedures, the breasts are positioned on a table to allow tangential x-ray exposures to be taken from various angles without exposing the rest of the body to radiation. The developed films are then interpreted for the presence of any abnormality.

The use of mammography as a mass screening tool has been investigated. One drawback that has emerged is that an unfavorable cost: benefit ratio has resulted. In a study of nearly 44,000 unselected women over 35 years of age, 69 carcinomas were detected by mammography during the initial examination, a rate of 1.6 per 1,000.[4] This is approximately a cost: benefit ratio of $22,000 per detected breast cancer, calculated from a cost of $35 per patient's mammogram. At the second annual screening in this study, 9 carcinomas detected in 13,361 patients reduce the return to 0.6/1,000, or about $59,000 per detected cancer. Economically speaking, the use of mammography as a mass screening tool for unselected women appears unfeasible. Its greatest contribution is in its use in high risk populations, such as those who have had a previous breast malignancy, those with a positive family history of breast cancer, those whose breasts are difficult to examine clinically and for further evaluation of a suspicious breast mass.

Another aid has been developed for the detection of breast cancer. Thermography is an entirely innocuous procedure which involves no radiation exposure and is based upon the detection of minute differences in temperature patterns in the skin overlying the breasts. A malignant mass with its increased vascularity and metabolism very often is as much as 1 or 2 °C warmer than surrounding tissue. Unfortunately, several nonmalignant conditions, such as fibrocystic disease, acute inflammation, abcesses and benign masses also may give rise to a positive thermogram. Similarly, false negatives have been noted. The venous pattern which is displayed is also important in the interpretation of

TABLE 40.1
Relationship of Delay in Seeking Medical Attention and Axillary Node Involvement

Length of Delay	Patients with More Than 3 Axillary Nodes Microscopically Involved
months	%
< 1	14
1-2	26
6-11	29
24-35	32

a thermogram. Asymmetrical patterns or changes in subsequent yearly thermograms may constitute a positive test. It is important to realize, however, that thermography can not and does not diagnose breast cancer. It does suggest the need for further investigation, either by mammography or biopsy, in patients with an abnormal result. Because of the absence of radiation and the less time and expense involved in thermography as compared to mammography, thermography may play an important role in the preliminary screening of large populations of patients for breast cancer.

These diagnostic aids mentioned are meant to select patients for biopsy who have some breast abnormality suggestive of a carcinoma. Microscopic examination of biopsy material is still the only method of absolutely diagnosing a breast malignancy.

Once the diagnosis of breast cancer is confirmed, the patient should undergo an extended diagnostic work-up to detect the presence of distant metastases. This is important in determining the stage of disease at initial presentation to eliminate women as candidates for potentially curative radical surgery who already have disseminated disease. Examination of the organs most frequently involved should include a chest x-ray, brain scan, bone scan and liver scan.

STAGING

The greatest single factor determining the fate of a patient with breast cancer is the extent of involvement, or stage of her disease, at the time of diagnosis. Breast cancer metastasizes from the primary tumor site by two routes. Tumor cells escape into the circulation and lodge in distant sites, providing entry for lung, liver, sketetal and brain metastasis among others. These tumor emboli may be present in the blood stream by the time the disease is first clinically evident, as demonstrated by Handley. Also, enormous numbers of these cells may be liberated during the trauma inflicted by surgery. The competency of the patient's defense mechanisms responsible for the destruction of these cells may be a critical factor in their ability to survive. The second route of tumor spread is through the lymphatic drainage of breast tissue to two primary lymph node chains, the axillary and the internal mammary

lymph nodes. Tumor cells reaching these lymph nodes should be filtered and destroyed by the body's defense mechanism, thereby preventing further spread. They may, however, proliferate in these nodes rather than be destroyed and allow release of cells which can involve the next higher node, etc. In this manner, the axillary and internal mammary lymph nodes retard the progress of the disease but become metastatic foci of tumor cells themselves. When this process has occurred for a sufficient period of time, the nodes become clinically enlarged and are palpable.

The location of the primary tumor has a direct anatomic relationship to the nodes which are likely to become involved. Thus, the internal mammary nodes are more likely to be involved if they are responsible for a greater proportion of the lymphatic drainage from the area of the primary tumor. The presence of involved lymph nodes at surgery serves as a prognostic indicator of survival. A precipitous fall in 10-year survival rates, as shown by Handley's study, Table 40.2, demonstrated the significance of lymph node involvement.[5] Two other factors that also relate to nodal involvement and survival are the size of the primary lesion and the number of involved lymph nodes. The larger the presenting tumor mass is, the greater the chance of nodal involvement. In one study, only 1/3 of all patients with primary lesions less than 3 cm in diameter had axillary node involvement, while ½ of the patients with a primary lesion greater than 3 cm in diameter had axillary involvement.[6] The number of nodes involved similarly plays a prognostic role.

TABLE 40.2
Relationship between Degree of Nodal Involvement and Survival

Degree of Nodal Involvement	Patients Alive and Well after 10 Years
	%
No nodes involved	67
Only axillary node(s) involved	41
Only internal mammary node(s) involved	37
Both axillary and internal mammary node(s) involved	6

The fewer the number of nodes involved the better the patient's chance of survival.[7] All of these interrelated factors concerning the size of the primary lesion and the presence and the extent of lymph node involvement serve to emphasize the importance of early diagnosis and treatment.

Documentation of extensive local breast involvement is important in the adequate staging of breast cancer, as it conveys a poorer prognosis. This may be evidenced by several clinically apparent signs. Extensive edema of the skin of the breast, called *peau d'orange* because of its characteristic orange skin-like pitting, is caused by tumor emboli blocking lymphatic drainage of the skin and subcutaneous tissues. Satellite nodules are multiple skin lesions resulting from direct infiltration of the tumor from the primary lesion which has spread along lymphatic channels to reach the skin. Skin ulceration is caused by direct growth of the primary lesion through breast tissue to the surface of the skin. This locally advanced stage is preceded by immobility of the skin over the tumor and localized areas of redness. Immobile fixation of the tumor to the chest wall is another sign of extensive local tumor involvement.

These criteria of lymph node involvement and local extension of disease are characteristics important in the staging procedure necessary in breast cancer. The course of therapy most beneficial to each patient is dependent upon the degree of advancement present at the time of diagnosis. For example, radical surgery would not be indicated in a patient presenting with evidence of distant metastases as it could not possibly provide a cure. From a research standpoint, staging is necessary to standardize collection of data, to evaluate therapy and to allow uniform end result reporting.

Several staging systems have been developed based on clinical and/or pathological findings at the time of diagnosis. One representative system is the Columbia Clinical Classification System,[8] Table 40.3.

Distant metastases result when tumor cells escape from the primary tumor site in the breast and travel by means of the circulatory system to another organ system where they lodge and proliferate. The most frequent sites of metastases from cancer of the breast are to the lungs, bones and liver, in that order, with

TABLE 40.3
Columbia Clinical Classification System for the Staging of Breast Cancer

Stage A	No skin edema, ulceration or solid fixation of tumor to chest wall; axillary nodes not clinically involved
Stage B	No skin edema, ulceration or solid fixation of tumor to chest wall; clinically involved nodes, but less than 2.5 cm in transverse diameter and not fixed to overlying skin or deeper structures of axilla
Stage C	Any one of grave signs of advanced breast carcinoma: 1. Edema of skin of limited extent (involving less than 1/3 of the skin over the breast) 2. Skin ulceration 3. Solid fixation of tumor to chest wall 4. Massive involvement of axillary lymph nodes (measuring 2.5 cm or more in transverse diameter) 5. Fixation of the axillary nodes to overlying skin or deeper structures of axilla
Stage D	All other patients with more advanced breast carcinoma, including: 1. A combination of any 2 or more of the 5 grave signs listed under stage C 2. Extensive edema of skin (involving more than 1/3 of the skin over the breast) 3. Satellite skin nodules 4. The inflammatory type of carcinoma 5. Clinically involved supraclavicular lymph nodes 6. Internal mammary metastases as evidenced by a parasternal tumor 7. Edema of the arm 8. Distant metastases

metastases also presenting in other organ systems, such as skin, brain, ovaries, adrenals and other sites less frequently. The reason for the high percentage of lung metastases in breast cancer, present in approximately 65% of autopsied cases, is that there are three routes of venous drainage from the breast to the lungs. The lungs, therefore, are the first organs exposed to many of the tumor emboli being disseminated into the circulation.

Lung metastases are diagnosed by the appearance of areas of increased density or nodules on chest x-ray. Patients are usually asymptomatic until these nodules either become grossly enlarged or produce an airway obstruction. Lung metastases may progress to the pleural cavity, the membrane-lined space which surrounds the lungs. When this occurs, fluid is produced and accumulates in this cavity and the patient becomes progressively more dyspneic. Removal of this fluid by thoracentesis produces symptomatic relief.

Metastasis to bone occurs in a high percentage of cases of advanced breast cancer and arises either from tumor cells entering the systemic circulation from the lungs or directly from the intercostal veins which drain the chest wall. The latter route allows direct access to the spine, pelvis and skull. The most frequent sites of bone metastases are in the lower vertebrae and pelvic bones. Unfortunately, x-rays do not visualize many of these lesions well and other diagnostic techniques, such as bone scanning with a Technetium 99m-labeled phosphate compound is necessary. The intertrabecular lesions where the bone marrow is replaced by carcinoma are not detectable on x-ray. Osteolytic lesions are areas of decreased density owing to bone trabeculae destruction and are detectable on x-ray. Osteoblastic lesions are evidenced by increased density owing to thickening of the trabeculae and are also detectable by x-ray. More than one type of bone metastases may be present in a patient. Often the first evidence of bone involvement is a painful or tender area due to pressure or involvement of the periosteum. Pathological fractures occur in about 25% of patients with bone metastases. It is possible to rejoin the bone in these patients utilizing local immobilization and radiation.

The third most frequent site of metastases in breast cancer is the liver. Approximately 60% of autopsied cases demonstrate liver metastases. Access to this organ from the circulation is from the hepatic artery. Often the patient has few, if any, symptoms of liver involvement until the lesions become grossly enlarged, at which time the patient may show evidence of functional liver failure. Serial liver function tests are useful in evaluating the status of patients with liver metastases.

Symptoms of central nervous system involvement are either those associated with an increase in intracranial pressure, such as headache, vomiting, visual disturbances and seizures or those associated with some focal sign of central nervous system disturbance. Therapy for these brain lesions is primarily radiotherapy with corticosteroids used for symptomatic relief by reducing cerebral edema.

TREATMENT

Once the patient is properly diagnosed and staged, treatment may be begun. Great variations exist in the characteristics of breast cancers from patient to patient, especially factors of growth rate and hormonal sensitivity, and they require that each patient's course of therapy be individually planned. Following initial treatment for localized disease, breast cancer may lie dormant and undetected for 5, 10 or 20 years in some patients and then recur locally or with distant metastases. Other patients may not be so fortunate as to be disease free for this long an interval, experiencing disease recurrence within months of initial therapy. A third, and most fortunate group, are those whose disease never recurs following initial treatment. For this reason, the standard disease free interval of 5 years which is spoken of as a cure for many other malignancies is invalid when discussing breast cancer. A more realistic figure of 10 years has been accepted and, realizing exceptions are possible, is the disease free interval required to be considered cured of breast cancer. Most studies, however, report results in terms of survival rather than cure. For the same reason as cited above, the importance of 10-year survival figures, rather than 5-year survival figures, is evident.

The two main factors which determine the general treatment approach in most patients are the extent of the disease and the menopausal status of the patient. Patients whose work-up indicates limited local disease only, that is stage A or B, are considered candidates for surgery. Postoperative radiotherapy may be included, depending upon, among other things, the facility at which the patient is being treated. Patients presenting with advanced disease, stage C or D, have inoperable cases and are considered for any of the various other modalities of treatment, including radiotherapy, hormonal therapy or antineoplastic chemotherapy.

Following surgery, treatment of recurrences in premenopausal women very often is attempted initially with castration. Women 10 or more years postmenopausal frequently respond well to estrogen therapy. Women at or near (up to 10 years after, in some cases) the age of menopause do not respond as predictably as the other two groups mentioned, but therapy may also be initiated with castration if there is evidence of ovarian function remaining. The patient's response to initial hormonal therapy is an important factor in determining the subsequent therapeutic approach.

SURGERY

Surgery is the best single agent in producing a cure for breast cancer. Based on the staging system described, only a certain population of patients with breast cancer are considered candidates for surgery. Stage C involvement is a relative contraindication to surgical intervention due to the very poor results demonstrated in these patients. Stage D involvement eliminates a patient as a potential surgical cure. Once a patient has been selected for surgery, the extent of the operation to be performed must be decided.

The pioneer in the area of mastectomy was William Steward Halsted, who designed the classical radical mastectomy. His first paper on this subject was published in 1894. With only minor changes, it is still the most widely performed surgical procedure with curative intent in the therapy of breast cancer. Several alternative operations have been in use in recent years in an attempt to improve upon the results achieved with radical mastectomy. The important fact to remember is that the purpose of surgery is to cure the disease by removing all disease present while retaining appearance and function as close to normal as possible. The most limited operation that is performed for breast cancer is the removal of the primary lesion and a limited amount of breast tissue immediately surrounding the mass. This method produces the least disfigurement, as frequently only a dimple in the normal breast contour is detectable and no loss of function or mobility results.

A simple mastectomy involves removal of much of the breast tissue with preservation of the pectoral muscles and significant breast tissue and no axillary intervention.

A modified radical mastectomy is again a compromise toward a less extensive operation than the radical mastectomy, but it includes more than the "lumpectomy" or simple mastectomy. Nearly all breast tissue is removed and the lower 3/4 of the axillary contents are resected to remove axillary lymph nodes for immediate histological examination. The pectoral muscles are preserved, giving the patient an improved appearance with the normal pectoral fold. The axillary nodes should be histologically examined while the patient is still on the operating table. If they are positive, a Halsted radical mastectomy may be performed which includes a complete axillary dissection and removal of the pectoral muscles.

Operations more extensive than the radical mastectomy include the extended radical mastectomy where the internal mammary nodes are excised. This operation might be selected in a patient who had a relatively greater likelihood for involvement of these nodes, i.e., a patient with a large lesion located in the central or medial portion of the breast.

A super radical mastectomy is the most aggressive operation proposed and includes dissection of the supraclavicular lymph nodes which are located at the base of the neck.

It will be several more years before adequate controlled clinical trials comparing these various surgical procedures can be evaluated for survival rates, recurrences and complications. Until that time, many experts recommend that the more standard and accepted radical mastectomy be performed. Early data from several studies already suggest that, in certain groups of patients, limited surgical intervention may produce results identical to more radical procedures.

Whatever operation is performed, the surgeon must be acutely aware of the psychological impact a mastectomy may have. He must be prepared to support both the emotional and medical needs of the patient. A physician-patient relationship based on trust and understanding is crucial to achieving an uncomplicated adjustment and adaptation to postmastectomy life. Detailed discussion of this field is beyond the scope of this chapter. Refer to Reference 9 for a more thorough presentation.

A major postoperative complication of mastectomy is edema of the arm due to partial obstruction of lymphatic drainage. There is usually some edema immediately postoperatively. This should disappear within 1 month with the development of collateral lymphatics to provide adequate drainage. Approximately 5% of the patients develop permanent edema which may be massive and severely debilitating in some cases. This is directly due to the surgical technique and may be aggravated by infectious complications. A secondary delayed edema may occur at any time following mastectomy when an infection of the hand or arm occurs. This may result in permanent edema in some patients. Mastectomized patients are susceptible to this complication for the rest of their lives and must be very cognizant of even what appears to be a minor infection on the limb of the affected side. An active program of rehabilitation and patient education is encouraged to regain maximal function and mobility and minimize unnecessary morbidity.

The frequency and degree of postoperative edema appear directly related to the extent of axillary dissection performed during the procedure. A superradical mastectomy is accompanied by a more frequent and greater degree of edema than a more limited operation. Patients who receive postoperative radiation to the axilla also have greater problems with edema owing to the development of fibrosis causing restricted lymphatic drainage.

RADIOTHERAPY

Radiation therapy for breast cancer has been an important method of treatment both as a single agent and when combined with surgery. Just as there is much controversy among surgeons concerning the optimal operation to be performed, radiotherapists differ in opinion as to when and how radiotherapy should be employed in the treatment of primary breast cancer.

Patients who are not candidates for surgery because of the presence of locally advanced disease should receive radiotherapy to the primary lesion and to local areas likely to be involved, such as the axillary and internal mammary lymph node chains. This produces results approximately equal to that achieved from radical mastectomy in these stages and is the preferred initial therapy in advanced localized breast cancer. The results of radiotherapy alone in stage A or B disease, however, are significantly inferior to those of radical mastectomy. Radiotherapy, therefore, should never be

used alone as initial treatment of patients with limited local involvement, unless surgery is absolutely contraindicated for other medical reasons or is refused by the patient.

Radiotherapy has been combined with surgery in an attempt to improve the results achieved with mastectomy. Both pre- and postoperative radiation has been used.

The theory behind administering preoperative radiation is that it prevents viable tumor cell dissemination from occurring during surgery. The physical manipulation of excising breast tissue, including lymphatic and circulatory drainage routes, may liberate tumor cells into the circulation. Disadvantages credited to the use of preoperative radiation are that it delays the surgery 6 to 8 weeks; it increases the incidence of postoperative complications, specifically edema; and it renders many lymph node specimens removed during surgery falsely negative.

Postoperative radiation is used extensively following all of the various surgical techniques previously described. Some physicians feel less extensive surgery can be performed if radiotherapy is employed. The McWhirter method, for example, uses a simple mastectomy followed by 3,750 rads delivered through 4 ports over a 3-week period. Neither of these two components is considered aggressive therapy if used alone. (Several studies, however, show this method to be inferior to the radical mastectomy alone when the disease is confined to early stages. In advanced disease, it is a reasonable alternative to radiation alone.) Several disadvantages have been cited to the use of postoperative radiotherapy. Firstly, a significant number of women will be permanently cured by the surgical procedure alone and will never need the radiation exposure to cure their disease. Thus, the side effects and complications associated with radiation exposure, such as esophagitis, pulmonary fibrosis, skin reactions and potential carcinogenicity, are unwarranted. Secondly, the body's host defense mechanisms responsible for destruction of tumor cells remaining locally following surgery are inhibited by radiation. This may explain why some studies show patients treated with radiotherapy following radical mastectomy actually do worse than patients treated with radical mastectomy alone.[10]

For these reasons, postmastectomy patients

should be carefully evaluated to select for radiotherapy only those most likely to benefit. This selection is based on degree of local tumor involvement and the extent of surgery performed.

RECURRENT DISEASE

Once a patient has received primary treatment for localized breast cancer, there is usually a disease free interval. Approximately ½ of all such patients will remain clinically free of recurrent disease for the rest of their lives. The other half, however, will develop recurrent disease anywhere from a few months to over 20 years after the initial treatment. For this latter group of patients, several therapeutic directions are available depending upon factors particular to each case.

Many patients have their disease recur locally. These lesions occur most frequently along the suture sites of the previous mastectomy and are probably due to failure to remove all viable tumor cells during surgery. They generally respond well to local radiation.

Disease appearance in the opposite breast may be either a metastatic lesion or a second primary malignancy and, if not accompanied by involvement elsewhere, may be treated by the same therapy that was used for the initial presentation.

Breast cancer also may recur in remaining axillary or internal mammary lymph nodes after surgery. Treatment of these nodes is also with radiation.

One additional group of patients is those whose disease recurs not locally but metastasizes to some distant organ. For these women, this signals the beginning of a series of palliative therapeutic attempts to halt the progression of a disease which now is considered beyond the curable stage.

HORMONAL THERAPY

The first therapy utilized for these women is usually in the field of hormonal management. Many advanced breast cancers are sensitive to the changes in environmental chemistry brought about by alteration of hormonal factors. Women who are premenopausal or within 1-year postmenopausal may undergo surgical removal of the ovaries (oophorectomy) to remove the ovarian source of estrogenic hormones. This produces objective regression of disease in 30 to 50% of premenopausal women with advanced breast cancer and also serves as an indicator of the hormonal responsiveness of the tumor. Women who respond to castration are said to have a hormonally responsive tumor and are probable candidates for future hormonal manipulations. Some additional method of endocrine/hormonal manipulation will be attempted in most women who relapse following a response to oophorectomy because a tumor, which initially was responsive to this mode of therapy, will be responsive to additional hormonal changes in approximately 40 to 50% of the cases. Premenopausal women who fail to respond to castration historically experience little chance of responding to subsequent hormonal therapy and may proceed to antineoplastic chemotherapy. The duration of response to therapeutic castration averages 10 to 14 months.

Disease recurrence in postmenopausal women frequently is treated initially with estrogen or androgens. Generally reserved for women 5 or more years postmenopausal, additive hormonal therapy produces regressions in about 20% of cases with androgens and 30% with estrogens, the chance of improvement increasing with age. It is most effective in patients with pleural effusions, skin lesions, pulmonary nodular disease and bone metastases and least effective in brain and liver metastases. An expected survival of several months is optimal, since 6 weeks or more may be required to demonstrate a response to additive hormonal therapy.

Diethylstilbestrol is the estrogen almost exclusively used and is usually well tolerated at the standard dose of 15 mg a day. Gastrointestinal (GI) symptoms of nausea and vomiting may accompany initial therapy and are usually alleviated with antiemetics. In contrast with the situation in selecting an estrogen, several androgens are being considered as acceptable alternatives to the parent compound used, testosterone propionate. The disadvantages inherent in using testosterone propionate are its virilizing property and its necessity for parenteral administration. It has been demonstrated that the masculinizing effect and the antitumor effect of androgens are distinct. Research has been directed at developing non-virilizing androgens effective in the management of advanced breast cancer which may be given orally. Several compounds have resulted and appear most promising. Conclusive studies demonstrating their toxicity, side effects and above all, usefulness in breast cancer are awaited.

In patients who have demonstrated responses to initial hormonal manipulation and then relapsed, further endocrine control of the tumor may be obtained with either of two ablative procedures, adrenalectomy or hypophysectomy. The mode of action of these two procedures is removal of endogenous substances which appear to exert some influence over the growth of breast cancer. Adrenalectomy removes a significant extraovarian source of estrogen and would be indicated only after ovarian function has stopped, either naturally or artificially. Hypophysectomy abolishes the secretion of several factors arising from the pituitary, including adrenocorticotrophic hormone (ACTH), growth hormone, prolactin, thyroid-stimulating hormone and posterior pituitary hormone. Of these, the removal of the first three is considered significant in the treatment of breast cancer. Elimination of ACTH secretion results in adrenal atrophy, giving a therapeutic effect similar to that of adrenalectomy, with the exception of preservation of the zona glomerulosa, that area of the adrenals responsible for aldosterone production. Hypophysectomy may be useful in either pre-or postmenopausal women and may occasionally be utilized following a relapse after an adrenalectomy response. The response rate approximates 30% for either adrenalectomy or hypophysectomy, with a much higher response percentage occurring in those patients who initially responded to castration (45%) compared to those who initially failed with castration (10%). Since most comparative studies fail to show a significant difference between these two operations with respect to remission and survival, major factors determining which operation a woman would receive are the technical capabilities and preferences of the surgeon and hospital involved.

Endocrine replacement therapy is necessary following either of these ablative procedures. Following adrenalectomy, glucocorticoid and mineralocorticoid replacement is required, as would be satisfied by a regimen of dexamethasone 1 to 2 mg every day plus fluorocortisone 0.1 mg every day or every other day, respectively. Following hypophysectomy, replacement therapy would include dexamethasone 1 to 2 mg every day, thyroid hormone 100 mg every day, and posterior pituitary hormone. In either case, requirements must be individually determined and re-evaluated constantly to adjust for changing conditions of stress and environment.

ANTINEOPLASTIC CHEMOTHERAPY

The field of antineoplastic chemotherapy has been explored in recent years with the hope of finding agents effective in breast cancer. Chemotherapy generally is reserved for premenopausal women who have failed castration, patients who have either failed or relapsed from hormonal therapy, patients with organ involvement (especially liver and brain) and those women with rapidly advancing disease in whom hormonal therapy would not be indicated owing to the apparent lack of time required to demonstrate a response. Chemotherapy is not used in early breast cancer because it is only palliative therapy, not curative. The premise behind administering antineoplastic drugs is that the cells incorporate the drug into their cell cycle metabolism where the drug exerts its cytotoxic effect, killing the cell. Malignant neoplastic tissue, by virtue of its relative increased growth rate, preferentially incorporates the drug compared to nonmalignant cells. Unfortunately, since this drug effect depends only on a quantitative factor to separate malignant from nonmalignant cells, certain normal rapidly dividing tissues, such as bone marrow, GI epithelia and hair follicles receive cytotoxic quantities of these drugs as well. Consequently, the primary toxicities of antineoplastic drugs as a class are granulocytopenia, thrombocytopenia, anemia, stomatitis, GI ulceration and alopecia. Specific agents differ in their tendency to produce one or more of these toxicities in addition to other toxicities they may have.

When we speak of response of breast cancer to chemotherapy, we refer to the relative improvement of certain parameters, but we do not require complete disappearance of all aspects of disease. Most studies define response as at least a 50% reduction in size of measurable tumor masses, skin nodules, or lymph nodes, recalcification of osteolytic lesions and the appearance of no new lesions during this time interval.

The chemotherapeutic approach to malignant disease began with investigation of single agents to determine which drugs demonstrated an antitumor effect. These agents were then studied in various combinations to find the optimal drug combination and dosage schedule. All classes of antineoplastic agents have been tried in breast cancer with some measure of success being demonstrated by one or more members of each class.

Several alkylating agents have been shown effective in treating breast cancer. Of these, cyclophosphamide (CTX) appears the most impressive. The mechanism of action of an alkylating agent involves the liberation of highly reactive electrophilic carbonium ions which react (alkylate) with nucleophilic substances of deoxyribonucleic acid (DNA) to disrupt normal cell growth and proliferation. Other alkylating agents, including mechlorethamine (nitrogen mustard), melphalan, chlorambucil and thioTEPA have been investigated in varying doses and schedules and collectively exhibit approximately a 25% response rate. Considering either chronic daily oral administration or an intravenous loading dose followed by daily oral dosage, CTX has given a response rate of approximately 35%. CTX appears to be the alkylating agent of choice in the treatment of breast cancer.[11]

Of the antimetabolites tested against breast cancer, 5-fluorouracil (5-FU), a pyrimidine analogue, and methotrexate (MTX), a folic acid antagonist, have shown the greatest success. 5-FU, probably the most commonly used single agent in breast cancer, inhibits the enzyme, thymidylate synthetase, which converts uridylic acid to thymidylic acid, thereby interfering with pyrimidine synthesis necessary in the formation of DNA. Several intravenous dosage schedules have been investigated, including a loading dose of 15mg per kg per day for 5 days followed by a half-dose every other day to toxicity, weekly administration of 15mg per kg and others with an overall response rate of approximately 25%.[11] Response rates appear practically the same with either the loading dose schedule or the weekly schedule, but toxicity appears to be less severe with weekly administration. Controlled studies are necessary to substantiate this early observation.

In contrast to the similarity of results obtained with varied dosage schedules of CTX or 5-FU, the results obtained with MTX appear to be schedule dependent. Summarizing different levels of single daily, divided daily and twice weekly dosage schedules, MTX gives a response rate of approximately 40% in breast cancer. Using a monthly loading dose, however, results in a 21% response rate.[11] MTX's action as a folic acid antagonist prevents the enzyme, dihydrofolate reductase, from reducing folic acid to folinic acid, the biologically active form necessary to transfer one-carbon fragments to nucleic acids in the synthesis of DNA. This inhibition of DNA synthesis explains its cytotoxic action on neoplastic tissue as well as its toxicity to bone marrow and GI epithelium. Two other antimetabolites, 6-mercaptopurine, a purine analogue, and cytosine arabinoside, a pyrimidine analogue, have been investigated for activity in breast cancer but have not matched the response rates reported with 5-FU and MTX.

Two alkaloids obtained from *Vinca rosea,* vinblastine and vincristine, have each shown approximately a 20% response rate when used as single agents in breast cancer. These drugs are thought to work during cell division by destroying the mitotic spindle and arresting the cell in metaphase. It is interesting that vincristine does not share the same degree of bone marrow and GI toxicity observed with vinblastine and most other antineoplastic agents. Its primary toxicity is neurotoxicity, usually manifested by loss of deep tendon reflexes, numbness, paresthesia and constipation. Prophylactic stool softeners and/or laxatives are advisable in patients to be treated with either vinca alkaloid.

A few antineoplastic antibiotics have been tried in patients with advanced breast cancer. Of these, preliminary results with adriamycin appear promising.

One final class of agents to be presented in the treatment of breast cancer is the corticosteroids. There are four indications for the use of corticosteroids in breast cancer. They are intracranial lesions, lymphangitic pulmonary involvement, an alternative to adrenalectomy for adrenal suppression and acute hypercalcemia. It is postulated that corticosteroids exert a local dehydrating action in the brain to reduce the cerebral edema associated with intracranial lesions. The mechanism of action of corticosteroids in lymphangitic pulmonary involvement is unknown, but it may be related to the lympholytic property of corticosteroids. Patients considered poor surgical risk for an adrenalectomy may receive corticosteroids to produce adrenal suppression through interference with the feedback system which releases ACTH from the anterior pituitary. Results obtained with this method are inferior to those obtained with surgical adrenalectomy but may be an acceptable alternative in patients too ill to undergo an endocrine ablative procedure. The mechanism of action of corticosteroids in treating an acute hypercalcemic episode associated with breast cancer is unclear. It appears exogenous steroids play a role in diminished GI absorption of calcium, facilitate renal excretion and increase bone incorporation of calcium.[12]

In combining agents effective against a certain malignancy, one must bear in mind two factors. Each agent employed should work through a different mechanism of action, i.e., as an alkylating agent, a pyrimidine analogue, a folic acid antagonist, etc. Secondly, the drugs, doses and scheduling should be arranged so that the dominant toxicity of each agent does not overlap. Several research centers currently are investigating various drug combinations and schedules, attempting to find an effective regimen with tolerable toxicity. One of the significant combinations reported is that by Cooper which showed a 90% response rate among 60 patients with advanced breast cancer.[13] Other investigators, however, have been unable to confirm this initial response rate. His induction regimen, as shown in Table 40.4, did produce serious toxicity. Consequently, studies modifying the doses of these five agents are underway hoping to approach his response rate with significantly less toxicity. One representative study is that of Ansfield *et al.* which produced 11 responses in 17 evaluable patients with relatively minor toxicity.[14]

SUMMARY

Certain risk factors have been identified which increase a woman's chance of developing breast cancer. Of these, positive family history and a previous breast malignancy in the patient in question are most significant. The over-all risk for a woman in the United States is about 6% during her lifetime.

Increased public education and awareness should continue to reduce the delay women have displayed in seeking medical attention

TABLE 40.4
The Cooper Regimen of Combination Chemotherapy for Hormone-resistant Breast Cancer

Vincristine	35µg/kg	IV	Weekly
Cyclophosphamide	2.5 mg/kg	PO	Daily
Prednisone	0.75 mg/kg	PO	Daily
Methotrexate	25-50 mg	IV	Weekly
5-Fluorouracil	12 mg/kg	IV	Daily X 4,
	500 mg	IV	followed by weekly

thus allowing treatment to begin at an earlier stage of disease. Early diagnosis and treatment are important factors responsible for the improved prognosis of breast cancer today.

An important influence on prognosis is the stage of disease at the time of initial presentation. For this reason, the patient should be thoroughly staged to allow her to receive the best therapy for her disease.

The treatment of breast cancer utilizes four disciplines: surgery, radiotherapy, endocrine manipulation and antineoplastic chemotherapy. Curative surgery is attempted as initial therapy in operative candidates. Several operations of varying magnitude have been proposed, with none yet proven to produce a higher cure rate than the radical mastectomy. Radiotherapy may be employed either pre- or postoperatively and may be considered primary initial therapy for locally advanced cases. Radiotherapy is useful in controlling local recurrences. Hormonal manipulation may produce gratifying results in patients who relapse from primary therapy. Depending on the menopausal status of the patient, either an oophorectomy or estrogen therapy may be useful. Subsequent ablative hormonal therapy such as adrenalectomy or hypophysectomy or additive therapy with androgens is frequently beneficial in those patients who initially responded to hormonal therapy and then relapsed. Chemotherapy is reserved for patients who have failed all other forms of treatment, those patients whose disease is rapidly progressing and those with organ metastases. Single agents which have been shown to be relatively effective in breast cancer include adriamycin, cyclophosphamide, MTX, 5-FU, vincristine and prednisone. Research to identify other effective single agents, as well as effective drug combinations, is in progress in many cancer research centers throughout the world.

REFERENCES

1. Culter, S. J., Christine, B. and Barclay, T. H. C.: Increasing incidence and decreasing mortality rates for breast cancer, Cancer, 28: 1376, 1971.

2. Haagensen, C. D.: Diseases of the Breast, Ed. 2, p. 466. W. B. Saunders Co., Philadelphia, 1971.

3. Galante, M., Minimal breast cancer: a surgeon's dilemma, Cancer, 28: 1516, 1971.

4. Stevens, G. M. and Weigen, J. F.: Survey mammography as a case finding method for routine and postmastectomized patients, Cancer, 24: 1201, 1969.

5. Handley, R. S.: A surgeon's view of the spread of breast cancer, Cancer, 24: 1231, 1969.

6. Haagensen, C. D.: Diseases of the Breast, Ed. 2, p. 401. W. B. Saunders Co., Philadelphia, 1971.

7. Fisher, B., Ravdin, R. G., Ausman, R. K., Slack, N. H., Moore, G. E.. and Noer, R. J.: Surgical adjuvant chemotherapy in cancer of the breast: results in a decade of cooperative investigation, Ann. Surg., 168: 337, 1968.

8. Haagensen, C. D.: Diseases of the Breast, ed. 2, p. 630. W.B. Saunders Co., Philadelphia, 1971.

9. Bard, M., and Sutherland, A. M.: Psychological impact of cancer and its treatment, IV. Adaptation to radical mastectomy, Cancer, 8: 656, 1955.

10. Farrow, J. H., Fracchia, A. A., Robbins, G. F., and Castro, E.: Simple excision or biopsy plus radiation therapy as the primary treatment for potentially curable cancer of the breast, Cancer, 28: 1195, 1971.

11. Carter, S.: Single and combination nonhormonal chemotherapy in breast cancer, Cancer, 30: 1543, 1972.

12. Rosenfeld, M. G. (editor): Manual of Medical Therapeutics, Ed. 20. p. 61. Little, Brown and Co., St. Louis, 1971.

13. Cooper, R.: Combination chemotherapy in hormone-resistant breast cancer, Proc. Am. Assoc. Cancer Res., 10: 15, 1969.

14. Ansfield, F. J., Ramirez, G., Korbitz, B. C., and Davis, H. L. Jr.: Five-drug therapy for advanced breast cancer: a phase I study, Cancer Chemother, Rep., 55: 183, 1971.

Infectious diseases

chapter **41**

URINARY TRACT INFECTION

Joseph L. Hirschman, Pharm.D.
Eric T. Herfindal, Pharm.D.

Infections of the urinary tract have always been cause for great concern. Yet paradoxically in this age of antimicrobial chemotherapeutics, this concern has been intensified. For one thing, urinary tract infections are the most common urological disease. But despite specific antibiotic therapy, pyelonephritis often becomes chronic and nearly impossible to cure. Contrast this with the remarkable success of antibiotic therapy in respiratory infections, which once constituted the majority of refractory infections, and one can readily understand why a large proportion of clinically and research-oriented urologists spend the major portion of their time dealing with this disease.

In the therapy of urinary tract infection, the pharmacist's main contribution, in most cases, will derive from monitoring his patients. Adequate patient records should enable one to determine whether appropriate dosages are prescribed, if the patient is taking the medication as directed, the possibility of drug interactions and when an inappropriate drug selection has occurred because of hypersensitivity or other contraindications.

Urinary tract infection in the context used throughout this discussion refers to cystitis, urethritis and pyelonephritis of nonspecific origin. Infections of the urinary tract caused by specific organisms, *e.g.*, gonococcus and the tubercle bacillus, produce clinically unique diseases and will be discussed elsewhere (Chapters 42 and 44). Even though such descriptive terms as cystitis and pyelonephritis imply spe-

cific, localized infections, we prefer to consider all urinary tract infections as potentially involving the entire urinary collective system. Approaching therapy on the basis that one is treating a limited infection exposes the practitioner to the risk of converting an acute, treatable infection into a chronic refractory disease with a great deal of concomitant morbidity. Indeed, chronic pyelonephritis is the leading cause of uremia and a significant factor in the etiology of secondary cardiovascular disease.[1]

ETIOLOGY AND PATHOGENESIS

The etiological common denominator in urinary tract infections is the presence of infecting organisms. The difference between easily curable infections and more refractory cases is the presence of other factors such as obstruction of urine flow by stones, tumors or anatomic anomalies; decreased host resistance; and the source and method of entry into the urinary tract by the infecting organism. If these factors go unevaluated and failure to correct them persists, no amount of antibiotic therapy will permanently eradicate the infection.

Although many organisms can be pathogenic for the urinary tract, the Gram-negative bacilli are the most commonly found. In fact, up to 90% of first diagnosed infections are due to *Escherichia coli* and around 50% of recurrent infections are also due to this organism. Other organisms found are such species as *Enterobacter, Klebsiella, Proteus, Pseudomonas, Enterococcus, Staphylococcus* and, in extraordinary circumstances, *Candida.* Many of these organisms are normal flora of the large intestine.[2]

Staphylococcus is a relatively minor infectant whereas *Proteus* and *Pseudomonas* are stubborn infections and, more often than not, are iatrogenically induced. Mixed infections occur almost entirely in patients who have a history of previous antimicrobial therapy or catheterization or both. Naturally occurring infections are almost always the result of a single species.

Normal urine is sterile because homeostatic mechanisms prevent infections even on repeated contamination. However, even slight alteration in host defenses will allow entrenchment of bacteria and subsequent infection. Thus general debility, as well as systemic diseases such as diabetes mellitus, will render the urinary tract much more susceptible to invasion by infecting microbes. Pharmacists should be especially cognizant of the possibility of drug-induced alterations of host immunity. Glucocorticoid and antineoplastic therapy, for example, can profoundly suppress normal defense mechanisms making the likelihood of infection much greater and its therapy more difficult.[3]

Just how the offending organism manages to find itself in the urine-collecting system can be of utmost therapeutic importance in terms of preventing recurrence. The organisms usually gain access to the bladder via the urethra.[4] "Honeymoon cystitis," for example, is often the result of the mechanical transferring of bacteria from the female's perineum by the male during sexual intercourse. Urinary tract infection in women may follow intercourse in those already suffering with vaginitis or cervicitis. Urethral contamination in women may also occur simply as a result of poor personal hygiene of the analperineal areas.

A majority of infections are caused by bacteria ascending the urinary tract via the urethra. Bacteria entering via the bloodstream are less frequent and are said to be causing secondary infections.[4] Primary infections such as osteomyelitis, carbuncles, endocarditis and empyema may seed organisms into the blood which find their way to the kidneys. Treating the primary infections will prevent recurrence of the secondary urinary tract infection, although once established, the latter must also be treated.

We have previously mentioned iatrogenic infections briefly. These infections are induced through the urethra by catheters, especially in the indwelling variety and various instruments, such as cystoscopes.

Urinary stasis is frequently a prime factor in the development of infection. Urine is a good culture medium and a slow passage of urine allows time for bacteria to multiply. Kidney stones, besides other concomitant problems, produce obstruction of the urinary tract and thus are commonly accompanied by infections. Other obstructive influences include strictures and tumors which produce similar sequelae. Chronic bacterial prostatitis is a common cause of relapsing urinary tract infection.[5] Low fluid intakes and infrequent voidings may also contribute to urinary stasis, encouraging infection. No matter how specific antimicrobial therapy might be, if obstruction is present and not relieved, even the most vigorous drug therapy will be unsuccessful.

Anatomical or functional defects of the urinary tract greatly increase the chances for infection but are not necessarily essential for infection. One could characterize the short (relative to males) urethra of the female as an anatomical factor predisposing women to infection. Other anatomical variances such as urethral and bladder diverticula serve as a reservoir for bacterial growth with continual relapsing of infection. Surgical correction of these lesions is necessary to achieve lasting results.

INCIDENCE

Urinary tract infections are predominantly a feminine pathology. About 4% of all women of childbearing age will acquire an infection of the urinary tract. When they reach 60 years of age, their liability to infection increases to about 10%. On the other hand, urinary tract infections are rare in men under the age of 50.

Pregnancy, enough of a burden in itself, increases the liability to urinary tract infection. The over-all incidence of infection during pregnancy is about 8%, twice that for the nonpregnant woman of the same age. Also, catheterization at delivery carries its own risk, contributing to the higher incidence reported.

Hypertension and diabetes mellitus are both associated with higher rates of bacteriuria and pyelonephritis than is present in the general population.

DIAGNOSIS AND CLINICAL FINDINGS

Most authorities agree that significant numbers of bacteria in the urine constitute an infection. The accepted criteria of "significant" is the presence of 100,000 organisms per ml of urine. In actuality, most patients with infection will have counts in excess of 1,000,000. Bacteria counts between 10,000 and 100,000 are not definitive; however, repeated demonstration of equivocal counts should be considered evidence of infection. Relatively lower counts are more common with Gram-positive organisms.

In the vast majority of cases, pyuria will also be found. A few urologists believe that finding a minimum of 10 pus cells per high power field in the centrifuged urine is pathognomonic for urinary tract infection. Generally, the more severe the infection, the more intense is the pyuria. However, relying solely on the demonstration of pyuria as the criterion for diagnosis is a questionable practice because pyuria may be present in nonbacterial inflammatory conditions or may even be absent when substantial bacteriuria exists.

There are a number of acceptable techniques for collecting urine for colony counts and culture and sensitivity determination. Those most commonly used are the clean catch midstream specimen, suprapubic needle aspiration of the bladder and urethral catheterization.[6] If contamination occurs, colony counts of less than 10,000 probably will be found. Mixed cultures should also be viewed with skepticism as they are uncommon and may be the result of contamination. In either case, new specimens must be obtained to arrive at an unequivocal diagnosis.

In addition to careless technique in obtaining urine samples, such factors as recent antimicrobial therapy, dilute urine and frequent voiding may produce artifacts in the bacterial count. However, while prior treatment may impede the growth of organisms, it will not diminish any pyuria already present, making the latter a valid criterion for diagnosis in these circumstances.

Other diagnostic procedures include a white blood count, blood urea nitrogen (BUN) determinations, complete urinalysis and assorted radiographic studies. An elevated white blood count is frequently found in acute pyelonephritis but less often in cystitis and chronic infections. The BUN tends to rise if there is extensive renal tissue destruction. The use of x-ray diagnostic studies will uncover structural and functional anomalies that may predispose the patient to infection.

In addition, there are several screening tests which can be done easily while one is awaiting definitive results from the laboratory. The commonly used screen for bacteriuria is the familiar Gram stain. Other tests include Stat-Test, Testuria, Microstix, Bacta-Uria and Uro-screen. Of this latter group of proprietary tests available for use in the physician's office, only Testuria and Bacta-Uria offer any real advantage over the simple Gram stain since they provide reliable quantitative bacterial culture of the urine. The others are only qualitative tests and not entirely reliable.[7]

Up to now we have been describing mostly the laboratory approach to diagnosis. Although there is a wide variety of physical signs and symptoms, none provide a reliable basis for definitive therapy. With this in mind, consider that many infections may be asymptomatic; then one can readily appreciate the importance of a laboratory work-up of a patient suspected to have an infection. Signs and symptoms that might indicate infection include fever, flank pain, gross pyuria, suprapubic and perineal pain, dysuria and urgency to void.

Some symptoms may be specific for infections of localized portions of the urinary tract. Flank pain, for example, may indicate upper tract involvement. However, the cardinal rule of diagnosis is never to assume specificity of syndromes, e.g., cystitis or pyelonephritis. Infected urine presumes present or potential involvement of the kidney and should be treated accordingly.

COMPLICATIONS

The greatest danger of urinary tract infections is their tendency to become chronic. Once chronic infection of the kidney tissue becomes established, precise treatment is no longer applicable and the risk of uremia and its associated morbidity becomes very real. Every effort should be made by the clinician to relieve obstructions and anatomical defects that lead to stasis or refluxing of urine up the tract. Unrelieved obstruction may lead to chronic renal infections. Any patient with a history of recurrent infections should be evaluated thoroughly as to the presence of these abnormalities.

There are, however, defects that may prove to be unremediable. Permanent cure of these patients is infrequent. The best that can be done is to provide long term therapy in the hope that symptomatic recurrences can be prevented.

TREATMENT—PHARMACOLOGY OF URINARY ANTIMICROBIAL DRUGS

All urinary tract infections should be actively treated with drugs. The drugs used in the treatment of urinary tract infections fall into these classes: systemic antibiotics, sulfonamides and the various urinary antiseptics (Table 41.1).

Systemic Antibiotics

A number of antibiotics are useful in the treatment of urinary tract infections. Most of these will produce good tissue levels in addition to urine levels. They are thus useful in treating infections with tissue involvement.

Ampicillin. This antibiotic is found unchanged in the urine in relatively high concentrations after oral or parenteral administration. As well as being active against most penicillin-sensitive organisms, it is also effective against many Gram-negative enteric bacteria such as *E. coli* and *Proteus mirabilis.* However, it is not reliable against *Enterobacter, Pseudomonas* or *Klebsiella.* Since ampicillin is also excreted in the bile, it can be used safely in the presence of a moderate degree of renal impairment, *i.e.,* a creatinine clearance of 10 ml per min or above.[8] As with penicillin G, ampicillin is not effective against penicillinase-producing organisms.

Cephalosporins. This class of antibiotics is active against many Gram-positive and some Gram-negative species. The cephalosporins can be found in high concentrations in the urine. *Pseudomonas* and *Enterobacter* are generally resistant to these drugs. Cephalothin and cephaloridine have clinically identical spectrums and can only be utilized by the parenteral route. Cephalexin and cephaloglycine are orally effective cephalosporins. Cephaloglycine produces therapeutic concentrations in the urine, not in the serum. Cephalexin, however, produces adequate tissue levels for most infections. Of the two oral agents, cephalexin is the preferred drug. It should be kept in mind that patients who are allergic to penicillins may also demonstrate an allergy to the cephalosporins, but the incidence of true cross-sensitivity is relatively low.[9] As a consequence, these drugs can be used prudently in patients who have a history of allergic reactions to a penicillin.

Chloramphenicol. This drug is highly active against most urinary pathogens after oral or parenteral administration and is primarily bacteriostatic. However, since most of the drug is metabolized by the liver, only a small percentage (5 to 10%) is found in the biologically active form in the urine, making it a less efficient agent than ampicillin for sterilizing the urine.[11] Because of the rare occurrence of irreversible aplastic anemia with this drug, it should not be used until other drugs of less potential toxicity have been tried.

Carbenicillin. This semisynthetic penicillin derivative is effective against *Pseudomonas* and *Proteus* urinary tract infections. Because the other agents that are effective against *Pseudomonas* are nephrotoxic, carbenicillin which does not cause kidney damage has an important advantage. A disappointing development with this drug, however, has been the rapid emergence of resistant organisms.[12] Also, high doses or use in the presence of renal dysfunction tends to cause an abnormality in platelet function, resulting in some undesirable hemorrhagic manifestations.[13] A combination of carbenicillin and gentamicin is believed by many clinicians to be the best current therapy for *Pseudomonas* infections.[14]

Gentamicin. Gentamicin is related chemically and structurally to kanamycin and neomycin. Gentamicin shares the nephrotoxicity and ototoxicity of this class of drugs. It is poorly absorbed after oral ingestion and can only be used parenterally. Gentamicin, however, appears to be relatively less toxic than its congeners and, in addition, has the distinct advantage of being effective against *Pseudomonas*—a virtue not shared with kanamycin. The ototoxicity of gentamicin is more likely to be vestibular in nature rather than actually affecting hearing acuity as is the case with kanamycin.[15]

Kanamycin. Like gentamicin, this bactericidal drug is only effective by the parenteral route and is both ototoxic and nephrotoxic. Unlike gentamicin, however, it is not effective in urinary *Pseudomonas* infections. *Proteus, Enterobacter* and *Klebsiella* are often sensitive to kanamycin. Kanamycin is almost completely excreted by the kidney and doses must be carefully altered in renal insufficiency in order to prevent toxicity.[16] For optimal activity, the urine should be neutral or slightly alkaline.[17]

Penicillin G and Other Penicillins. In doses of 100,000 to 300,000 units per kg every 6 hr intravenously, penicillin G has been effective in clearing up coliform infections of the urinary tract. Penicillin is a relatively nontoxic drug and these extremely high doses are well tolerated. However, this use of penicillin obviously requires hospitalization, limiting its usefulness in these infections.

In addition, it should be kept in mind that the cation (potassium or sodium) that accompanies the penicillin may have undesirable effects in these doses. Sodium penicillin G contains 2 mEq of sodium per 1,000,000 units, and potassium penicillin G contains 1.7 mEq of potassium per 1,000,000 units. There are very few real differences between the penicillinase-resistant penicillins. Any one of these agents could be used for staphylococcal infections. We prefer, however, cloxacillin or dicloxacillin for oral use and oxacillin for parenteral administration.

Polymyxins. Polymyxin B and polymyxin E (colistin) are polypeptide antibiotics that are active against coliform (except *Proteus*) and *Pseudomonas* organisms. These potent bactericidal agents are not absorbed from the GI tract and require parenteral administration. Because the polymyxins are nephrotoxic and neurotoxic and are excreted primarily by the kidneys, the dose must be altered in renal impairment.[18] Polymyxin and colistin have identical spectrums and there is complete cross-resistance between the two.[19] The parenteral from of colistin is colistimethate, which must be converted to the active colistin base *in vivo*. How rapidly and completely this conversion takes place is not clear. Polymyxin B, however, is active as such. Thus, since in equipotent doses there are no differences between the two drugs therapeutically or in toxicity, polymyxin B would seem to be the better agent.[20]

Tetracyclines. Because of the relatively rapid emergence of resistant strains, the tetracyclines have limited usefulness in urinary tract infections.[21] Theoretically, these agents should be effective against most urinary tract pathogens with the exception of *Proteus* and *Pseudomonas*. The widespread use of tetracyclines has created a situation where the drug is now ineffective in recurring urinary infection where it was formerly effective.[22] The tetracyclines are bacteriostatic, a relative disadvantage since phagocytic mechanisms do not operate well in the urine.

Sulfonamides

The sulfonamides are widely used in the therapy of initial acute urinary tract infections. All are bacteriostatic and are effective against the gram-negative coliform bacteria with the exception of *Pseudomonas* and *Proteus*. The sulfonamides vary in pharmacokinetic properties but have the same spectrum of activity.[23] The soluble sulfonamides are absorbed well from the GI tract and are effective by the oral route. Sodium salts of the sulfonamides are used by the parenteral route. Varying amounts of free (active) and acetylated (inactive) sulfonamides are found in the urine. In order to prevent precipitation of sulfonamides in the urine which can produce hematuria and even obstruction, a highly soluble sulfonamide, such as sulfisoxazole or triple sulfas, should be selected.[24] Resistance to sulfonamides should be suspected if therapeutic results are not seen in 24 to 48 hr.

Urinary Antiseptics

Methenamine. Methenamine is excreted in the urine after oral absorption. When exposed to a strongly acidic urine, formaldehyde is released. No tissue levels are produced. In order to ensure the production of an acidic urine, an acidifying agent such as ammonium chloride, ascorbic acid, methionine or hippuric acid (from cranberry juice) may be employed.[25] Preparations such as methenamine mandelate, methenamine hippurate and methenamine sulfosalicylate provide acids that acidify the urine and are mildly antiseptic in themselves. In certain patients it may be necessary to add another acidifying agent to the above preparations, as the latter may not produce the degree of acidification necessary. The patient should be instructed to measure the urine pH with nitrazine or hydrion paper. If sulfonamides are given concurrently, insoluble compounds may form in the urine owing to the acidity.

Nalidixic Acid. Nalidixic acid is a urinary antiseptic which is initially effective against most coliform bacteria with the exception of

TABLE 41.1
Antimicrobial Therapy of Urinary Tract Pathogens[a]

Pathogen	Drugs of Choice	Adult Dosage	Comments
E. coli	Ampicillin	0.5 g q 6hr po; 1.0 g q 4-6hr IV	Diarrhea and rashes are common
	Cephalothin	1.0 g q 4-6hr IV	Alternative parenteral therapy to ampicillin
	Cephalexin	0.5 g q 6hr po	Should only be used when ampicillin contraindicated or as follow-up to parenteral cephalosporin therapy
	Kanamycin	15 mg/kg/24hr in 2 doses IM	Reserve for severe infection unresponsive to less toxic drugs
	Sulfonamide	1 g q 6hr	Resistant organisms are common
Klebsiella	Cephalothin	1.0 g q 4-6hr IV	Resistant organisms are common; sensitivity determinations are mandatory; other cephalosporins can be used with the same restrictions
	Kanamycin	15 mg/kg/24hr in 2 doses IM	Resistance is becoming more prevalent; combination therapy with cephalothin is sometimes more effective; reserve for severe, unresponsive infections
	Gentamicin	3 mg/kg/24hr in 3 doses IM	Reserve for severe infection unresponsive to less toxic drugs
Proteus	Ampicillin	See above	See above; *P. mirabilis* only
	Cephalexin; cephalothin	See above	See above; *P. mirabilis* only
	Kanamycin	See above	See above
	Carbenicillin	50-100 mg/kg/day in divided doses q 4-6 hr IM or IV; 500 mg-1 g q 6 hr po (indanyl sodium salt)	Useful in ampicillin-resistant species
	Gentamicin	See above	See above

Pseudomonas	Carbenicillin	50-200 mg/kg/day in divided doses q 4-6hr IM or IV; 1 g q 6hr po (indanyl sodium salt)	Combination therapy with gentamicin may be synergistic
	Gentamicin	See above	Combination therapy with carbenicillin may be synergistic
	Polymyxin B	1.5-2.5 mg/kg/24hr in 2 doses IM	Should be considered only as alternative therapy; never first choice
Enterococcus	Ampicillin-kanamycin	See above	Combination therapy necessary because of demonstrated synergism
Staphylococcus	Cloxacillin; dicloxacillin	250 mg q 6hr po	Other penase-resistant penicillins can be used equally well either orally or parenterally
	Cephalothin	See above	See above

[a] Empirical therapy should only be used when sensitivity testing is not readily available.

Pseudomonas. After oral absorption, about 20% is excreted unchanged in the urine and 80% is found as a glucuronide conjugate. It has no systemic activity. The major drawback to this drug is that resistance develops very rapidly, limiting the duration of effective treatment.[26]

Nitrofurantoin. This member of the very useful nitrofurans is effective for most urinary pathogens after oral administration. Approximately 40% of the drug is excreted unchanged in the urine. The spectrum of activity includes most coliform bacteria with the exception of most strains of *Proteus* and all strains of *Pseudomonas*. Fortunately, the development of resistance is very slow, thus making the drug suitable for prolonged administration. The mechanism of nitrofurantoin activity is not clear.[27]

Phenazopyridine. This dye has little or no antibacterial activity in the urine, but it has some local anesthetic activity on the urinary tract mucosa. It is frequently prescribed in combination with sulfonamides and other urinary antimicrobial agents, although its efficacy is of a dubious nature.

Methylene Blue. Methylene blue is a weak urinary antiseptic that has been replaced by more effective compounds.

Trimethoprim. Trimethoprim is a synthetic compound that has both antimalerial and antibacterial properties. The drug interferes with bacterial purine synthesis (dihydrofolic acid reductase) at a stage immediately after the point of interference by sulfonamides (dihydrofolic acid synthesase) making the combination of trimethoprim and sulfonamide synergistic.[28] Trimethoprim is active against most urinary tract pathogens (except *Pseudomonas*) and is excreted unchanged in the urine.[29] Since there appear to be no other major pathways of excretion, the use of this drug in renal failure could lead to toxic accumulation. The combination of trimethoprim and a sulfonamide can be of significant value in treating resistant urinary tract infections unresponsive to older, safer and cheaper drugs. At the present, trimethoprim-resistant strains of usually sensitive strains are uncommon; however with increased clinical use, acquired bacterial resistance will undoubtedly increase. Gastrointestinal symptoms seldom occur with currently used doses, and a reversible bone marrow depression consisting of leukopenia, anemia and thrombocytopenia has been noted in some studies.[30] It is advisable to perform regular blood counts during long term trimethoprim therapy.[29]

TREATMENT—CLINICAL USE OF URINARY ANTIMICROBIAL DRUGS

The primary therapeutic goal is seemingly simple, *i.e.*, sterilize the urine. Unfortunately, it takes more than just appropriate antimicrobial therapy. Many of the additional therapeutic modalities have already been mentioned. For example, it is impossible to render urine permanently sterile in the presence of any type of obstruction, regardless of the period of treatment, amounts or combination of drugs used. Good hygiene in the genital-urinary area will also contribute to successful therapy. Forcing fluids is generally advisable as well. This will not only correct any pre-existing fluid imbalances but also ensure an adequate urine volume and frequent voiding. The latter minimizes stasis of urine flow which might encourage bacterial growth. The pH of the urine may enhance the effectiveness of certain antimicrobials (Table 41.2).

The selection of the appropriate antimicrobial agent is based on a number of considerations. It is known that drugs that produce inhibitory concentrations in the blood but not the urine are ineffective in treating urinary tract infections, and drugs that only produce urine concentrations have been shown to be effective.[31] Studies have not clearly demonstrated any superiority of drugs that produce both blood and urine levels.[32]

The effectiveness of bactericidal agents as compared with bacteriostatic agents has been the subject of considerable controversy. There is no compelling evidence to indicate that the cidal agents are more effective than static agents, but on a theoretical basis there seems to be some reason to select bactericidal agents. This is particularly true in treating infections with tissue involvement when there is reason to believe that host defense mechanisms are compromised. Other points that must be considered in selecting a drug are: always assume that it will be difficult to eliminate the organisms and that recurrence is possible, consider the infection to be one of the whole urinary collecting

TABLE 41.2
Drugs More Active in Acid and Alkaline Urines

Those More Active in Acid Urine	Those More Active in Alkaline Urine
Teracyclines	Streptomycin
Methenamine (inactive if pH is above 5.5)	Gentamicin
	Kanamycin
Nitrofurantoin	Erythromycin

system and that there is always the possibility of progression of the disease to chronicity.

In acute urinary tract infections, treatment is initiated after appropriate work-up and collection of urinary samples. If the sensitivity is known, the most likely agent is used that is compatible with the patient. However, pending sensitivity results, empiric therapy with ampicillin or cephalexin is initiated and continued for 14 days. Improvement should be dramatic and prompt. If not, culture and sensitivity studies should be repeated and further diagnostic work-up is required. In most first, acute infections, sulfisoxazole works as well as the suggested antibiotics, but these authors feel that the latter more closely fits the description of the ideal drug. Consequently, the antibiotics offer greater assurance of sterilizing the urine and preventing tissue involvement in the greatest number of patients in the long run.

Any case of recurrent infection requires thorough searching for predisposing and complicating factors as well as identification of the responsible organisms and their antibiotic sensitivities. Two-week therapy with the selected drug is the minimal therapeutic requirement. Cultures and sensitivity testing should be repeated after 3 or 4 days of therapy and any necessary drug changes made accordingly. Once the urine becomes sterile, some clinicians prefer to maintain the patient on chronic therapy with nitrofurantoin, methenamine or a sulfonamide. Compelling evidence, however, for the effectiveness of this prophylactic procedure is minimal. In any event, follow-up of the patient with urine cultures at intervals is advisable and should be continued for several years.[33]

There are times when the therapeutic response is not at all what it should be. Some of the explanations for this occurrence are given in Table 41.3.

TABLE 41.3

Factors Contributing to a Poor Therapeutic Response

1. Ineffective drug
2. Drug interactions
3. Inaccessibility of organisms to the action of the drug
4. Mixed infection
5. Iatrogenic re-infection
6. Selecting out of resistant organisms during therapy
7. Poor host defenses

PROGNOSIS

In acute urinary tract infections without complications, quick cures are common. At present, 75% of the cases treated with the drug of choice are cleared of infection in the first course of treatment. However, prevention of smoldering asymptomatic infections which may ultimately destroy the kidney must be ensured. Obviously, this is where the real therapeutic challenge lies. We are convinced from our own practice and experiences that the cure rates can still be improved if this challenge is pursued with more vigor by clinicians.

CONCLUSIONS

The primary emphasis in the treatment of urinary infections must be on the accurate identification of the infecting organisms, the use of intensive specific bactericidal drug therapy, the elimination of primary foci that are seeding the urinary tract with pathogenic organisms, the search for and elimination of predisposing functional or anatomic defects and the prompt treatment of any complicating secondary manifestations of infection. Pharmacists can contribute to the management of these infections through patient monitoring. Vigilant monitoring can uncover such detrimental elements as inappropriate drug selection, inadequate dosage, insufficient duration of treatment and drug interactions.

REFERENCES

1. Kagan, J. M. (editor): Antimicrobial therapy. In Antimicrobial Therapy of Urinary Tract Infections, Ed. 1, Chap. 27. Edited by C. W. Daeschner, Jr., W. B. Saunders Co., Philadelphia, 1970.
2. Hoeprich, P. D.: Urethritis and cystitis. In Infectious Diseases, Ed. 1, p. 457. Edited by P. D.: Hoeprich. Harper and Row, New York, 1973.
3. Weinstein, L. and Dalton, A. C.: Host determinants of response to antimicrobial agents. N. Engl. J. Med., 279: 580, 1968.
4. McCabe, W.: Pyelonephritis. In Infectious Diseases, Ed. 1, p. 507. Edited by P. D. Hoeprich. Harper and Row, New York, 1973.
5. Meares, E. M., Jr.: Bacterial prostatitis vs. prostatosis. J.A.M.A., 224: 1372, 1973.
6. Pfau, A., Sacks, T. G.: An evaluation of midstream urine cultures in the diagnosis of UTI in females. Urol. Int., 25: 326, 1970.
7. Anon.: Bacta-uria. Med. Lett. Drugs Ther., 11: 75, 1969.
8. Kirby, W. M. M., and Kind, A. C.: Clinical pharmacology of ampicillin and hetacillin. Ann. N.Y. Acad. Sci., 145: 791, 1967.
9. Scholand, J. F., Tennenbaum, J. I., and Cerilli, G. J.: Anaphylaxis to cephalosporin in a patient allergic to penicillin. J.A.M.A., 206: 130, 1968.
10. Rahal, J. J., Jr., Meyers, B. R., and Weinstein, L.: Treatment of bacterial endocarditis with cephalothin. N. Engl. J. Med., 279: 1305, 1968.
11. Lindberg, A. A., Nilsson, L. H., Bucht, H., and Kallings, L. O.: Concentration of chloramphenicol in the urine and blood in relation to renal function. Br. Med. J., 2: 724, 1966.
12. Holmes, K. K., Clark, H., Silverblatt, T., and Turck, M.: Emergence of resistance in pseudomonas during carbenicillin therapy. Antimicrob. Agents Chemother., p. 391, 1969.
13. Lurie, A., Ogilvie, M., Townsend, R., Gold, C., Meyers, A. M., and Goldberg, B.: Carbenicillin-induced coagulopathy. Lancet, 1: 1114, 1970.
14. Smith, C. B., Wilfert, J. N., Dans, P. E., Kurrus, T. A., and Finland, M.: In-vitro activity of carbenicillin and results of treatment of infections due to pseudomonas with carbenicillin singly and in combination with gentamycin. J. Infect. Dis. Suppl., 122: 14, 1970.
15. Wersäl J., Lundquist, P. G., and Björkroth, B.: Ototoxicity of gentamycin. J. Infect. Dis., 119: 410, 1969.
16. Kunin, C. M.: Absorption, distribution, excretion and fate of kanamycin. Ann. N.Y. Acad. Sci., 132: 811, 1966.
17. Sabath, L. D., Gerstein, D. A., Leaf, C. B., and Finland, M.: Increasing the usefulness of antibiotics: treatment of infections caused by gram-negative bacilli. Clin. Pharmacol. Ther., 11: 161, 1970.
18. Kunin, C. M.: A guide to use of antibiotics in patients with renal disease. Ann. Intern. Med., 67: 151, 1967.
19. Kucers, A.: The Use of Antibiotics, Ed. 1, p. 237. J. B. Lippincott Co., Philadelphia, 1972.
20. Goodwin, N. J.: Colistin and sodium colistimethate. Med. Clin. North Am., 54: 1267, 1970.
21. Kucers, A.: The Use of Antibiotics, Ed. 1, p. 292. J. B. Lippincott Co., Philadelphia, 1972.

22. Sabath, L. D.: Current concepts: drug resistance of bacteria. N. Engl. J. Med., 280: 91, 1969.
23. Garrod, L. P., and O'Grady, F.: Antibiotics and Chemotherapy, Ed. 3, p. 13. Williams and Wilkins Co., Baltimore, 1972.
24. Lehr, D.: Clinical toxicology of sulfonamides. Ann. N.Y. Acad. Sci., 69: 417, 1957.
25. Gandelman, A. L.: Methenamine mandelate: antimicrobial activity in urine and correlation with formaldehyde levels. J. Urol., 97: 533, 1967.
26. Roland, A. R., Turck, M., and Petersdorf, R. G.: A critical evaluation of nalidixic acid in urinary-tract infections. N. Engl. J. Med., 275: 1081, 1966.
27. Kucers, A.: The Use of Antibiotics, Ed. 1, p. 362. J. B. Lippincott Co., Philadelphia, 1972.
28. Kucers, A.: The Use of Antibiotics, Ed. 1, p. 339. J. B. Lippincott Co., Philadelphia, 1972.
29. Darrell, J, H., Garrod, L. P., and Waterworth, P. M.: Trimethoprim: laboratory and clinical studies. J. Clin. Pathol,, 21: 202, 1968.
30. Kahn, S. B., Fein, S. A., and Brodsky, I.: Effects of trimethoprim on folate metabolism in man. Clin. Pharmacol. Ther., 9: 550, 1968.
31. McCabe, W.: Pyelonephritis. In Infectious Diseases, Ed. 1, p. 507. Edited by P. D. Hoeprich. Harper and Row, New York, 1973.
32. Stamey, T. A., Govan, D. E., and Palmer, J. M.: Localization of treatment of urinary tract infection: role of bactericidal urine levels as opposed to serum levels. Medicine, 44: 1, 1965.
33. McCabe, W.: Pyelonephritis. In Infectious Diseases, Ed. 1, p. 519. Edited by P. D. Hoeprich. Harper and Row, New York, 1973.

chapter 42

SYPHILIS AND GONORRHEA

Richard deLeon, Pharm.D.

More than 624,000 cases of gonorrhea, over 23,000 cases of infectious syphilis and more than 71,000 cases of noninfectious syphilis were reported by physicians, hospitals and venereal disease clinics in the United States during 1971.[1] These figures represent significant increases over the number of cases reported in 1970. However, only about 1 in 4 cases of syphilis or gonorrhea is reported and adjustment of the above figures indicate that over 2,000,000 cases of gonorrhea and more than 80,000 cases of infectious syphilis actually occurred in 1971.[2] Additionally, it is estimated that there are about 800,000 American women who have undetected gonorrhea.[3]

The venereal disease situation in the rest of the world is just as grim. After a high incidence of both gonorrhea and syphilis at the end of World War II, the occurrence of both diseases decreased at a steady rate to new lows during 1958, 1959 and 1960 owing to the introduction of penicillin and other antibiotics. It is difficult to compare case incidences between countries because of variables in the reporting systems but, in general, there has been a rise in the occurrence of reported primary and secondary syphilis throughout the world. However, there has been a decline in early congenital syphilis in almost all countries. Gonorrhea has not declined in incidence. In fact, there has been a tremendous increase in the rate of occurrence of gonorrhea in many countries during the past 20 years.

The reasons for the increased incidence of syphilis and gonorrhea are numerous and all contribute to the present epidemic.[4] The host is more mobile and, owing to the adoption of the sexual mores of the "new morality," is more likely to have indiscriminate sexual encounters than his counterpart of previous years, increasing his chances of acquiring or transmitting syphilis or gonorrhea. Changes in the virulence of the organism and decreased sensitivity to antibiotics are among the factors that tend to increase the incidence of venereal disease.

EPIDEMIOLOGY

Syphilis and gonorrhea occur at the greatest rate in patients between the ages of 20 and 24.[3,5] The national case rate is 42 cases and 1,615 cases per 100,000 population, respectively. The 25- to 29-year-old group is the next most affected group with rates of 34 cases per 100,000 population for syphilis and 845 cases per 100,000 population for gonorrhea.[3] Over 60% of the cases of syphilis occur in persons between the ages of 15 and 25, and 70% of all cases of gonorrhea occur in persons under 24 years old.

Twice as many males as females are reported to have syphilis while 3 times as many males as females are reported with gonorrhea.[5] The disparity in reporting ratios for men and women is a· reflection of the fact that many women have asymptomatic infections and remain subclinical in terms of disease evidence. Indeed, the asymptomatic infected female patient is one of the main contributors to the resurgence of the incidence of gonorrhea.

When the incidence of syphilis and gonorrhea is related to the degree of urbanization of cities, it is evident that the greater the population of an area the greater the rate of occurrence of syphilis and gonorrhea.[3] For example, cities with population greater than 200,000 have much higher incidences of gonorrhea and syphilis than small cities or rural areas of less than 50,000 population, when compared on the basis of case rates per 100,000 population. Obviously, syphilis and gonorrhea strike hardest in the cities. Nationally, there are 12 cases of syphilis per 100,000 population; yet Newark with a rate of 124 led the list in 1971, followed closely by Atlanta and San Francisco. Also in 1971, Atlanta had a gonorrhea case rate of 2,510 per 100,000 population in contrast to a nation-wide incidence of 308 gonorrhea cases per 100,000 population.

In general, the person between 20 and 24 years of age who lives in a city with a population greater than 200,000 runs the greatest risk of contracting syphilis or gonorrhea.

ETIOLOGY

The Gram-negative diplococcus, *Neisseria gonorrhoeae,* is the organism that causes gonorrhea. *N. gonorrhoeae* requires moisture, a medium with a pH of 7.2 to 7.6 and a temperature range of 33 to 39°C in order to survive. Because of these physical requirements, it is virtually impossible to acquire gonorrhea from toilet seats, drinking glasses and the like. Decreasing sensitivity of *N. gonorrhoeae* to antibiotics is causing mounting concern. The resistance is not absolute; rather, it is a relative condition—it takes more penicillin to effect a cure today than it did 20 years ago.[6,7] Reports of the introduction of "killer strains" of *N. gonorrhoeae* to the American public by servicemen returning from southeast Asia have caused concern. The connotation is that after infection with a "killer strain," death or severe disability will ensue in spite of treatment. However, this

is not the case. The strains of *N. gonorrhoeae* imported from southeast Asia exhibit a relative resistance to penicillin that is slightly higher than our own indigenous strains but they can be treated successfully with antibiotics.

Complicating the picture is the fact that strains of gonococcus that are resistant to penicillin are usually resistant to tetracycline, erythromycin and streptomycin.[8,9] This cross-resistance to antibiotics has forced the use of higher doses of tetracycline and erythromycin in an effort to achieve higher blood levels. However, the resistance to streptomycin is so high that sufficient blood levels can not be achieved safely. Fortunately, strains of *N. gonorrhoeae* that are resistant to penicillin, erythromycin and tetracycline are sensitive to spectinomycin.[10]

Treponema pallidum, a spirochete, is the causative organism of syphilis. *T. pallidum* can invade any tissue or organ of the body causing acute, chronic or contagious syphilis. Infection usually occurs through sexual activity, but a fetus may become infected during childbearing if the mother has syphilis (congenital syphilis) or a patient may become infected if he received donated blood contaminated with *T. pallidum.* The organism can not survive outside of body tissues or fluids, and infection by means other than personal contact are rare.

PATHOGENESIS

A gonorrheal infection is manifested in males after a 4- to 10-day incubation period after contact with an infected source. The first signs are usually a milky urethral discharge associated with meatal pain, especially on voiding, and frequency of urination. As the disease progresses, the discharge becomes more profuse and may be blood-tinged. The discharge is caused by the irritating endotoxin released by the gonococcus when it dies.

The infection may extend into the seminal vesicles, epididymis and prostate, resulting in inflammation, pain and sometimes fever. Untreated gonorrhea often subsides over a period of weeks with only a small amount of persistent morning urethral discharge left as a reminder. Urethral stricture after repeated attacks and sterility after epididymitis are complications of gonococcal infection.

In women, the disease may often remain

asymptomatic (about 75% of infected women are asymptomatic), but there is usually a purulent urethral discharge. Dysuria, frequency and urgency occur, as do involvement of the cervix and Bartholin's and Skene's glands. Symptoms of lower genital tract involvement may last for only a month. However, the patient may remain an asymptomatic carrier of gonorrhea—a major contributor to the rising incidence of gonorrhea. Spread of the infection to the upper genital tract can cause salpingitis. The salpingitis may lead to fibrosis and scarring of the fallopian tubes resulting in sterility. Pelvic inflammatory disease (PID) is manifested by acute onset of fever and lower abdominal pain and is a result of the extension of infection with abscess formation in the peritoneal cavity. PID tends to be a recurrent problem.

The most common manifestation of gonorrhea in infants is a destructive conjunctivitis that frequently caused blindness before antibiotics were introduced. Infection with *N. gonorrhoeae* takes place during birth as the baby passes through the birth canal or by the hands of infected persons with poor personal hygiene. Acute purulent conjunctivitis develops 3 to 4 days after infection. If untreated, the disease causes corneal ulceration, perforation, scarring and possible blindness.

Gonococcal arthritis occurs in about 1% of patients with a genital infection and is manifested by fever, arthralgia and painful arthritis. The arthritis involves more than one joint in about 80% of the cases with the knee the most frequently involved joint. Following the knee in order of frequency of involvement are the wrists, ankles, hands, elbows, hips and shoulders. Before antibiotics became available, permanent joint damage was a common occurrence because of the muscle wasting around the joint.

Gonococcal bacteremia, endocarditis and perihepatitis are rare complications of gonorrhea.

Syphilis has a more complicated pathogenesis than gonorrhea. Like gonorrhea, syphilis is transmitted by direct contact. *T. pallidum* invades the body by penetrating the epithelium. The site of penetration is usually on the genitals but may occur in the rectum, mouth or any other cutaneous tissue. After penetration, *T. pallidum* spreads through the lymphatics, and the regional lymph nodes may become tender. The spirochete also travels to the lungs by way of the venous circulation and through the arteries. During this sojourn, *T. pallidum* leaves the small vessels and sets up numerous metastatic foci along the way. This dissemination of the disease occurs within a few days after the initial implantation of *T. pallidum.* Up to this point, the syphilitic's infection is characterized by focal infection near the site of implantation, metastatic infection foci and a spirochetemia.

A chancre usually appears near the site of invasion within 10 to 90 days and is evident at about 3 weeks. The primary chancre, which is not typical in nature, may be inconspicuous and missed altogether. However, when evident, the chancre may be single or multiple in number, indurated, painless, and heal slowly with or without scarring. The appearance of the chancre is usually accompanied by enlargement of the regional lymph nodes without suppuration unless there is a secondary infection. The primary lesion usually heals in 2 to 6 weeks. The lymph node involvement may resolve or persist and worsen if the syphilitic metastases are widespread. The period from the time of implantation of *T. pallidum* in the tissues at the primary site of infection until the disease becomes generalized comprises the primary stage of the syphilitic process.

The secondary stage of syphilis commences about 6 weeks to 6 months after the appearance of the primary chancre. This stage is characterized by generalized involvement of the skin and mucous membranes. The maculopapular skin rash that develops may be confused with many other rashes, causing confusion and incorrect diagnosis. The rash is usually widespread and frequently involves the palms of the hands and the soles of the feet in addition to the trunk and extremities. The mucous membranes may be involved simultaneously or independently of the skin. The lesions that develop in the mucous membranes of the mouth and genitalia are usually superficial and painless and may be covered with a gray exudate. Lesions of the palate and tonsillar area may cause a persistent sore throat. The "split papule," a tiny moist papule at the corner of the mouth, may be the only demonstrable lesion of a syphilitic infection, yet it can easily be overlooked because of its location and the frequent occurrence of innocuous lesions in this area. The "split papule" is especially dangerous because, like all cutaneous and mucous lesions of early syphilis, it teems with infectious *T. pallidum*. During the secondary stage, the patient may complain of fatigue, malaise, headache and fever. A generalized lymphadenopathy may occur. Some patients lose their hair in clumps, giving them a moth-eaten appearance. An iritis or neuroretinitis occurs in about 4% of syphilis cases. Skeletal lesions may occur causing arthralgia, hydroarthrosis, swelling and tenderness of joints. Proteinuria, edema and hypercholesterolemia indicate a syphilitic nephrosis.

If untreated, the lesions of the secondary stage of syphilis heal in about 4 to 12 weeks, heralding the beginning of the latent stage of the syphilitic process. The latent stage is characterized by the absence of clinical lesions, a negative dark field examination, a normal cerebrospinal fluid (CSF) examination and positive serological tests. Patients with abnormal CSF findings but who are without other signs and symptoms have a more serious prognosis and are classified as having asymptomatic neurosyphilis rather than latent syphilis. The latent stage is arbitrarily divided into early and late phases. The early latent phase, which is less than 4 years' duration, is considered to be potentially infectious following relapse to the secondary stage, while the latent phase, which is greater than 4 years' duration, is considered noninfectious.

Syphilis may be transmitted to a fetus through the placenta by the infected mother after the 5th month of pregnancy. As a result of infection, the pregnancy may result in spontaneous abortion, a stillborn infant or a premature or full term infant with syphilis. A serological examination for syphilis should be a routine test taken at the first prenatal visit of every pregnant woman.

Congenital syphilis is often a severe disease manifested by dehydration and malnutrition. The infants also display skin lesions, persistent rhinitis, tenderness over the long bones and pseudoparalysis. X-ray of the long bones may demonstrate areas of bone destruction and osteochondritis. Late congenital syphilis often is manifested 20 years after birth with signs of central nervous system (CNS) involvement. Eighth nerve deafness, optic atrophy and juvenile paresis occur. Hutchinson's teeth are an unusual manifestation of late congenital syphilis; the peg-like teeth are widely spaced, small and notched. Congenital neurosyphilis poses a serious prognosis owing to a lack of response to therapy.

The lesions of late syphilis are manifested in virtually every organ system and tissue in man. Late syphilis of the skin and the mucous membranes is demonstrated by the appearance of small nodules or ulcerating gummas. The gumma begins as a painless sore that swells and eventually ruptures, exuding a thick gummy material. Gumma formation in the mucous membranes of the nose and throat may lead to painful destruction of the palate and nasal septum.

The skeletal system is affected in about 5% of patients with late syphilis. The skull and tibia are most frequently involved; however, the clavicle, humerus and ribs may also be affected. Pain, tenderness and inflammation over the affected area are common complaints. The Charcot joint is a common manifestation of bone involvement and is a result of the destruction of proprioceptive nerves in tabes dorsalis. The knee, ankle, hip and occasionally the spine are the areas most affected. The joint swells and becomes hypermobile. Disintegration of the joint surface follows, leaving fragments of bone and connective tissue behind. Antisyphilitic therapy is of little use, and so orthopedic measures must be pursued. Differentiation between osseous syphilis and other diseases is obtained by serological tests, roentgenographic examination, biopsy and response to antisyphilitic therapy. A negative Venereal Disease Research Laboratory (VDRL) is strong evidence against the diagnosis of osseous syphilis.

Syphilitic involvement of the cardiovascular system and CNS are the most serious complications of the disease and account for 90% of the deaths due to syphilis. Cardiovascular manifestations usually appear 20 to 30 years after the original infection. The fundamental lesion is an inflammation of the ascending aorta. *T. pallidum* invades the media of the aorta causing a destruction of the tissues and a subsequent loss of elasticity which may lead to the formation of an aneurysm. The aneurysm can subsequently enlarge and rupture, causing death.

The clinical symptoms of neurosyphilis may range from a reversible meningitis to irreversible paralysis and insanity. The mildest symptoms, such as headache, vomiting and malaise, are manifestations of a meningitis that is usually reversible upon institution of appropriate therapy. However, invasion of the nervous system tissues by *T. pallidum* may lead to general paresis, tabes dorsalis or optic atrophy. General paresis, or dementia paralytica, usually occurs 10 to 25 years after the primary lesion and is first evidenced by loss of memory, confusion and impaired judgment. The disease process rapidly progresses to the point where the patient is physically, mentally and socially disabled. General paresis is fatal, usually within 3 years. Tabes dorsalis, or locomotor ataxia, may become evident 10 to 20 years after the primary lesion. Destruction of portions of the nervous system affect the patient's sense of joint position and cause stumbling while walking. A characteristic gait is developed as the disease progresses. Sharp jabs of pain may appear anywhere in the body; these "lightning pains" are experienced by most patients with tabes dorsalis. Optic atrophy occurs in 1% of untreated syphilitics and eventually leads to blindness.

DIAGNOSIS

Dark field microscopic examination is an important tool used in the diagnosis of syphilis. It provides the earliest means of diagnosing syphilis. The object of dark field examination is to obtain serous material from a suspected syphilitic lesion, place the material on a slide and view it through a compound microscope fitted with a dark field condenser. Objects viewed through such equipment appear to be brightly illuminated when placed against a black background. Positive identification can be made by observing organisms of the characteristic morphology and motility of *T. pallidum*. The identification of *T. pallidum* with dark field microscopy is a positive diagnosis of infectious syphilis.

The serological tests used for the diagnosis of syphilis are divided into treponemal and nontreponemal types. The treponemal tests utilize antigen from *T. pallidum* and detect antibodies to that pathogen. Reagin titers may result from infections or conditions other than those caused by *T. pallidum;* hence, nontreponemal tests are less specific than treponemal tests. Nontreponemal tests may be further divided into complement fixation and floccula-

tion forms. The most widely used complement fixation test is the Kolmer. The VDRL slide test is the most commonly used flocculation test. Reagin titers are usually negative or low during early primary syphilis but continue to rise as the disease progresses. The majority of patients treated for primary syphilis return to a negative VDRL within 6 to 12 months after treatment. The VDRL in patients with secondary syphilis usually becomes negative within 12 to 24 months after treatment. However, some patients remain positive for life but do not require further treatment.

One of the problems of the nontreponemal test is the occurrence of the false positive reaction. Since reagins are nonspecific antibodies and may result from conditions other than syphilis, such as autoimmune diseases, the nontreponemal tests do not confirm the diagnosis of syphilis. The diagnosis must be made with the aid of a complete and careful history coupled with physical and dark field examinations. It may be necessary to corroborate laboratory tests and physical findings with a treponemal test in order to make the final diagnosis of syphilis.

The treponemal test of choice is the FTA-ABS (fluorescent treponemal antibody absorption) test. Killed *T. pallidum* in suspension is used as the antigen. The reaction indicator is a fluorescein-labeled antihuman globulin. When the antigen, indicator and patient's serum are combined, the antibody in the patient's serum, if present, fluoresces under a microscope that utilizes an ultraviolet light source. The FTA-ABS test has essentially replaced the Treponema Pallidum Immobilization test as a diagnostic tool. The FTA-ABS test is sensitive, has high specificity for the treponematoses, and manifests only infrequent false positive reactions.

The diagnosis of gonorrhea is made more easily in males than in females. The history of recent sexual contact combined with positive clinical findings and the microscopic demonstration of Gram-negative diplococci in urethral exudate smears constitutes a positive diagnosis of gonorrheal infection. If the history and clinical picture are suggestive of gonorrhea, but no diplococci can be seen on microscopic examination, a culture specimen from the anterior urethra should be obtained and inoculated on Thayer-Martin (TM) medium. TM medium is a medium that contains vancomycin, colistimethate and nystatin and is selective for *N. gonorrhoeae* and *N. meningitidis.* Specimens from the anal canal and pharynx may also be inoculated on TM medium. The diagnosis of gonorrhea in the females is difficult and presents major obstacles to control programs. Direct smears taken during the acute phase of the disease are fairly reliable; however, they become unreliable as the disease progresses or if the patient is asymptomatic. Specimens from the cervix and anal canal can be inoculated on TM medium for diagnosis. The culture procedure must be repeated after treatment as a test-for-cure. Gram staining with microscopic examination is recommended only as an adjunct to TM culture because of the likelihood of obtaining false negative and positive reactions. Gonococcal infections in women must be differentiated from leukorrhea due to *Trichomonas* vaginitis, monilia or physical or chemical irritants.

TREATMENT

The successful treatment of syphilis and gonorrhea requires the recognition and application of several principles. First, the antibiotic used for treatment should be effective against both diseases, since syphilis and gonorrhea may simultaneously infect the host. Second, high serum levels of the antibiotic should be achieved with the proper dosage regimen. This aspect of antibiotic therapy is most important when treating gonorrhea. Third, the prescriber should know the local resistance patterns of gonorrhea to avoid prescribing ineffective doses of the antibiotic. And fourth, the antibiotic used should be inexpensive and effective in a single dose so that the patient's compliance will not be a factor in the therapeutic result.

Compliance is a major factor in treatment failures. Patients simply fail to adhere to dosage regimens because they are too complicated or require frequent dosing. Conversely, a patient is more likely to be willing to follow a single dose regimen because it requires little effort and memory on his part.

The drug of choice for the treatment of syphilis at any stage is parenteral penicillin G (Table 42.1).[11,12] Unlike gonorrhea, there is no evidence to indicate that *T. pallidum* is becoming resistant to penicillin; hence, treat-

ment regimens are relatively straightforward. Patients with primary, secondary and latent syphilis with negative CSF findings may be treated with either 1.2×10^6 units of aqueous procaine penicillin G (APPG) given intramuscularly daily for 10 days or with a single intramuscular dose of 2.4×10^6 units of benzathine penicillin G given in two sites.[11,12] Patients with late syphilis and those with cardiovascular and neurological involvement are treated with 1.2×10^6 units of APPG given intramuscularly each day for 15 days;[12] alternative therapy may be instituted with 3×10^6 units of benzathine penicillin G given intramuscularly at once and repeated twice at 7-day intervals.[12]

Pregnant women are treated in the same manner as other infected individuals. Monthly serological tests should be done until delivery to determine the adequacy of therapy as indicated by a fall in titer. If there has been a rise in serological titer, retreatment of the mother is necessary.

The treatment of infants over 2 months old with congenital syphilis is best accomplished with APPG. Children under 2 months of age should receive aqueous crystalline penicillin G to avoid abscess formation. Children under 2 years of age may be given 100,000 units of APPG for each kg of body weight divided into daily doses for 10 days with a 3,000,000-unit maximal total dosage.[12]

Tetracycline and erythromycin are alternative drugs to penicillin for the treatment of syphilis. Either drug may be substituted for penicillin in case of penicillin allergy, but tetracycline should be avoided in pregnant patients because of the potential for adverse effects on the teeth and bones of the developing fetus. For the same reasons, tetracycline should not be given to children under 8 years of age. Tetracycline 500 mg may be given orally every 6 hours for 15 days with a total dose of 30 g.[12] Erythromycin 750 mg orally every 6 hours for 15 days may be given to pregnant patients who are allergic to penicillin.[12]

Gonorrhea presents drug treatment problems because of the relative resistance to multiple antibiotics that *N. gonorrhoeae* has acquired. The objective of drug therapy is to attain and maintain high serum levels of antibiotic. In order to attain these high levels, it has become necessary to administer large doses of drugs and adopt the use of probenecid to maintain effec-

TABLE 42.1
Drug Regimens for the Treatment of Syphilis

Drug	Dose	Route	Frequency	Special Considerations
Procaine penicillin G[a] [1] [2] or Benzathine penicillin G	600,000–1.2×10^6 units 2.4x10^6 units	IM IM	Daily for 10 days Single dose	For primary, secondary and latent syphilis with negative CSF findings
Procaine penicillin G[1] [2] or Benzathine penicillin G[1] [2]	600,000–1.2×10^6 units 3x10^6 units	IM IM	Daily for 15 days Once weekly for 3 weeks	for late syphilis, neurosyphilis, cardiovascular syphilis
Procaine penicillin G[1] [2]	100,000 units/kg	IM	Daily for 10 days with maximal total dose of 3x10^6 units	for congenital syphilis for infants under 2 years of age; use crystalline penicillin G for newborns less than 2 months of age
Tetracycline[1] [2]	500 mg	PO	QID for 15 days	Useful for penicillin-sensitive patients; do not use in pregnant patients or children under 8 years old
Erythromycin[1] [2]	750 mg	PO	QID for 15 days	Useful for pregnant patients allergic to penicillin.

[a]Penicillin is the drug of choice.

tive serum levels of penicillin and its derivatives (Table 42.2).[13,14] Probenecid blocks the renal excretion of the penicillin. This blocking effect allows the penicillin to accumulate in the body, producing peak serum levels that are 25 to 100% higher than if the penicillin were administered alone. However, the use of probenecid is not without risk. For example, hemolytic anemia can occur in those patients with glucose 6-phosphate dehydrogenese deficiency.[15] Also, a drug rash that develops during therapy with a penicillin and probenecid presents diagnostic problems because either drug may be responsible.

Although the dose of penicillin G used and recommendations for the use of probenecid vary from one area of the world to another, penicillin is still the drug of choice for the treatment of gonorrhea.[12,16] At present, recommendations for the United States specify that 4.8×10^6 units of APPG should be given intramuscularly in 1 dose to patients with gonorrhea.[16] Both men and women should receive 1 g of probenecid 30 min prior to the APPG injections to provide for drug absorption and to insure effective inhibition of penicillin excretion. Benzathine penicillin G should not be used for the treatment of gonorrhea because adequate serum levels can not be attained.

Ampicillin may be given instead of penicillin in single doses of 2 g intramuscularly with 2 g of probenecid or 3.5 g orally with 1 g of probenecid.[16] The oral dose of ampicillin seems to be well tolerated and effective, but nausea, vomiting and diarrhea may occur.

Tetracycline is an effective antigonococcal when 1.5 g are given as an oral loading dose and followed by 500 mg every 6 hr for a total dose of 9g.[16] Doxycycline or minocycline may also be used if 200 mg are taken by mouth immediately, followed by 100 mg at bedtime and then 100 mg twice daily for three days; a single 300-mg dose is less effective.[17] Doxycycline and minocycline are more expensive than tetracycline but are no more effective.[17] However, the convenience of 12-hr dosing may favorably influence patient compliance.

The use of kanamycin should be avoided in those patients with compromised renal function because of the tendency of the drug to accumulate and cause ototoxicity. However, if necessary, the dose can be adjusted to avert this problem. A single intramuscular dose of 2 g is usually sufficient to eradicate infection.[12] Kanamycin should be used only if other drugs are ineffective or cause adverse reactions.

Spectinomycin is a new antibiotic derived from *Streptomyces spectabilis*. It is offered as a single dose injectable alternative to penicillin in the treatment of gonorrhea. Spectinomycin, unlike penicillin, is not effective against syphilis. There is no gonococcal cross-resistance between spectinomycin and penicillin nor is there any cross-allergenicity. Spectinomycin, while not a drug of first choice for the treatment of gonococcal infections, may be used in patients who have not responded to penicillin therapy or who are allergic to penicillin.[18] The usual dose is a single 2-g intramuscular injection for men and 4 g for women.[16] Spectinomycin appears to be ineffective in treating gonococcal pharyngitis.[19]

Cephaloridine may also be used as a single dose alternative to penicillin if 2 g are given intramuscularly. Cephaloridine is less effective than penicillin in the treatment of gonococcal infections and should not be used as a drug of first choice.[20–22]

The Jarisch-Herxheimer reaction is usually a benign complication of antitreponemal therapy with an antibiotic, usually penicillin. Six to 10 hr after an injection of penicillin, the skin lesions of the syphilitic may become intensified and the patient may complain of fever and malaise. The exacerbation of lesions is thought to be due to the sudden release of antigenic substances from lysed treponemes. Symptoms of the reaction may be controlled with antipyretics or corticosteroids.

Retreatment of the male patient is indicated if a Gram-stained smear from the anterior urethra is positive. If the smear is negative, a TM-culture specimen should be taken and the decision to treat the patient based upon culture results. Culture specimens should be taken from the endocervical *and* anal sites in female patients to determine the need for retreatment.

PREVENTION, PROPHYLAXIS, AND THE PHARMACIST

The prevention of gonorrheal ophthalmia neonatorum may be achieved with local instillation of tetracycline or choramphenicol ophthalmic drops, systemic penicillin G or with Crede's

TABLE 42.2
Drug Regimens for the Treatment of Gonorrhea

Drug	Dose	Route	Frequency	Special Considerations
Procaine penicillin G[a] [16] plus Probenecid [16]	4.8x10⁶ units 1.0 g	IM PO	Single dose Single dose	Give probenecid 30 min before penicillin
Ampicillin[a] [12] plus Probenecid [12]	2.0 g 2.0 g	IM PO	Single dose Single dose	Give probenecid 30 min before ampicillin
Ampicillin plus Probenecid [16]	3.5 g 1.0 g	PO PO	Single dose Single dose	May cause GI distress Give simultaneously
Spectinomycin [16]	2.0 g	IM	Single dose	Dosage for males; ineffective against syphilis and gonorrheal pharyngitis [19]
Spectinomycin [16]	4.0 g	IM	Single dose	Dosage for females; ineffective against syphilis and gonorrheal pharyngitis [19]
Tetracycline [16]	500 mg (1.5 g at once then 0.5 g every 6 hr for total of 9 g)	PO	QID for 4 days	Do not give to pregnant patients or children under 8 years of age
Doxycycline or Minocycline [21,23]	200 mg at once then 100 mg every 12 hr for 3 days	PO	Bid for 3 days	Same as tetracycline; no more effective than other tetracyclines; more expensive than tetracycline
Cephaloridine [20–22]	2.0 g	IM	Single dose	Less effective than other drugs listed
Kanamycin [12]	2.0 g	IM	Single dose	Potentially ototoxic and renal toxic

[a]Penicillin and ampicillin are the drugs of choice.

1% silver nitrate ophthalmic drops. However, these procedures are not without problems. The use of local antibiotics may cause a decrease in symptoms without effecting a cure. If allowed to progress, opthalmia neonatorum due to a gonococcal infection may lead to blindness. Systemic antibiotics, such as penicillin G may induce a hypersensitivity. Silver nitrate drops cause a chemical conjunctivitis after ophthalmic instillation. Because of these undesirable effects, there is much disagreement as to what procedure constitutes the best method for the prevention of gonorrheal ophthalmia. While the use of the Crede method has been on the wane, the trend appears to be a return to the instillation of 1% silver nitrate drops in both eyes of the newborn immediately after birth for the prevention of gonorrheal ophthalmia neonatorum.

The value of the condom as an effective barrier to venereal infection has been debated at length. Evidence acquired during World Wars I and II indicates that the condom is an effective device for preventing the spread of venereal disease. However, instruction on the use of the condom is an essential part of any effective preventive program.

The mainstay element of venereal disease control has been the case finding and treatment programs carried out by public health departments. The purpose of the programs is to find all persons who had sexual contact with the infected patient and provide all contacts with effective treatment. These programs, while effective, are hampered because all physicians do not report every case of venereal disease that they treat. Without a 100% reporting program, there can not be 100% control of venereal disease.

Pharmacists can instruct patients on the use of prophylactics and proper personal hygiene. The condom can be an effective mechanical barrier to infection and can greatly decrease the possibility of acquiring a venereal disease. Urination after intercourse or douching will also decrease the chances of infection as will the liberal application of soap and water to the genitals. In order to insure compliance, the pharmacist should instruct the patient in the proper way to self-administer antigonococcal and antisyphilis medications and stress the reasons for adhering to prescribed dosage regimens. The pharmacist's role in the prevention and treatment of venereal disease centers around education. It is important for the pharmacist to realize that many of the problems associated with venereal diseases are the result of ignorance. It is extremely important to educate the public to the disease processes of syphilis and gonorrhea so that old wives' tales and half-truths may be dispelled.

CONCLUSION

By any measurement, the world situation with respect to venereal disease presents us with a rather dismal outlook for the future. There is no sign of a decrease in the rate of infection. Ignorance, fed by complacency, about venereal disease is probably at an all time high. Unless some rather ambitious efforts are made to educate the lay public and the practitioner, attempts to control the rising incidence of the venereal diseases will be futile.

REFERENCES

1. Anon.: VD Fact Sheet, Ed. 28, 1971. Center for Disease Control, Atlanta, Georgia.
2. Fleming, W. L., Brown, W. J., Donohue, J. R., and Branningan, P. W.: National survey of venereal disease treated by physicians in 1968. J.A.M.A., 211: 1827, 1970.
3. Lucas, J. B.: The national venereal disease problem. Med. Clin. North Am., 56: 1073, 1972.
4. Willcox, R. R.: The current status of gonorrhoea control. Br. J. Clin. Pract., 25: 215, 1971.
5. Anon.: Morbidity and mortality annual supplement summary, 1971. Center for Disease Control, Atlanta, Georgia, 20: 15, 1972.
6. Lucas, J. B.: Gonococcal resistance to antibiotics. South. Med. Bull., 53: 22, 1971.
7. Amies, C. R.: Sensitivity of N. gonorrhoeae to penicillin and other antibiotics. Br. J. Vener. Dis., 45: 216, 1969.
8. Phillips, I., Rimmer, D., and Ridley, M.: In-vitro activity of twelve antibacterial agents against Neisseria gonorrhoeae. Lancet, 1: 263, 1970.
9. Reyn, A., and Bentzon, M. W.: Relationships between the sensitivities in vitro of Neisseria gonorrhoeae to spiramycin, penicillin, streptomycin, tetracycline and erythromycin. Br. J. Vener. Dis., 45: 223, 1969.
10. Martin, J. E., Jr., Samuels, S. B., and Peacock, W. L., Jr.: Neisseria gonorrhoeae and Neisseria meningitidis sensitivity to spectinomycin, lincomycin, and penicillin G. Antimicrob. Agents Chemother., 1964: 437, 1965.
11. Venereal Disease Program, Center for Disease Control: Syphilis: a synopsis. U.S. Public Health Service Publication No. 1660, p. 1, 1968.

12. Anon: Treatment and prevention of syphilis and gonorrhea. Med. Lett., 13: 85, 1971.
13. Holmes, K. K., Johnson, D. W., and Floyd, T. M.: Studies of venereal disease. I. Probenecid-procaine penicillin G combination and tetracycline hydrochloride in the treatment of "penicillin resistant" gonorrhea in men. J.A.M.A., 202: 461, 1967.
14. Johnson, D. W., Kuale, P. A., Afable, V. L., Stewart, S. D., Halverson, C. S., and Holmes, K. K.: Single dose antibiotic treatment of asymptomatic gonorrhea in hospitalized women. N. Engl. J. Med., 283: 1, 1970.
15. Williams, H. E.: Genetic disorders. In Clinical Pharmacology: Basic Principles in Therapeutics, p. 534, edited by K.L. Melmon and H.F. Morelli. The MacMillan Co., New York, 1972.
16. Anon.: Recommended treatment schedules for gonorrhea. Ann. Intern. Med., 76: 991, 1972.
17. Lucas, J. B.: Gonococcal resistance to antibiotics. South. Med. Bull., 53: 22, 1971.
18. Pedersen, A. H. B., Wiesner, P. J., Holmes, K. K., Johnson, C. J., and Turck, M.: Spectionmycin and penicillin G in the treatment of gonorrhea: a comparative evaluation. J.A.M.A., 220: 205, 1972.
19. Wiesner, P. J., Tronca, E., Bonin, P., Pedersen, A. H. B., and Holmes, K. K.: Clinical spectrum of pharyngeal gonococcal infection. N. Engl. J. Med., 288: 181, 1973.
20. Molin, L., and Mystrom, B.: A comparison between cephaloridine and penicillin in the treatment of gonorrhea. Chemotherapy, 15: 384, 1970.
21. Lucas, J. B., Thayer, J. D., Utley, P. M., Billings, T. E., and Hackney, J. E.: Treatment of gonorrhea in males with cephaloridine. J.A.M.A., 195: 919, 1966.
22. Keys, T. F., Halverson, C. W., and Clerke, E. J.: Single-dose treatment of gonorrhea with selected antibiotic agents. J.A.M.A., 210: 857, 1969.
23. Fiumara, N. J.: The diagnosis and treatment of gonorrhea. Med. Clin. North Am., 56: 1105, 1972.

chapter 43

UPPER RESPIRATORY INFECTIONS

Robert H. Levin, Pharm. D.

An upper respiratory tract infection (URI) is defined as one that involves the head and neck above the vocal cords or larynx. Any respiratory infection below the larynx in the trachea or bronchial tree is considered a lower respiratory infection, such as bronchitis and pneumonia. Upper respiratory infections represent a major health and economic problem to our society. For example, the loss of man-hours of work due to URI's costs approximately $5,000,000,000 annually.

ETIOLOGY

Krugman and Ward[1] have stated that greater than 90% of all acute respiratory infections are probably viral in origin. Hable[2] has shown that viruses (19%) and group A beta hemolytic streptococci (38%) account for most URIs in children from birth to 16 years of age. The viruses Hable reported responsible were influenza A_2/Hong Kong (5.5%), adenovirus (4.9%), parainfluenza (4.7%), rhinoviruses (1.2%), and Herpes simplex (1.8%). Respiratory syncytial virus (RSV), coxsackie B, cytomegalovirus (CMV) and polio account for less than 1% each. Mufson[3] identified specific viruses 34% of the time in a group of adults with URIs. The most predominant were rhinoviruses, found in 18% of the cases. Influenza A virus, parainfluenza virus type 1 or 3 and herpes virus each occurred in 2 to 5% of patients. Coxsackie virus, adenovirus and RSV accounted for less than 1% each in Mufson's study. There are more than 100 different viruses that can cause URIs (Table 43.1). The major viral groupings are the orthomyxoviruses, picornaviruses, adenoviruses, herpes virus, poxvirus and paramyxoviruses.[4] Nonviral causes of URI are Mycoplasma pneumonia, other bacteria, such as streptococci, Hemophilus influenza, some fungi and some rickettsia. However, these nonviral agents are much more commonly associated with lower respiratory tract infections.

GENERAL CHARACTERISTICS OF VIRUSES

Viruses are characterized by a lack of metabolism and only proliferate in living host cells in the animal body, in tissue culture medium or in the developing chick embryo. The size of viruses is quite variable. For example, the picornavirus is extremely small and can be seen only with an electron microscope. More complex viruses such as the poxvirus, however, can be visualized with a light microscope. The nucleus

TABLE 43.1

Viruses and Nonviral Agents in Acute Respiratory Disease[a]

Group	Nucleic Acid	Size	Subgroups	Total Number	Clinical Syndromes
		mμ			
Adenovirus	DNA	70-90	Adenoviruses, human	31	URI, pneumonia, bronchitis, croup, influenza-like illness
Herpesvirus	DNA	120-180	Herpes simplex 1, 2	2	Acute tonsillopharyngitis with vesicles or ulcers
			Varicella-zoster virus	1	Pneumonia
			Cytomegalovirus (CMV)	1	Pneumonia
			Mononucleosis (EBV)	1	URI
Poxvirus	DNA	230-300	Variola (smallpox)	1	Severe URI
Picornavirus	RNA	15-30	Rhinoviruses	>90	URI mainly in adults; bronchitis and pneumonia in children
			Enteroviruses		
			Coxsackie virus A	24	URI, tonsillopharyngitis, influenza-like illness
			Coxsackie virus B	6	URI, influenza-like illness, bronchitis, pneumonia
			Echovirus	33	URI, croup
			Poliovirus 1, 2, 3	3	URI
Togavirus	RNA	20-70	Rubella	1	URI
Orthomyxovirus	RNA	80-120	Influenza A, B, C	3	Influenza, croup, URI
Paramyxovirus	RNA	100-200	Rubeola	1	Measles, laryngitis, bronchitis pneumonia
		100-300	Parainfluenza 1, 2, 3, 4	4	URI, croup, bronchitis
		120-300	Respiratory syncytial	2+?	URI, croup, bronchitis, pneumonia
Nonviral agents (included because historically considered virus) Mycoplasma (PPLO)		125-150	*M. pneumoniae*	1	URI, pneumonia
			Other mycloplasmas	7	

[a]Others causing disease are reoviruses, psittacosis-ornithosis virus, lymphocytic choriomeningitis virus.

of a virus has either a core of ribonucleic acid (RNA) or deoxyribonucleic acid (DNA). DNA and RNA are nucleic acids that govern viral replication since they carry the genetic codes which determine all hereditary characteristics.

There are three current hypotheses to help explain the origin of viruses:[5]

1. Viruses originated as parasites of the first cellular organisms. These first viruses gradually developed into present viruses as new organisms and animals evolved.

2. Viruses are not individual organisms but only components of normal cells which occasionally and inexplicably get out of hand. In this sense, viruses may be likened to genes which have gotten out of control and continue

to replicate as long as there is building material available. A corollary to this hypothesis is that viruses are derivatives of normal cellular genes (nucleic acids) which centuries ago developed the capability of reproducing by themselves and forming a protective envelope to stabilize the structure as it passed from cell to cell.

3. Viruses have evolved from pathogenic bacteria through a retrograde evolutionary process. There is no evidence to support this theory. However, it remains viable because there are bacteria which have developed a parasitic existence and grow only with great difficulty outside host cells.

Most viruses, for example, measles, mumps, rubella and polio, have remarkably stable immunological characteristics so that after countless replication cycles, they have little or no genetic change. In contrast, a few are unstable and change continuously, such as the influenza viruses, rhinoviruses and adenoviruses. This instability poses a large problem to developing effective immunizations against the latter group. The protective envelope of the virus plus the other structured proteins have several important functions: they protect the virus from inactivation by enzymes (the nucleases), participate in the attachment of the virus particle to susceptible cells and are responsible for the structural symmetry of the virus. The proteins in the viral envelope are also responsible for the antigenicity of the virus: this is important when considering vaccine production.

PATHOGENESIS

The viruses causing URI gain entrance to the human host through the respiratory or gastrointestinal (GI) tract. Discharges from the mouth and nose of infected persons are transmitted to susceptible people by direct contact or droplet infection or by recently contaminated articles. Those viruses causing colds, flu or croup have a short incubation period of approximately 1 to 3 days, while measles and mumps, where viral replication occurs in the lymph nodes rather than in the respiratory tract, have a long incubation period. The incubation period in these diseases may be as long as 3 weeks. After the primary viremia seeds these sites with virus, a lag period occurs as the virus propagates in lymph tissue. Upon rupture of the lymph cells, numerous virus are released causing a secondary viremia. The viremia disseminates the virus into target tissues, such as the lungs and skin, which results in systemic disease. Even longer incubations are encountered with the so-called "slow" viruses. For example, reactivation of latent measles virus may occur 2 to 17 years after a measles infection and lead to Dawson's encephalitis (subacute sclerosing panencephalitis), a slowly debilitating and fatal disease. Other "slow" viruses are CMV and herpes virus; both are implicated as causative agents of disease many years after the primary infection.

As the virus replicates and disseminates, the human body responds to the foreign invader. The body produces an inflammatory condition in affected areas to increase blood perfusion. The increased perfusion brings lymphocytes to fight the infection and allows circulating antibodies, if present, to come in contact with the virus and inactivate it. Other physiological changes which occur in the affected areas and aid the body in combating infection are pyrexia, lowered cellular pH, and hypoxia. A cell-mediated immunity, which is not clearly understood, is also present[6-8] and consists of sensitized lymphocytes, activated macrophages and interferon, a nonspecific antiviral protein. Most viruses are potent stimulators of interferon production. Also a viral infection generally results in antibody production that aids in preventing reinfection.

Viral infections induce both local and systemic antibody production. Those viruses which invade the respiratory tract and proliferate in the superficial respiratory epithelium induce a local antibody response. Secretory gamma globulin A (IgA) is produced in the mucous cells and is secreted into the mucous blanket to act locally to inhibit viruses.[6,9] Unfortunately, there is a rapid turnover of these resistant epithelial cells and they are replaced with cells that are susceptible to reinfection. The IgA is very specific for each viral agent so that protection is afforded only upon reinfection with the same virus. Furthermore, only secretory IgA is of any benfit in fighting local infection. Circulatory serum gamma globulins are only partially protective for these local infections.

Serum gamma globulin G (IgG), gamma globulin M (IgM) and IgA afford complete protection only when systemic viremia occurs. These gamma globulins are produced after systemic viral infection. Serum levels of IgG afford excellent protection against those diseases with long incubation periods, such as measles, rubella and smallpox. The difference between local and systemic antibody production can be illustrated with polio vaccine. The parenteral inactivated polio vaccine (Salk, IPV) achieves high serum levels of immunity. However, no local immunity in the GI tract is produced. During a polio epidemic, a person adequately immunized with IPV can act as a carrier of the wild polio virus.[9] The poliovirus gains entrance to the host's intestine, proliferates and is excreted via the mouth and feces to infect others; but because of immunity, it causes no systemic disease in the host. However, when the oral polio vaccine (Sabin, OPV) is used to induce immunity, both local antibodies in the GI tract and systemic antibodies are produced. Thus, a person adequately immunized with OPV cannot act as a carrier or contract the disease during epidemics. Similar differences in the types of antibodies produced by natural rubella infection and immunization may account for the carrier state associated with immunized individuals during epidemics.[10-13] Individuals with protective serum antibodies asymptomatically harbor and transmit wild rubella virus to susceptible individuals. To correct this, Puschak utilized intranasal rubella vaccine and reported very promising results.[14]

The exogenous reinfection state,[6] as mentioned with polio and rubella, is an interesting phenomenon. With reinfection there is a presence of antibody, a decreased amount and duration of viral excretion by the host, usually no clinical manifestations and difficulty in isolating the virus. This is in sharp contrast to the initial infection where there are no antibody levels, viral excretion is heavy, clinical manifestions are present and isolation of the virus is relatively easy. The quantitative amount of antibody in the serum will determine the host's response to reinfection. With low levels of antibody, the host, upon asymptomatic reinfection, will respond by producing high serum levels. It is important to remember that even low levels protect the host from disease because only a small amount of the virus is present during the initial viremia. This, in a sense, is equivalent to receiving a booster dose of an immunization and is probably responsible for the lifetime immunity against diseases such as measles, rubella, mumps and others. If the host has high antibody levels, reinfection will not occur and antibody levels will remain unchanged. At times, owing to low levels of antibody, reinfection can occur with symptoms apparent.

There is also an endogenous reinfection state[6] which may or may not be clinically apparent. Cold sores and shingles from herpes virus can remain dormant or unapparent for many years in the host and suddenly appear and become symptomatic. CMV and measles virus can also exhibit this phenomenon.

INCIDENCE

Respiratory tract infections constitute more than half of all illnesses reported in the United States. From 1957 to 1962 there were 1,000,000,000 acute respiratory illnesses or about 227,000,000 per year.[1] This figure has been steadily rising so that currently there are approximately 1,000,000,000 cases of respiratory disease each year of which a majority are URIs.[15] About 52% of the time the patient is required to spend at least 1 day at home in bed. This corresponds to a loss of productivity of 2 days per person per year.

The incidence of acute URI in childhood has been reported to be 7 or more episodes per year per child.[16,17] The incidence is age-dependent with very little difference in sexes. Most cases occur in the age group of less than 1 year to 2 years old and then steadily decrease with age to about 4 to 6 episodes of acute URI per year for adolescents and adults. The frequency of infection in the last 40 years has remained relatively unchanged.[18]

DIAGNOSIS AND CLINICAL FINDINGS

Many of the viruses can cause all or none of the many symptoms of URI. The same virus may cause one illness in one individual and another illness in others.[19] Also, many viruses cause the same symptoms in many individuals. The common cold in children and adults and croup in children are the most common forms of upper respiratory infections and can be caused by most of the viruses discussed. Viral cultures to ascertain the etiological agent are seldom done because of the difficulty in culturing viruses and the time period involved in receiving an answer. Two weeks are required to report the results of a culture so that standard cultures are done only with epidemics. New techniques are being developed which are capable of determining the identity of viral agents in 24 hr. The use of immunofluorescent staining is one very promising method.[20] In this procedure, a patient's nasal secretion is mixed with fluorescent conjugated horse anti-parainfluenza antibody. If there is para-influenza virus in the nasal secretions, this antibody attaches to the virus and fluoresces in 24 hr giving a positive identification.

COMMON COLD

The etiological agents of colds and croup can be divided into groups of viruses which cause similar symptoms. Picornaviruses, adenoviruses, orthomyxoviruses and paramyxoviruses, with few exceptions, cause nearly identical disease states.

General Virus Groups

Picornaviruses. The picornaviruses derived their name from their physical characteristics, *i.e.,* a very small size (pico) and nucleic acid core (RNA). This group is composed of two diversified subgroups: the rhinoviruses and the enteroviruses—coxsackie, enteric cytopathogenic human orphan (ECHO) and polio.

Rhinoviruses. The rhinoviruses are appropriately named for they were first isolated from the nasal discharge of colds. Many of the 63 variants are the main cause of colds or coryza in adults,[1] especially during the months of March through June. They are destroyed by stomach acid which differentiates them from the acid-stable enteroviruses.

Enteroviruses. The enteroviruses are predominately associated with GI complaints since they primarily propagate in and infect the intestinal tract; but they also cause URI. Many of the 30 varieties of coxsackie groups A and B and many of the 33 ECHO variants cause a large number of respiratory symptoms in children and adults.

Adenoviruses. The adenoviruses were recovered from adenoid tissue in 1953. The 28 variants may account for as much as 23% of viral URI in young children,[21] but it affects all ages with an over-all incidence of 5 to 10%.[1] Some recently published articles[22-24] have included the observation that adenoviruses may either exactly mimic or cause pertussis (whooping cough) or make the patient more susceptible to secondary bacterial invasion. History sometimes repeats itself. For years it was thought that the bacteria *H. influenza* was the cause of influenza. Now influenza is known to be viral in origin. Now we see that much of pertussis may actually be viral. Adenoviruses have also been implicated in causing cancer in laboratory animals[25] a finding which brought research on adenovirus immunizations to a standstill.

Orthomyxovirus. *Influenza.* Influenza is the only member of this group that causes URI symptoms. Influenza, when it reaches epidemic proportions, accounts for a large majority of viral infections. Influenza viruses occur in three antigenically different types: A, B and C. Types A and B cause epidemics, such as the A_2/Hong Kong epidemic, whereas type C causes only sporadic disease. The incidence of infection varies from year to year. These cyclic epidemics are caused by either a periodic waxing and waning of the general immunity of the population or a periodic change in the antigenic composition of the influenza virus.

Paramyxovirus. This group contains the subgroups of parainfluenza, RSV, measles and mumps. The paramyxoviruses are medium-sized viruses with a RNA core.

Parainfluenza. Parainfluenza virus accounts for a large percentage of viral URI infections in children less than 4 years old. There are 4 antigenically separate groups classified as 1, 2, 3 and 4. The primary infection in children is usually severe or "croupy," but reinfection is generally mild because of protective antibody titers.

Respiratory Syncytial (RS). The ubiquitous RS virus probably occurs in at least two strains and is the agent primarily responsible for causing lower respiratory disease in infants less than 6 months old.[1,26] As with parainfluenza virus, the primary RS infection is severe but later reinfections are mild because of protective antibody levels.

Symptoms

The common cold encompasses a number of entities—URI, coryza, rhinitis, rhinopharyngitis, acute catarrh and tonsillopharyngitis with or without exudate, vesicles or ulcers. The incubation period is short, being from 1 to 6 days with an average of 2 days. Colds are spread by direct person-to-person contact through contaminated droplets in the air or by touching contaminated personal items.

The common cold causes a wide range of symptoms which are all too familiar to each of us. Varying degrees of nasal congestion and discharge will occur. Initially, this discharge is clear and watery but, with progression of the disease, it becomes thicker and opaque. It may also become purulent if secondarily infected with bacteria. A conjunctivitis and watering eyes, a sore throat and unproductive cough are also rather common manifestations of the cold. If a lower respiratory infection complicates a cold, the increased pulmonary secretions will lead to a productive cough. A redness of the pharynx and tonsils without an exudate commonly occurs and is usually accompanied by a sore throat. If an exudate is present on the tonsils, bacterial agents such as streptococci or diptheria are suspected, although some forms of adenoviruses and herpes virus can also cause exudates. Herpes virus is also the probable causative agent (coxsackie has also been implicated) when vesicles or ulcers are seen. Temperature usually is not elevated to more than 101°F. Chilly sensations are common, as are sneezing and headache. Infection with influenza virus also causes marked prostration, muscular aches and a high incidence of lower respiratory symptoms.

In patients, especially children, with repeated colds, it is important to differentiate an infectious process from an allergic one. The symptoms of both a cold and allergic rhinitis are clinically indistinguishable. Fortunately, a patient with allergic rhinitis does have some characteristic symptoms. A constant watery rhinorrhea is noted with frequent sneezing and nasal itching. Wheezing is generally heard and night cough is a frequent occurrence. The allergic child also has a higher incidence of skin rashes.

The common cold is usually a short-lived benign disease. Although the symptoms can be very discomforting, they seldom cause serious complications. The complications they do cause are exacerbations of the primary disease. The usual complications which are more common in children are secondary bacterial infection, chiefly in the pulmonary tree because of mucous plugging of the bronchioles, otitis media and croup. Bacterial agents and some viral agents will cause bronchitis, bronchiolitis, pneumonia and other lower respiratory tract infections. Pharyngitis caused by streptococci (strept throat) is an important disease to differentiate from a viral sore throat because it can cause numerous serious sequela, such as rheumatic fever, kidney damage and scarlet fever.

Acute otitis media is almost always associated with an URI. Infectious agents enter the middle ear through the eustachian tube. Normally these agents are excreted from the ear via the eustachian tubes. However, children have short horizontal eustachian tubes which are prone to obstruction from inflamed tonsils, adenoids or mucous plugging. If a tube is obstructed, the infectious agents will progate in the middle ear and cause otitis media. To prevent damage to the ear and a possible loss of hearing, it is important to treat probable bacterial otitis media with medications.

There are some interesting observations that can be made about colds. Cold weather *per se* does not increase the probability of getting colds. Chilling of the body and wet feet will not in themselves induce colds; however, a chilly body will result in a decrease in body temperature. The nose, which is especially sensitive to cold, becomes irritated when chilled, and sneezing and a serous discharge follow. This ensuing rhinitis is frequently confused with actual viral infections. Susceptibility to infection does not appear to be affected by the general state of a person's health but a poor state of nutrition is a large factor for increasing the severity of colds or developing complications. Fatigue or emotional disturbances may temporarily lower one's resistance to infection. Allergic people develop colds more easily after exposure than nonallergic people, 45 and 30% incidence, respectively.[27] Finally, women in the middle third of their menstrual cycle (10 to 20 days after menstruation) are more susceptible to colds after being chilled and exposed to cold than at any other time in their cycle.[27]

Medicinal Treatment

The treatment of colds is carried out on a completely symptomatic basis. With the plethora of medications on the market,[28,29] it seems more of an art than a science to select the proper treatment. The growing number of combination products not only "boggles the mind" because of sheer numbers but also from the standpoint of efficacy. This large number of products plus the reported high placebo response to cold medications leads one to believe that effective treatment is difficult to quantify. The inclusion of many pharmacological agents in one preparation, some of which negate the action of others, makes it difficult to understand the rationality of the formulation. The combination "shotgun" preparations containing antihistamines, decongestants, expectorants and antitussives seem to alleviate some symptoms of colds but no one has shown why or how. We have come to this enigma because people desire and manufacturers have produced one pill or liquid to cure all symptoms. Cold formulas should be kept simple with the judicious use of a few drugs to treat a limited number of specific symptoms (Table 43.2).

Analgesics. Analgesics, such as aspirin and acetaminophen, are commonly used for the minor aches, pains and fever associated with colds. Aspirin is the drug of choice for adults and older children but not for children under 2 years old. This young age group is particularly sensitive to the toxic effects of aspirin and small overdoses can cause serious problems. Acetaminophen is an excellent substitute for aspirin in this age group. It is equivalent to aspirin as an analgesic and antipyretic and is much less toxic.[28] Its availability in liquid and chewable form is a definite advantage. Acetaminophen is also commonly substituted for aspirin in those older children and adults who can not tolerate aspirin.

Antibiotics. Antibiotics should not be used prophylactically for colds but only for proven or highly suspected bacterial infections.[30,31] The indiscriminate use of antibiotics has not changed the incidence of respiratory infections[18] and can only lead to the development of more resistant strains of micro-organisms, which remain a major problem. The proper antibiotic should be used for suspected bacterial otitis media, pneumonia or other pulmonary disease.

Nose Drops and Sprays. Nose drops and sprays containing decongestants sometimes provide impressive and immediate relief of congestion. Unfortunately, this relief does not last unless the drops or sprays are used continuously.

The drops and spray are equally efficacious, but the spray is easier to use and has a better distribution in the nasal mucosa. Tolerance to these preparations is common. Upon withdrawal of the drops, it is not uncommon to get a rebound congestion which may be as severe as the original congestion. Because of this, it is not unusual for adults and young children to abuse the use of drops and get into a nose drop habit. In short, nose drops or sprays should be used judiciously, as infrequently as possible and not for sustained periods of time.

Nose drops in oily vehicles should not be used because infants frequently choke and aspirate the drops, which may result in a lipoid pneumonia. Those containing antibiotics and antiseptics are not efficacious and should not be used. Antiseptics like eucalyptus and thymol can paralyze the cilia and prevent the clearing of mucous. This causes more problems than the disease.[1] The cilia can also be paralyzed if hypotonic or very hypertonic solutions are used. If a physician requests a mother to prepare normal saline drops for her infant, she can do more harm than good if she incorrectly prepares the solution. A solution prepared by a pharmacist, though, would be isotonic and relatively sterile. Decongestant nasal drops have been utilized in otitis media; however, their value in preventing otitis media is questionable. Because infants less than 6 months of age breath only with their nose, drops may be helpful just prior to meals in those congested infants who are having difficulty feeding. The 2 most common drops used for infants are phenylephrine and xylometazoline. The fact that phenylephrine is available over-the-counter (OTC) may be an advantage. Phenylephrine causes more rebound congestion than xylometazoline, but the latter is more toxic causing profound sedation when absorbed systemically. Other nasal preparations used by adults have little difference in efficacy except for providing possibly longer effects with less frequent dosing.

Ear Drops. Ear drops containing local anesthetics have been used to reduce the pain of otitis media by anesthetizing the tympanic membrane. Most pediatricians, however, prefer to use systemic acetaminophen or aspirin for pain relief. The use of ear drops containing antibiotics and/or corticosteroids for otitis media is irrational. There is no effective penetration of these agents across the tympanic membrane into the middle ear. However, a perforated ear drum secondary to a case of otitis media can discharge purulent material into the external canal. This discharge can lead to an otitis externa which is amenable to local therapy with an antibiotic otic solution. One consideration that has not been studied with otic solutions is the problem of local absorption through the perforated ear drum of neomycin, an ototoxic drug and a common constituent in otic solutions. The perforated drum could allow a significant absorption of neomycin to occur and possibly cause ear damage.

Oral Decongestants. The most frequently used oral decongestants are ephedrine, pseudoephedrine, phenylpropanolamine and phenylephrine (Table 43.3). These agents are used either alone or in combination with antihistamines and other agents. Because these agents may increase blood sugar and raise blood pressure, people with diabetes mellitus, heart disease, hypertension, hyperthyroidism or cardiovascular disease and geriatric patients or infants should be appropriately cautioned regarding these products. The geriatric patient is much more sensitive to the effects of these agents. Nasal secretions in the infant less than 6 months of age with rhinorrhea can become so viscous after decongestant use as to cause obstruction of the nasal passages and extreme difficulty in breathing.

Oral decongestants have certain advantages over the nasal decongestants.

1. They reach all the respiratory membranes via the blood and are not dependent on absorption through the thick mucous layer in the nose as are the drops.

2. They generally have a longer duration of effect.

3. They cause no rebound nasal congestion.

4. There is no nose drop habit.

5. They are easily administered with an accurate dosage which is not easily achieved with drops.

6. They cause no pathological changes in the cilia or nasal mucosa.

The oral decongestants also have disadvantages:

1. Systemic side effects are common, such as nervousness, increased heart rate and insomnia.

Such side effects are unusual with normal doses of the nasal decongestants.

2. Tolerance develops so that increasing doses must be given.

3. They have not been conclusively proven to be efficacious in the treatment of nasal congestion. They are used traditionally and empirically as a rational way to treat rhinorrhea.

Ephedrine is probably the best orally absorbed of these agents. Phenylephrine is the most poorly absorbed since it is readily destroyed in the stomach by the enzyme monoamine oxidase. It is so readily inactivated that an adequate oral dose is very difficult to achieve, making its use in oral preparations at best questionable. Ephedrine causes the most central nervous system (CNS) stimulation and phenylephrine the least (Table 43.3). Phenylpropanolamine has a greater vasopressor effect than ephedrine or pseudoephedrine but less than phenylephrine. Antihistamines are sometimes combined with these agents in an effort to counteract their central stimulating effect.

Combination Products. Because of their sedative properties, the antihistamines do counteract some of the stimulant effects of the oral decongestants. This theoretical balancing of effects does not always achieve the anticipated results. Some people are more sensitive to the effects of either the antihistamines or the decongestants and react accordingly. Not surprisingly, parents seek those products which produce sedation in children. The combination products are more attractive to mothers because they want to give as few different doses of medications as possible to their sick, cranky and obstinate children. Successful combinations for each individual are usually found only after considerable trial and error using many products. This combination also has an additive effect in decreasing rhinorrhea—the decongestant due to vasoconstriction there by decreasing edema and the antihistamine due to its anticholinergic effect of mucous drying.[32] The combination products, however, reduce flexibility in dosing. It is not possible to recommend one combination oral decongestant and antihistamine preparation over another. Minimal side effects, symptomatic relief and palatability will determine the product used by each individual. Children or adults with asthma, acute

TABLE 43.2
Pediatric Preparations[a]

Preparation	Ingredients[b]				Miscellaneous
	Expectorant	Antihistamine	Decongestant	Antitussive	
Cough preparations (OTC with dextromethorphan)					
Arrestin cough medicine	GG, sodium citrate, chloroform			10 mg D.M.	10% alcohol
Cerose-DM expectorant	Ipecac, glycerin, potassium guaiacosulfonate, sodium citrate, citric acid	5 mg phenindamine tartrate	Phenylephrine	10 mg D.M.	
Cheracol-D cough syrup	GG, chloroform, NH_4Cl, antimony potassium tartrate, white pine, wild cherry bark			10 mg D.M.	
Children's Romilar	GG			7.5 mg D.M.	
Coldene cough & cold	Chloroform, GG, sodium citrate	1 mg Chlorpheniramine	11 mg phenylpropanolamine	7.5 mg D.M.	11.4% alcohol 120 mg acetaminophen
Contotuss antitussive syrup	100 mg GG, chloroform	3.5 mg doxylamine		15 mg D.M.	10% alcohol
Coryban-D cough syrup	Chloroform, GG	1 mg chlorpheniramine	5 mg phenylephrine	7.5 mg D.M.	120 mg acetaminophen
Cosanyl-DM cough syrup	Tr. euphorbia, Syr. wild lettuce, Tr. cocillana, Syr. squill, cascarin, menthol		5 mg phenylephrine	15 mg D.M.	6% alcohol

TABLE 43.2
Pediatric Preparations[a]

Preparation	Ingredients[b]				
	Expectorant	Antihistamine	Decongestant	Antitussive	Miscellaneous
Dextrotussin cough syrup	NH₄Cl	2 mg chlorphenir-amine	5 mg phenylephrine	15 mg D.M.	
Diacof cough syrup	GG, ether	0.75 mg chlorphenir-amine		7.5 mg D.M.	
Dorcol pediatric cough syrup	GG		8.75 mg phenylpro-panolamine	7.5 mg D.M.	5% alcohol
Dristan cough formula	Sodium citrate, GG, chloroform	1 mg chlorphenir-amine	5 mg phenylephrine	7.5 mg D.M.	12% alcohol
Endotussin NN pediatric syrup	NH₄Cl, citric acid			5 mg D.M.	0.15 mg homatropine
Endotussin NN syrup	Sodium citrate, NH₄Cl	7.5 mg pyrilamine		10 mg D.M.	0.25 mg homatropine
Naldetuss syrup	Terpin hydrate	7.5 mg phenyltol-oxamine	17.5 mg phenylpro-panolamine	15 mg D.M.	160 mg acetaminophen
Orthoxicol cough syrup	Sodium citrate		17 mg methoxy-phenamine	10 mg D.M.	
Pertussin 8 hour formula	NH₄Cl, chloroform, sodium citrate			7.5 mg D.M.	9.5% alcohol
Pertussin wild cherry cough syrup	NH₄Cl, chloroform, sodium citrate			3.5 mg D.M.	
Pyraldine expectorant	NH₄Cl, citric acid	12.5 mg pyrilamine		15 mg D.M.	
Pyraldine pediatric cough syrup	NH₄Cl, citric acid	12.5 mg pyrilamine	5 mg phenylephrine	7.5 mg D.M.	

[a]Tabulation by Claudia Swenson, Pharm. D., University of Washington.
[b]All ingredients are tabulated per 5-cc dose. Abbreviations: GG = glycerol guaiacolate; D.M. = dextromethorphan; NH₄Cl = ammonium chloride; Tr = tincture; Syr. = syrup.

TABLE 43.2
Pediatric Preparations[a]

Preparation	Ingredients[b]				Miscellaneous
	Expectorant	Antihistamine	Decongestant	Antitussive	
Quelidrine syrup	Ipecae, NH$_4$Cl	2 mg chlorphenir-amine	5 mg ephedrine, 5 mg phenylephrine	10 mg D.M.	2% alcohol
Robitussin-DM syrup	100 mg GG			15 mg D.M.	1.4% alcohol
Romilar cough formula	Ipecac, chloroform	1 mg chlorphenir-amine		15 mg D.M.	120 mg acetaminophen, 10% alcohol
St. Joseph's cough syrup for children	Ipecac, sodium citrate, menthol			7.5 mg D.M.	
Thormal syrup	Potassium guaiacol-sulfonate, citric acid, sodium citrate, thymol, tolu, chloroform, menthol	12.5 mg pyrilamine	5 mg phenylephrine	10 mg D.M.	
Triaminicol syrup	NH$_4$Cl	6.5 mg pyrilamine and pheniramine	12.5 mg phenyl-propanolamine	15 mg D.M.	
Trind-DM syrup	GG		2.5 mg phenylephrine	7.5 mg D.M.	150 mg acetaminophen, 15% alcohol
Tussagesic suspension	Terpin hydrate	6.25 mg phenir-amine, 6.25 mg pyrilamine	12.5 mg phenyl-propanolamine	15 mg D.M.	120 mg acetaminophen
Tussi-Organidin DM expectorant	Iodinated glycerol	2 mg chlorphenir-amine		10 mg D.M.	15% alcohol

TABLE 43.2
Pediatric Preparations[a]

Preparation	Ingredients[b]					
	Expectorant	Antihistamine	Decongestant	Antitussive	Miscellaneous	
Cough syrups (OTC with noscapine)						
Conar liquid	Chloroform, menthol	2 mg chlorphenir-amine	10 mg phenyleph-rine	10 mg noscapine	5% alcohol	
Conar-A suspension	GG	1 mg chlorphenir-amine	5 mg phenylephrine	5 mg noscapine	120 mg acetaminophen	
Conar expectorant liquid	GG, menthol, chloroform	2 mg chlorphenir-amine	10 mg phenyleph-rine	10 mg noscapine	5% alcohol	
Cough preparations (containing codeine)						
Actified-C expectorant	100 mg GG	2 mg tripolidine	30 mg pseudoephe-drine	10 mg codeine phosphate		
Acutuss expectorant with codeine	GG, chloroform	2 mg chlorphenir-amine	5 mg phenylephrine, 5 mg phenylpropan-olamine	10 mg codeine phosphate	5% alcohol	
Ambenyl expectorant	NH$_4$Cl, menthol, potassium guaia-colsulfonate	3.75 mg bromo-diphenhydramine, 8.75 mg diphen-hydramine		10 mg codeine sulfate	5% alcohol	
Calcidrine syrup	Calcium iodide		4.2 mg ephedrine	8.4 mg codeine	6% alcohol	
Cerose expectorant	Chloroform, sodium citrate, citric acid, ipecac, potassium guaia-colsulfonate, glycerine	10 mg phenind-amine	5 mg phenylephrine	10 mg codeine phosphate	2.5% alcohol	

TABLE 43.2
Pediatric Preparations[a]

| Preparation | Ingredients[b] | | | | | |
	Expectorant	Antihistamine	Decongestant	Antitussive	Miscellaneous
Cetro-Cirose	NH_4Cl, ipecac, sodium citrate, citric acid, potassium guaia-colsulfonate			5 mg codeine	1.5% alcohol
Cheracol syrup	NH_4Cl, tartar emetic, chloroform, wild cherry, white pine, potassium guaiacolsulfonate			11 mg codeine	3% alcohol
ChlorTrimeton expectorant with codeine	GG, NH_4Cl, sodium citrate, chloroform		10 mg phenylephrine	10 mg codeine phosphate	19% alcohol
Codimal PH syrup	Potassium guaia-colsulfonate, sodium citrate, citric acid, chloroform, menthol thymol, tolu	8.3 mg pyrilamine	5 mg phenylephrine	10 mg codeine phosphate	1% alcohol
Cosadein	Chloroform, wild cherry, white pine, eriodictyon, poplar bud, glycerine			11 mg codeine	20% alcohol
Cosanyl cough syrup	Tr. Cocillana, Syr. wild lettuce, cascarin, Tr. euphorbia, menthol, Syr. squill comp.		5 mg phenylephrine	11 mg codeine	6% alcohol

TABLE 43.2
Pediatric Preparations[a]

Preparation	Ingredients[b]				
	Expectorant	Antihistamine	Decongestant	Antitussive	Miscellaneous
Cotussis syrup	Menthol, chloroform glycerine, terpine hydrate		5 mg phenylephrine	11 mg codeine	6% alcohol
Dimetane expectorant D.C.	100 mg GG	2 mg bromopheniramine	5 mg phenylephrine, 5 mg phenylpropanolamine	10 mg codeine phosphate	3.5% alcohol
Emeracol	Potassium guaiacolsulfonate, NH_4 Cl chloroform, potassium antimony tartrate			5 mg codeine	3% alcohol
Ephedrol with codeine	Tolu, potassium guaiacolsulfonate, menthol, Syr. of squill		Ephedrine	10 mg codeine phosphate	
Histadyl E.C. syrup	NH_4Cl, chloroform, menthol	13.5 mg methapyrilene	5 mg ephedrine	10 mg codeine phosphate	5% alcohol
Isoclor expectorant	GG, sodium citrate citric acid	2 mg chlorpheniramine	12.5 mg pseudoephedrine	10 mg codeine phosphate	
Mercodol with decapryn	Sodium citrate	6 mg doxylamine	5 mg phenylephrine, 10 mg etafedrine	10 mg codeine phosphate	5% alcohol
Mercodol cough syrup	Sodium citrate		10 mg etafedrine, 5 mg phenylephrine	10 mg codeine phosphate	5% alcohol
Novahistine DH	Chloroform	2 mg chlorpheniramine	10 mg phenylephrine	10 mg codeine phosphate	5% alcohol

TABLE 43.2
Pediatric Preparations[a]

Preparation	Ingredients[b]				
	Expectorant	Antihistamine	Decongestant	Antitussive	Miscellaneous
Novahistine expectorant	100 mg GG, chloroform	2 mg chlorpheniramine	10 mg phenylephrine	10 mg codeine phosphate	5% alcohol
Phenergan expectorant with codeine	Ipecac, potassium guaiacolsulfonate, citric acid, sodium citrate, chloroform	5 mg promethazine		10 mg codeine phosphate	7% alcohol
Phenergan VC expectorant with codeine	Ipecac, potassium guaiacolsulfonate, citric acid, sodium citrate, chloroform	5 mg promethazine	5 mg phenylephrine	10 mg codeine phosphate	7% alcohol
Prunicodeine	Terpin hydrate, pinus strobus, prunus virginiana, sanguinaria			10 mg codeine	
Pyribenzamine expectorant with codeine	NH₄Cl, menthol, chloroform	37.5 mg tripelennamine	12.5 mg ephedrine	10 mg codeine phosphate	5% alcohol
Robitussin AC syrup	100 mg GG	7.5 mg pheniramine		10 mg codeine phosphate	3.5% alcohol
Sedatole expectorant	Wild cherry bark, sanguinaria, squill, gilead, phosphoric acid, menthol			5 mg codeine phosphate	6% alcohol

TABLE 43.2
Pediatric Preparations[a]

Preparation	Ingredients[b]				
	Expectorant	Antihistamine	Decongestant	Antitussive	Miscellaneous
Semcof syrup	Sodium citrate, NH₄Cl, tartar emetic		5 mg ephedrine	10 mg codeine phosphate	
Synephricol	Potassium guaiacolsulfonate, menthol, NH₄Cl, chloroform	4 mg thenyldiamine	5 mg phenylephrine	10.85 mg codeine	8% alcohol
Terpin hydrate with codeine elixir	85 mg Terpin hydrate			10 mg codeine phosphate	
Tussi-Organidin expectorant	Iodinated glycerol	2 mg chlorpheniramine		10 mg codeine phosphate	15% alcohol
Tussar-2 syrup	GG, sodium citrate, citric acid, chloroform	2 mg chlorpheniramine		10 mg codeine phosphate, 7.5 mg carbetapentane citrate	5% alcohol
Tussar S.F. cough syrup	GG, sodium citrate, citric acid, chloroform	2 mg chlorpheniramine		10 mg codeine phosphate, 7.5 mg carbetapentane citrate	12% alcohol
Prescription cough preparations (containing miscellaneous narcotics) Citra Forte syrup	Potassium citrate	3.3 mg pyrilamine, 2.25 mg pheniramine		5 mg hydrocodone bitartrate	2% alcohol
Citra syrup	Potassium citrate	3.33 mg pyrilamine, 2.5 mg pheniramine	2.5 mg phenylephrine	1.67 mg hydrocodone bitartrate	2% alcohol

TABLE 43.2
Pediatric Preparations[a]

Preparation	Ingredients[b]				
	Expectorant	Antihistamine	Decongestant	Antitussive	Miscellaneous
Codimal DH syrup	Potassium guaia-colsulfonate, sodium citrate, citric acid, chloroform	8.3 mg pyrilamine	5 mg phenylephrine	1.67 mg hydroco-done bitartrate	1% alcohol
Coditrate syrup	Sodium citrate, citric acid, potassium guaia-colsulfonate			1.67 mg hydroco-done bitartrate	1% alcohol
Combi-Tuss expectorant	Potassium guaia-colsulfonate		10 mg phenyleph-rine	0.83 mg hydroco-done, 7.5 mg D.M.	5% alcohol
Hycodan syrup				5 mg hydrocodone bitartrate	1.5 mg homa-tropine MBr
Hycomine syrup	NH$_4$Cl	12.5 mg pyrilamine	10 mg phenyleph-rine	5 mg hydrocodone bitartrate	1.5 mg homa-tropine
Hycomine pediatric syrup	NH$_4$Cl	6.25 mg pyrilamine	5 mg phenylephrine	2.5 mg hydroco-done bitartrate	0.75 mg homa-tropine
Tussend liquid		4 mg chlorphenir-amine	20 mg phenyleph-rine	5 mg hydroco-done bitartrate	5% alcohol
Tussionex suspension		10 mg phenyltolox-amine (in resin complex)		5 mg hydrocodone	
Cough preparations (containing miscellaneous non-narcotics) Novrad suspension				50 mg levopropoxy-phene	

TABLE 43.2
Pediatric Preparations[a]

Preparation	Ingredients[b]				Miscellaneous
	Expectorant	Antihistamine	Decongestant	Antitussive	
Rynatuss suspension		4 mg chlorpheniramine	5 mg ephedrine tannate	30 mg carbetapentane tannate	
Ulo syrup				25 mg chlophedianol	
Cold preparations (OTC, antihistamine-decongestant combinations)					
Coricidin cough formula	NH$_4$Cl, GG	2 mg chlorpheniramine	12.5 mg phenylpropanolamine		
Covangesic liquid		1 mg chlorpheniramine, 6.25 mg pyrilamine	3.75 mg phenylephrine, 6.25 mg phenylpropanolamine		120 mg acetaminophen
Ryna-Tussadine expectorant liquid	NH$_4$Cl	1 mg chlorpheniramine, 6.25 mg Pyrilamine	6.25 mg phenylpropanolamine, 3.75 mg phenylephrine		
Triaminic syrup		6.25 mg pyrilamine, 6.25 mg pheniramine	12.5 mg phenylpropanolamine		
Trind syrup	GG		2.5 mg phenylephrine		150 mg acetaminophen, 15% alcohol
Ventilade syrup		4.17 mg pyrilamine, 4.17 mg pheniramine, 4.17 mg methapyrilene	12.5 mg phenylpropanolamine		5% alcohol

TABLE 43.2
Pediatric Preparations[a]

Preparation	Ingredients[b]				
	Expectorant	Antihistamine	Decongestant	Antitussive	Miscellaneous
Cold preparations (prescription antihistamine-decongestant combinations)					
Actified syrup		1.25 mg tripolidine	30 mg pseudoephedrine		
Co-Pyronil suspension		7.5 mg pyrrobutamine, 12.5 mg methapyrilene	6.25 mg cyclopentamine		
Demazine syrup		1.25 mg chlorpheniramine	2.5 mg phenylephrine		
Dimetapp elixir		4 mg bromopheniramine	5 mg phenylephrine 5 mg phenylpropanolamine		
Isoclor liquid		2 mg chlorpheniramine	12.5 mg D-isoephedrine		
Naldecon syrup		2.5 mg chlorpheniramine, 7.5 mg phenyltoloxamine	20 mg phenylpropanolamine, 5 mg phenylephrine		
Nethaprin syrup		6 mg doxylamine	25 mg etafedrine		60 mg theophylline aminoisobutanol
Phenergan expectorant, plain	Ipecac, citric acid, potassium guaiacolsulfonate, chloroform	5 mg promethazine			7% alcohol
Phenergan VC expectorant, plain	Ipecac, citric acid, potassium guaiacolsulfonate, chloroform	5 mg promethazine	5 mg phenylephrine		7% alcohol

TABLE 43.2
Pediatric Preparations[a]

| Preparation | Ingredients[b] | | | | |
	Expectorant	Antihistamine	Decongestant	Antitussive	Miscellaneous
Polaramine expectorant	100 mg GG	2 mg dexchlorphen-iramine	20 mg D-isoephe-drine		7.2% alcohol
Pyribenzamine expectorant	NH$_4$Cl	37.5 mg tripelen-namine	12.5 mg ephedrine		
Ronec-D drops		5 mg carbinoxamine	150 mg pseudo-ephedrine		
Ronec-S syrup		2.5 carbinox-amine	60 mg pseudo-ephedrine		
Rynatan suspension		2 mg chlorphenir-amine tannate, 12.5 mg pyrilamine tannate	5 mg phenylephrine tannate		
Triaminic concentrate oral infant drops		50 mg pyrilamine, 50 mg pheniramine	100 mg phenyl-propanolamine		
Tuss-Ornade liquid		2 mg chlorphenir-amine	15 mg phenylpropan-olamine	5 mg caramiphen	0.75 mg isopropamide

TABLE 43.3
Common Decongestants

Drug	Equivalent Adult Dose mg	Frequency	Pediatric Dose mg/kg/24 hr	CNS Stimulation
Ephedrine	50	tid-qid	3	+++
Phenylephrine	10-25	tid-qid	4	−
Phenylpropanolamine	50	tid-qid	3	+
Pseudoephedrine	60	tid-qid	1-2	++

otitis media or sensitivity to antihistamines are probably better served with decongestants alone.

Furthermore, the usual practice is to put numerous drugs in cold preparations to treat cough symptoms as well. It is not uncommon to find antitussives, expectorants, decongestants, anticholinergics, vitamins and antihistamines together in the same preparation. This combination of ingredients increases the incidence of adverse effects. These products also pose a major treatment problem when accidently ingested in toxic quantities. Some ingredients in combination products are in a suboptimal dose, requiring doses above the recommended ones to achieve therapeutic results. The use of the larger doses may provide sufficient doeses of the other ingredients to cause serious side effects or toxicity. This lack of flexibility in dosing is an obvious drawback to the use of combinations. Finally, there is no convincing evidence that combination products are any better than placebos in treating the common cold.

When recommending products and doses, a pharmacist must carefully check the quantity of each ingredient in the product against its recommended dose. Most combination products, especially those sold OTC are labeled with directions that result in gross underdosing. An OTC product should be initially given at the recommended dose level to ascertain whether the patient will react adversely. If no adverse effects ensue, the recommended dose generally must be doubled before any therapeutic effect becomes evident. In some products, even higher doses must be given. In general, the dose should be increased until a therapeutic effect is achieved or until side effects become evident.

Antihistamines. The antihistamines are most effective for allergic reactions, such as allergic rhinitis, angioneurotic edema and others where their primary action is to block the effect of histamine.[33,34] They have equivocal effects in asthma and many exacerbate the wheezing because of their mucous drying effect. There is little difference between the antihistamines based on their efficacy as histamine blockers. Finally, the antihistamines are most effective as drying agents only in the initial stages of a cold.

The preference of one product over another rests purely on the side effects each produces (Table 43.4). The prominent side effects produced are anticholinergic in nature—mucous drying, sedation, tachycardia and decreased GI motility. Since the differences in products are based on side effects and somewhat on cost, the antihistamine chosen should be inexpensive and cause only desired side effects. For example, if a daytime dose is needed, a product with a low incidence of sedation, *e.g.*, chlorpheniramine, should be chosen so as not to interfere with one's routine. If a nighttime medication is needed, the reverse would be true—use the antihistamine with the highest incidence of sedation, *e.g.*, diphenhydramine. If one antihistamine does not achieve the desired effects after being given in doses large enough to elicit side effects, another product, preferably in a different chemical class, should be tried.

Cough and Throat Preparations. The cough associated with URI is usually brief, self-limiting and does not require an arsenal of medication to treat. If the cough is nonproductive and

TABLE 43.4
Common Antihistamines

Drug	Equivalent Adult Dose[a]	Pediatric Dose[a]	CNS Sedation
	mg	*mg/kg/24 hr*	
Ethanolamines			
Bromodiphenhydramine	25	2.5	+++
Carbinoxamine	4	0.4	+
Diphenhydramine	50	5.0	+++
Doxylamine	12-25	2.0	+++
Ethylenediamines			
Methapyrilene	50-100	5.0	+
Pyrilamine	50	2.5	++
Tripelennamine	50	5.0	++
Alkylamines			
Brompheniramine	4	0.5	+
Chlorpheniramine	4	0.35	+
Triprolidine	2.5[b]	0.2[b]	+
Phenothiazines			
Promethazine	25[b]	1.5[b]	+++

[a] All taken tid-qid, except as noted.
[b] Taken bid-tid.

is caused by irritation to the respiratory tract from inflammation or a postnasal drip, the treatment objective should be to ameliorate the cough. A rational approach would dictate the use of demulcents for the irritation with or without an antitussive. If a postnasal drip complicates the picture, a decongestant with or without an antihistamine could be separately added and individually titrated. If the patient has a lower respiratory infection and has a nonproductive cough, the aim of treatment should be to produce a productive cough to facilitate the removal of pulmonary secretions. Dehydration, a common problem in infections with high fever and patients with poor appetite, causes mucous to become viscous and tenacious. This is not reversed with medications until the patient is rehydrated. Expectorants are available and utilized to decrease mucous viscosity and facilitate its removal. Cool mist and steam vaporizers are also effective in loosening mucous, providing they are capable of significantly increasing the relative humidity of the air in the room.

Demulcents. A demulcent is any product that will coat the throat and soothe the irritated mucous membrane, *e.g.,* compound tincture of benzoin, elm bark or linseed. These products can be in the form of liquids, pastilles or lozenges. The liquids are thick and act as a protective blanket. Normal oral secretions act as the diluting liquid when pastilles or lozenges are used. In order to properly employ these agents to relieve sore throats, they must be able to coat the inflamed area—the back of the throat. The most effective way to achieve this with lozenges is for the patient to lie on his back and allow the lozenge to dissolve and slowly coat the back of his throat. This procedure can also be utilized with liquids but care must be taken in order not to aspirate them.

Gargles and Sprays. Most gargles and sprays are combinations of antiseptics and/or local anesthetics. Neither of these is effective for fighting viral or bacterial infections. The gargles, in addition, do not reach the pharynx— the painful area of a sore throat. Some local pain relief can be achieved from the local anesthetics in the sprays, but it is transient in nature. Importantly, a sore throat that lasts longer than 3 days should be seen and treated by a physician, for it may be a streptococcal infection.

Expectorants. There are a number of expectorants utilized in cough medications which are of little or no value, *e.g.,* ammonium citrate and other ammonium compounds, terpin hydrate, creosote, chloroform and squill.[35] There are three commonly used expectorants which in proper doses do seem to have value although this is unproven:[35] glyceryl guaiacolate, syrup of ipecac and iodide salts.

Blanchard[36] reported in 1954 that glyceryl guaiacolate with desoxyephedrine is an effective antitussive-demulcent-expectorant. The definition used here of an antitussive is one which reduces cough by facilitating the removal of mucous. The addition of desoxyephedrine is of doubtful efficacy in this preparation, however. Also, the subjectivity of this study makes the results difficult to interpret. Other studies done during the 1950's could be cited, but all suffer from being subjectively done with few or no controls. If glyceryl guaiacolate is to be effective at all, it must be given in therapeutic doses. Chodosh[37] stated that only at doses of 300 to 600 mg 4 times daily is there a definite decrease in sputum viscosity. Thus, the commonly recommended dose of 100 mg (usually 1 teaspoonful) 4 times daily is a substantial underdose. A therapeutic dose of glyceryl guaiacolate cough syrup for adults should be 10 to 30 ml 4 times daily with a proportional increase also for children. Generally, hydration alone is sufficient for children with URI.

Syrup of ipecac can be utilized as an expectorant in doses that are lower than the 15-ml emetic dose. Traditionally, 1 to 2 teaspoonsfuls were given to children with croup to induce emesis and force up tenacious sputum.[36] This proved to be efficacious but was usually only temporary in nature and unpleasant for the patient and family. The doses recommended now of 5 drops for a 1-year-old with a drop added for each year is an underdose. Furthermore, most commercial preparations contain less than 10% of the therapeutic dose.

Potassium and sodium iodide are the most commonly used iodides. They are effective in adults when given in therapeutic doses of at least 300 mg (0.3 ml saturated solution of potassium iodide) every 2 to 4 hours and in children at doses of 100 mg per year of age per 24 hr. Most preparations containing iodides have considerably less than these therapeutic doses. More important is that long term usage of iodides has caused goiters and symptoms of hypothyroidism, and so only short term usage should be considered.

Antitussives. The antitussives are considered to be medications which depress the cough reflex either centrally in the medulla or locally in the respiratory tree. The narcotics used (codeine, hydrocodone and ethylmorphine) work centrally as do the non-narcotics, dextromethorphan, noscapine and levopropoxyphene. Other non-narcotics,, such as chlophedianol HCl, dimenthoxanate HCl, benzonate HCl, or pipazethate, act as local anesthetics in the respiratory tree to produce their antitussive effect. The high cost and dubious value of the non-narcotic drugs other than dextromethorphan make their use questionable.

Codeine is by far the most commonly employed antitussive in adults. The recommended dose of 10 mg every 3 to 4 hr can usually be safely increased to 20 to 40 mg every 3 to 4 hr to achieve effects.[38,39] Occasionally 60 mg every 4 hr may be needed.[35] The usual dose range for children is 5 to 15 mg.[35] Dextromethorphan, however, is the drug of choice for children.

Dextromethorphan is recommended especially for children, but it is also popular with adults because it does not have the sedative, analgetic, gastric irritating, constipating or habituating properties of codeine. It is as effective as codeine when used in adequate doses. The recommended dose in children of 1 mg per kg every 24 hr has been exceeded 4-fold without causing any apparent ill effects.[38] Adult doses of 20 mg every 4 hr are minimal doses but 45 to 60 mg every 4 hr is a good therapeutic dose.[39] A prudent policy a pharmacist could follow when recommending doses would be to start with the recommended dose. If no cough suppression is noted, a careful increase in dose is warranted until the cough abates or side effects occur.

General Treatment

Bed rest and sufficient fluids, especially with fever, are very important for treating colds. Hydration is extremely important and must be achieved either through oral or respiratory intake. The steam vaporizers are somewhat effective in increasing room humidity and, therefore, fluid intake occurs via the lungs; however, they must be used in a small closed room to achieve this effect. They have the disadvantage of causing serious burns when tipped over—a decided problem where small ambulatory children are being treated. The cool mist vaporizers do not have this disadvantage but they also must be used in a small closed room to be effective. Generally, the most effective humidifier is the steam from a hot shower. A croupy child is frequently put to sleep in the bathroom near the shower, in his bed, with the hot water running. Heat lamps have also been used to treat colds. The warmth they produce feels good but has a dubious value in ameliorating the symptoms of a cold.

Prevention of Colds

Numerous panaceas have been proposed in the hopes of preventing the incidence of colds. Combined bacterial catarrhal vaccines,[29] antihistamines, ultraviolet radiation and vitamins have all been tried and have proved worthless. One vitamin, vitamin C, has recently received a wide press coverage for its proposed effects on colds. Linus Pauling has claimed large doses (1 to 5 g per day) can prevent colds and 15 g a day can cure colds.[40] *The Medical Letter*[41,42] carefully reviewed his book and concluded, "In the absence of convincing evidence of its effectiveness and safety, the *Medical Letter* does not recommend the use of large doses of Vitamin C for the prevention or treatment of the common cold". Recent studies done by Hornick[43] and Charleston[44] shed little new light on this subject.

Hornick used only 21 patients, ½ of which were controls, and found no difference between the test group and controls in preventing experimental rhinovirus infection in adults. The test subjects received 1 g of ascorbic acid 3 times a day starting 2 weeks before the infection and continued for 1 week past the infection. A placebo was given to the control group. He found no difference between groups in onset of illness, in the peak illness, virus excretion, antibody levels or nasal mucous flow. He did find that the test group on day 4 of the illness had less severe rhinitis and rhinorrhea than did the control group. Because of the lack of patients, this study is not too meaningful. Charleston with 47 patients and 43 controls and using 250 mg of ascorbic acid 4 times daily for 15 weeks did find a reduction in the incidence of colds in the test group. The average number of colds per person in the test group was 0.94 compared to 1.86 in the control group. He also found a significant reduction in the average duration of cold symptoms (3.5 days compared with 4.2 days). This study was reported in a letter to the editor so very little information about control procedures is known. This study also is difficult to interpret but does indicate additional research needs to be done to elucidate the role of vitamin C in the prevention of colds.

A number of killed viral vaccines have been utilized and have been somewhat effective. Influenza vaccines are efficacious if the patient receives the immunization 1 month before exposure occurs. Unfortunately, the Hong Kong flu and the more recent London flu were epidemic in the United States 6 months after the virus was initially isolated. It now takes approximately 1 year to produce a new vaccine. This lag time severely diminishes the prophylactic effect of the vaccine. Additionally, the rapid mutation of influenza virus makes production of an effective immunization for all influenza strains all but impossible. The influenza A_2/Hong Kong vaccine was used for the London flu and proved to be about 50% effective because of the mutation of the virus. Recently the lay press has reported a possible major breakthrough in developing a somewhat permanent influenza vaccine. Professor Claude Hannoun of the Pasteur Institute in Paris[45] has reported the development of an influenza vaccine to protect people from the present strain plus all its proposed mutant forms (produced experimentally in his lab) for the next 5 years.

They reported their new vaccine is ready for use and is 84% effective against the London flu. Killed parainfluenza vaccine has also been produced and has proven somewhat efficacious when used intranasally.[46]

In addition to vaccines, one medication has been produced to be used specifically for prophylaxis against influenza A_2. Amantadine given for 10 days after an exposure has been somewhat effective in preventing infection and is recommended only for high risk influenza patients—those with chronic debilitating disease or the elderly.

Chemotherapeutic agents can attack the virus in a number of different ways.[15] Drugs may be effective in attacking the virus extracellularly during its attachment to host cells, during penetration of the cells by the virus, during the uncoating of the virus in the cells, during the synthesis of certain critical enzymes by the virus, by inactivating certain viral components, during assembly of virus particles by the host cell or during the release of virus particles from the cell. As can now be appreciated, drugs can interfere and destroy viruses in a variety of ways. Additionally, chemotherapeutic agents do not always destroy viruses but may only suppress symptoms of a viral infection. They may only stimulate natural defenses such as interferon production or antibody production, or they may only act to slow down the infectious process and allow the body's own defenses to work. Each agent, however, is rather specific for only certain viruses; e.g., amantadine works only on the RNA-containing influenza A_2 virus by preventing the virus from penetrating the host cell.[15]

CROUP

Croup is a clinical syndrome of multiple etiologies characterized by inspiratory stridor or difficulty when inhaling. A high-pitched sound is emitted when coughing or inspiring owing to a narrowing of the larynx. This narrowing is caused by inflammation, edema or infection and can be quite serious. The more pronounced the narrowing of the larynx the more difficulty the patient has in breathing. Complete closure necessitating lifesaving procedures seldom occurs, but the potential of this sequela makes croup a serious disease. In addition to the inspiratory stridor and difficulty in breathing, hoarseness and a seal-like barking cough are other common symptoms seen with this malady. A child with croup must be closely watched by his parents in order for them to gauge the difficulty the child has with breathing. If the child has become fatigued with the effort of breathing, is becoming cyanotic and suffers from respiratory embarrassment, he should be immediately rushed to an emergency room. A physician there will watch the patient closely and be prepared to do a tracheostomy or place an endotracheal tube if needed. The use of oxygen is contraindicated because it may actually decrease the patient's respiratory effort.

Viral croup, which is less severe than bacterial (H. influenza) croup, seldom requires a tracheostomy or the placement of an endotracheal tube. Croup caused by H. influenza is a severe debilitating disease and frequently requires hospitalization. The large cherry-red epiglottis seen with H. influenza can easily fall into the trachea and completely obstruct respiration. A very careful examination of the pharynx is required in order to avoid this sequela. In fact, many pediatricians suspecting H. influenza croup will not examine the child until he is in an emergency room so that if the swollen epiglottis falls into the trachea an emergency tracheostomy can be performed. Croup can also occur with diphtheria infection. Fortunately, this disease has been largely eliminated through effective immunization programs. Other causes of croup are a foreign body lodged in the trachea, spasmodic croup or angioneurotic edema causing laryneal swelling.

The treatment of choice for croup is high humidity. Dehydration must be prevented to insure the maintenance of a patent airway. Vaporizers or hot showers, as mentioned before, should be utilized. Oral fluids must also be given and in large quantities. Expectorants usually have little or no effect. Antibiotics are utilized only to treat bacterial infections.

Corticosteroids can be lifesaving in both viral and bacterial infections. They should, however, be used cautiously and concomitantly with antibiotic therapy to prevent the occurrence of serious secondary infections.[1] Croup caused by a foreign body is treated by removal of the foreign body. After removal, symptoms will disappear without further treatment. Spasmodic croup responds well to the induction of emesis with clearing of all croupy symptoms. Croup caused by angioneurotic edema will respond to treatment with epinephrine and antihistamines. With proper treatment of croup, the prognosis is excellent.

POLIO

Only a short time ago, poliomyelitis was a deservedly feared disease. The advent of an effective immunization has almost eliminated this disease. Endemic areas, however, still exist in the United States and accounted for 23 cases in 1972.[47] Poliomyelitis has the ability to cause mild URl symptoms in addition to serious paralysis. Muscle weakness, headache, stiff neck, fever and sore throat are not uncommon signs of early polio. Since there is no specific treatment for this disease, prevention is the goal.

The Sabin vaccine or live attenuated OPV is the immunization of choice. The vaccine confers local antibody immunity in the gastrointestinal tract in addition to systemic antibody production. OPV bestows lifetime immunity, whereas the Salk or IPV requires boosters every 2 years after the initial immunization period. Because of its effectiveness, OPV has replaced IPV for immunizations (Table 43.5). Furthermore, it is extremely difficult, if not impossible, to obtain IPV in the United States.

A new development in culture media has been commercially introduced. Human diploid cells[48] have been successfully and safely employed as a culture media for polio. The Hayflick WI-38 cell line[49] is extremely promising and will probably be the media for future vaccines. The original human fetal lung cells have been grown and studied for 10 years and possess the following advantages over animal or egg cultures:[49]

1. Negligible cost.
2. Lack of extraneous virus with little chance of finding any in the future.
3. Unlimited cells available from a single cell source.
4. Successive vaccine lots easily produced.
5. Easily preserved.
6. No tumorgenicity.
7. Pretesting of cells done prior to their use.
8. Standardized cells.
9. Use of cloned cells.
10. No oncogenic viruses found.

TABLE 43.5
Revised Schedule for Active Immunization and Tuberculin Testing of Normal Infants and Children in the United States[a]

2 months	DTP[b]	TOPV[c]
4 months	DTP	TOPV
6 months	DTP	TOPV
1 year	Measles[d]	Tuberculin test[e]
1-12 years	Rubella[d]	Mumps[d]
1½ years	DTP	TOPV
4-6 years	DTP	TOPV
14-16 years	Td[f]	And thereafter every 10 years

[a]Routine smallpox vaccination is no longer recommended. Approved by the Committee on Infectious Diseases October 17, 1971.

[b]DTP—diphtheria and tetanus toxoids combined with pertussis vaccine.

[c]TOPV—trivalent oral polio virus vaccine. The above recommendation is suitable for breast-fed as well as bottle-fed infants.

[d]May be given at 1 year as measles-rubella or measles-mumps-rubella combined vaccines.

[e]Frequency of repeated tuberculin tests depends on risk of exposure of the child and on the prevalence of tuberculosis in the population group.

[f]Td—combined tetanus and diphtheria toxoids (adult type) for those over 6 years of age in contrast to diphtheria and tetanus (DT) containing a larger amount of diphtheria antigen. Tetanus toxoid at time of injury: For clean, minor wounds, no booster dose is needed by a fully immunized child unless more than 10 years have elapsed since the last dose. For contaminated wounds, a booster dose should be given if more than 5 years have elapsed since the last dose.

Other viruses also have been successfully propagated on diploid cells: adenoviruses, rhinoviruses, measles, rubella, smallpox and varicella.

HERPES VIRUS

There are five main subgroups of herpes virus: the hominus virus (simplex), the B virus (simiae), varicella-zoster (chicken pox and shingles), the CMV and the Epstein-Bar virus [(EBV), infectious mononucleosis]. Herpes virus is one of the most common causes of vesicular or ulcerative acute tonsillopharyngitis.

Varicella-zoster

Varicella-zoster virus is believed to be the cause of chickenpox and shingles. Zoster or shingles is thought to be a latent form of herpes infection and occurs inexplicably on the skin overlying nerves. Shingles does not have any respiratory symptoms as does chickenpox or varicella.

Although predominately a dermatological disease, chickenpox does manifest some prodromal symotoms such as slight malaise and fever. Pneumonia, however, is the major respiratory sequela of chickenpox and can be serious in patients with compromised respiratory function. Chickenpox can manifest severe enough symptoms to be confused with smallpox in patients with immunoglobin deficiency states, malignancies or those undergoing steroid or antimetabolite therapy. The treatment available is very limited. Zoster immune globin is available and, if given early, will modify severe manifestations of the disease.[50] Research to develop a successful prophylactic vaccine is continuing slowly.

Herpes Simplex

Herpes manifested as cold sores is a common infection in many people. This opportunistic organism can also cause acute tonsillopharyngitis with vesicles and ulcers. The disease is painful and largely untreatable. Local use of idoxuridine (IDU) has been successfully employed for ophthalmic infections.[15,48] Systemic use of IDU has been employed for disseminated infections with equivocal results.[15,51] IDU works only with DNA-containing viruses like herpes by becoming incorporated into the nucleus of the virus in place of thymidine.[15] This causes a different viral DNA to be produced which is incompatible with viral replication mechanisms so that the virus is unable to reproduce. IDU also inhibits the enzymes needed to make DNA. Additionally, the recent dermatological use of topical neutral red dye with fluorescent light exposure is effective and looks very promising.[52]

Cytomegalovirus

CMV is a ubiquitous agent which quite probably causes a lot of common infections[53–55] not readily associated clinically with this virus. It can cause an infectious mononucleosis-type disease with symptoms of sore throat, fever, cough and occasionally pneu-monia. Treatment of this virus is largely symptomatic. In severe cases, such as congenital CMV infection, medications such as cytosine arabinoside (cytarbrine) have been employed with some success and work by blocking DNA synthesis.[15,56]

Epstein-Bar Virus

This virus is the main cause of infectious mononucleosis, the "kissing disease," so called because of the close contact needed to spread infection. This disease usually occurs in children and young adults producing sore throat, fever, cough, extreme tiredness and enlarged spleen. Mononucleosis can be confused with measles, rubella or leukemia so it is imperative to diagnose it correctly.

There is little available for specific treatment. Corticosteroids and chloroquin have been shown to be beneficial in severe cases.[1] Symptomatic treatment with aspirin and codeine is usually employed. Bed rest is mandatory and is usually continued for a number of weeks. EBV has also been implicated in causing Burkitt's lymphoma, a form of cancer.[25]

SMALLPOX

Smallpox is a very serious disease with a high morbidity and a 40% mortality associated with it. It causes a high fever, severe backache, prostration and severe respiratory difficulties, leading to secondary infections. Thankfully, there have been no reported cases of smallpox in the United States since 1949. There are, however, endemic areas in parts of Africa, Asia and South America. Jenner introduced the first vaccine in 1798 which was very effective, but because of the many adverse reactions associated with the vaccine, its routine use has now been abandoned.[51,57–59] New vaccines are now being studied[60] in the hopes of decreasing the high incidence of these adverse reactions. Smallpox vaccine is only currently indicated for health care workers, border personnel, travelers to endemic areas and armed services personnel. The symptoms of smallpox can be ameliorated if prophylactic measures are taken immediately after exposure. Vaccinia immune globulin is available and effective in preventing or altering the symptoms of smallpox[51] and works by inhibiting viral synthesis of messenger RNA.[15]

MEASLES (RUBEOLA)

The measles virus is remarkably stable in its immunological make-up, having only a single strain in humans and two in animals. Before immunizations were available to prevent measles, there were hundreds of thousands of cases each year. The incidence has decreased to 31,425 cases in 1972.[47]

Measles virus can cause the following symptoms during its prodromal period: fever, conjunctivitis, coryza, photophobia and a barking, harsh cough. The exanthematous phase of the disease is a characteristic maculopapular confluent rash.[51,61] Koplick spots are the enanthemous phase of measles and are pathognomonic for this disease.[51,61] Measles is often severe and produces complications like encephalitis in 1 of 1,000 cases and death in 1 of 10,000 cases. There is no specific treatment, only symptomatic. Preventative immunization is the recommended procedure.

The use of live attenuated measles vaccine is strongly recommended in an effort to eradicate the disease.[62] The killed measles virus vaccine has been withdrawn because of its propensity to cause "atypical measles" (fever, an exanthem, frequent pneumonia, pleural effusion and peripheral edema).[63] The live vaccine has been free of this problem although a recent study by Cherry[64] cast some doubt on this premise. Current immunization practices recommend the vaccination of all children over 1 year old (Table 43.5). Children less than 1 year old, when given measles vaccine (rubella, mumps and smallpox also), do not become adequately immunized because of interference from maternally derived antibodies.[51] The immunizations routinely used are either the more attenuated Schwartz strain or the Moraton strain. Both are more attenuated, Edmonston B strains and are used because they cause less incidence of rashes and fever than the older Edmonston B strain vaccines. It is advisable to test the child for tuberculosis with purified protein derivative (PPD) prior to the immunization because measles or measles vaccine can exacerbate active tuberculosis.[51] If the child has tuberculosis and PDD is used after the immunization, a false negative may result owing to depression of the reaction by the measles vaccine.[65] This has also occurred with other vaccines and diseases[65] and could obscure the diagnosis of tuberculosis.

TOGAVIRUS

This is a new classification of a group of viruses which contain a RNA nucleus and are small in size, 20 to 70 mμ. Rubella (German measles) is the only member of this group to cause URI symptoms.

German measles is occasionally confused with regular measles, or misdiagnosed as other viral diseases. It is however, a benign 3-day disease in children producing only a characteristic rash, lymphadenopathy, mild fever, headache, malaise, coryza, sore throat and cough. This is to be compared with the severe symptoms from the 7-day measles. Some children and many adults who contract rubella experience some arthralgia, arthritis symptoms and some joint swelling. It is, however, the fetus in the pregnant woman which suffers most.[1,66] Congenital rubella causes heart defects, cataracts, deafness and death. It has been estimated by the USPHS that the 1964 rubella epidemic resulted in a $2,000,000,000-loss to the economy. In an effort to eradicate rubella, many immunizations and viral strains have been tested and utilized.[14,67-70]

Rubella vaccination is recommended after the 1st year of life (Table 43.5). It can be used in combination with mumps and/or measles or given singly.[51,62] The use of rubella vaccine in children to prevent disease in adult women is a novel approach to vaccination. Two questions arise: "Will this immunity last until the young girl is of child-bearing age?" and "Does this vaccination create a population immunity and wipe out the disease?" There is a tremendous amount of controversy concerning these subjects. It may well be that these female children will have to be revaccinated when they reach child-bearing age. A better method, it would seem, would be to immunize only women of child-bearing age.[51] The present immune status of adult women is reported to be about 75%,[11] so that only 25% of the female population needs to be vaccinated. Perhaps every woman should be tested for antibody titers and immunization be given after puberty, after childbirth or before marriage if titers are absent. Even after immunization of most children in a community, rubella epidemics have still spread through the populace.[10-13,71] This asymptomatic reinfection in immunized individuals is of great concern. These individuals can act as carriers of the disease and possibly transmit it to others.[6] Farquhar[10] pointed out that "with presently licensed rubella vaccines it is not possible to produce a herd immunity; at least not in an institutional population." The effect of herd immunity on preventing infection has been challenged further by Fox *et al.*[71] Fox and his associates carried out a mathematical analysis of herd immunity and concluded "the important determinants of an epidemic were the number of susceptibles plus the number of opportunities for their exposure to the disease, and that if these two variables remained constant, the total number of immune persons in the population had no influence on the epidemic." These findings would strongly suggest that unless the disease can be totally eliminated, immunizations should be given only to women of childbearing age. In an effort to reduce this reinfection rate, intranasal preparations have been tested and found to be effective in inducing local and systemic antibody production.[67,69] Finally, the vaccine is teratogenic in females.[66,72,73] Before giving the vaccine, it must be ascertained that the woman is not pregnant and will remain so at least 2 to 3 months after the immunization.[51]

OTHER VIRAL DISEASES

The virus of psittacosis-ornithosis, the cause of parrot fever, can also manifest symptoms ranging from a mild influenza-like disease to severe atypical pneumonia. Lymphocytic choriomeningitis virus is usually an animal infection but can also produce human disease. Respiratory manifestations such as cough, sore throat, an influenza-like syndrome and occasionally pneumonia are not uncommonly produced.

NONVIRAL CAUSES

M.pneumonia is included here because historically it was thought to be a virus and to be the cause of "atypical pneumonia." In 1962, it was reclassified to pleuropneumonia-like organism, a bacteria. It may account for as much as 30 to 50% of lower respiratory disease of young adults.[1,51] In epidemics, as many as 10% of children with URI will be afflicted. Its incidence in younger children is about 1%. Other bacteria causing URI symptoms are streptococci, staphylococci, pneumococci, diphtheria and *H. influenza.* All of these are treated with

appropriate antibiotics and symptomatic treatment. Fungal agents like coccidioidomycosis and histoplasmosis and rickettsial agents, such as *Rickettsia burnetti,* the cause of Q fever, can also cause URI symptoms and are treated with appropriate antibiotics and symptomatic treatment.

DISCUSSION AND SUMMARY

A great deal of research is being done in the area of interferon inducers, new vaccines and chemotherapeutic agents in the hopes of eradicating viral diseases.[15,48]

Interferon

Interferon is a protein made by white cells in the spleen, liver, thymus and lymph nodes in response to viral infection.[15,74-76] It is a nonspecific entity so that it is active against virtually all viruses, some bacteria and some protozoa.[74-76] There are five known human varieties of interferon which probably are produced by at least two specific genes in white blood cells. Interferon has a rapid onset and is produced shortly after the onset of illness. It is effective both before and during an infection. In addition to viruses[74-78] activating these genes, at least 30 synthetic chemical inducers[74-77] of interferon have been produced. Because of cost, induction of endogenous interferon is preferable to isolation, purification and administration of exogenous interferon. It has been estimated that it would require $5,000 worth of parenteral interferon to treat one case of the common cold.[48]

Vaccines

Vaccines on human diploid cells, varicella-zoster vaccine, intranasal vaccines for rubella and improved smallpox vaccines are being tested. Other vaccines in the testing stage, such as measles used intranasally, may prove to be very efficacious. Future vaccines, such as influenza, will undoubtedly be developed as live attenuated vaccines and probably will be given through the portal of entry of the disease; that is, intranasally for respiratory diseases. Some viruses such as RSV and adenovirus have been utilized to prepare vaccines but are now discarded. RSV caused a number of atypical reactions in humans and the adenovirus was found to be carcinogenic in animals.[15] The combination of different viruses in the same preparations, *e.g.,* measles, mumps and rubella will be pursued. This has obvious advantages in requiring fewer immunizations. The hopeful breakthrough in Paris with the development of a 5-year influenza vaccine is very encouraging.[45] Finally, new adjuvants to increase antigenicity are being developed, *e.g.* emulsified oils like peanut and mineral oil.[48]

Chemotherapy

Research on treatment for cancer has produced many chemotherapeutic agents. Recently, some cancers have been shown to be caused by viruses, spurring on the use of many chemotherapeutic agents to treat various viral infections. In addition to amantadine, cytarbrine, methisazone and IDU, there seems to be little doubt that many other drugs will shortly be utilized to treat other viral infections.

CONCLUSIONS

The causes of upper respiratory disease are many, but the symptoms are largely similar. The treatment of choice is generally symptomatic with specific therapy for only a few indicated infections. Diseases that have been largely eliminated by the use of immunizations can only remain so if vaccinations are routinely done. Work on interferon, new vaccines and chemotherapeutic agents will continue with further research being done with lymphocyte transfusions, lymphocyte mediator substances and other immunological preparations. The next few years should herald major breakthroughs in the discovery and treatment of many viral induced illnesses.

REFERENCES

1. Krugman S., and Ward, R.: Infectious Diseases of Children, Ed. 5, p. 221. C. V. Mosby Co., St. Louis, 1972.
2. Hable, K. A., Washington, J. A., and Herrmann, E. C.: Bacterial and viral throat flora, comparison of findings in children with acute upper respiratory tract disease and in healthy controls during winter. Clin. Pediatr., 10:199, 1971.
3. Mufson, M. A., Webb, P. A., Kennedy, H., Gill, V., and Chanock, R. M.: Etiology of upper-respiratory-tract illnesses among civilian adults. J.A.M.A., 195: 91, 1965.
4. Melnick, J. L.: Classification and nomenclature of animal viruses. Prog. Med. Virol., 13: 462, 1971.
5. Jawetz, E., Melnick, J. L., and Adelberg, E. A.: Review of Medical Microbiology, Ed. 10, p. 279, Lange Medical Publications, Los Altos, California, 1972.
6. Chang, T. W., Recurrent viral infection (reinfection). N. Engl. J. Med., 284: 765, 1971.
7. Craddock, C. G., Longmire, R., and McMillian, R.: Lymphocytes and the immune response, Part I. N. Engl. J. Med., 285: 324, 1971.
8. Craddock, C. G., Longmire, R., and McMillan, R.: Lymphocytes and the immune response, Part II. N. Engl. J. Med., 285: 378, 1971.
9. Tomasi, T. B.: Secretory immunoglobins. N. Engl. J. Med., 287: 500, 1972.
10. Farquhar, J. D.: Follow up on rubella vaccinations and experience with subclinical reinfection. J. Pediatr., 81: 460, 1972.
11. Klock, L. E., and Rachelefsky, G. S.: Failure of rubella herd immunity during an epidemic. N. Engl. J. Med., 288: 69, 1973.
12. Horstmann, D. M., Liebhaber, H., Le Bouvier, G. L., Rosenberg, D. A., and Malstead, S. B.: Rubella reinfection of vaccinated and naturally immune persons exposed in an epidemic N. Engl. J. Med., 283: 771, 1970.
13. Chang, T. W., Des Rosiers, S., and Weinstein, L.: Clinical and serologic studies of an outbreak of rubella in a vaccinated population. N. Engl. J. Med., 283: 246, 1970.
14. Puschak, R., Young, M., McKee, T. V., and Plotkin, S. A.: Intranasal vaccination with RA 27/3 attenuated rubella virus. J. Pediatr., 79: 55, 1971.
15. Stevens, D. A., and Merigan, T. C.: Approaches to the control of viral infections in man. Ration. Drug Ther., 5: 1, 1971.
16. Loda, R. A., Glezen, P. E., and Clyde, W. A.: Respiratory disease in group day care, Pediatrics, 19: 428, 1972.
17. Hope-Simpson, E. E., and Higgins, P. G.: A respiratory virus study in Great Britain: review and evaluation. Prog. Med. Virol., 11: 354, 1969.
18. McCammon, R. W.: Natural history of respiratory tract infection patterns in basically healthy individuals. Am. J. Dis. Child., 122: 232, 1971.
19. Kempe, H.: Current Pediatric Diagnosis and Treatment, Ed. 2, Lange Medical Publications, Los Altos, California, 1972.
20. Marks, M. I., Nagahama, H., and Eller, J. J.: Parainfluenza virus immunofluorescence in vitro and clinical application of the direct method. Pediatrics, 48: 73, 1971.
21. Moffet, H., Siegel, A. C., and Doyle, H. K.: Nonstreptococcal pharyngitis. J. Pediatr., 73: 51, 1968.
22. Connor, J. E.: Evidence for an etiological role of adenoviral infection in pertussis syndrome. N. Engl. J. Med., 283: 390, 1970.
23. Klenk, E. L., Gaultney, J. V., and Bass, J. W.:

Bacteriologically proved pertussis and adenovirus infections: possible association. Am. J. Dis. Child, 124: 303, 1972.

24. Olson, L. C., Miller, G., and Honshau, J. E.: Acute infection-lymphocytosis presenting as a pertussis-like illness: its association with adenovirus type 12. Lancet, 12: 200, 1964.

25. Allen, D. W., and Cole, P.: Viruses and human cancer. N. Engl. J. Med., 286: 70, 1972.

26. Jacobs, J. W., Peacock, D. B., Corner, B. D., Caul E. O., and Clarke, S. K. R.: Respiratory synctyial and other viruses associated with respiratory disease in infants. Lancet, 1: 871, 1971.

27. Dowling, H. F., Jackson, G. G., and Inouye, T.: Transmission of the experimental common cold in volunteers. J. Lab. Clin. Med., 50: 516, 1957.

28. Griffenhagen, G. B. and Hawkins, L. L.: Handbook of Non-prescription Drugs, Ed. 3, p. 19, American Pharmaceutical Assocation, Washington, D.C., 1971.

29. Kastrup, E.: Facts and Comparisons, Ed. 4, edited by G. M. Schwach. Facts and Comparisons, Inc., St. Louis.

30. Lexomboon, Y., Duangmani, C., Kusalasai, V., Sunakorn, P., Olson, L., and Noyes, H.: Evaluation of orally administered antibiotics for treatment of upper respiratory infections in Thai children. J. Pediatr., 78: 772, 1971.

31. Anon.: Antimicrobial cold remedies. Med. Lett. Drugs Ther., 9: 30, 1967.

32. Callaghan, R. P., Cox, A. J., Boulder, R. V. M., Lawrence, N., Lazarus, S., Mahon, D., Owen, W. L., Russell, L., and Sievers, I. M.: Combination therapy in hay fever and allergic rhinitis. Practitioner, 198: 713, 1967.

33. Hartman, M. M.: Capabilities and limitations of major drug groups in allergy: their role within current theories. Ann. Allergy. 27: 164, 1969.

34. Feinberg, S. M.: The antihistamines: pharmacologic principles in their use. Pharmacol. Physic. 1: 1, 1967.

35. Anon.: Cough remedies. Med. Lett. Drug Ther., 13: 9, 1971.

36. Blanchard, K., and Ford, R. A.: Effective antitussive agent in the treatment of cough in childhood. Lancet. 74: 443, 1954.

37. Chodosh, S.: Newer drugs in treatment of chronic bronchitis. Med. Clin. North Am., 51: 1177, 1967.

38. Carter, C. H.: Evaluation of the effectiveness of Novrad and acetysalicylic acid in children with cough. Am. J. Med. Sci. 245: 713, 1963.

39. Calesnick, B., and Christensen, J. A.: Latency of cough response as a measure of antitussive agents. Clin. Pharmacol. Ther., 8: 374, 1967.

40. Pauling, L.: Vitamin C and the Common Cold, Ed. J. W. H. Freeman and Co., San Francisco, 1970.

41. Anon.: Vitamin C: were the trials well controlled and are large doses safe? Med. Lett. Drugs Ther., 13: 46, 1971.

42. Anon.: Vitamin C and the common cold. Med. Lett. Drugs Ther., 12: 105, 1970.

43. Hornick, R. B.: Does ascorbic acid have value in combating the common cold? Med. Count., 4: 50, 1972.

44. Charleston, S. S., and Clegg, K. M.: Ascorbic acid and the common cold (Letter to the Editor). Lancet. 1: 1401, 1972.

45. Anon.: Anticipating the flu virus. Time. 101: 68, 1973.

46. Wigley, F. M., Fruchtman, M. H., and Waldman, R. H.: Aerosol immunization of humans with inactivated parainfluenza type 2 vaccine. N. Engl. J. Med., 283: 1250, 1970.

47. Center for Disease Control: Morbidity and mortality weekly report, 21: 445, 1968.

48. Meyer, H. M.: The control of viral disease: problems and prospects viewed in perspective. J. Pediatr., 73: 653, 1968.

49. Hayflick, L.: The choice of the cell substrate for human virus vaccine production. Lab. Pract., 19: 58, 1970.

50. Brumell, P. A., Gershon, A. A., Hughes, W. T., Riley, M. D., and Smith, J.: Prevention of varicella in high risk children: a collaborative study. Pediatrics, 50: 718, 1972.

51. Top, F. M. (editor): Report of the Committee on Infectious Disease, Ed. 16. American Academy of Pediatrics, Evanston, Ill., 1970.

52. Felber, T. D.: Photodynamic inactivation of herpes simplex, J.A.M.A., 223: 289, 1973.

53. Weller, T. H.: The cytomegaloviruses: ubiquitous agents with protean clinical manifestation, Part I., N. Engl. J. Med., 285: 203, 1971.

54. Weller, T. H.: The cytomegaloviruses: ubiquitous agents with protean clinical manifestations, Part II., N. Engl. J. Med., 285: 267, 1971.

55. Hayes, K., Danks, D. M., and Gibas, H.: Cytomegalovirus in human milk. N. Engl. J. Med., 287: 177, 1972.

56. Kraybill, E. N., Sever, J. L., Avery, G. B., and Movassaghi, N.: Experimental use of cytosine arabinoside in congenital cytomegalovirus infection. J. Pediatr., 80: 485, 1972.

57. Anon.: For and against smallpox vaccination. Br. Med. J., 2: 311, 1970.

58. Anon.: Routine smallpox vaccination: a dilemma. Lancet, 1: 1270, 1970.

59. Center for Disease Control: Morbidity and mortality weekly report. 18: 43, 1969.

60. Galasso, G. J.: Projected studies on immunization against smallpox. J. Infect. Dis., 121: 575, 1970.

61. Suringa, D., Bank, L. J., and Ackerman, B. A.: Role of measles virus in skin lesions and Kopliks spots. N. Engl. J. Med., 283: 1139, 1970.

62. Krugman, S.: Present status of measles and rubella immunization in the United States: a medical progress report. J. Pediatr., 78: 1, 1971.

63. Fulginiti, V. A., Eller, J. J., Downie, A. W., and Kempe, C. M.: Altered reactivity to measles virus: atypical measles in children previously immunized with inactivated measles virus

vaccines. J. A.M.A., 202: 1075, 1967.
64. Cherry, J. D., Feigin, R. D., Lobes, L. A., and Shackelford, P. G.: Atypical measles in children previously immunizaed with attenuated measles virus vaccines. Pediatrics, 50: 712, 1972
65. Brody, J. A., Overfield, T., and Hammes, L. M.: Depression of the tuberculin reaction by viral vaccines. N. Engl. J. Med., 271: 1294, 1964.
66. Vaheri, A., Vesikari, T., Oker-Blom, N., Seppala, M., Parkman, P. D., Veronelli, J., and Robbins, F. C.: Isolation of attenuated rubella-vaccine virus from human products of conception and uterine cervix. N. Engl. J. Med., 286: 1071, 1972.
67. Ogra, P. L., Kerr-Grant, O., Umana, G., Ozierba, J., and Weintraub, D.: Antibody response in serum and nasopharynx after naturally acquired and vaccine-induced infection with rubella virus. N. Engl. J. Med., 285: 1333, 1971.
68. Cooper, L. Z.: Clinical trial with live attenuated rubella virus vaccine. Am. J. Dis. Child., 115: 639, 1968.
69. Davis, D. J., and Murray, R.: Proceedings of the international conference on rubella immunizations. Am. J. Dis. Child., 118: 1, 1969.
70. Hilderbrandt, R. J., and Weber, J. M.: Immunization of young adult females with cendehill strain of rubella vaccine. Am. J. Obstet. Gynecal., 107: 645, 1970.
71. Fox, J. P., Elveback, L., Scott, W., Gatewood, L., and Ackerman, E.: Herd immunity: basic concept and relevance to public health immunization practices. Am. J. Epidemiol., 94: 179, 1971.
72. Korones, S. B., Todard, J., Roane, J. A., and Sever, J. L.: Maternal virus infection after the first trimester of pregnancy and status of offspring to 4 years of age in a predominately Negro population. J. Pediatr., 77: 245, 1970.
73. Phillips, C. A., Maeck, J. U. S., Robers, W. A., and Sauel, H.: Intrauterine rubella infection following immunization with rubella vaccine. J.A.M.A., 213: 624, 1970.
74. Grossberg, S. E.: The interferons and their inducers: molecular and therapeutic considerations, Part I. N. Engl. J. Med., 287: 13, 1972.
75. Grossberg, S. E.: The interferons and their inducers: molecular and therapeutic considerations, Part II. N. Engl. J. Med., 287: 79, 1972.
76. Grossberg, S. E.: The Interferons and their inducers: molecular and therapeutic considerations, Part III. N. Engl. J. Med., 287: 122, 1972.
77. Ho, M.: Interferon and herpes zoster (Editorial). N. Engl. J. Med., 283: 1222, 1970.
78. Armstrong, R. W., Gurwith, M. J., Waddell, D., and Merigan, T. C.: Cutaneous interferon production in patients with Hodgkins disease and other cancers infected with varicella or vaccinia. N. Engl. J. Med., 283: 1182, 1970.

chapter 44

TUBERCULOSIS

David S. Tatro, Pharm. D.

The incidence of tuberculosis has been decreasing over the last 2 decades; however, it still represents one of the leading causes of death due to infectious disease. Since drugs play an important role in any therapeutic regimen of tuberculosis, it is essential that the practicing pharmacist have a thorough knowledge of the disease as well as its treatment. He is in an ideal position to monitor drug usage and may be the first to learn of an adverse reaction that a patient is experiencing as a result of drug therapy.

Tuberculosis is an infection caused by *Mycobacterium tuberculosis*. The disease derives its name from the characteristic lesion that is formed—the tubercle. When infection occurs, the host response leads to the formation of cells around bacilli in an attempt to keep the reaction localized. In most instances, infection stops at this point, leaving its characteristic scar. If the host response is unable to halt the infection, growth continues and an active case of infectious tuberculosis develops.

ETIOLOGY AND PATHOGENESIS

Any infection caused by *M. tuberculosis* is referred to as tuberculosis. Three types of tubercle bacilli are pathogenic to man—human, bovine and aviary. Aviary tuberculosis is extremely rare in the U.S. and with the advent of pasteurization of milk and testing of cows, the human type has become the more significant. The most prevalent means of spreading tuberculosis between individuals is by coughing and sneezing. The sputum of actively infected patients is contaminated with many bacilli. These droplets are airborne and may be inhaled by unsuspecting individuals.

Since the tuberculous bacillus is an aerobe, the high oxygen tension of the lungs offers an ideal environment for harboring tuberculosis as a respiratory disease: however, even though pulmonary infection is most common, tuberculosis may strike any organ in the body. With few exceptions, the infecting organism gains entry into the body via the lungs. It is here that primary tuberculosis is established. From the lungs, infection spreads to other organs by way of the lymphatic system and the blood stream.

At this stage, the infection usually becomes dormant, and immunity, on the part of the host, prevents further spread. The lesions may become walled off by the production of fibrous tissue and calcification. The time during which tuberculosis remains dormant varies greatly. Organisms may remain inactive for the life of the host or they may become reactivated at any time.

Following the period of dormancy, reactivation of a latent infection may take one of two courses—chronic tuberculosis or miliary tuberculosis. The factors allowing recurrence of infection are not completely understood; however, a breakdown in the host's immune mechanism is an important factor. Thus, reactivation is more common in patients suffering or recovering from another illness. Reactivation may also occur in a patient receiving immunosuppressive drugs or steroid therapy.

CHRONIC TUBERCULOSIS

Although chronic tuberculosis may develop in any organ of the body, the most frequently encountered sites are those with the greatest oxygen tension. Therefore, the kidneys and brain provide a suitable environment in which *M. tuberculosis* may grow.[1] When the primary infection occurs during childhood, the epiphysis of the long bones (wrist, elbow, knee) and spine is undergoing rapid growth. The oxygen tension at these sites is high and may harbor the tubercle bacilli. Tuberculosis may remain dormant in these areas for many decades only to manifest itself in the elderly patient. Other organs involved in tuberculosis include lymph nodes, meninges, skin, peritoneum, eyes, larynx, pericardium, adrenal glands and gastrointestinal tract.

The infection of these sites by the invading organism results from the spread of small quantities of tubercle bacilli by hematogenous dissemination.

MILIARY TUBERCULOSIS

It is also possible for large numbers of bacilli to be released from a primary focus, spreading throughout the body. The occurrence of this is referred to as miliary tuberculosis.

Like chronic tuberculosis, miliary tuberculosis may occur any time after primary infection. However, the occurrence of this form of tuberculosis is seen most frequently in children under 4 years of age. It is most feared by clinicians since death may rapidly occur.

INCIDENCE

Presently, the incidence of tuberculosis is steadily declining. Although many adults still demonstrate a positive tuberculin test, the prevalence of these adult reactors is much less than it was in 1900. In many instances, adults showing positive reactions to the tuberculin skin test acquired their primary infection as children; however, few children (less than 10%) show positive tests today.[2]

Many factors are responsible for the declining rate of tuberculosis in today's society. Some of these considerations are listed in Table 44.1. Tuberculosis now tends to occur within a family, rather than in the epidemic proportions of the past. Thus, several children living under the same roof may become infected owing to a common contact (parent, grandparent) with an infectious adult.

DIAGNOSIS AND CLINICAL FINDINGS

Signs and symptoms that may be present in tuberculosis include malaise, fever, anorexia, fatigue, nausea, night sweats and weight loss. However, it should be noted that in either pri-

TABLE 44.1
Factors Contributing to the
Decreasing Incidence of Tuberculosis

1. Adequate antitubercular drugs
2. Rapid identification of disease
3. Adequate nutrition
4. Less crowded living conditions
5. Declining rate of infection in adults
6. Vaccination
7. Isolation of infectious cases

mary or chronic tuberculosis, patients may be asymptomatic. Indeed, symptoms may be absent even in the presence of extensive infection. Most cases of asymptomatic childhood infections are uncovered during routine physical examinations.

Skin Tests

Intradermal injection of tuberculin or its purified protein derivative (PPD) to individuals infected with *M tuberculosis* will elicit a positive skin test. This reaction represents a cutaneous hypersensitivity to bacterial protein from the culture media.

Test materials are isolated from a broth in which human strains of *M. tuberculosis*, are cultured. Tuberculin and PPD are used for the diagnosis of tuberculosis. Following the intracutaneous injection of the appropriate dilution of test material, one waits 48 to 72 hr before interpreting the results.

A positive reaction is indicated by a palpable induration of greater than 5 mm diameter. A positive reaction to very low concentrations of material supports a diagnosis of active tuberculosis. A slight reaction or no reaction to a low concentration of test substance is an indication for retesting with the next highest concentration (*e.g.*, PPD second strength). Positive test results on either test dosage are an indication for further diagnostic testing.

The greatest value of tuberculin testing probably can be attributed to a negative test. With very few exceptions, a negative test, with both solutions, rules out active tuberculosis. It should be noted, however, that a negative test may be seen in severe tuberculosis (*i.e.*, miliary tuberculosis) where the body's defense mechanisms are overwhelmed. Patients receiving corticosteroids or immunosuppressive therapy may also show false negative skin tests.

As of January 1973, PPD used in tuberculin skin tests are stabilized solutions. Recent literature.[3,5] demonstrates that previously used preparations requiring the addition of a diluent lose significant amounts of test material by adsorption to the walls of glass and plastic syringes or vials. Tween 80 has been shown to be an effective stabilizing agent minimizing the loss of tuberculoprotein to containers.[4] Therefore, less false negative skin tests occur with stabilized PPD.[5]

In an *in vitro* comparison betwen stabilized (5 ppm of tween 80) and nonstabilized PPD, a much greater loss of tuberculoprotein to the container occurred with the latter preparation (Table 44.2).[4] It can be seen that with nonstabilized PPD, patients would receive considerably less than the intended amount of test material.

When 115 patients with known active tuberculosis were simultaneously tested with 5 TU of commercial PPD-nonstabilized, U.S. Public Health Service standard tuberculin 346, and commercial PPD-stabilized (with tween 80), the greatest number of nonpositive results occurred with nonstabilized PPD (Table 44.3).[5]

Since the initial preparations of stabilized PPD were of a greater concentration than the reference standard, more false positive tests occurred.[3] The Division of Biological Standards and the manufacturers are taking action to insure uniform potency, stability and bioequiv-

TABLE 44.2

PPD (STU)	Loss to Container						
	Glass Vials		Plastic syringe				
	8 hr	24 hr	20 min	60 min	4 hr	8 hr	24 hr
	%	%	%	%	%	%	%
Nonstabilized	33	40	60	70	80	90	97
Stabilized	No significant loss						

TABLE 44.3
Comparison of PPD

	Nonstabilized Commercial PPD	U.S.P.H.S. Standard	Stabilized Commercial PPD
	%	%	%
Negative (0-4 mm induration)	49	34	17
Doubtful (5-9 mm induration)	10	3	2
Positive (10+mm induration)	41	63	81

alency of products labeled as 5-TU PPD.[6] PPD should be used within 30 min of reconstitution; however, to insure uniformity in testing in tuberculosis control programs and private practice, a stabilized form of PPD is recommended.

Bacterial Infection

Isolation of *M. tuberculosis* from an infected site provides positive proof of tuberculosis in the patient. The most frequent souce of the bacillus is sputum and tracheal or gastric washings. Material from washings or biopsy should be cultured for identification of the bacillus.

Mycobacterial infections by organisms other than tuberculosis are also possible. These have been categorized as unclassified or "atypical" mycobacterial infections. Examples of mycobacterium other than tuberculosis include *Mycobacterium kansasii, Mycobacterium scrofulaceum, Mycobacterium batteyi* (Battey Bacillus) and *Mycobacterium fortuitum.* Infections by these organisms are not known to be communicable, and it is, therefore, not necessary to isolate patients. Although some of the infections are very similar to *M. tuberculosis,* response to drug therapy is frequently unpredictable, and surgical excision is necessary. These other mycobacterial infections may give a positive skin test for tuberculosis.

X-rays

Chest x-rays are valuable in the identification of pulmonary tuberculosis. Repeated films are usually necessary to establish the presence of the disease. X-rays are essential in evaluating the progress of therapy.

COMPLICATIONS

The complications associated with tuberculosis are dependent on the organ involved. A complete discussion covering every conceivable complication in conjunction with each vulnerable organ is beyond the scope of this chapter. However, the most frequent and serious complications will be considered.

In active pulmonary tuberculosis, necrosis with liquefaction develops. As this fluid empties, cavities remain. Arteries leading to the resulting cavities may burst, causing frank pulmonary hemorrhage. Atelectasis is a further complication associated with respiratory lesions.

A similar process occurs with renal involvement. When lesions are in the kidney, cavitation may also occur. Ruptured blood vessels in this area lead to hematuria.

When tuberculosis strikes the lining of organs in the body, such as peritoneum, pleura and pericardium, several types of complications may result. Tuberculous peritonitis may take two forms—wet or dry. In the wet form, serous fluid is present in the abdominal cavity and numerous white tubercles are spread over the peritoneal surface. The dry form of peritonitis is characterized by little effusion of fluid. However, a great deal of adhesions may form between peritoneal surfaces or fibrous membranes which will lead to constriction and impair intestinal motility. In infants and children, if the abdominal lymph nodes are infected with tuberculosis, the consequence may be life-threatening. When the lining of the heart is involved, its function can be seriously impeded by the formation of inelastic fibrous tissue. However, once again, the course of infection is variable and one may find large amounts of fluid accumulating in the pericardium.

Two very serious complications are miliary tuberculosis and tuberculosis meningitis. Miliary tuberculosis (discussed earlier) is a hematogenous disease, allowing wide spread infection throughout the body. In tuberculosis meningitis, fluid collects around the base of the brain causing adhesion. Since these lesions are in the area of hypothalamus, fatal brain damage may be encountered. There is a high incidence of tuberculosis in patients with Addison's disease. Progressive destruction of the adrenal gland with resulting adrenal cortical insufficiency occurs when the adrenal is infected with tuberculosis. Patients with Addison's disease must be routinely tested for tuberculosis.

TREATMENT

Drug therapy is indicated for all forms of tuberculosis. Patients will receive antitubercular therapy for long periods, usually in excess of 1 year. Because of the long duration of treatment, special attention must be given to dose-related side effects (Table 44.4).

In many instances the selection of drugs to be used in tuberculosis is based on their tox-

TABLE 44.4
Drugs Used in the Treatment of Tuberculosis

Drug	Dosage	Duration	Special Considerations
Aminosalicylic acid K+ = 25% Ca++ = 30%	Adult: 4 g tid PO. (25% higher if salts are used) Child: 200 mg/kg/24 hr	24 months	Gastrointestinal side effects are frequent
Capreomycin (Capastat)	Adult: 1.0 g/24 hr I.M. Child: 15 mg/kg/24 hr	24 months	Monitoring of renal and eighth nerve function is indicated
Cycloserine (Seromycin)	Adult: 250 mg 2-4 times daily PO. (1.0 g maximal) Child: 15 mg/kg/24 hr PO. (500 mg maximal)	18-24 months	Reduce dosage in renal impairment
Ethambutol (Myambutol)	Adult: 25 mg/kg/24 hr P.O., then 15 mg/kg/24 hr P.O. Child: 20 mg/kg/24 hr P.O., then 15 mg/kg/24 hr P.O.	For up to 2 months then for remainder of therapy Up to 2 months, then remainder of 2 years	Frequent tests for occular changes are indicated
Ethionamide (Trecator)	Adult: 250 mg tid or qid P.O. or recal Child: 20 mg/kg/24 hr P.O. or rectal	24 months	Measure liver function tests frequently
Isoniazid (INH)	Adult: 300 mg daily Child: 20 mg/kg/24 hr	24 months	Administer with pyridoxine 10/mg/ 100 mg isoniazid
Kanamycin (Kantrex)	Adult: 7.5-15 mg/kg/24 hr I.M. Child: 7.5-15 mg/kg/24 hr I.M.	18-24 months	Audiometric tests should be performed
Pyrazinamide	Adult: 2 g/24 hr P.O. (maximal 35 mg/kg/24 hr, but not more than 3.0 g) Child: 20-30 mg/kg/24 hr, (Maximal 2.0 g)	18-24 months	Fatal hepatic reactions may occur; liver function should be monitored
Rifampin (Rifampin, Rimactane)	Adult: 600 mg/24 hr P.O. Child: 10-20 mg/kg/24 hr P.O.	18-24 months	Complete blood counts should be performed
Streptomycin	Adult: 1 g/24 hr I.M., then 1 g 2-3 times/week Child: 20-40 mg/kg/24 hr (Maximal 551	Until 1 month after negative culture, then for remainder of therapy	Audiometric tests and tests of vestibular function are important
Viomycin (Viocin)	Adult: 0.5-1.0 g q 3 days Child: Rarely used 30 mg/kg/3 days, if no suitable alternative	18-24 months	Periodic electrolyte panels should be performed; in addition, renal tests are advisable

icity. Medication with the most serious and frequent side effects is generally reserved for treatment of resistant organisms.

Aminosalicylic Acid

In combination with isoniazid and streptomycin, aminosalicylic acid (PAS) delays the emergence of resistant strains of tuberculosis. Although PAS is widely distributed in body fluids following oral administration, drug levels within cells are low and therapeutic concentrations are not achieved. Like isoniazid, PAS is metabolized by acetylation. Therefore, concurrent administration of the two drugs will increase the plasma levels of isoniazid.[7] However, at this point, clinical data are lacking as to whether this elevation is of any beneficial effect. The most frequently encountered adverse reactions are nausea, vomiting, diarrhea and anorexia. These untoward effects may be circumvented by careful adjustment of dosages. In some instances, where gastrointestinal reactions persist, it may be necessary to discontinue therapy. Aminosalicylic acid-induced hepatitis and blood dyscrasias may also occur. Potassium loss and other electrolyte disturbances have also been seen with administration of PAS. Because these complications are dependent upon the manner in which PAS is excreted in the urine when given as the acid *per se,* the drug is usually given as the salt which will minimize these reactions. However, patients with cardiovascular disease can not tolerate the increased sodium load. Thus, other salts or drugs should be selected for these patients.

Capreomycin

This drug has recently been released for treatment of tuberculosis. Because of its poor absorption following oral administration, capreomycin is given by intramuscular injection. Tubercle bacilli resistant to capreomycin are also resistant to viomycin and kanamycin. Like streptomycin, this antitubercular drug may cause vestibular damage. Since capreomycin is excreted by the kidneys, the dose must be reduced in renal impairment to prevent loss of hearing.

Cycloserine

Absorption occurs readily following oral administration. This drug is well distributed throughout body fluids and tissue, including the cerebrospinal fluid. However, in the treatment of tuberculosis, cycloserine appears to be less effective than streptomycin.[8] Serious side effects include neurological manifestations such as depression, convulsions and psychoses. Since cycloserine decomposes in the presence of moisture, it must be dispensed and stored under dry conditions.

Ethambutol

Ethambutol is available for oral use in the therapy of tuberculosis. Though it has had limited clinical trials, the early findings indicate ethambutol to be a valuable drug in managing this disease.[9,10] Ocular side effects have limited the widespread use of this compound. Two types of retrobulbar neuritis are manifest. In one instance, there is a constriction in peripheral vision, while in the other there is a loss of visual acuity. In the latter instance, central scotoma and green color blindness may also occur. Monthly eye examinations should accompany therapy.

Therapeutic doses of ethambutol have been shown to cause an elevation in serum uric acid levels.[11] In one study the majority of significant increases occurred between the 1st day and 3rd week of therapy. Fifty percent of the patients studied were classified as hyperuricemic—none demonstrated symptoms of gout. Elevated serum uric acid levels were seen in patients receiving ethambutol alone and in combination with isoniazid and pyridoxine. The results of this investigation are equivocal since in earlier studies ethambutol did not alter plasma uric acid.[12,13] Until further controlled trials are available, drug regimens containing ethambutol should be suspected when hyperuricemia occurs.

Ethionamide

The greatest incidence and variety of side effects occur with this drug. The most frequently encountered untoward effects are those affecting the gastrointestinal tract. These include nausea, vomiting and diarrhea. In addition, loss of appetite and cramps may be experienced. These adversities appear to be mediated through the central nervous system and occur even with parenteral administration of ethionamide. Other adversities experienced are gynecomastia, peripheral neuritis, impotence and hepatitis. Dermatological reactions consist of photosensitivity, alopecia and acneform eruptions. Though ethionamide is absorbed orally and is distributed to all body tissues and fluids, its use should be limited to that of a second line drug when no preferable alternative is available.

Isoniazid

To date, isoniazid (INH) is the most effective drug for the treatment of tuberculosis. It may be given as either a 100-mg dosage 3 times daily, or a 300-mg dosage once daily. Neither drug regimen alters the efficacy of isoniazid.[14,15] However, a single daily dose offers greater convenience to the patient and possibly results in better compliancy.

Rapid absorption occurs after oral administration of this drug. Isoniazid is widely distributed in the body, with therapeutic levels being achieved in all tissue and fluid including skin, feces, urine and saliva. Though patients vary in the rate at which they metabolize (acetylate) this drug, this does not appear to be of therapeutic significance. However, it is noteworthy that slow metabolizers appear to develop pyridoxine deficiency anemia with a greater frequency than normal acetylators. Peripheral neuritis resembling pyridoxine deficiency is also encountered with high doses of this antitubercular agent. Concomitant administration of pyridoxine in a dosage of 10 mg of isoniazid will prevent these adverse reactions. Other side effects which have been encountered are optic neuritis and skin rashes.

Both retrospective and prospective studies indicate that isoniazid can cause liver damage.[16,17] The mechanism of isoniazid-induced hepatitis remains ill defined. In one study 2,321 tuberculin reactors received 300 mg of isoniazid daily.[16] Nearly 1% developed acute hepatic disease. In another investigation, it was necessary to discontinue isoniazid in 10% of the patients being treated because of side effects; however, none became jaundiced.[17] At the same time, over 20% of the patients demonstrated abnormal liver function tests but were free of symptomatic hepatic disease. During one trial, a patient developed hepatitis 1 month after the initiation of therapy with normal isoniazid dosage.[17] Two months after the drug was discontinued a liver test proved normal. A

new course of isoniazid therapy was followed by recurrence of hepatitis. Signs and symptoms of hepatitis include nausea, vomiting, fever, chill, loss of appetite, tiredness and dark urine. Most reactions occur in the first 6 months of therapy, and patients should be monitored most closely during this period.[16-18]

An interesting interaction may occur when diphenylhydantoin and isoniazid are administered concurrently. The incidence of diphenylhydantoin toxicity is increased 10-fold when normal dosages of the two drugs are given simultaneously.[19,20] A possible mechanism for this reaction is the inhibition of diphenylhydantoin metabolism, allowing plasma concentration to increase to toxic levels. Monitoring the patient and reduction of anticonvulsant dosage will lead to adequate drug therapy.

Kanamycin

This antitubercular drug is administered parenterally. The long term use of kanamycin is limited by the various resulting side effects that include vestibular damage, ototoxicity and nephrotoxicity. Ethacrynic acid can also produce ototoxicity. Thus, patients receiving concurrent therapy with kanamycin and ethacrynic acid should be monitored closely to avoid deafness.[21] Respiratory paralysis may result when kanamycin and curareform skeletal muscle relaxants are administered jointly.[22,23] These drugs should be used with particular caution in surgical patients. Since kanamycin is excreted by the kidney, dosage must be carefully adjusted to avoid toxic reactions in patients with renal insufficiency.

Pyrazinamide

This drug can be administered orally. However, since fatal hepatic reactions have occurred, the use of this drug in the treatment of tuberculosis has been limited. Liver function tests should be performed on all patients receiving therapy with this drug. Elevated plasma uric acid levels and gout may also result from the administration of pyrazinamide.

Presently, pyrazinamide is only available for distribution from the manufacturer directly to hospitals. Therapy is to be initiated in hospitalized patients and frequent tests of liver function are to be performed.

Rifampin

Rifampin is the most recently released antitubercular agent. Initial findings indicate that this drug may have an efficacy similar to that of isoniazid.[24-27] Rifampin is available for oral administration. It has wide distribution in the body reaching most organs, body fluid and cerebrospinal fluid. Though adequate clinical trials with rifampin are lacking, the incidence of side effects is apparently low. Reported side effects include gastrointestinal disturbances such as nausea, vomiting, diarrhea, "heartburn" and loss of appetite. More serious side effects encompass blood dyscrasias and hearing defects. Patients should be warned that rifampin causes an orange discoloration of the urine.

The high cost of rifampin has led to the investigation of alternative dosing schedules.[28] An intermittent regimen consisting of rifampin once or twice weekly results in lower total weekly doses of rifampin. Evaluation of the efficacy and toxicity of such regimens is warranted since intermittent therapy has been associated with a higher incidence of hypersensitivity reactions.[28] Adversities consist of cutaneous reactions, abnormal liver function tests, renal failure and jaundice.[28-30] Rifampin-dependent antibodies have been demonstrated by an indirect antiglobulin test in a patient experiencing prolonged, acute renal failure after a single 600-mg dose.[29] Two months previously, the patient had completed a 10-month course of rifampin therapy (600 mg per day).

Streptomycin

Like kanamycin and capreomycin, streptomycin is poorly absorbed from the gastrointestinal tract. It is therefore administered by intramuscular injection. Streptomycin will not cross the blood-brain barrier unless the meninges are inflamed. Its use, for this reason, is limited in tuberculosis involving the central nervous system. The most serious side effect encountered with streptomycin therapy is eighth nerve damage leading to loss of vestibular function. Deafness may also be encountered, though less frequently than with kanamycin.

As with kanamycin therapy, ethacrynic acid should be administered with caution to patients receiving streptomycin since loss of hearing may result. Neuromuscular blockage leading to respiratory paralysis can occur when curareform skeletal muscle relaxants are given concurrently with streptomycin therapy. Thorough drug histories are essential in patients about to receive preoperative relaxants.

Dosage adjustments are necessary in patients with impaired renal function since streptomycin is excreted via the kidneys. Vestibular damage and deafness occur more frequently in patients with renal insufficiency, unless the dose of streptomycin is reduced. Resistant strains of *M. tuberculosis* develop rapidly if streptomycin is used alone. It should, therefore, always be administered in combination with another antitubercular drug.

Viomycin

Viomycin is less effective than streptomycin and must also be given by the intramuscular route. Organisms resistant to kapamycin and capreomycin show cross-resistance to viomycin. Side effects include eighth nerve damage, nephrotoxicity and electrolyte disturbances, especially loss of potassium.

Corticosteroids

In the treatment of certain life-threatening and severe infections, steroids are administered. Prednisone is the most frequently used oral agent, though therapeutically equivalent dosages of other corticosteroids may be substituted with the same clinical response. When used, these medications are given for their anti-inflammatory action.

Once the diagnosis of tuberculosis is established, prompt treatment with antituberculosis agents is instituted (Table 44.4). The drugs used in tuberculosis are bacteriostatic. As such, they exert their action by arresting the growth of *M. tuberculosis*, while relying on host response to eradicate the infection and repair tissue. Because this process is slow, medication is administered on a long term basis. It will be necessary for patients to continue their medication for 18 months to 2 years.

As in choosing any anti-infective agent, drugs should be selected on the basis of culture and sensitivity testing in order to insure optimal therapeutic response. Tuberculosis is no exception. However, *M. tuberculosis* grows slowly and up to 6 weeks may elapse before results of these cultures are available. Therapy should be initiated prior to receiving results of culture and sensitivity tests. Following the outcome, appropriate adjustments in the drug regimen can be made. Drugs to which the bacilli are resistant should be discontinued, and effective drugs substituted.

Of the agents discussed in the preceding section, only three are widely used for tuberculosis. Over the years, iosoniazid, aminosalicylic acid and streptomycin have proven to be the most efficacious. The high rate of clinical success and relatively low incidence of toxicity with these agents have made them the drugs of choice in this disease. Isoniazid is the single most effective drug, and all treatment regimens should contain this medication. The newly FDA-approved drug, rifampin, shows great promise of joining these three agents as a first line drug. The initial studies utilizing rifampin confirm its effectiveness. However, more clinical trials are needed to evaluate adequately the drug's toxicity. Since rifampin inhibits RNA synthesis and is widely distributed in body tissues and cells, clinical trials should focus on the incidence of gastrointestinal and hematological side effects that may occur. These adversities are yet to be evaluated fully. Another new agent, ethambutol, has been shown to be quite effective. However, the drug's ocular side effects have limited its usefulness as a first line drug.

The remaining antituberculosis agents are viewed as back-up drugs or second line therapy by clinicians. Their use is limited to the treatment of patients with *M. tuberculosis* resistant to isoniazid, PAS and (or) isoniazid. Resistance may be evidenced by culture and sensitivity tests as well as failure of the infection to respond during the treatment period. These drugs are also indicated when toxicity or hypersensitivity make it impossible to continue with one or more of the first line drugs.

Resistance develops rapidly to treatment with any single drug, though less frequently with isoniazid. For this reason, therapy of active disease should always be instituted with a minimum of two drugs. This will minimize the emergence of resistance. However, there are situations such as the prophylactic use of INH where one drug alone may be used efficaciously.

Varying drug regimens consisting of one to three or more drugs may be indicated, depending on the nature and severity of infection (Table 44.5).

If a suitable alternative drug is needed, rifampin, kanamycin, ethambutol, capreomycin, ethionamide, pyrazinamide, viomycin or cycloserine should be considered. When a single drug is to be utilized, isoniazid is the drug of choice. PAS and streptomycin should never be used as sole agents to treat tuberculosis. The former has little bacteriostatic action, and with either drug, resistance develops rapidly. For the two-drug regimen, isoniazid with PAS or isoniazid with streptomycin is the combination of choice. Severe infections calling for the administration of three drugs should include one of the following combinations (listed in order of decreasing preference):

isoniazid-aminosalicylic acid-streptomycin
isoniazid-aminosalicylic acid-rifampin
isoniazid-streptomycin-rifampin
isoniazid-aminosalicylic acid-ethambutol
isoniazid-ethambutol-streptomycin

When possible, each drug regimen should include isoniazid. Few populations of tuberculosis are totally resistant to this drug.[31,32] If drug toxicity or bacterial resistance prevents use of isoniazid, either rifampin or ethambutol should be considered as an alternative to be used in combination with streptomycin.

TABLE 44.5
Drug Regimen Indicated in Tuberculosis

One Drug	Two Drugs	Three Drugs
Asymptomatic primary	Skin	Miliary
Children with positive skin test	Joints and bones	Meningitis
Prophylaxis	Lymph nodes	Renal
	Chronic pulmonary	Pleural effusion
		Severe pulmonary

In certain instances, it is necessary to add corticosteroids to the treatment protocol. An inflammatory response is part of the host's normal defense against tuberculosis infection. Since corticosteroids have an anti-inflammatory action, they have no role in the chronic treatment of tuberculosis. However, in certain acute situations where the loss of either life or permanent function of an organ may result, steroid therapy is indicated.[33] Clinical manifestations for which steroids may be administered are listed in Table 44.6. When necessary, corticosteroids are given concurrently with anti-tuberculosis therapy. Steroids are administered only for short term use until beneficial effects are achieved. At this point, steroid therapy is discontinued by tapering the dosage to circumvent serious adverse reactions that may occur from sudden drug withdrawal.

The patient's reliability in taking his medication is not a matter to be taken lightly. A serious factor leading to drug-resistant tuberculosis is failure on the part of the patient to follow a prescribed drug regimen. Side effects, long duration of treatment and frequency of dosage are all factors that may contribute toward the patient's poor compliance in following the drug regimen.

The pharmacist is in an ideal position to advise the patient of the importance of following directions as prescribed, since (s)he is physically involved in the distribution of the medication. His/her contribution in this area is invaluable. Further, (s)he has access to drug records and can discern whether or not the time proximity for prescription renewals is consistent with the dosing regimen. Something is obviously amiss when the patient receiving 100 tablets to be taken 3 times a day returns for a renewal after a 6-month period. The patient-centered pharmacist should not hesitate to discuss his/her findings with both the patient and physician.

Prophylaxis

The most common prophylactic measure used worldwide to prevent tuberculosis is the administration of bacillus Calmette-Guerin (BCG) vaccine. However, for a number of reasons, this vaccine has not gained wide acceptance in the United States. BCG vaccine is a suspension of living cells of the BCG strain of

TABLE 44.6
Indications for Administration of Corticosteroids

1. Treatment of allergic reactions to antitubercular agents
2. Prevent permanent loss of function in an organ, *e.g.,* ocular tuberculosis
3. Life-threatening tuberculous infections
   A. Miliary
   B. Meningitis
   C. Pleurisy with effusion
   D. Severe pulmonary

bovine *M. tuberculosis*, maintained so as to preserve its power of sensitizing man to tuberculin while maintaining a relative non-pathogenicity to man.

Vaccination with BCG, at best, provides 80% protection against tuberculosis.[34] Its routine use is not advocated. However, administration is offered to high risk patients. These individuals are in an environment where contact with tuberculosis is unavoidable. Circumstances under which this arises include children of parents with tuberculosis, family and friends of a tuberculosis patient and hospital and rest home employees where contact is likely to occur. Vaccination converts tuberculin negative reactors to positive reactors. This is a disadvantage because skin testing of vaccinated individuals becomes meaningless.

In addition to the use of BCG vaccine, the administration of INH to household contacts of tuberculosis patients and positive skin test reactors in endemic areas and, of course, the isolation of patients with infectious tuberculosis have also proved to be effective preventive measures against tuberculosis. The usual prophylactic dose of INH is 5 mg per kg per day. At this dosage level, good protection is afforded those individuals exposed to active tuberculosis.

CLINICAL DILEMMAS

Pregnancy

There is a striking paucity of information regarding the safe clinical use of antitubercular drugs in pregnancy. This is in part due to the fact that: the populations studied are too small to allow adequate statistical handling, certain defects may not manifest for many years, fetal abnormalities occur with some frequency even in the absence of drugs, and tuberculosis itself may have adverse effects on the fetus.

The incidence of malformations associated with the use of PAS, isoniazid and streptomycin in pregnancy has been reported to be 2 to 3 times higher than normally occurs.[35] However, the possibility that tuberculosis or some other undefined variable may have caused the abnormalities was not ruled out. A review of side effects of drugs on the fetus indicates eighth nerve damage and impaired psychomotor activity may be present in the newborn when streptomycin and isoniazid, respectively, are administered during pregnancy.[36] Reports, though, are too infrequent to be conclusive.

Of the drugs used in treating tuberculosis, only isoniazid has been cleared for use. It may be administered in the last trimester of pregnancy to treat previously untreated inactive tuberculosis. With respect to all other antitubercular drugs, their safety has not been established. Physicians must weigh the benefits to the mother against the potential harm to the unborn child in making a decision.

Renal Function

The dosages of the antitubercular drugs listed in Table 44.4 are for patients with normal kidney function. There is ample evidence indicating that the occurrence of adverse reactions to drugs increases in patients with abnormal renal function.[37-39] Unless appropriate adjustment in dosage is made, certain of the drugs used to treat tuberculosis may accumulate in the body and lead to more frequent or serious side effects. This cumulative effect of drug administration can often be circumvented by reduction in dosage, an increase in the dosing interval or a combination of these. Dosage adjustments which should be made in patients with abnormal renal function are listed in Table 44.7. Although patients with impaired renal function may be receiving lower dosages of drugs, they must still be closely observed for signs of toxicity.

Tuberculosis Meningitis

Not all drugs will pass the blood-brain barrier. Ionized and lipid-insoluble drugs do not readily transfer into the cerebral spinal fluid (CSF), whereas therapeutic concentrations of lipid-soluble compounds may be achieved. In addition, the rate of penetration is inversely related to the size of the molecule; *i.e.*, small molecules enter more freely than do large.[7] The picture is further complicated in that, although some drugs may not gain access into the CSF of healthy individuals, they do enter in patients with inflamed meninges (tuberculosis meningitis). The drugs used in treating tuberculosis differ in the degree with which they cross the CSF (Table 44.8).

Although PAS does not enter the CSF, it is still used in combination with isoniazid to treat tuberculosis meningitis. This is because the former drug is believed to cause higher and prolonged blood levels of isoniazid. Cycloserine, ethionamide, isoniazid and rifampin enter the CSF of healthy patients and those with tuberculosis meningitis.[7,44] However, therapeutic concentrations of ethambutol and streptomycin are encountered only in meningitis.[7,45,46] Only low levels of kanamycin and viomycin can be achieved.[7]

When treating tuberculous meningitis in adults and children, a three-drug regimen consisting of isoniazid, aminosalicylic acid and streptomycin should be utilized. The dose and duration of treatment are listed in Table 44.4, except isoniazid, which should be given as 600 mg daily.[8]

PROGNOSIS

The prognosis for patients with tuberculosis is variable and dependent on several factors. Drug therapy is the single most important consideration in the outcome of tuberculosis. Prior to the advent of chemotherapy for tuberculosis, mortality figures were high. However, today few people die of this disease. Early identification and prompt treatment with the correct drug regimen are usually sufficient to render patients free of active infection. Periodic examinations should be routine since reactivation has been shown to occur in a small percentage of cases. The most serious danger exists in miliary tuberculosis where the infecting organisms are spread rapidly in the blood. Even in this instance, therapy usually results in striking clinical improvement within 2 months.

CONCLUSION

There is no simple cure for tuberculosis. In its present stage, therapy is complicated and

TABLE 44.7
Dosing of Antitubercular Drugs in Abnormal Renal Function

Drug	Dosage
Aminosalicylic	When the creatinine clearance is less than 50 ml/min, aminosalicylic acid should not be used;[40] if clearance is greater, 2-4-g may be administered 3 times daily[40,43]
Capreomycin	This drug is renal toxic; more data are needed before recommending doses in patients with poor kidney function
Cycloserine	Since most of this drug (60%) is excreted unchanged in the urine, the dose should be reduced in patients with renal insufficiency[42]
Ethambutol	As much as 80% of ethambutol is eliminated unchanged in the urine; dosage adjustments may be needed in patients with renal impairment[42]
Isoniazid	If the creatinine clearance is less than 50 ml/min, the dosing interval should be increased from 100 mg 3 times daily to 100 mg every 12-24 hr[40]
Kanamycin	Following a normal loading dose of kanamycin, clinically therapeutic levels may be maintained by administering 7 mg/kg every 3 half-lives,[43] the serum half-life (in hours) may be estimated by multiplying the serum creatinine concentration (mg/100 ml) by 3
Pyrazinamide	Not enough clinical data available to allow a recommendation
Rifampin	Only about 13% of a dose is eliminated unchanged in the urine; the major route of elimination is biliary; therefore, problems would not be expected in patients with decreased renal function[42]
Streptomycin	Doses of 500 mg twice weekly should be adequate for patients with a creatinine clearance below 50 ml/min[40,41]
Viomycin	The dosage should be reduced in patients with impaired function; however, guidelines are not established; a noteworthy consideration is that viomycin is nephrotoxic

TABLE 44.8
Passage of Antitubercular Drugs into the CSF

	Healthy and TB Meningitis	TB Meningitis	Low Levels	Not at All
Aminosalicylic acid				X
Cycloserine	X			
Ethambutol		X		
Ethionamide	X			
Isoniazid	X			
Kanamycin			X	
Rifampin	X			
Streptomycin		X		
Viomycin			X	

treatment involves long term administration of medication. Drug selection must often be made despite possible serious adverse reactions. Additionally, at a time when the trend is toward simple treatment, using a minimum of drugs, there exists a disease requiring multiple drug therapy. A comprehensive understanding of the disease and its treatment places the pharmacist in a situation where he can effectively discuss the therapy of tuberculosis with both physician and patient. With this understanding, the pharmacist may make a valuable contribution to rational drug usage.

REFERENCES

1. Stead, W. W.: The importance of changes in diagnostic standards and classification of tuberculosis. Ann. Intern. Med., 71: 424, 1969.
2. Wintrobe, N. M.: Principles of Internal Medicine, Ed. 6, p. 867. McGraw-Hill Book Co., New York, 1970.
3. Anon: Tuberculin tests. Med. Lett. Drugs Ther., 14: 70, 1972.
4. Landi, S., Held, H. R., and Tseng, M. C.: Disparity of potency between stabilized and non-stabilized dilute tuberculin solutions. Am.

Rev. Respir. Dis., 104: 385, 1971

5. Holden, M., Dubin, M. R., and Diamond, P. H.: Frequency of negative intermediate-strength tuberculin sensitivity in patients with active tuberculosis. N. Engl. J. Med., 285: 1506, 1971.

6. Houck, V. N.: Tuberculin: past, present and future (editorial). J.A.M.A., 22: 1421, 1972.

7. Goodman, L. S., and Gilman, A.: The Pharmacological Basis of Therapeutics, Ed. 4, p. 1319. MacMillan Company, New York, 1970.

8. Kendig, E. L., Jr.: Tuberculosis. Pediatr. Clin. North Am., 15: 213, 1968.

9. Bobrowitz, I. D.: Ethambutol compared to streptomycin in original treatment of advanced pulmonary tuberculosis. Chest. 60: 14, 1971.

10. Lees, A. W., Allan, G. W., Smith, J., Tyrrell, W. F., and Fallon, R. J.: Isoniazid and ethambutol in previously untreated patients with pulmonary tuberculosis. Am. Rev. Respir. Dis., 105: 135, 1972.

11. Postlethwaite, A. E., Bartel, A. G., and Kelley, W. N.: Hyperuricemia due to ethambutol. N. Engl. J. Med., 286: 761, 1972.

12. Place, B. A., Peets, E. A., and Buyske, D. A.: Metabolic and special studies of ethambutol in normal volunteers and tuberculosis patients. Ann. N.Y. Acad. Sci., 135: 775, 1966.

13. Bobrowitz, I. D.: Ethambutol in the retreatment of pulmonary tuberculosis. Ann. N.Y. Acad. Sci., 135: 796, 1966.

14. Reisner, D.: Comparison of single and divided dosages of isoniazid and PAS in the treatment of tuberculosis. XV A report of the Veterans Administration-Armed Forces Cooperative Study on the chemotherapy of tuberculosis. Am. Rev. Respir. Dis., 94: 849, 1966.

15. Hawkins, J. A., Arrington, C. W., Morse, W. C., and Hansen, J. E.: Once versus twice daily administration of antituberculosis drugs. Dis. Chest, 48: 573, 1965.

16. Garibaldi, R. A., Drusin, R. E., Ferebee, S. H., and Gregg, M. B.: Isoniazid-associated hepatitis: report of an outbreak. Am. Rev. Respir. Dis., 106: 357, 1972.

17. Byrd, R. B., Nelson, R., and Elliott, R. C.: Isoniazid toxicity: a prospective study in secondary chemoprophylaxis. J.A.M.A., 220: 1471, 1972.

18. Martin, C. W., and Arthaud, J. B.: Hepatitis after isoniazid administration. N. Engl. J. Med., 282: 433, 1970.

19. Hutt, H., Brennan, R., Dehejia, H., and Verebely, K.: Diphenylhydantoin intoxication: a complication of isoniazid therapy. Am. Rev. Respir. Dis., 101: 377, 1970.

20. Brenna, R., Dehejia, J., Kutt, H., Verebely, K., and McDowell, F.: Diphenylhydantoin intoxication attendant to slow-inactivation of isoniazid. Neurology, 20: 687, 1970.

21. Mathog, R. H., and Klein, W. J.: Ototoxicity of ethacrynic acid and aminoglycoside antibiotics in uremia. N. Engl. J. Med., 280: 1223, 1969.

22. Pittinger, C. B., Eryasa, Y., and Adamson, R.: Antibiotic-induced paralysis. Anesth. Analg., 49: 487, 1970.

23. McQuillen, M. P., Cantor, H. E., and O'Rouke, J. R.: Myasthenic syndrome associated with antibiotics. Arch. Neurol., 18: 402, 1968.

24. Raleigh, J. W.: Rifampin in treatment of advanced pulmonary tuberculosis. Am. Rev. Respir. Dis., 105: 397, 1972.

25. Newman, R. Doster, B., Murray, F. J., and Ferebee, S.: Rifampin in initial treatment of pulmonary tuberculosis. Am. Rev. Respir. Dis., 103: 461, 1971.

26. Vall-Spinosa, A., and Lester, T. W.: Rifampin: characteristics and role in the chemotherapy of tuberculosis. Ann. Intern. Med., 74: 758, 1971.

27. Lees, A. W., Allen, A. W., Smith, J., Tyrell, W. F., and Fallon, R. J.: Rifampin and isoniazid in previously untreated patients with pulmonary tuberculosis. Am. Rev. Respir. Dis., 105: 132, 1972.

28. Aquinas, M., Allan, W., Horsfal, P., Jenkins, P. K., Hung-Yan, W., Girling, D., Tall, R., and Fox, W.: Adverse reactions to daily and intermittent rifampicin regimens for pulmonary tuberculosis in Hong Kong. Br. Med. J., 1: 765, 1972.

29. Kleinknecht, D., Homberg, J. C., and Decroix, G.: Acute renal failure after rifampicin (letters to the editor). Lancet, 1: 1238, 1972.

30. Poole, G.: Potentially serious side effects of high-dose twice-weekly rifampicin. Br. Med. J., 3: 343, 1971.

31. Mitchell, R. S.: Control of tuberculosis. N. Engl. J. Med., 276: 842, 1967.

32. Mitchell, R. S.: Control of tuberculosis. N. Engl. J. Med., 276: 905, 1967.

33. Horne, N. W.: Advances in the treatment of tuberculosis. Practitioner, 199: 465, 1967.

34. Miller, F. J.: The prevention and treatment of tuberculosis in childhood. Practitioner, 204: 117, 1970.

35. Varpela, E.: On the effect exerted by first-line tuberculosis medicines on the foetus. Acta Tuberc. Scand., 35: 53, 1964.

36. Takata, A.: Adverse effects of drugs on the fetus. Hosp. Form. Manag., 4: 25, 1969.

37. Smith, J. W., Seidl, L. G., and Cluff, L. E.: Studies on the epidemiology of adverse drug reactions. V. Clinical factors influencing susceptibility. Ann. Intern. Med., 65: 629, 1966.

38. Richet, G., Lopez de Novales, E., and Verroust, P.: Drug intoxication and neurological episodes in chronic renal failure. Br. Med. J., 2: 394, 1970.

39. Erlanson, P., and Lundgren, A.: Ototoxic side effects following treatment with streptomycin, dihydrostreptomycin, and kanamycin. Acta Med. Scand., 176: 147, 1964.

40. Bennett, W. M., Singer, I., and Coggins, C. H.: A practical guide to drug usage in adult patients with inpaired renal function. J.A.M.A., 214: 1468, 1970.

41. Finegold, S. M., Davis, A., Ziment, I., and Jacobs,

I.: Medical progress; chemotherapy guide. Gal. Med., 111: 362, 1969.

42. Reidenberg, M. M.: Renal Function and Drug Action, Ed. 1, p. 73. W. B. Saunders Co., 1971.

43. Cutler, R. E., and Orme, B. M.: Correlation of serum creatinine concentration and kanamycin half-life, therapeutic implications. J.A.M.A., 209: 539, 1969.

44. Doliveira, J. J. G.: Cerebrospinal fluid concentrations of rifampin in meningeal tuberculosis. Am. Rev. Respir. Dis., 106: 432, 1972.

45. Piheu, J. A., Maglio, R., Cetrangolo, R., and Pleus, A. D.: Concentrations of ethambutol in the cerebrospinal fluid after oral administration. Tubercle, 52: 117, 1971.

46. Bobrowitz, I. D.: Ethambutol in tuberculosis meningitis. Chest, 61: 629, 1972.

index